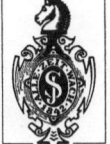

N. Nakamura · T. Hashimoto
M. Yasue (Eds.)

Recent Advances in Neurotraumatology

With 225 Figures

Springer-Verlag
Tokyo Berlin Heidelberg
New York London Paris
Hong Kong Barcelona
Budapest

Norio Nakamura, Chaiman and Professor
Takuo Hashimoto, Associate Professor
Masaharu Yasue, Assistant Professor
Department of Neurosurgery, The Jikei University School of Medicine,
3-25-8 Nishi-Shinbashi, Minato-ku, Tokyo, 105 Japan

ISBN-13:978-4-431-68233-2   e-ISBN-13:978-4-431-68231-8
DOI: 10.1007/978-4-431-68231-8

Printed on acid-free paper

Preface

The dawn of neurosurgery can be traced back to the first description preserved in the Edwin Smith papyrus (3000 BC) which dealt with head and spinal injury. In the course of 5000 years, since the first record in Egypt, advances in lifestyle and technology have brought about our modern civilized society. However, as a result of civilization, currently the total number of severe head injuries worldwide is believed to exceed 10 000 000 and the number of severe spinal injuries is believed to be more than 75 000 each year. This means that central nervous system injury is not only the oldest topic in neurosurgery, but that it is also of critical importance in modern life.

Taking these problems into consideration, the International Neurotraumatology Committee was organized in 1965 as an affiliated Committee of the World Federation of Neurosurgical Societies. The first scientific meeting was convened by the Committee in Marseilles in 1970. Nine further meetings were subsequently held, in Europe, Africa, and South America. The meeting was first named "International Conference on Recent Advances in Neurotraumatology" (ICRAN) by Professor Phillip Harris, when the scientific meeting was held in Edinburgh in 1982.

The tenth meeting, (ICRAN 1992), the first one in Asia, was held at Karuizawa, Japan, from September 23rd to 26th, 1992.

For the more than 20 years since the first meeting in Marseilles, our senior neurosurgeons have made enthusiastic efforts to promote the development of world neurosurgery, including the treatment of neurotrauma. Startling progress has recently been made in neuroimaging and basic neuroscience. Consequently, pathomechanisms in brain injuries have become clearly understood and both structural transformation and functional disarrangement in the injured brain have been elucidated to a remarkable extent at the cellular level. Nevertheless, we must recognize that there are still advances to be made in the saving of life and in minimizing posttraumatic disorder in cases of severe head and spinal injury. At present, nothing is more crucial than the prevention of central nervous system trauma.

Thus, it had been suggested by the International Neurotraumatology Committee that in ICRAN 1992 we should have a seminar on "Prevention of Neurotrauma". Another seminar "Disaster Assistance and Neurotrauma" was also a timely theme, in the light of the numerous castrophic earthquakes, volcanic eruptions, and air accidents that have occurred all over the world in recent years.

As expected, the tenth meeting was a milestone in the history of ICRAN. Keeping the significance of this meeting in mind, three topics were proposed as the main themes for ICRAN 1992:

— Chronic subdural hematoma, an old but still relevant topic.
— Neuroimaging as the frontline in advanced research.

— Cell damage and repair in the central nervous system, a developing topic of which great things are expected.

All three of these topics were discussed earnestly in the Conference Symposia.

In addition, Professor Jean Brihaye kindly agreed to make a presentation on the history of the International Neurotraumatology Committee, and the President of this Conference described the effectiveness of protective safety helmets on the basis of his longstanding experimental and clinical investigations.

A total of 190 well-researched presentations were of much interest to all participants over the two and a half days of the Conference.

In this publication, all 190 presentations are listed in the Table of Contents, but about half of them have been chosen to be published in the form of a compact book of three-page summaries.

We would like to express our sincere gratitude to all those who contributed to making ICRAN 1992 so worthwhile and these proceedings possible.

NORIO NAKAMURA

Table of Contents

---

*Paper not available at time of going to press

4—Chronic Subdural Hematoma

5—Neuroimaging in Central Nervous System Injury

6—Cell Damage and Repair in Central Nervous System Injury

7—Experimental Studies

8—Monitoring

9—Focal Injury

10—Acute Epidual and Subdrual Hematoma

11—Diffuse Axonal Injury and Severe Head Injury

12—Pediatric Head Injury

13—Spinal Cord Injury

14—Epidemiology, Miscellaneous

Some Notes on the History of the Committee on Neurotraumatology (CNT) of the World Federation of Neurosurgical Societies (WFNS) from 1965 to 1979

Jean Brihaye[1] (Brussels), Historian of the CNT

I would like to dedicate this short history of the initial years of the CNT to its first and past-chairman, Professor Antonio de Vasconcellos Marques (Fig.1). He was and remained, even when he became the past chairman, an inspiring and moderating colleague, deeply involved in all aspects of neurotraumatology but mainly being concerned with the important problem of prevention. Professor Marques ran the activities of the committee in a great spirit of friendship and devotion. For all of us, he remains a reliable and hearty friend.

From the start, neurosurgical societies were confronted with the medical and socio-economical problems caused by injuries, mainly head trauma.

When the first International Congress of Neurological Sciences took place in Brussels (1957), the neurological surgery section placed the subject of traumatology on its agenda. At this meeting, the World Federation of Neurosurgical Socieites (WFNS) was founded and Sir Geoffrey Jefferson became its first President.

In 1965, a special ad hoc committee on head injuries was appointed during the third Congress of Neurological Surgery in Copenhagen in order "...to continue studies on the ways and means of maintaining interest and activity in the resolution of the problem of head injury." (A. Earl Walker*). Antonio de Vasconcellos Marques (Lisbon) was elected chairman of the committee with the following members: K.O.C. Elliot (Canada), R. Frowein (Germany), E.S. Gurdjian (USA), K.J. Jamieson (Australia), K. Kristiansen (Norway), J.M. Potter (UK), K. Sano (Japan), R. Vigouroux (France), and as ex-officio members, E. Busch (President — Denmark), D.W.C. Northfield (Secretary of Congress Affairs — UK), A.E. Walker (Secretary of Federation Affairs — USA). (Fig. 2).

During this third congress, stress was laid on head and spinal injuries, emphasizing the seriousness with which the Federation was considering the problem. Besides, in his introductory address during the opening ceremony, President Busch declared "...one of the greatest problems of modern society — that of traumatic injury to the nervous system, especially by traffic accidents — is one of our main themes at this meeting, and for the first time we shall have an overall picture of the magnitude and seriousness of this world problem, which every year claims an ever greater number of victims. Neurosurgery must assume an increasingly important part in meeting this challenge". Therefore, the decision to write to all national governments was taken unanimously; the letter shown in Fig. 3 was dispatched to the Belgian Prime Minister as well as to other governments worldwide.

---

[1] 98 Av. des Franciscains, 1150 Bruxelles, Belgium

*A.E. Walker: The History of the World Federation of Neurosurgical Societies. Edited and distributed by the WFNS (1985)

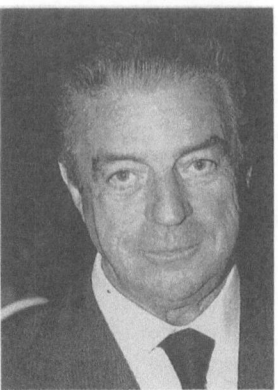

Fig.1. Antonio de Vasconcellos Marques

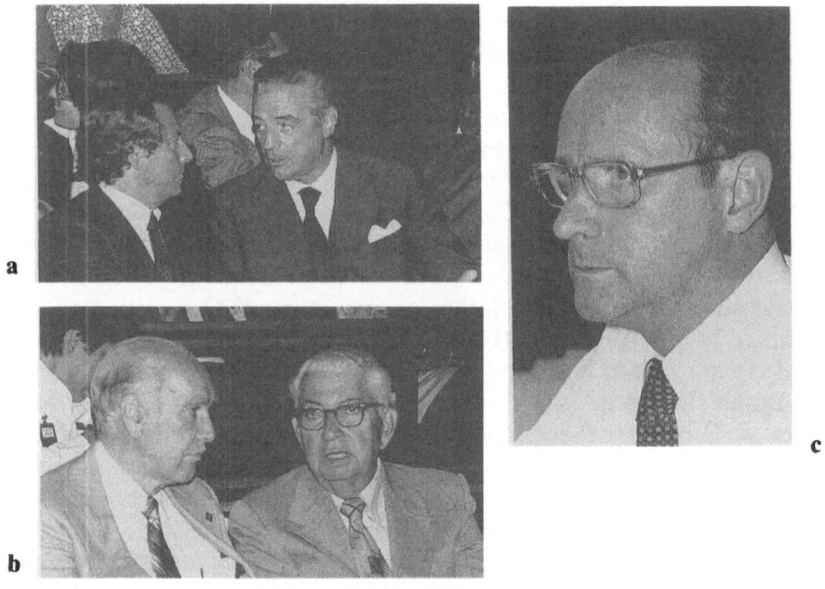

Fig.2. a A. de Vasconcellos Marques and R. Vigouroux **b** A.E. Walker and E.S. Gurdjian **c** R. Frowein

In the 4-year interval between the congress in Copenhagen (1965) and the following one in New York (1969), the chairman, A. de Vasconcellos Marques, established contact with the officers and members of the committee in order to strengthen the committee for further activity. In New York, new members came to reinforce the team; they were: J. Brihaye (Belgium), J.C. Christensen (Argentina), A. El-Banhawy (Egypt), J.P. Evans (USA), B. Guidetti (Italy), S. Ishii (Japan), Sten Lindgren (Denmark), AT.K. Ommaya (USA), A.R. Taylor (Ireland), and E. Zander (Switzerland) (Fig. 4). Study groups were also established within the committee to consider intensive care, lesions caused by cars, transportation-first aid, and terminology. A limited number of members were in charge of these study groups.

World Federation of Neurosurgical Societies

THIRD INTERNATIONAL CONGRESS OF NEUROLOGICAL SURGERY

Copenhagen, August 23 - 28, 1965

November 2, 1965

OFFICE OF THE SECRETARY FOR FEDERATION AFFAIRS

DR. A. EARL WALKER,
601 *North Broadway*
Baltimore 5, Maryland
U.S.A.

OFFICERS

Prof. Eduard Busch
President

Prof. Kentaro Shimizu
Vice-President

Dr. A. Earl Walker
Secretary for Federation Affairs

Mr. D. W. C. Northfield
Secretary for Congress Affairs

Dr. Bendt Broager
Asst. Secretary for Congress Affairs

Prof. Hugo Krayenbühl
Treasurer

Prof. Richard Malmros
Asst. Treasurer

Dr. Arnold C. De Vet
Editor of Publications

HONORARY PRESIDENTS
Dr. Percival Bailey
Dr. Paul C. Bucy
Dr. Paul Martin
Dr. Herbert Olivecrona
Dr. Wilder Penfield
Dr. Daniel Petit-Dutaillis

His Excellency Pierre Harmel
Prime Minister of Belgium
Brussels

My dear Mr. Prime Minister:

At the Third International Congress of Neurological Surgery held in Copenhagen, August 21-27, 1965, the primary theme was trauma to the nervous system. Reports were made by representatives of many nations of the world regarding the frequency, severity and sequelae of injuries to the nervous system. On the basis of these reports which indicated that injuries were the most common cause of death in people between the ages of 1 and 44, that head injuries were responsible for approximately 2/3 of these deaths and that the frequency and severity of head injuries was progressively increasing in all countires of the world, the World Federation of Neurosurgical Societies, unanimously passed the following resolution which they asked that I bring to your attention.

"The World Federation of Neurosurgical Societies, having devoted the first day of the III International Congress of Neurological Surgery to the subject of Acute Head Injuries, wishes to draw the attention of all appropriate Government authorities, Universities and centres of medical education to the increasing frequency and severity of head injury due to traffic, industry, sport and home accidents and the consequent mortality and economic disability.

The World Federation of Neurosurgical Societies recommends that the appropriate Government authorities, the Universities and centres of medical education explore ways and means of meeting this problem by:

1. Energetic propaganda for prevention (for instance improved designs of both vehicles and roads, research into the mechanics of crash-injuries).

Page 2

2. Improving and expanding accident services.

3. Creating and expanding the facilities for neurosurgical care and here the Neurosurgical Societies are in a particularly favourable position to offer specific and detailed recommendation."

Fig.3. Letter to the Prime Minister of Belgium *(continued)*

The representative of the World Federation of Neurosurgical Societies in your country and its delegate or delegates is given below, in case you would wish to communicate with them in setting up a national program related to head injuries.

Sincerely yours,

A. Earl Walker, M. D.

AEW/ke

Groupement Belge de Neurochirurgie-Belgische Vereinigung voor Neurochirurgie
Delegates: Dr. G. R. Hoffman
Park Plein
St. Denis-Westrem
Ghent

Dr. J. Brihaye
Brussels

Fig. 3. Continued

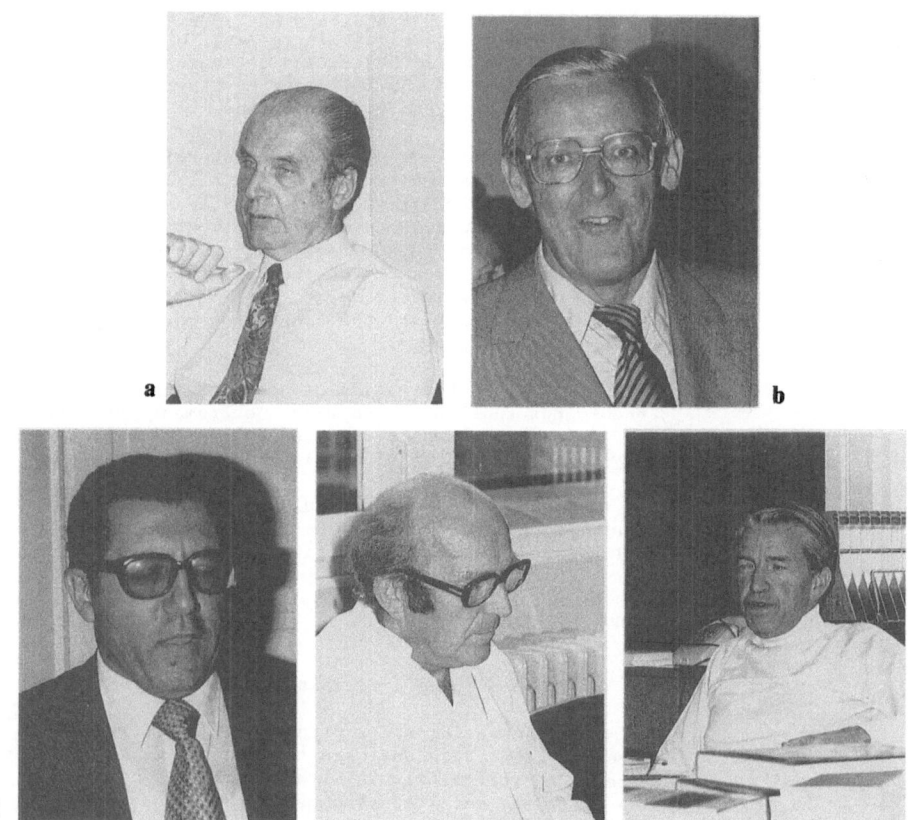

a   b

c, d   e

Fig. 4. a J.C. Christensen **b** Eric Zander **c** A. El-Banhawy **d** J. Brihaye **e** Sten Lindgren

At the same meeting in 1969, the need was felt by the officers to have rules of procedure. Four years later, during the World Congress in Tokyo, the constitution of the committee, prepared in the meantime by Eric Zander, was referred to the Executive Committee of the WFNS for approval and was adopted on the 9th of October, 1973. In the following years (Oxford, 1975; Sao Paulo, 1977) some minor changes were made which were considered appropriate In Paris (July, 1979), during the European Congress, E. Zander was again in charge of revising the constitution; a first draft was discussed in Sitges (Spain) during the European course (September, 1979) by a restricted number of members, including A. de Vasconcellos Marques, R. Frowein, J. Brihaye, W. Luyendijk, R. Vigouroux and E. Zander. These changes were submitted to the WFNS Committee on Constitution and were officially accepted on April 20, 1980, in New York; they were approved by the Executive Committee of the WFNS in Munich, 1981. The written constitution of the NTC is shown below, with the original version on the left of the page and the amended text on the right.

BY-LAWS OF THE COMMITTEE OF NEURO-TRAUMATOLOGY (CNT) OF THE WFNS adopted by the Executive Committee in Tokyo on 9th of October 1973

BY-LAWS OF THE COMMITTEE OF NEURO-TRAUMATOLOGY (CNT) OF THE WFNS adopted by the Executive Committee of the WFNS in Tokyo on October 9, 1973 and amended in 1975 in Oxford, in 1977 in Sao Paulo; revision already submitted to the Committee on Constitution (April 1980, New York) and accepted by this Committee

1. The CNT is a *scientific Committee* of the WFNS and is based on its Constitution (Art. VI, Section 12):
"Section 12 — Scientific Committees
Scientific Committees must have a clearly defined purpose accepted by the Executive Committee on the grounds of submitted By-Laws. These Committees nominate their members and their officers and submit the list of nominees to the Administrative Council for election by the Executive Committee.
The chairman must deliver a written report to the Executive Committee at each of its meetings".

1. Main purpose of the CNT
   1.1. To collect and exchange epidemiological information; to organize the collection and correlation of research findings; and to prepare critical evaluations of this material. To standardize definitions and terminology in neurotraumatology (NT).
   1.2. To develop policies through which prevention and management of NT and necessary research can be improved.
   1.3. To disseminate this information to all members of the WFNS — especially through international meetings on NT and during special sessions of the WFNS international congresses.

2. *Main purpose of the CNT*
   2.1. To collect and exchange epidemiological information; to organize the collection and correlation of research findings; and to prepare critical evaluations of this material. To standardize definitions and terminology in neurotraumatology (NT).
   2.2. To develop policies through wihch prevention and management of NT and necessary research can be improved.
   2.3. To disseminate this information to all members of the WFNS and continental committees for NT, especially through international, regional, and national meetings on NT and during special sessions of the WFNS international congresses.

Original version *(cont.)*

1.4. To communicate and exchange information with organisations such as:
- WHO, EE, and ILO
- Governments (through individual members of societies)
- Other organizations concerned with neurotrauma in the broadest sense

1.5. The CNT should prepare a list on the priorities of the problems to be dealt with (e.g., terminology, intensive care, prehospital care, epidemiology, chronic care, and rehabilitation).

2. Functions of the CNT

2.1. Being an international committee, it should chiefly function by correspondence.

2.2. There should be at least a biennial meeting of the whole CNT (for example, during the WFNS international congress or continental meetings, or international conferences, symposia, etc. on NT).

2.3. The CNT should establish *working parties* on special topics by choosing a group of members of the CNT, on individual members, or members of national societies of the World Federation. The object of these working parties would be to draft a preliminary report which should be circulated among all the members of the CNT for criticism and then be returned to the working parties for redrafting as agenda items for the next CNT meeting.
It is important that, for limited or specialized studies, members other than those of the Committee should be co-opted with the aim of enlarging our contacts, without having to increase the actual number on the Committee.

2.4. *Agenda items* should be called for 6 months before the meeting and a draft agenda should be circulated among the CNT members 3 months before the meeting. The final agenda should be sent 1 month before the meeting. All agenda items should have supporting documentation.

2.5. *Committee meetings* should be formal and follow the usual rules. Minutes should be kept by the secretary and should be circulated among the members of the CNT as soon as possible after the meeting.

Amended version *(cont.)*

2.4. To communicate and exchange information with organizations such as:
- WHO.
- Governments (through individual members of societies)
- Other organizations concerned with neurotrauma in the broadest sense

2.5. The CNT should prepare a list of the priorities of the problems to be dealt with (e.g., terminology, epidemiology, prevention, prehospital care, intensive care, chronic care, and rehabilitation).

3. Functions of the CNT

3.1. Being an international committee, it should chiefly function by correspondence. The secretary should receive reports from the members visiting related congresses and involved in activities; suitable material should be circulated between the members.

3.2. There should be at least a biennial meeting of the whole CNT (for example during the WFNS international congress or continental meetings, or international conferences, symposia, etc., on NT.).

3.3. The CNT should establish *working parties* on special topics by choosing a group of members of the CNT, or individual members, or members of national societies of the World Federation. The object of these working parties would be to draft a preliminary report which should be circulated among all the members of the CNT for criticism and then be returned to the working parties for redrafting as agenda items for the next CNT meeting.
It is important that, for limited or specialized studies, members other than those of the Committee should be co-opted with the aim of enlarging our contacts, without having to increase the actual number on the Committee.

3.4. *Agenda items* should be called for 6 months before the meeting and an agenda should be sent to the CNT members 4 months before the meeting. All agenda items should have supporting documentation.

3.5. *Committee meetings* should be formal and follow the usual rules. Minutes should be kept by the secretary and should be circulated among the members of the CNT as soon as possible after the meeting.

3.6. A written report of the activity of the CNT should be delivered to the Executive Committee of the WFNS at each of its meetings by the President of the CNT.

3. Structure of the CNT
   3.1. *Committee members* should be selected for one or more of the following reasons:
      – Ability and good reputation in NT
      – Willingness to cooperate in working parties and to attend meetings with reasonable frequency
      – Interest in specific fields of NT
      – Geographical distribution of membership communities
   3.2. The President and the Secretary of the WFNS will be ex officio members.
   3.3. *The total number of members of the CNT* should not be less than 12 and not more than 18. A quorum should consist of three-quarters of the members of the CNT voting personally or by "proxy". Members of the executive committee of the WFNS may be invited to participate in meetings of the CNT.
   3.4. *Length of office* shall be 4 years with possible reappointment for two further terms of 4 years. Members should be appointed by the WFNS executive committee on nomination by the CNT. No nomination shall be accepted unless notice be given on the agenda paper.
   Four or five members should retire in rotation every 4 years so that the Committee changes gradually and progressively. The advisability for active members to serve for more than 4 years should be insisted on.
   3.5. *The executive committee of the CNT:*
   shall consist of a *chairman*, a *deputy-chairman*, and a *secretary*, together with such other members as the CNT shall appoint (liaison officer to WHO, etc.)
   In the year of the WFNS congress, an election should be held for all office bearers by secret vote.
   3.6. *Power of the executive of the CNT*
   Postal ballots may be sought by the executive on any subject with a closing date. An affirmative vote by three-quarters of those replying shall empower the executive to take action.

4. *Accounts*
   4.1. Annual audited accounts shall be submitted to the secretary of the CNT for all moneys received by members or working groups.
   4.2. An annual audited account shall be submitted each year to the treasurer of the WFNS by the secretary of the CNT.

4. Structure of the CNT
   4.1. *Committee members* should be selected for one or more of the following reasons:
      – Ability and good reputation in NT
      – Willingness to cooperate in working parties and to attend meetings with reasonable frequency
      – Interest in specific fields of NT
      – Geographical distribution of membership communities
   4.2. The President and the Secretary of the WFNS will be ex officio members.
   4.3. *The total number of members of the CNT* should not be more than 25 with voting rights. A quorum should consist of a majority of the members, voting personally or by "proxy".
   4.4. *Length of office* shall be 4 years with possible reappointment for two further terms of 4 years. Members should be appointed by the WFNS Executive Committee on nomination by the CNT. No nomination shall be accepted unless notice be given on the agenda paper.
   Four or five members should retire in rotation every 4 years so that the Committee changes gradually and progressively. The advisability for active members to serve for more than 4 years should be insisted on.
   Outgoing members of the CNT who wish to continue their work in NT may remain as associated members, but without voting power.
   4.5. *The Executive of the CNT*:
   shall consist of a *chairman*, a *deputy chairman*, and a *secretary*.
   These officers shall be appointed by the President of the Federation after nomination by the CNT.
   During the International Congress of the WFNS all officers should be selected for nomination by secret vote.
   4.6. *Power of the executive of the CNT*:
   Postal ballots may be sought by the executive on any subject with a closing date. An affirmative vote by three-quarters of those replying shall empower the executive to take action.

5. *Accounts*
   5.1. Annual audited accounts shall be submitted to the secretary of the CNT for all monies received by members or working groups.
   5.2. An audited account shall be submitted every 2 years to the treasurer of the WFNS by the secretary of the CNT before the meeting of the Executive Committee of the WFNS.

From 1969 on, the CNT strove to have a scientific and an associated business meeting each year, organized by one of its members in their own country, giving the opportunity for a national or continental conference there and then. In addition to these business meetings, whenever possible, the members of the CNT used to hold unofficial gatherings at other meetings or occasions provided that a significant number was present. This was the case in Sitges when a draft of the constitution was discussed and drawn up.

Robert Vigouroux, who became the secretary of the committee in 1969, organized the first major meeting, in Marseilles on October 2 and 3, 1970, within the framework of a large "Colloque de Neurotraumatologie". The topics for discussion were; localized traumatic lesions of the cerebral hemispheres, atypical extradural hematomas, associated injuries of head and limbs, metabolic disturbances in head trauma, and neurotraumatology in traffic and industrial accidents. Furthermore, the members had the opportunity to visit a modern neurosurgical intensive care unit in the "Hôpital de la Conception". This Marseilles meeting was very successful and was attended by a large number of neurosurgeons and the members of the Committee, confirming that an annual meeting of the members of the CNT was useful and necessary.

During this convention in Marseilles, an administrative meeting of the CNT took place on the 1st of October. Three relevant matters were considered: legislation on alcoholism in different countries, the organization of intensive care units, and terminology in head injuries. The question of terminology had already been raised by a few members, mainly J.P. Evans, J.C. Christensen and Sten Lindgren, on previous occasions in Edinburgh and Madrid.

On September 13-15, 1971, some officers (A. de Vasconcellos Marques, K. Sano, W. Luyendijk, J. Brihaye, and S. Lindgren, who was temporarily acting as secretary at this business meeting) attended the International Symposium on Rehabilitation after head injuries in Göteborg (Sweden); they took this opportunity to discuss the program for the session on traumatology in Tokyo (October 1973), including the reports by the subgroups on first aid, intensive care units, terminology, types of collisions, and types of injuries. In regard to this last topic, Sten Lindgren made a summary of the present state of knowledge concerning correlations between types of collisions and the resulting injuries. Keiji Sano and T. Hayashi presented a paper on a cooperative study on calculations for various mechanical models and produced evidence from experiments with human dummies, monkey dummies, and monkeys for comparison.

During the European Congress in Prague, June 28 – July 2, 1971, in addition to free communications on neurotraumatology, there was also a panel discussion on brain death and a session on posttraumatic and degenerative disorders of the spinal cord. Besides, the participants in this convention, including those of the CNT, were strongly involved in the official foundation of the European Association of Neurosurgical Societies (EANS), for which one of the members of the CNT (J. Brihaye) was elected general secretary.

In Buenos-Aires on August 27-30, 1972, J.C. Christensen arranged a large "Conferencia Internacional de Neurotraumatologia". In his opening address, Dr. Christensen declared "This conference represents a further step in the strenuous work initiated by the WFNS when, in 1965, it appointed a head injury committee... Lately, the committee enlarged the scope of its interests to spinal and peripheral nerve injuries, changing its name to the neurotraumatology committee". Fifteen members of the CNT took part in this important Argentinian Conference: J.C. Christensen, E. Zander, P. Benedek, J.P. Evans, J. Brihaye, K.J. Jamieson, E.S. Gurdjian, AT. K. Ommaya, R.A. Vigouroux, A. de V. Marques, W. Luyendijk, A.R. Taylor, A. El-Banhawy, S. Ishii, and K. Sano (Fig. 5). In addition,

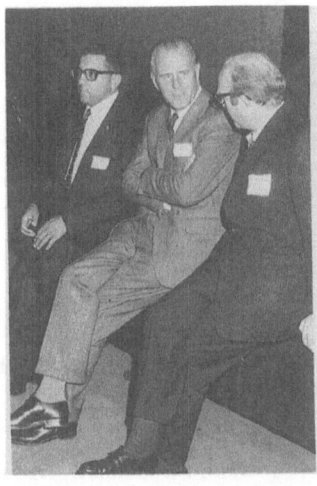

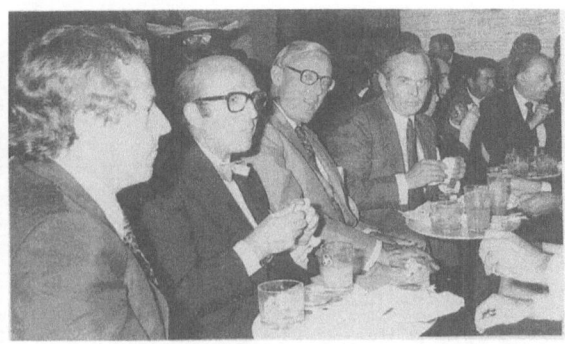

b

a

Fig.5. a Conferencia Internacional de Neurotraumatologia. Reunion of Head Injuries Committee of the World Federation of Neurosurgical Societies. Buenos Aires, Argentina, August 27-30, 1972. Drs. El-Banhawy, Luyendijk, and Brihaye. **b** Drs. Vigouroux, Brihaye, Zander, Jamieson, and de Mattos Pimenta

three other colleagues, who were later to become members of the CNT, attended the meeting: P. Niemeyer (Brazil), A. Lasierra (Spain), and Norio Nakamura (Japan). A full day was devoted to the discussion of psychological, somatic, socioeconomic, and mechanical predisposing factors to head injuries. First aid was also discussed and it was clearly demonstrated that much more had been done, particularly in the more developed countries, to repair damage than to prevent accidents.

The fifth International Congress of Neurosurgery was held on October 7-13, 1973, in Tokyo. A symposium on neurotraumatology was arranged on October 12 by A. de V. Marques. AT. K. Ommaya correlated the biomechanics of head injuries with the clinico-pathological findings; U. Ponten discussed biochemical alterations in brain injuries; H. Pia presented his studies on disregulation of the brain stem in brain injuries; I. Klatzo discussed the pathological findings; R. Vigouroux spoke about the posttraumatic sequellae, and J. Ransohoff demonstrated the biochemical alterations in spinal cord trauma. Once more new colleagues joined the committee: Ph. Harris (Scotland), P. Niemeyer (Brazil), I. Oprescu (Romania), and B. Ramamurthi (India) (Fig. 6). Doctors Evans, Elliott, Potter, and Guidetti wished to withdraw from the committee, saying how happy they were to have worked in collaboration with the officers and members for several years.

It was also in Tokyo that a special committee on glossary terms in neurotraumatology was instituted. In fact, already in 1969, an international head injury terminology study group of the WFNS had been created. J.P. Evans played a leading role in this group, together with Drs. Lindgren, Frowein, Luyendijk, Christensen, and Brihaye. J.P. Evans made a first report in Prague (1971) on the work acomplished by the study group*. At this stage, the group

---

* Proceedings of the Fifth International Congress of Neurological Surgery (1973), Excerpta Medica, 293: 225-245 (A.E. Walker quoted above)

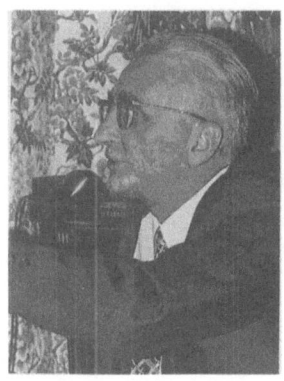

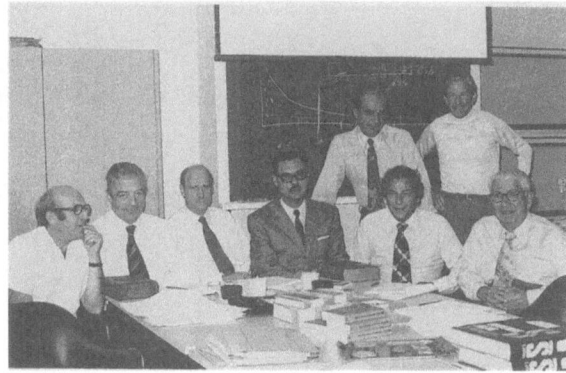

Fig.6   Fig.7

Fig.6. Ion Opresou

Fig.7. Group at work, from left to right: Drs. Brihaye, Marques, Frowein, Stroobandt, Vigouroux, and Gurdjian; standing: Drs. Christensen and Lindgren

had received much help and many suggestions from Drs. Pevehouse, Voris, and Walker and it used much of the Head Injury Nomenclature prepared by a committee of the Congress of Neurological Surgeons that was published in *Clinical Neurosurgery*, vol 12, 1966. But Dr. Evans retired from the CNT in Tokyo (1973), where, at this time, the glossary committee was settled officially; it was composed of Dr. Gurdjian as chairman, with Drs. Brihaye, Christensen, Frowein, Lindgren, and Ommaya as members, and with Drs. W. Luyendijk, G. Norlen, A. de Vasconcellos Marques and R. Vigouroux as ex-officio members. This committee was very active under the guidance of Dr. Gurdjian and remained in close contact by correspondence and with several working meetings, a 1-day meeting in Oxford in October 1975, three days in Brussels (Fig. 7) in October 1976, and two days in Sao Paulo in June 1977. The final result was published in 1979 in four languages (English, French, Spanish, and German) as supplementum 25 to *Acta Neurochir [Suppl.] Wien*. Subsequently, this hardworking team was discharged of its duties.

In July 1974, A. de Mattos Pimenta organized a meeting on neurotraumatology in Sao Paulo and invited a number of members of the CNT to take an active part in it. Eight committee members (Drs. Marques, Vigouroux, Brihaye, Zander, Christensen, Ishii, Luyendijk, and Niemeyer) attended the symposium and presented papers. We remember with amusement that, in order to entertain his guests in an unusual way, Dr. de Mattos Pimenta arranged a neurosurgical prize in a horse race; we gambled a very small amount of money, listening to the advice of our host, but no one carried off the prize!

In the same year (September 15-22, in Brussels), J. Brihaye organized the first European training course with the cooperation of the CNT. The general topic of the course, which lasted for the whole week, was head injuries. The following members made prominent contributions: Drs. Oprescu (who died in December 1987), Lindgren, Vigouroux, Taylor, Luyendijk, Zander, Frowein, and Marques. The chairman A. de Vasconcellos Marques, gave the concluding remarks at the end of the course.

The same year also, Sten Lindgren was advised by E.O. Backlund, who had just returned from travelling with a delegation in China, and who believed that Chinese doctors could be interested in participating in the CNT, and that this could lead to an exchange of experiences with neurosurgeons in the Peoples Republic of China. Letters were thus sent by Sten

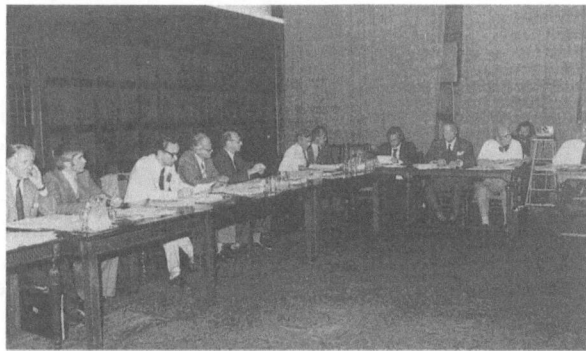

a

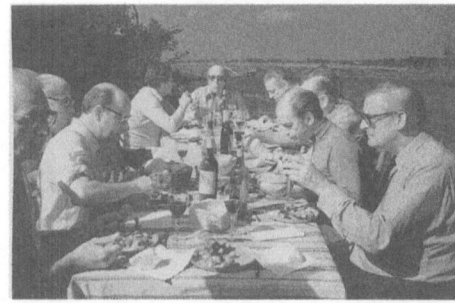

b

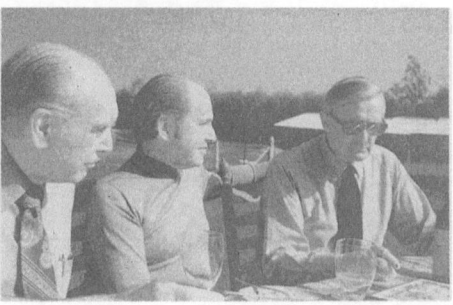

c

Fig.8. a Part of a large working group: one recognizes among others Drs. Harris, Loew, and Frowein.
b some rest is taken and some strength regained at the Brihaye's country house. Around the table:
Drs. Opresou, Frowein, Gurdjian, Vigouroux, Brihaye, Marques, Christensen, and Zander. **c** Drs.
Walker, Christensen, and Zander

Lindgren to professors of neurosurgery in Beijing and Shanghaï, but unfortunately, these
efforts were not successful.

The fifth European Congress was held September 15-20, 1975, in Oxford, with a business
meeting of the CNT, as well as a meeting of the glossary group, being held on Saturday
September 13. Dr. T. Pentelenyi, who later became a member of the committee, participated
in a panel on head injuries. A special session was also devoted to coma, with particular reference to prognosis and treatment, and a debate on design and equipment for intensive care
units was organized, with neurosurgical nurses being present. In all, we had four working
meetings, with Dr. Brihaye acting as chairman. Drs. Christensen, El-Banhawy, Frowein,
Gurdjian, Harris, Lindgren, Oprescu, Vigouroux, and Zander participated in the discussion
of Dr. Frowein's report on the definition of coma states. Furthermore, the financial affairs
and the committee's participation in the forthcoming Sao Paulo congress in June 1977 were
planned, as well as other projects for joint clinical research work in the field of traumatology.

During 1975, a meeting of the CNT was also planned to be held in Madras, along with
the Silver Jubilee celebrations of the Institute of Neurology, organized by B. Ramamurthi.
However, unfortunately, no formal meeting of the NTC could be carried out, although
neurotraumatology was discussed in some papers.

On September 19-23, 1976, a symposium was held in Brussels, devoted to coma (chairperson: J. Brihaye), to injury scaling (chairpersons: S. Lindgren and G. Stroobandt), and to
brain death (chairperson: E.A. Walker and E. Pillen). A great number of neurosurgeons

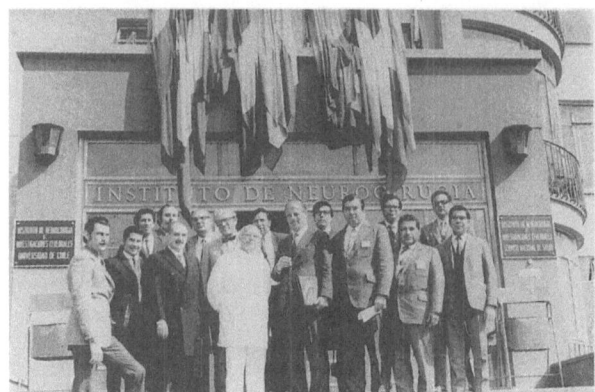

Fig.9. a Group photographed in front of the Institute of Neurosurgery in Santiago de Chile. In front of the group: Professor Asenjo (in white); behind: Drs. Basauri, Columella, Brihaye, and Luyendijk, amid their Chilean colleagues. **b** Group composed of: Drs. Luyendijk, Basauri, Columella, Asenjo, Vigouroux, Nelly Chiofalo, Brihaye, and Mario Castro, neuroradiologist

a

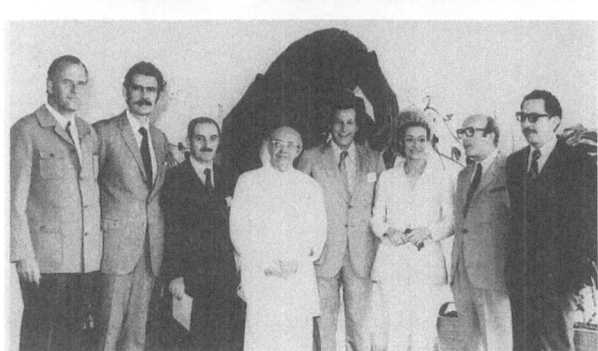

b

and many committee members took an active part in the discussion (Fig. 8). The final report of this symposium appeared in *Acta Neurochir* (Wien) (1978) vol 40, pp. 181-186.

In 1977, the CNT extended its activities mainly in South America. Prior to the International Congress of the WFNS held in Sao Paulo (June 19-25), a workshop on cerebral death was held in Santiago de Chile (June 12-17) on the occasion of a large multidisciplinary assembly of the Latin American Congress of Neurosurgery together with the Latin American Organization of Electroencephalography, the International Symposium of Neurological Sciences, and the Latin American Congresses of Neuroradiology, of Pediatric Neurosurgery, and of Neurosurgical Nurses. E.A. Walker, together with Nelly Chiofalo of the Latin American EEG Congress, was in charge of organizing this workshop as a supplementary conference to the symposium which had been held the year before in Brussels, and as a preliminary to the report to the WFNS in Sao Paulo. Drs. Benedek, Christensen, Vigouroux, and Brihaye played an active part in this workshop. (*Neurochirurgia* (Stuttg) (1978), vol 36, no. 3 (Fig. 9).

During the CNT business meeting in Sao Paulo, new members were accepted: Drs. A. Lasierra from Spain, P. Benedek from Uruguay (Fig. 10), A. Rakotobe* from Madagascar, R.C. McLaurin from the USA, and G.K. Vanderfield from Australia. Drs. Gurdjian and Taylor left the committee, and unfortunately Dr. Jamieson passed away the year before. Nearly all members of the CNT attended the Sao Paulo meetings and

---

* Sadly, our colleague, A. Rakotobe died a few months ago.

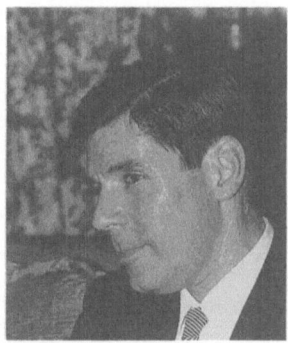
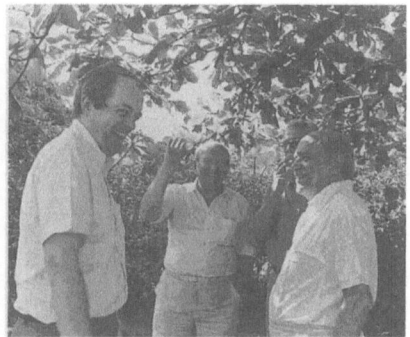

Fig.10   Fig.11

Fig.10. P. Benedek

Fig.11. Drs. Dohrmann, Brihaye, Vigouroux, and Paolo Niemeyer in the garden of the Niemeyer's residence

several of them participated in presentations and discussions on the topic "Injuries of the Cervical Spine and Cord".

After the Sao Paulo congress, a third meeting was held in Rio de Janeiro (June 28-29), arranged by Paulo Niemeyer, with the assistance of the Brazilian College of Surgeons. Drs. Marques, Vigouroux, Christensen, Luyendijk, Harris, and Brihaye were invited to participate actively in the main subject "The organization of emergency transportation within cities. An international exchange of experiences with special regard to neurosurgical emergency cases". (Fig. 11)

On March 2-4, 1978, Dr. Marques organized, in the department of neurosurgery and neurotraumatology of the civil hospitals in Lisbon, a "Simpósio Nacional de Traumatismos Crânio-encefálicas". Some officers of the CNT presented papers at this meeting.

In 1978, 11 members of the CNT attended an international conference on neurotraumatology organized by the Egyptian Society of Neurology, Psychiatry, and Neurosurgery in Cairo on April 17-19, under the Presidency of Ahmed El-Banhawy, and with Sayed El Gindi as secretary. Three topics (posttraumatic neuroses and psychoses, posttraumatic epilepsy, and cranial nerve injuries) were presented and widely discussed by our Egyptian colleagues and the committee members present. Professor El-Banhawy*, a regular member of the CNT, succeeded in creating a warm and welcoming atmosphere during the entire gathering. Moreover, this joint cooperative conference in Cairo between neurosurgeons from the Arab countries and officers of the CNT conformed in spirit to and was in full agreement with the official decision, taken the year before, during the WFNS congress in Sao Paulo, i.e., that the Pan Arab Union of Neurological Sciences would be affiliated to the European Association of Neurosurgical Societies.

The sixth European Congress was held in Paris on July 16-20, 1979. As usual, the CNT had a business meeting, held in the department of Professor B. Pertuiset the day after the congress (Fig. 12), where it was decided to establish five working groups, on rehabilitation (J. Brihaye), prevention (S. Lindgren), epidemiology (R. Frowein), posttraumatic epilepsy (R. Vigouroux), and spinal and medullary trauma (Ph. Harris). Those officers responsible

---

* Professor El-Banhawy passed away in 1986.

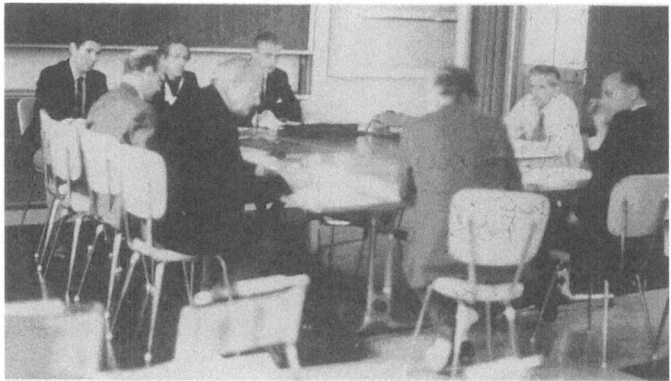

Fig.12. Working team in Paris: Drs. Zander, Frowein, Benedek, Vigouroux, Marques, Lindgren, Luyendijk, and Harris (viewed from back)

for the groups delivered their manuscripts to the committee members in 1980, but unfortunately, these were never published.

On November 11-16, 1979, a second meeting took place in Buenos Aires, on the occasion of the 18th Latin American Congress of Neurosurgery. Juan Carlos Christensen was in the chair for the "Conferencia Internacional de Traumatologia", which was held on Friday the 16th. The program consisted of: discussions of complications and sequellae of head injuries, advances in the treatment of spinal trauma, and free communications. The following doctors participated actively in these panels: Marques, Sano, Lasierra, Vigouroux, Brihaye, Harris, Luyendijk, Mc Laurin, Niemeyer, Oprescu, Rakotobe, Benedek, Ramamurthi, and Nakamura. Once again, this conference, like the others, was a great success, and the members were enthusiastic, seeing that the CNT was one of the most effective scientific committees in the WFNS.

In 1980, the CNT moved to New York with Dr. Mc Laurin as organizer, this history will be told another time.

Brussels   Prof. JEAN BRIHAYE

I respectfully apologize for possible omissions of names or of documents and statements, but this report is essentially based upon by personal notes or memories; it was indeed no easy task to collect the data. I want to thank W. Luyendijk and S. Lindgren for their assistance.

List of Organizers

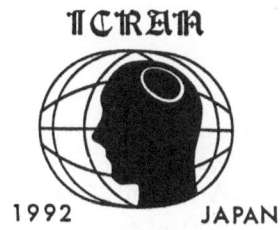

ICRAN

1992   JAPAN

Honorary President
Keiji Sano, M.D.
Shozo Ishii, M.D.
Hiroyasu Makino, M.D.

President
Norio Nakamura, M.D.

Organizing Committee

Hiroshi Abe, M.D.	Keizoh Matsumoto, M.D.	Hideo Terao, M.D.
Tetsuhiko Asakura, M.D.	Shozo Nakazawa, M.D.	Takashi Tsubokawa, M.D.
Masashi Fukui, M.D.	Akira Nishimoto, M.D.	Akira Yamaura, M.D.
Toru Hayakawa, M.D.	Syuro Nishimura, M.D.	Yukichi Yonemasu, M.D.
Kimiyoshi Hirakawa, M.D.	Haruo Sakai, M.D.	Takashi Yoshimoto, M.D.
Haruhiko Kikuchi, M.D.	Hiroaki Sekino, M.D.	
Shinken Kuramoto, M.D.	Kintomo Takakura, M.D.	

Secretary
Takuo Hashimoto, M.D.

Local Committee

Toshiaki Abe, M.D.	Tsutomu Koyama, M.D.	Satoshi Tani, M.D.
Takaharu Fuse, M.D.	Shigehiro Nakahara, M.D.	Masaharu Yasue, M.D.
Ryuzo Ishiyama, M.D.	Shoichi Sanada, M.D.	Kenji Yuhki, M.D.
Masami Kamio, M.D.	Jun Sato, M.D.	
Ryuichi Kanda, M.D.	Soji Shinoda, M.D.	

Neurotraumatology Committee

Chairman:	G. Dohrmann, M.D., U.S.A.
Deputy Chairman:	M. Sambasivan, M.D., India
Secretary:	D. Stålhammer, M.D., Sweden
Deputy Secretary:	P. Niemeyer, Jr., M.D., Brazil
Historian:	J. Brihaye, M.D., Belgium
Ex-Officio:	L. Symon, M.D., U.K.
Past Chairman:	A.V. Marques, M.D., Portugal
	R. Vigouroux, M.D., France

Supported by:
Japan Brain Foundation
The Japan Neurosurgical Society
Japan Foundation for Emergency Medicine
Japanese Society of Neurotraumatology
The Commemorative Association for the Japan World Exposition (1970)
Inoue Foundation for Science

1—Presidential Lecture

Protective Effectiveness of a Safety Helmets – Its Limitations in Preventing Diffuse Brain Injury

NORIO NAKAMURA[1], SATOSHI TANI[2], and SHIGEYUKI MURAKAMI[2]

[1]Professor and Chairman Department of Neurosurgery, The Jikei University, School of Medicine, Minato-ku, Tokyo, 105 Japan, and [2]Department of Neurosurgery, The Jikei University, School of Medicine, Minato-ku, Tokyo, 105 Japan

SUMMARY

The first step of the study was animal experiments using eighty-five monkeys in close cooperation with engineers from the Japan Automobile Research Institute (JARI).The dynamic mechanism of craniocerebral injury was investigated which resulted in development of the JARI Human Head Impact Tolerance Curve (JHTC). The second step consisted of a series of drop tests using a dummy head wearing a safety helmet. Dynamic data recorded at the moment of impact to the head were evaluated on the basis of JHTC. A crush mark left on the helmet which reflected hight of drop was investigated, too. It was concluded that an impact of approrimateley 21 Km/h was the upper limit under which a helmet could protect a human head from danger.
The third step was a field study of traffic accidents. One hundred and twenty damaged helmets were collected immediately after motorcycle accidents. The extent of crush marks on a shells and liners of the helmets did not always correspond to the severity of brain injury suffered by the riders.
A series of these studies emphasizes that one must not overestimate the advantages of helmet use in preventing craniocerebral injury. That means, in terms of protective effectiveness of a helmet, it appears that a helmet does not sufficiently protect against diffuse brain injury induced by rotational acceleration impact to the human head at the moment of impact.

KEY WORDS: head injury, animal experiment, helmet,safety threshold, motocycle accident

INTRODUCTION

According to clinical studies which were undertaken in the University of Pennsylvania Head Injury Center, the two worst types of head injury were subdural hematoma and severe diffuse axonal injury[1]. These two are thought to be produced by different dynamic mechanisms at the moment of impact to the head. From a neurosurgical viewpoint, surgical and conservative treatment to severe head injuries have played a limited role in saving life and minimizing posttraumatic neurological deficits.In addition,such injuries as subdural hematoma or diffuse axonal injury are induced primarily at the moment of impact. Under these circumstances nothing is more impotant than the prevention of severe head injury itself.

A helmet is believed to protect the head from injury by altering the dynamic nature of the impact to the head making it less destructive. This is qualitatively true though it is not certain to what extent a helmet reduces the impact by its cushioning characteristics. We conducted a series of experimental as well as field studies to elucidate the protective effectiveness of a helmet quantitatively.

Our study had three steps.
The first step consisted of animal experiments.
The second step was the dropping of a dummy human head, firstly helmeted and then unprotected.
The third step was the analysis of damaged-helmets involved in traffic accidents.

This series of studies revealed both qualitatively and quantitatively the limited capacity of a helmet in protecting the human head from injury. Its capacity depended on the force of impact to the head as well as the dynamic mechanism producing brain injury.

STEP 1 : ANIMAL EXPERIMENTS

Under close co-operation with engineers, two experimental projects were scheduled over the course of ten years. The purpose of the first project was to answer primarily the question of which contributes more in producing brain injury, translational acceleration impact or angular acceleration impact. The second project was to elucidate the different features of brain injury as a consequence of different impact sites on the head. The final goal of these animal experiments was to estimate the tolerance limit of the human head on the basis of experimentally determined safety thresholds in monkeys

Experimental Apparatus and Impact Method

To deliver translational acceleration impact to the monkey's head, experimental apparatus was specially designed(Fig.1). The whole system was composed of a sled, a sled rail and an impactor. A monkey was fixed to the hard head restraint mask which was suspended on the slider guide of the sled. When the sled was pushed by the thrust column powered by compressed air, the slider on the sled moved along the slider guide and impinged against the lead block and the whole sled system with the animal ran straight along the rail. Thus, purely translational acceleration impact was delivered to the monkeys head.[2][3][4]

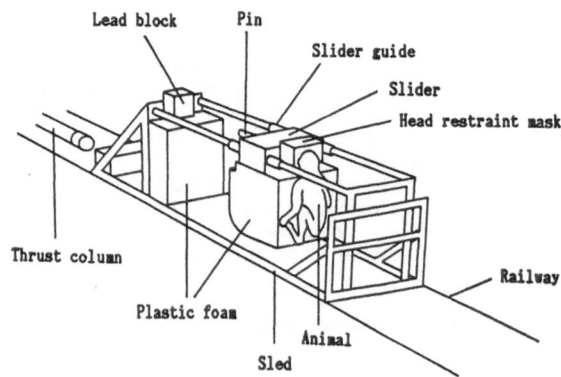

Fig.1 Illustration of the impacter system for translational acceleration impact.

To deliver angular acceleration impact, further experimental apparatus was designed. This system was composed of a monkey chair and an impactor ejection device.(Fig.2) The impactor ejection device was driven by compressed air and gave impact to the head of the monkey seated on the chair. In the first experiment, the head of the animal was restrained in an metal cap. However,in the second experiment the head was positioned and fastened loosely to the supporting poles.[5][6][7][8]

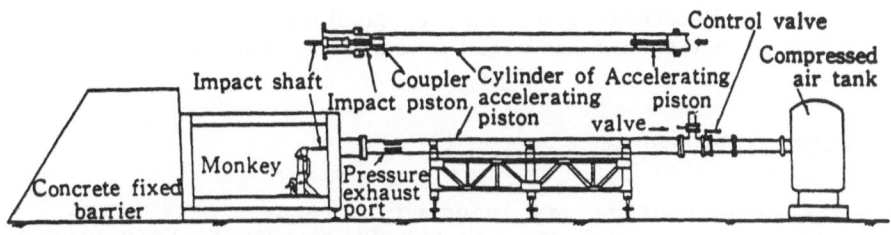

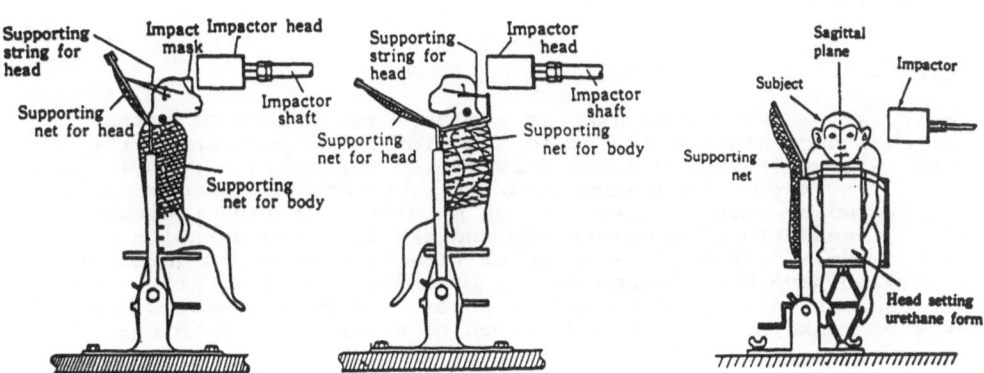

Fig.2 Illustration of the impactor system for rotational acceleration impact.

Table 1 and Table 2 shows physical measurements and medical examinations.

Table 1   Physical examinations
　　　　　　Acceleration—duration(X,Y,Z axes)
　　　　　　　Head, slider, sled
　　　　　　Volocity
　　　　　　　Head (4000 f/s)
　　　　　　　Body (2000 f/s)

5

Table 2

Medical observations

Physiological survey (respiration, pulse rate, blood pressure, EEG, ECG, auditory brain stem response)

Biochemical survey (blood gas analysis of O_2, CO_2 and PH)

Neurological survey (corneal reflex, light reflex, eye movement, oculocephalic response, pain response)

Radiological survey (chest XP, skull XP)

Pathological survey (autopsy, optical microscopic examinations)

Dimensional and weight measurements (skull, brain)

Experimental Procedure

Ketamine hydrochloride was injected intramuscularly about 2 hrs prior to the experiment and the scheduled sensors were placed in position on the subject.The impact was delivered to the head under light anesthesia.

When the monkey did not survive the experiment, an autopsy was performed immediately. Monkeys that survived were sacrificed within a week and autopsied.

Results

Twenty-six monkeys were used to evaluate the effect of translational acceleration impact to the midfrontal portion of the head. Eleven monkeys did not survive the experiment. Surprisingly enough, no gross brain contusion or intracerebral hemorrhage was discovered by autopsy, even though magnitude of impact exceeded 1100G translational acceleration and 4millisecond duration at the most. From a pathological point of view, the monkey's death appeared to have been caused mainly by chest injuries. After ardent discussions on these experiments we decided posttraumatic alertness of monkeys to be an indication of safety limits in head injury.[4]

The criteria of concussion in our series of animal experiments is shown on the Table3. Fifty-nine monkeys were used to evaluate the effect of angular acceleration impact alone or in conjunction with translational acceleration impact to the midfrontal, midoccipilal or lateral part of the head.

Table 3 Criteria of concussion.

a. Loss of the corneal reflex persists for at least 20 seconds after the impact.
b. Respiration ceases for at least 20 seconds after the impact.
c. Two levels of severity of blood pressure disturbance occurs: "absent-mild" on one level, and "severe" on another level. These level are distinguished according to three indices, namely, the bradycardia, the duration and the overall patterns of the blood pressure.
These three criteria were used to grade the level of concussion as follows:
0: none of the three criteria applies.
I: one of the three criteria applies.
II: two of the three criteria apply.
III: all three criteria apply.

The angular and rotational acceleration impact to the monkey's head produced a variety of brain injuries, which were subarachnoid hemorrhage, brain contusion, brain stem hemorrhage, subdural hematoma etc in conjunction with concussion.

Rough results are shown on the Fig.3.

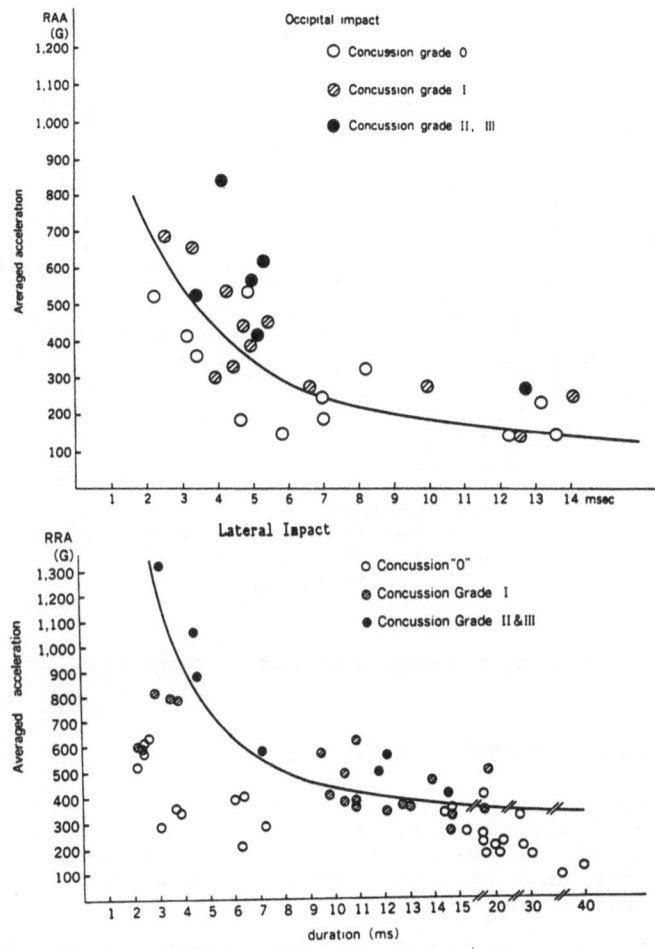

Fig.3 Results of animal experiments (Frontal impact omitted).

The X-axis shows duration of impact and the Y-axis averaged acceleration of impact. An open circle represents no concussion, a shaded one grade 1 concussion, a closed one severe concussion. A curved line shows the estimated safety limit with regard to the manifestation of concussion.

By applying the dimensional analysis method of Stalnacker et al. to the experimentally determined concussion threshold in monkeys,

it was possible to estimate the concussion threshold in humans[9]
[10]. Upon extrapolation of the data from monkeys to humans, it
was assumed that geometric forms of monkey and human's heads are
analogous and biological tissues are the same.
Thus, the Human Head Tolerance Curve of frontal or occipital
impact and lateral impact based on the animal experiments are
obtained.(Fig.4)[11]

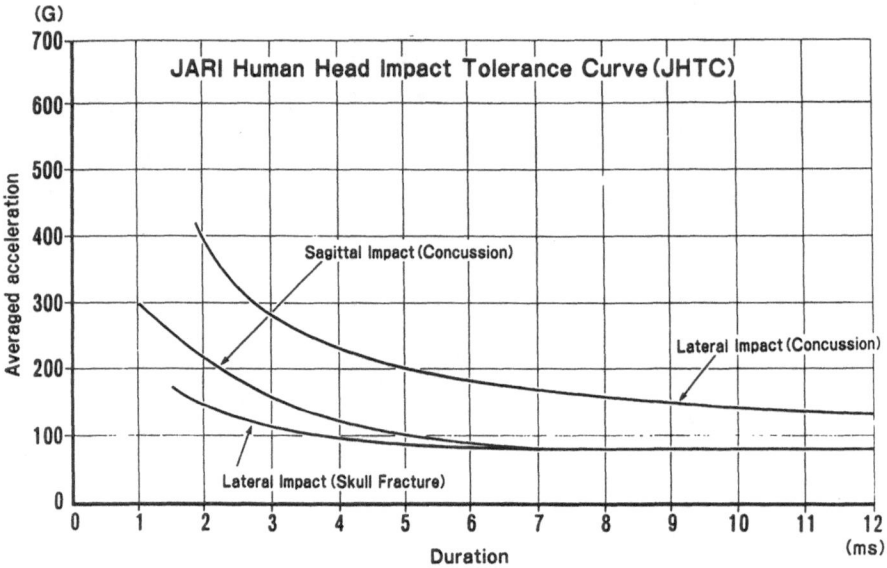

Fig.4 JARI Human Head Impact Tolerance Curve (JHTC).

STEP 2 : SAFETY HELMET DROP TEST

Since 5th july, 1986, wearing of helmet has been made obligatory
by road traffic laws for all motocycle riders in Japan. And quality standard of the helmet is set by japanese Industrial Standard since 1961, and is quite similar to standards in the U.S.A.
or Britain except for details.

This second step of the study had two objectives. The first was
to know quantitatively to what extent a helmet reduces the force
of impact by its cushioning. The second was to determine safety
limits of a helmeted human head in terms of collision velocity
ona hard plane, by applying the dynamic results of the drop test
tothe previously mentioned Head Tolerance Curve.

Experimental Apparatus and Impact Method.

A drop test apparatus is shown on Fig.5. The maximum possible
hight of the first crane was 200 cms. Another crane was used in
tests exceeding 200cms drop tests. Steel floor was used. The
helmets examined were made in Japan and passed the Japanese Industrial Standard C type, and had an average weight of 1270 gram-
ms.

The dummy head was made in the U.S.A, a NHTSA Hybrid 2type containing a three dimensional accelerometer inside, and covered with artificial rubber skin. Its total weight was 4655gramms(Fig. 6)

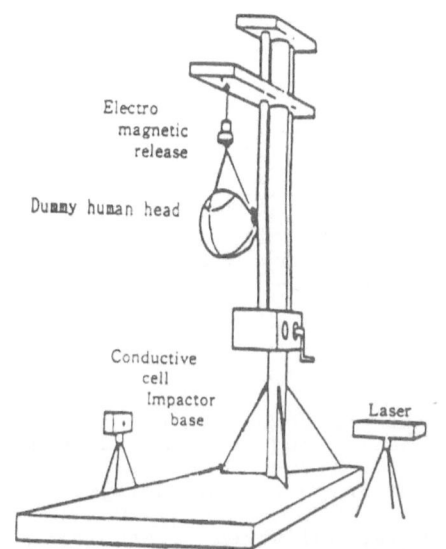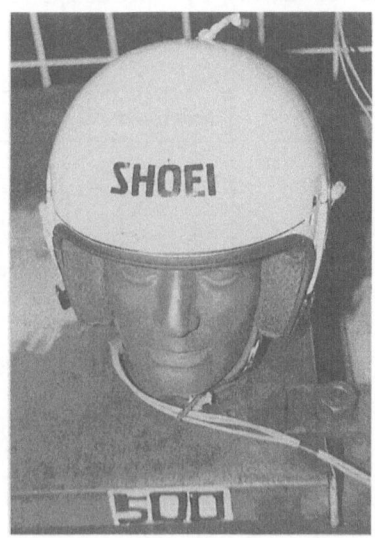

Fig.5 Drop test appratus.

Fig.6 Helmeted human dummy head.

Experimental Procedure.

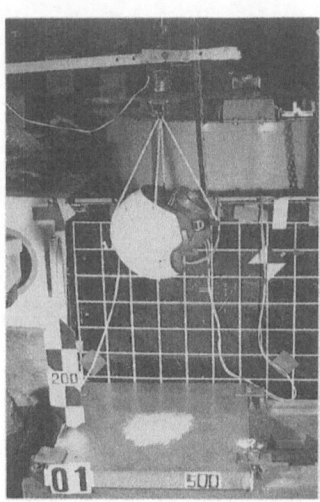

Fig.7 Drop test.(Midfrontal impact).

9

The impact sites were midfrontal, midoccipital and temporal.(Fig. 7)The dummy head was suspended from the drop test apparatus with an electromangnetic connecter and fell freely after disconnection from the connector. A diagram of dynamic measurement is shown on Fig.8. Velocity of the dummy head at collision was measured using a high-speed camera in some of the drop tests,in conjuction with theoretical estimation. Average impact acceleration and duration were obtained by the composition of threedimensional dynamic measurements.

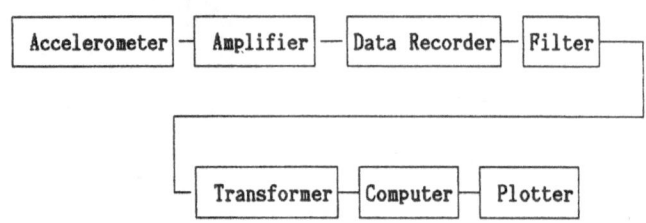

Fig.8 Test diagram

Prior to each test, blue colored-oil was spread on the floor surface. The contact area between helmet and floor could be measured by reference to the presense of oil on the helmet. After the drop tests, helmets were divided and inspected for damage.

Eighteen helmets were used. Impact was delivered to each area of the helmet only once. As a control test the unhelmeted dummy head was dropped in the same way(Fig.9).However, because we were afraid that the dummy head was not strong enough to withstand impact,the dropping distance was limited to a maximum of 75cms.

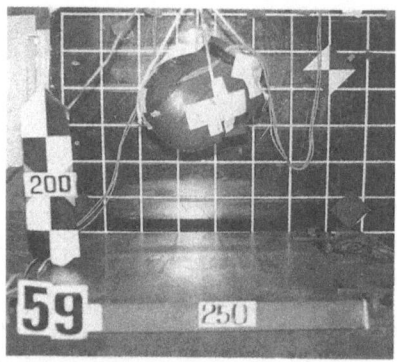

Fig.9 Drop test unhelmeted dummy.

Results

The principal results with regard to the efficiency of the helmet are shown on the Fig.10 and Fig.11. Fig.10 shows the results of frontal impact. Open circles represent the unhelmeted dummy head. Experiment No72 and No73 are shown to be on the safe side of the Tolerance Curve. The drop distance of these two tests was 75 cms.

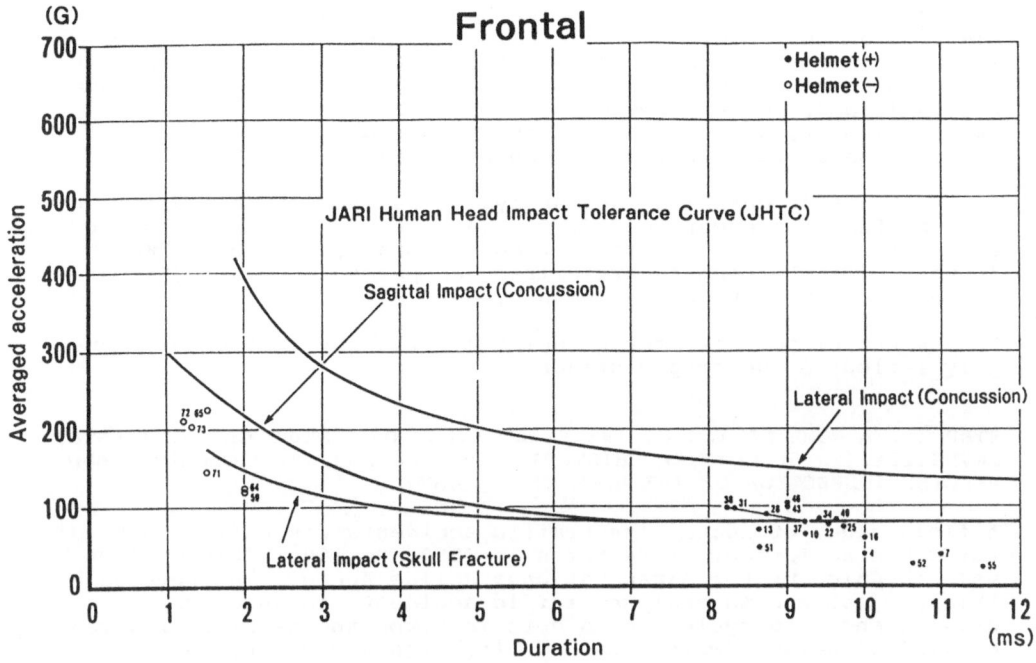

Fig.10 Results of drop tests.(Midfrontal impact)

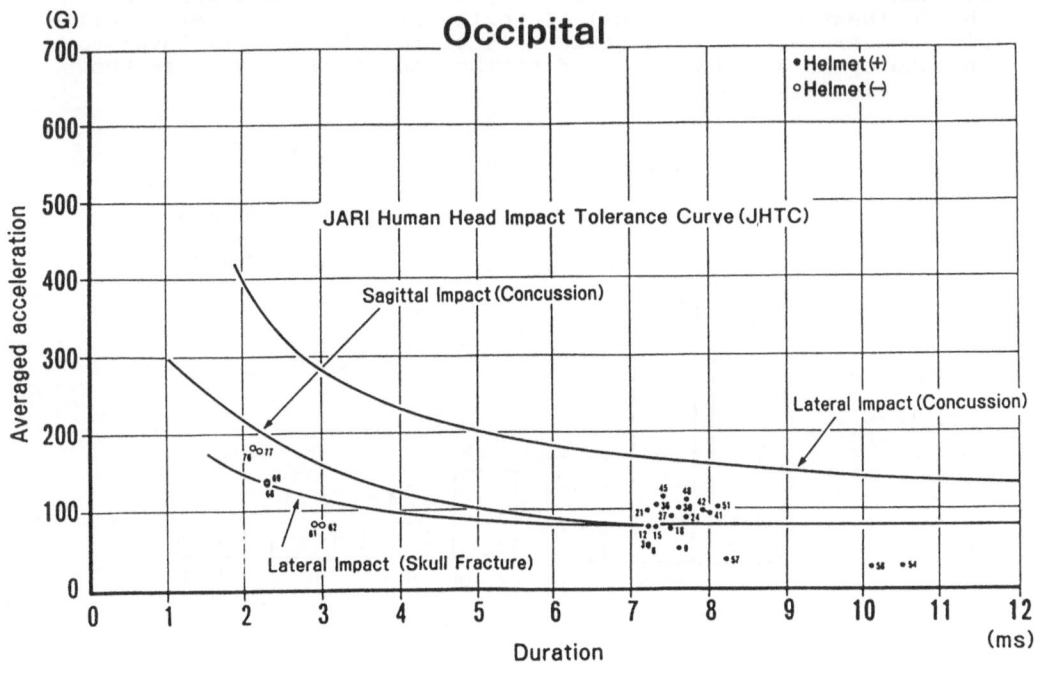

Fig.11 Results of drop test.(Midoccipital impact)

Closed circles represent the helmeted dummy head. Experiment No37
was just on the Tolerance Curve. Drop distance was 183cms. These
results demonstrate that the tolerance threshold of the unhelmeted human head to impact is estimated to be a little over to 75cms.
But is 183cms, for a helmeted head.In cases of occipital and
lateral impact,the threshold of the helmeted human head is estimated to be a little below a dropping distance of 150cms.

On the basis of detailed data analysis, we can estimate a helmet
will protect the human head from injury at a collision velocity
of about 21kms/hr at a maximum frontal impact, of about 19Kms h
in both occipital and lateral impact compared to about 12Kms hr
in cases of the unhelmeted human head.

The extent of contact area on helmets marked by colored oil roughly reflected the drop distance.

**STEP 3 : A COMBINATION OF THE FIELD STUDY OF MOTORCYCLE ACCIDENTS,
INVESTIGATION OF CLINICAL HISTORIES OF INJURIED MOTORCYCLISTS AND
PRECISION INSPECTION OF THE HELMETS INVOLVED.**

A field study of successive traffic accidents was carried out for
three months in four prefectures in 1990 and 1991. This project
was scheduled by the Japan National Police Agency. The purpose of
this project was to analyse traffic accidents in which car
drivers and motorcycle riders were involved and severely injured
or died.65 helmets were obtained after the accidents, and we
received clinical histories of the riders too, thanks to cooperation of riders involved and the doctors who gave them medical care. Besides these 65 helmets, we obtained 55 helmets over
the last 25 years, all of which had been worn in past motorcycle
accidents. With regard to these 55, both the circumstances of
the accident and the medical histories of the riders were available. Therefore, we investigated all of the 120 helmets involved
in motorcycle accidents. Age distribution of 111 riders is shown
on the Fig.12.

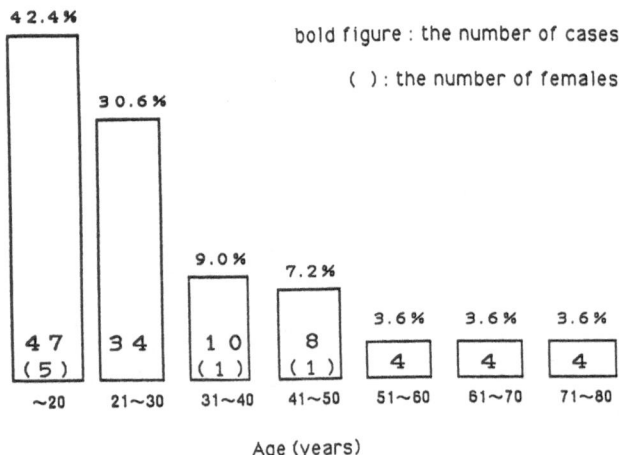

Fig.12 Age distribution of 111 motorcyclists

Data Analysis.

When an accident card indicated that the helmet came off at the
beginning of the accident and that the principal impact was
deliverd to the rider's uncovered head, the case was classified
in an "uncapped" group. Cases impacted to the face and showed
cerebral symptomes were classified in the same group.

Clinical severity of injuries was graded on the basis of Japanese
Abbreviated Injury Scale (J-AIS). JAIS Grade 0-2.5 represents
mild injury,3.0 to 5.0 severe and 6.0 to 9.0 death. When
posttraumatic initial loss of consciousness persisted for more
than 6hours, the case was diagnosed as diffuse axonal injury
after Gennarelli.

Inspection and Investigation of Helmets.

At first, the appearance of the outside and inside of the helmet
was deliberately inspected to find any crush or scratch mark on
the surface.(Fig.13,Fig.14,and Fig.15). The results were
recorded on a chart and photographed. Then the helmet was cut by
an electric saw and the inside of the shell and outside of the
plastic foam liner was inspected. The results were recorded.

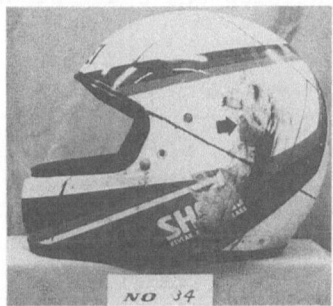

Fig.13 Damage mark on the outer surface of the shell.

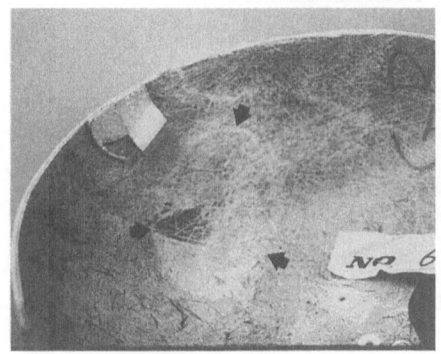 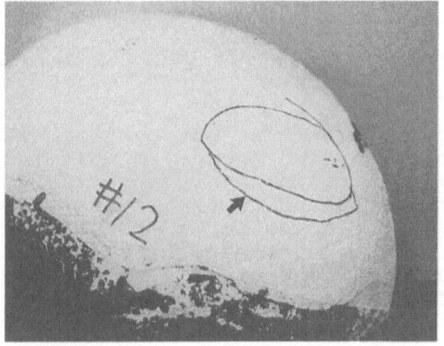

Fig.14 Damage mark on the inner surface of the shell.
Fig.15 Damage mark on the outer surface of the plastic
foam liner.

13

Severity of damage of helmets was graded into four categories.

Grade 0   no damage mark
Grade 1   mark on the shell but not on the liner.
Grade 2   mark on both the shell and liner.
          The area of the injury mark on the liner was less than
          30 square cms.
Grade 3   mark on both the shell and the liner.
          The area of mark is 30 square cm or larger.

Results and Discussion

It was to be expected that injuries were more severe in the uncapped group than in the helmeted group(Fig.16).Table 4 summarizes clinical diagnosis of riders in the two groups. It is clear
that skull fracture and focal brain damage were more frequent in
the uncapped group. Whereas, simple head injury without loss of
consciousness was frequent in the helmeted group.
These results mean that the hard shell of a helmet reduced deformation of the skull at the impact site which resulted less frequent skull fracture. Moreover, the plastic foam liner of a helmet had a cushioning effect to translational acceleration impact
as illustrated in the second step experiment, which resulted in
less frequent brain contusion and acute subdural hematoma

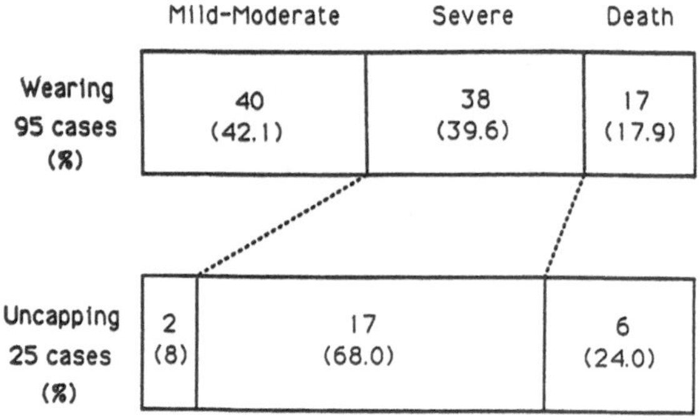

	Mild-Moderate	Severe	Death
Wearing 95 cases (%)	40 (42.1)	38 (39.6)	17 (17.9)
Uncapping 25 cases (%)	2 (8)	17 (68.0)	6 (24.0)

Fig.16 Overall severity of head injury.

However, we must not overlook the frequency of diffuse brain
injury in two groups in this analysis. As you can see on Table 4,
diffuse brain injury appeared to be more frequent among helmeted
riders, although statistcally insignificant. Diffuse brain injury is believed to be produced primarily by a shearing force in
consequence of angular acceleration movement in the brain[12][13]
[14][15]. Therefore, the cushioning effect of a helmet was possibly insufficientto protect the brain from shearing at the moment
of impact.

Table 4 Diagnosis head injury and its frequency in two groups.

	Wearing 95 cases (%)	Uncapping 25 cases (%)
Simple head injury	30 (31.6)	(0.0)
Fracture		
Vault	15 (15.8)	10 (40.0)
Basilar	11 (9.4)	6 (24.0)
Focal brain damage		
Acute subdural hematoma	9 (9.5)	6 (24.0)
Acute epidural hematoma	0 (0.0)	3 (12.0)
Cerebral contusion	25 (26.3)	12 (48.0)
Diffuse brain damage		
Concussion	10 (10.5)	4 (9.5)
Diffuse axonal injury	17 (17.9)	4 (9.5)

Here we have some further data.(Table 5) We investigated the severity of head injuries in connection with the extent of damage marks on helmets inspected. It is reasonable and understandable that more remarkable the damage mark,the more severe the head injury. However, I must emphasize that there are 9 cases on this table who suffered from severe or fatal head injury in spite of amild damage mark on the outer surface of the shell. The extent of damage marked on the helmet is believed to reflect the severity of impact force perpendicular to the helmet. Therefore, in these 9 cases it is possible that a shearing force was delivered to the surface of the helmet and left only a small damage mark on the surface, but gave severe rotational acceleration impact to the head which resulted in severe diffuse brain injury. In fact, the clinical histories of 6 of these 9cases recorded clinical diagnosis of severe diffuse axonal injury.

Table 5 Severity of head injury related to grade of helmet damage in "wearing"riders.

Severity of head injury related to grade of helmet damage in "wearing" cases

Severity	Helmet damage (%)		
	G0-G1	G2	G3
Mild-moderate	27 (28.6)	10 (10.5)	3 (3.2)
Severe	8 (8.2)	20 (21.1)	10 (10.5)
Death	1 (1.1)	4 (4.2)	12 (12.6)

Taking these results into consideration we are afraid the present
safety helmet is unsatisfactory to mitigate diffuse brain injury
at the moment of impact to the head. However,there may be some
other factors that would affect these results, and further investigations are indispensable in evaluating the use of the safety
helmet against rotational acceleration impact to the head.

CONCLUSION

1 Brain injury is produced by a combination of translational and
   angular acceleration impact but rarely by purely translational
   acceleration impact to the head.

2 The safety helmet is effective to protect the head from injury
   at collision velocity of less than about 21km/h.

3 The present helmet is useful to protect the human head from
   focal skull and brain injury but appears to be unsatisfactory
   to mitigate diffuse brain injury.

REFERENCES

[1]Gennarelli TA (1983) Head injury in man and experimental
   animals:Clinical aspects. Acta Neurochir Suppl 32:1-13

[2]Masuzawa H, Nakamura N, Hirakawa K, Sano K, Matsuno M, Sekino
   H,Mii K, Abe T(1976) Experimental head injury using pure
   linear acceleration impact. Neurol Med Chir (Tokyo) Part1 16:
   77-90

[3]Kikuchi A, Ono K, Kobayashi H, Nakamura N, Nakamura M(1980)
   Evaluation of head tolerance to sagittal impact by head
   acceleration and duration, and head velocity. JSAE Rev 3:85-93

[4]Ono K, Kikuchi A, Nakamura M, Kobayashi H, Nakamura N(1980)
   Human head tolerance to sagittal impact reliable estimation
   deduced from experimental head injury using subhuman primates
   and human cadaver skulls. In:Proceedings of 24th Stapp car
   crash conference. Society of automotive engineers,Inc.
   Warrendale. Pennsilvania.pp101-160

[5]Kanda R, Nakamura N, Sekino H, Masuzawa H, Mii K, Aoyagi T,
   Kono H, Sugimori T, Sugiura M, Mori N, Kikuchi A, Ono K,
   Kobayashi H(1981)Experimental head injury in monkeys concu-
   sion and its tolerance level. Neurol Med Chir.(Tokyo) 21:645-
   656

[6]Kikuchi A, Ono K,Nakamura N(1982) Human head tolerance to
   lateral impact reduced from experimental head injuries using
   primates. In:Ninth international conference on experimental
   safety vehicles. Japan Autmobile Instilute,Inc. Tsukuba.
   Ibaraki pp1-21

[7]Sakai H, Nakamura N, Sekino H, Kanda R, Taguchi Y, Kaneko D,
   Masuzawa H, Mii K, Aoyagi N, Aruga T, Sugimori T, Sugiura M,
   Mori N, Kikuchi A, Ono K, Ohashi H, Kobayashi H(1982)
   Experimental head injury with lateral impact using monkeys,
   Neurol Med Chir(Tokyo)22:491-498

[8]Nakamura N, Masuzawa H, Sekino H, Kono H, Kikuchi A, Ono,
   (1983) Which is the more severe impact on the head, sagittal
   or lateral? In: Proceeding of consensus workshop on head and
   necrk criteria. US Department of Transportation National
   Highway Traffic Safety Administration. Washington DC. PP61-68

[9] Stalnacker RL, Roberts VL, McElhaney JH (1973) Side impact tolerance to blunt trauma In:Proceedings of 17th Stapp car crush conference. Society of automotive engineers,Inc. Okurahoma city.Okurahoma.pp377-408

[10] Stalnacker RL, McElhaney JH, Snydes RG, Roberts VL (1971) Door Crashworthiness Criteria. U.S. Department of Transportation Report No HS-800-S34

[11] Nakamura N, Sekino H, Masuzawa H, Mii K, Kikuchi A, Ono K, Kobayashi H(1986) Experimental head injuries due to direct impact acceleration-head tolerance limit to impact.In:Sances Jr A, Thomas DJ, Euring CL, Larson SJ, Unterharnscheidt F, (eds) Mechanism of head and spine trauma. Aloray. Goshen New York. pp219-235

[12] Nakamura N,(1991) Diffuse brain damage in man : Diagnosis and investigation. In: Proceedings of 11th international congress of neuropathology. Kyoto.Japan. pp742-745

[13] Nakamura N (1991) Diffuse brain injury and brainstem dysfunction. In:Frowein R A (ed) Cerebral contusions, lacerations and hematomas. Springer. Wien New York.pp61-89

[14] Gennarelli TA, Thibault LE, Ommaya AK (1972) Pathophysiologic responses to rotational and translational acceleraions to the head. In:Proceedings of sixteenth stapp car crush conference. Society of automotive engineers,Inc. Two Pennsylvania plaza. New York.pp296-308

[15] Ommaya A, Gennarelli TA (1974) Cerebral concussion and traumatic unconsciousness.Brain 97:633-655

2—Prevention of Neurotrauma

The Management of Acute Neurotrauma in Rural and Remote Locations – A Set of Guidelines for the Care of Head and Spinal Injuries

GLEN S. MERRY

Chairman, Trauma Committee, Neurosurgical Society of Australasia, c/- Kenneth G. Jamieson Neurosurgical Unit, Royal Brisbane Hospital, Herston, Queensland, Australia

SUMMARY

The management of acute neurotrauma in rural and remote locations presents difficult and complex problems. Isolation and distance, medical facilities, level of neurosurgical training, specific epidemiological factors and administrative organisation can influence outcome. Acute neurotrauma treatment requires a consultative approach especially in the multiple injured patient and where transfer or retrieval is necessary. Adequate cerebral perfusion, oxygenation and control of intracranial pressure are essential for normal brain function. Preventable causes of death and disability such as delay in instituting primary resuscitation, delay in initiating definitive neurosurgical care and failure to prevent craniocerebral infections are discussed. As acute neurotrauma initially presents to General Practitioners, Rural Surgeons or Emergency Departments in country hospitals, a set of guidelines has been developed to assist in the early management of acute neurotrauma throughout Australasia. It is recognised that as a result of distance, regional geography, historical and philosophical concepts currently in place, a particular guideline may not be applicable in each instance. The guidelines include – epidemiological, mechanism of head injury, prehospital care, primary hospital care, i.e. early management of severe trauma, special neurosurgical assessment, C.T. head scan & skull, Xray guidelines, criteria for admission to hospital with head injury, criteria for neurosurgical consultation, neurosurgical indication for transfer, head injury triage scheme, consultation information for transfer, transport and retrieval, emergency surgical treatment, coma management, paediatric head injury, spinal injury, special issues, i.e. prevention of intracranial infection, restlessness and analgesia, post-traumatic epilepsy, status epilepticus, scalp wounds, minor head injury and discharge of a minor head injury patient, nursing management of acute neurotrauma, summary of major head injury management and neurotrauma - an integrated service.

KEY WORDS: rural, remote locations, management, guidelines, acute neurotrauma

INTRODUCTION

Rural and remote locations present difficulties and challenges in providing acceptable standards of treatment in acute neurotrauma. The aim is to provide care comparable as possible with that obtained in a neurosurgical centre. In Australia small areas of rural population are separated by vast distances with regional neurosurgical units distributed around the coastline where there is a population concentration. In a total population of 17 million, 4.6 million live in rural Australia; 1.9 million live in districts from 20,000 to 80,000 people and 2.7 million reside in districts of up to 20,000. An injured person may need to travel up to 3,000 kilometres to a neurosurgical unit.

This isolation has been referred to as the tyranny of distance. In New Zealand, due to the nature of the terrain and weather conditions, certain areas can present a special problem. Treatment, communications, transport and retrieval systems of trauma have been developed by various organisations in conjunction with regional neurosurgical units. Aerial transport either by fixed-wing or helicopter is an essential component, in addition to road transport. The aims are to minimise delay from the injury site to definitive care and to prevent the development of secondary injury to the brain.

As acute neurotrauma may present to General Practitioners, Rural Surgeons or Emergency Departments in country hospitals, a set of guide-lines has been developed to assist in the early management of acute neurotrauma throughout Australasia. It would be usual practice that operations and procedures for acute neurosurgical conditions normally would be performed by trained Specialist Surgeons. On occasions these operations and procedures may need to be performed by General Practit-ioners who have been trained appropriately. It is recognised that distance, geography, local demography and facilities available may make a particular guideline inapplicable in some instances.

DISCUSSION

The management of acute neurotrauma requires a consultative approach especially in the multiple injured patient and where transfer or re-trieval is necessary. Adequate cerebral perfusion, oxygenation and control of intracranial pressure are essential for normal brain function. Airway control, treatment of hypovolaemic shock, minimising delay from the accident site to definitive care, the development of effective communications, transport and retrieval systems and an appreciation of the mechanism of head injury should contribute to an improved outcome in the neurotrauma patient.

The first comprehensive study carried out by the Trauma Committee of the Neurosurgical Society of Australasia[1] compared a retrospective study of 1,161 cases of neurotrauma in New South Wales, 1977-78 and prospectively in 150 cases of neurotrauma occurring in country dis-tricts of South Australia, 1981-82. This showed that neurotrauma was responsible for 70% of all road fatalities and 50% of trauma deaths. Road crashes caused 50-60% of all head injuries. The highest incidence for hospital admissions in persons under 45 years of age was from trauma.

Three time frames are recognised in road trauma[2] - the first within minutes after the crash and often not compatible with survival, the second within 1-2 hours of injury and the third during the 30 day period following hospital admission. These authors emphasise that rural crashes are often associated with more severe forms of trauma,multiple casualties,time delays and a reduced level of primary care response.

FACTORS IN THE RURAL ENVIRONMENT

The following factors are significant in rural trauma[1,2,3],isolation and distance, medical facilities, level of neurosurgical competence, delay in definitive care, administrative organisation, rural crash pro-files, e.g. incidence of 40% fatality on admission, more severe in-juries, multiple injuries,higher incidence of single vehicle crashes, road and environmental conditions, driver competence and fatigue and compliance with preventative measures such as alcohol, seatbelts, hel-mets and speed. Isolation and population density is demonstrated in Table 1.

Table 1 - Comparison of countries in relation to population, area and population density.

COUNTRY	POPULATION (millions)	AREA km²	POP.density (per km²)
Australia	16.87	7,682.3	2
Canada	26.52	9,976.1	3
Japan	123.46	377.8	327
New Zealand	3.39	271.0	12
United Kingdom	57.24	244.1	234
United States of America	249.22	9,372.6	27

Clinical factors which adversely influence outcome (death and disability) are: severity of primary injury,intracranial complications, hypoxaemia, hypercarbia, hypotension, anaemia, multiple injuries, age, prolonged prehospital time, admission to inappropriate hospital,delayed or inappropriate interhospital transfer/retrieval and delay in definitive surgical treatment.

Preventable or avoidable causes of death or disability[4,5,6] include: delay in instituting primary resuscitation for hypoxia, hypercarbia and hypotension, delay in instituting definitive neurosurgical care especially for the rapidly developing intracranial haematoma and failure to prevent craniocerebral infections. In unplanned trauma systems between 20-25% of deaths possibly could be avoided. Marshall[7] has emphasised the adverse effect of increased distance from neurosurgical units on mortality, the importance of early treatment of shock and hypoxia and the need to develop strategies for improving regional organisation and to have firm linkages between neurosurgical units and rural hospitals.

Abnormal neurological signs involving level of consciousness,pupillary size and reaction to light, brain stem reflexes and motor response indicate the severity of cerebral dysfunction.[1] Children and elderly patients generally react adversely to trauma. Persons over 50 years of age can develop intracranial haematomas from an apparently minor head injury such as a fall.[8] (Table 2)

Table 2   Mortality from intracranial haematoma related to type of injury and age in Brisbane Neurosurgical Units - a prospective study of 3095 cases.

No Cases (1985-86)			3095
Primary admissions (Brisbane : 1 million)			2509
Secondary referrals (Rural : 3 million)			586 (17%)

Type of Injury	Age(years) < 60	Mortality (%) > 60
Road Trauma (1051)	5.3	14.9
Falls (1312)	1.2	18.6

A review of the literature on head and neck injuries in passenger cars [9] found that better first aid and primary care after car crashes may save lives.

PRIMARY HOSPITAL CARE

Primary Hospital Care is based on the early management of severe trauma programme[10]. This is adopted from the advance trauma life support programme in the U.S.A.[11]

The guidelines for computerised tomography scanning for head injured patients in country hospitals were based on a study carried out by Simpson and Worth [12]. The following indications is an example from the current guidelines.

Primary Hospital Care - Management Plan
  C.T. Head Scan Guidelines
  1.   GCS <9 after resuscitation
  2.   Neurological deterioration i..e. 2 points or more on the GCS,
            hemiparesis, squint
  3.   Drowsiness or confusion (GCS 9-12) persisting > 2 hours
  4.   Persistent headache, vomiting
  5.   Focal neurological signs
  6.   Fracture - known or suspected
  7.   Penetrating injury - known or suspected
  8.   Age - over 50 years or age
  9.   Post-operative assessment

Comment: A C.T. scan is the investigation of choice where available.
Except for a trivial injury, all patients ideally should have a C.T.
scan. This may involve a transfer.
Rapid deterioration may require an immediate operation rather than risk
delay in performing a C.T. scan.
As lesions may develop after an initial normal scan, serial C.T. scans
may be required should neurological deterioration occur.
A post-operative scan will demonstrate adequate removal of the
haematoma, reaccumulation or the development of a new lesion.

A Head Injury Triage Scheme was developed for consultation between the
primary hospital and the regional referral centre. This system is
based on level of consciousness (Glasgow Coma Score) size of pupils,
a lateralised neurological deficit, age of patient and presence of a
skull fracture and is modified on a flow chart outlining a systematic
approach to the triage of patients with head injury by Gennarelli. [13]

TRANSFER AND RETRIEVAL

The indications and timing for admission to a neurosurgical unit is a
decision taken in the light of any injury to other systems and with
particular attention to cardiopulmonary stabilisation.

The management options for intracranial haemorrhage include: 1. rapid
transfer under intensive care with or without Mannitol or Frusemide
and 2. immediate on-the-spot operation with neurosurgical support if
there is rapid deterioration and fastest transport time is greater
than 2 hours.

The decision on these options should follow neurosurgical consultation
based on: transfer time, clinical state i.e. level of consciousness
and pupillary size and light reflex, rate of deterioration and C.T.scan
(if available) or xray of skull.

A patient with a deteriorating head injury in a country hospital is
assessed and discussed with a neurosurgeon.[14] Should the fastest
transport time be greater than 2 hours distance, the patient is intubated, ventilated, given Mannitol and Frusemide and transferred to a
neurosurgical unit. If the transport is less than 2 hours, an
immediate burr hole exploration is advised with clot evacuation(extradural haematoma or subdural haematoma) via craniectomy or craniotomy
depending upon the level of neurosurgical expertise. The patient is
transferred to the regional unit by a retrieval team. Emergency
surgical treatment[15,16] for evacuation of acute EHD and acute SDH is
included in the guidelines together with an illustrated reference set
of instruments.

NEUROTRAUMA - AN INTEGRATED SERVICE

An integrated neurotrauma service is required for the management of
acute neurotrauma. This involves the early management of severe trauma,
communication systems, transport and retrieval systems, regional neurotrauma centre, uniform injury assessment, uniform data collection,
hospital accreditation, continuing medical education, rehabilitation
and long term support.

The increased availability of C.T. scanners and the development of
teleradiology[17,18] with access to a regional neurosurgery unit should
aid in improving the outcome in acute neurotrauma.

The guidelines were presented at the Annual Scientific Meeting of the
Royal Australasian College of Surgeons, Canberra 13th May 1992.[19]

REFERENCES

1. Trauma Subcommittee of the Neurosurgical Society of Australasia
    (1986) Neurotrauma in Australia. Report on Surveys in New South
    Wales and South Australia. Blackwell Scientific Publications,
    Melbourne.

2. Trinca GW, Johnson IR, Campbell BJ, Haight FA, Knight PR, Mackay GM,
    McLean AJ, Petrucelli E (1988) Reducing Traffic Injury - A Global
    Challenge. Royal Australasian College of Surgeons, AH Massina & Co.
    Melbourne pp 72-74

3. Traffic Safety Branch, Queensland Department of Transport, Traffic
    Safety Advisory Committee Seminar (1989) Innovative directions for
    Road Safety. Department of Transport, Brisbane.

4. Simpson D, North B, Gilligan J, McLean J, Woodward A, Antonio J,
    Altree P (1984) Neurological injuries in South Australia:
    The influence of distance on management and outcome. Aust. NZ. J.
    Surg. 54, 29-35 (Reprinted in Neurotrauma in Australia, Blackwell
    Scientific Publications, Melbourne).

5   Selecki BR, Berry G, Dan NG, Kwok B, Mandryk JA, North JB, Ring IT,
    Sewell MF, Simpson DA, Stening WA, Vanderfield G (1986)
    Preventable causes of death and disability from neurotrauma
    Aust. NZ. J. Surg 56, 529-534 (Reprinted in Neurotrauma in
    Australia, Blackwell Scientific Publications, Melbourne).

6. Deane SA, Gaudry PL, Woods P, Cass D, Hollands MJ, Cook RJ, Read C
    (1988) The Management of Injuries - A review of deaths in hospital.
    Aust. NZ. J.Surg 58, 463-469

7. Marshall L (1990) Preventable causes of bad outcomes - the neuro-
    surgeon's viewpoint. Abstract, Annual Scientific Meeting, Alice
    Springs Neurosurgical Society of Australasia, Symposium on Head
    Injuries in rural areas. pp 12

8. Stuart G (1992) - personal communications (paper in preparation)

9. McLean AJ, Simpson DA, Cain CMS, McCaul KA, Freund JR, Ryan GA (1987)
    Head and Neck Injuries in passenger cars : A review of the litera-
    ture. NH & MRC Road Accident Research Unit, University of Adelaide.
    Transport and Communications, Federal Office of Road Safety.
    Canberra, pp 6.10

10. Early Management of Severe Trauma Course Manual. Trauma Committee,
    Royal Australasian College of Surgeons.

11. Deane SA, Ramenofsky ML (1991) Advanced Trauma Life Support in the
    1980's : A decade of improvement in trauma care. Aust.NZ. J.Surg
    61, 809-813

12. Simpson DA, Worth RJ (1989) Neurotrauma in Country Hospitals :
    The role of Computerised Tomography Scanning (Editorial Comment)
    Aust. NZ. J.Surg 59, 1-3

13. Gennarelli TA (1986) Triage of Head Injured patients, Chapter
    author. Current Therapy of Trauma - 2, Trunkey DD, Lewis FR,
    BC Decer INC. Toronto. Philadelphia.

14. Simpson DA, Heyworth JS, McLean AJ, Gilligan JE, North JB (1988)
    Extradural haemorrhage strategies for management in remote places.
    Injury 19, 307-312

15. Oatey PE, Dinning TAR, Simpson DA (1983) Extradural haematomas in
    children, primary and secondary bleed intervals. Med J Aust 2,
    176-180

16. North JB (1992) - personal communication

17. Dohrmann PJ (1991) Low-cost teleradiology for Australia
    (original articles) Aust. NZ. J.Surg 61, 115-117

18. Richardson GD (1992) Management of Head Injuries in a country
    centre, teleradiology for neurosurgical consultation. Abstract
    Royal Australasian College of Surgeons' General Scientific
    Meeting, Canberra pp 211

19. Trauma Committee Neurosurgical Society of Australasia, Merry GS,
    Simpson DA, Fearnside M, Brazenor G, Chandran N, Dan N, Klug G,
    Liddell J, Newcombe R, North JB, Oatey P, Rosenfeld J, Stening W,
    Vanderfield G, Worth R (1992) The Management of acute neurotrauma
    in rural and remote locations - A set of guidelines for the care
    of head and spinal injuries.

Understanding Head Impact Tolerance as an Aid in Injury Prevention

A.J. McLean

NHMRC Road Accident Research Unit, University of Adelaide, Adelaide, Australia

SUMMARY:

Head injury prevention is best achieved by ensuring that there is no impact to the head. That is not always possible and so ways must be found to reduce the severity of the injuries that do occur when the head is hit. Protective headgear, such as the motorcyclist's crash helmet, can do this. However, in the design of crash helmets, and of vehicle components that are likely to be struck by the head in an accident, it is important to take into account the tolerance of the head to impact. This paper reviews the development and limitations of the most commonly used measure of head impact tolerance, the Head Injury Criterion, in the context of alternative tolerance criteria and research findings from experimental studies on human surrogates and the investigation of head injuries in actual crashes.

KEY WORDS: head, brain, impact tolerance, injury prevention, crash helmets.

INTRODUCTION:

This paper deals with the prevention of head injury from blunt impacts to the human head, with particular reference to injuries sustained in road accidents. Regardless of the characteristics of an impact, we know that it is desirable to spread its force over as wide an area of the head as possible. This has been recognised since ancient times, as we can see from helmets worn by warriors more than 1,000 years ago.

The coming of the motorised age increased the frequency of the type of head impact in which the moving head strikes an object, rather than a missile striking a stationary head. The first response to the recognition of the motorist's increased risk of head injury was to adapt the warrior's helmet to use as a crash helmet, with a composite fibrous material rather than steel plate for the shell. Helmets of this type were used in motorcycle racing before the first World War, but it was not until the 1950's that road going motorcyclists were seen wearing helmets. However it soon became apparent that although the hard shell provided substantial protection against skull fracture, particularly from concentrated impacts, it did not appear to significantly reduce the risk of brain injury in many cases.

The stiff shell of the early helmets was held away from the head by a webbing harness. This harness could absorb only a limited amount of the energy of an impact on the helmet and so inner liners, usually of compressed cork, were added. However in the 1960's the cork was replaced with rigid foam plastic, and liners covering most of the inside of the shell became common. During the 1980's helmets having no outer shell, but consisting almost entirely of a rigid plastic foam moulding, were introduced for use by pedal cyclists. This development has assumed that absorption of the energy of the impact is more important than distributing the impact load over a wider area of the head, and that most objects struck by the head of a cyclist involved in a crash are likely to impart a distributed load to the helmet rather than one concentrated in a small area.

THE TOLERANCE OF THE HEAD TO IMPACT

The best known of the early attempts to establish the tolerance of the head to impact was work carried out by Gurdjian and Lissner at Wayne State University in Detroit. The part of their work which is most relevant to this paper consisted primarily of impacts to the frontal bone of the cadaver head. The acceleration imparted to the head by the impact was measured and the outcome variable was the presence or absence of skull fracture. The results of the work indicated that very high accelerations or forces acting for a very short period of time were unlikely to be injurious in terms of skull fracture and that relatively low forces were similarly non-injurious even though they may have acted over a much longer time period. The researchers joined these two extremes of acceleration and time with a smooth curve which became known as the Wayne State Tolerance Curve. Gurdjian et al assumed that the presence of a linear skull fracture could normally be assumed to be accompanied by concussion in the living human. The Wayne State Tolerance Curve was therefore commonly referred to as indicating the threshold of concussion rather than skull fracture.[1]

The results of other experiments were added to the original data from the studies by Gurdjian and his co-workers. Human volunteer data obtained from the United States Air Force rocket sled, as exemplified by the pioneering runs by Colonel John Stapp, provided valuable input to the extreme right of the curve with comparatively low forces acting over relatively long periods of time. Studies using cadavers became more sophisticated, to the point where it was possible to pressurise the vascular system of the brain in such a way as to enable vascular lesions to be detected following an impact to the head.

Experiments on sub-human primates conducted in the United States by Ommaya [2] and later by Gennarelli [3] began to cast doubt on the adequacy of a tolerance measure which was based on the linear acceleration imparted to the head through an impact to the frontal bone. In particular both Ommaya and Gennarelli argued that impacts to the side of the head were more likely to result in brain injury than were impacts to the front of the head and that this difference could be explained by the much higher levels of angular acceleration in the lateral impacts. Gennarelli went on to claim that "Except for skull fracture and epidural hematoma, virtually every known type of brain injury can be produced by angular acceleration".[4]

Studies conducted in Japan by Nakamura, Ono and others using sub-human primates and human cadaver skulls demonstrated that "Fatal visible brain injuries could not be produced simply by means of the translational impact against the head with a gravity of acceleration around 1,000 G."[5] While rotational head acceleration was found to be an important factor in the causation of brain injuries, the investigators noted that "Deformation of the skull upon impact, and hence the contact area of the head upon impact, also play significant roles". They concluded that when concussion was taken as the outcome variable, lateral impacts were less likely to be injurious than saggital impacts. However when skull fracture was taken as the outcome variable, lateral impacts were significantly more likely to be injurious.

In the early 1980's the author initiated an on-going study of head impact characteristics and patterns of brain injury in living humans involved in road crashes in and around Adelaide, South Australia. The results of that work thus far are consistent with the finding by Gennarelli, based on studies conducted on sub-human primates, that impacts on the frontal bone are less likely to produce brain injury than are lateral impacts to the head. Most of the vascular lesions in the brain resulting from lateral impacts are not adjacent to the struck side of the head and hence are not directly related to contact phenomena at that location or to skull fracture.[6]

There has been considerable discussion of the extent to which it is valid to extrapolate from the results of tests conducted on sub-human primates and human cadavers to the living human. (See, for example, [7] and [8].) The Australian work mentioned in the previous paragraph suggests that, at least in general terms, such extrapolation is helpful. However there has been less attention devoted to the possible effects of differences between individual humans with respect to tolerance to head impact. Several researchers have reported that age has a very marked influence on the nature of injuries to the head.(See, for example, 9].) It is also possible that anthropometric differences in the shape of the cranial cavity may influence the pattern of brain injury resulting from an impact to a given location on the head.[10]

HEAD INJURY CRITERIA

With the development of the Wayne State Tolerance Curve it became possible to devise a simple mathematical expression to calculate the probability that a given impact to the head would result in "intolerable" injury to the brain. The Severity Index, developed by Gadd of General Motors in the 1960s, is a measure of the area under the acceleration/time curve for a given impact to the head but with particular emphasis given to the magnitude of the acceleration rather than the duration of the impact.[11] Today the Head Injury Criterion is the most widely used measure of the risk of severe or fatal brain injury resulting from an impact to the head.[12]   It was derived directly from the Gadd Severity Index.[13]

The Head Injury Criterion, or HIC as it is more generally known, removes from consideration relatively low levels of acceleration acting over an extended period because such impact conditions have been shown from human volunteer work to be non-injurious. However, as indicated above, the impact conditions which formed the original basis of the Wayne State Tolerance Curve, namely impacts on the frontal bone of the skull, are the least likely to be associated with brain damage or skull fracture. The limitations of HIC have been recognised for some years [14] but, largely because it is specified in motor vehicle safety legislation in the United States, it continues to be used. A tolerance curve based on the Japanese work referred to earlier in this paper appears to be more closely related to the actual risk of head injury in the human, particularly for saggital and lateral impacts.[5]

Other head injury criteria have been proposed which have been derived from mathematical models based on the frequency response of the human head to impact. The Mean Strain Criterion (MSC) devised by Stalnaker and McElhaney is one example.[15]   French and Australian researchers have recently demonstrated a consistent association between patterns of brain injury and brain injury mechanisms deduced from frequency response, or modal analysis, studies of the in vivo human head and impacted objects.[16]

One of the most comprehensive and detailed comparisons of head injury criteria was published by the Japan Automobile Research Institute, Inc. 16 years ago.[17] The fact that it is still a valuable reference work is testimony to its quality and to the comparative lack of progress in the development of head injury criteria since that time.

HEAD INJURY PREVENTION

The Head Injury Criterion is specified in United States' legislation for three reasons: it is, or was, thought to relate to the risk of an impact causing a severe or fatal head injury; at the time that it was introduced into legislation there was no other criterion that was demonstrably superior; and it is based on physical parameters which are readily measured in crash testing. Despite the generally acknowledged deficiencies in HIC, its use and practical importance have increased with time and that trend continues today. Australia has recently decided to adopt the U.S. safety standard for frontal impact protection in passenger cars (FMVSS 208) which includes HIC values for the crash test dummies in the driver's and front passenger's seating positions. Of greater significance is the use of HIC in the New Car Assessment Program (NCAP) in the United States. NCAP involves a barrier crash test at 35 mph rather than 30 mph as in FMVSS 208. The results of NCAP tests are publicised widely and so the car buying public is provided with a measure of the relative safety of cars in terms of the risk of severe head injury in this particular type of crash as estimated by HIC values derived from crash test dummies. This means that this program probably has more effect on vehicle frontal crashworthiness design than any other activity in the United States. A similar testing program has now commenced in Australia.

While the use of HIC has brought the prevention of head injury to centre stage in car design there are good reasons to be dissatisfied with the present situation. HIC takes no account of the location of an impact on the head. It includes no measure of angular acceleration of the head due to an impact. For these and other reasons there is an urgent need to develop a more realistic measure of the tolerance of the head to impact.

REFERENCES

1.   Anon. Human tolerance to impact conditions as related to motor vehicle design. (1964) Soc. Automotive Engrs.(SAE) Handbook Suppl. J885

2.   Ommaya AK, Rockoff DS, Baldwin M (1964) J. Neurosurg, 21: 249-265

3.   Gennarelli TA, Thibault LE, Ommaya AK (1972) SAE Paper No. 720970

4.   Gennarelli TA (1985) Proc. Amer. Ass. Automotive Med 29:447-463

5.   Ono K, Kikuohi A, Kobayashi H, Nakamura N (1985) In: Head injury prevention. Past and present research. Wayne State Univ., Dept. Neurosurg.

6.   Simpson DA, Ryan GA, Paix BR, McLean AJ, Kloeden CN (1991) Proc. Int. Res. Conf. on Biomechanics of Impacts, (IRCOBI), Bron, France, pp 89-100

7.   Ommaya AK, Hirsch AE, Harris E, Yarnell PR (1967) SAE Paper 670906, pp 47-52

8.   McElhaney JH, Stalnaker RL, Roberts VL (1973) In: King WJ, Mertz HJ (eds) Human impact response. Plenum Press.

9.   Schmidt G (1979) Proc. IRCOBI, Bron, France, pp 143-150

10. McLean AJ, Blumbergs PC, Kloeden CN, Palmer GJ, Ryan GA (1990) Proc. IRCOBI, Bron, France, pp 181-190.

11. Gadd CW (1966) SAE Paper No. 660793

12. National Highway Traffic Safety Admin. (1971) Occupant crash protection - Head Injury Criterion. FMVSS 208, S6.2.

13. Versace J (1971) SAE Paper No. 710881

14. Newman JA (1980) SAE Paper No. 801317

15. Stalnaker RL, McElhaney JH, Roberts VL (1971) MSC tolerance curve for human head impacts. Proc. Amer. Soc. Mech. Engrs. Biomechanical and Human Factors Conf.

16. Willinger R, Ryan GA, McLean AJ, Kopp CM (1992) Proc IRCOBI, Bron, France, pp 179-192

17. McElhaney JH, Roberts VL, Hilyard JF (1976) Handbook of Human Tolerance. Japan Automobile Research Institute, Inc. Tokyo

ACKNOWLEDGEMENT

The support of the Australian National Health and Medical Research Council in the preparation of this paper is gratefully acknowledged.

Countermeasures Against Head Injuries in Car Accidents

TOSHIMI YAMANOI

Engineer of Body Design Department, Nissan Motor Co., Ltd., Technical Center, Atsugi, Kanagawa, 243-01 Japan

SUMMARY

Since 1988,the number of death by traffic accidents in Japan has continued to exceed 10.000 each year. Especially, those who suffered death while riding on automobiles have rapidly increased year after year and today such fatalities occupy as high as about 40% of total vehicle casualties. As a result, improvement of safety coutermeasures for automobiles is now very strongly demanded in the society.

When body portion for serious injuries and fatalities of vehicle occupants are cheked, it is clearly noticeable that head is most frequently involved in such serious injuries or fatalities. Therefore,in terms of research and development of automobiles, emphasis is recently concentrated on coutermeasures to minimize head injuries.

These head injury preventive countermeasures can be broadly classified into two phases. In one phase, attempted is implementation of the coutermeasures to prevent "secondary contact" between heads and interior structual members or components at the time of collision of automobiles. In the other phase, tried is initiation of the coutermeasures to provide maximum shock absorbency on the structural section which may cause serious injuries when the secondary contact is inevitable. In connection with the countermeasures applied in these two phases, this paper reveals actual structural designs and clarifies relevant evaluation methods.

KEY WORDS: head injuries, vehicle accidents, countermeasures

1. INTRODUCTION

For 4 consecutive years since 1988, the fatalities by traffic accidents in Japan numbered more than 10,000 and this fact presents today a serious social problem (Fig. 1). Particularly, the persons who died in automobiles by accidents are quickly increasing in number and are accounting for approximately 40% of said total fatalities on all types of automobile accidents .

Under such social circumstances, various safety improvement countermeasures are being enforced in different fields for reducing automobile fatalities.Presently, activities and efforts in this direction can be classified into the prime areas of "people (namely, humen-related factors)", "environment (roads and other physical conditions)", and "automobiles themselves". In this paper, attention is focused onto the last area of "automobiles" or specifically to the topic of "safety countermeasures against head injureies in car accidents".

2.ACTUAL STATUS OF HEAD INJURIES ON DOMESTIC AUTOMOBILE ACCIDENTS

When distribution status of injury portions of body is reviewed for serious injuries and fatalities on domestic automobile accidents, we see the highest concentration in heads, followed by those in entire body sections and thoraxes (Fig. 2). Fatalities are often reported to be lower when seat belts are worn and therefore, correct wearing of seat belts may be one of effective basic countermeasures for prevention of head injuries.

When possibilities of belt wearers suffering head injuries are analyzed in terms of automobile collision types, frontal collisions are highest and side collisions are next (Fig3). Fig. 4 shows the status viewed on the basis of injury-inflicting structural members or components, indicating that head injuries are often caused by impact with exterior objects or opponent vehicles as a result of deformation.

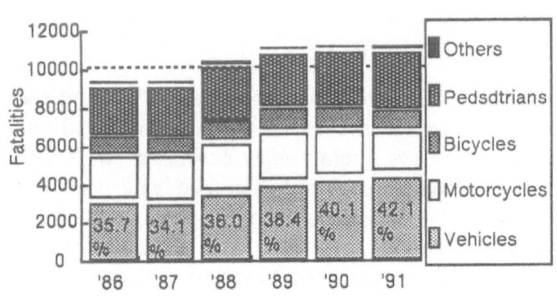

Fig.1 Status Categories of Accident Fatalities [1]

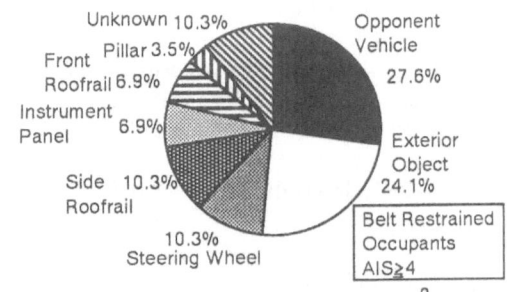

Fig.2 Analyses of Injury-receiving Body Portion [2]

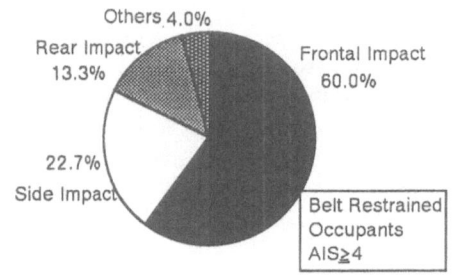
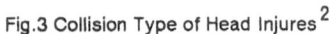

Fig.3 Collision Type of Head Injures [2]

Fig.4 Head Injury-causing Objects [2]

3. SAFETY COUNTERMEASURES OF AUTOMOBILES AGAINST HEAD INJURIES

Safety countermeasures for prevention of head injuries can be divided into two major areas. one area pertains to prevention of secondary contact between heads and car interiors and the other area concerns slackening of head impacting force at the time of secondary contact.

3.1 Preventive Countermeasures of Secondary Contact to Heads

We shall first review why the secondary contact to heads is caused. When extensive crushing of car body occurs as a result of partial collision or high-speed impact, the car compartments are deformed and the steering wheel or instrument panel is caused to intrude. On the other hand, the occupants restrained in the compartments with seat belts move forward by stretching the belts and contact is caused between forward-moving occupants and backward-retreating steering wheel or instrument panel. When the car is subjected to severe collision, extensive body deformation occurs and such deformation may sometimes cause intense impact of heads against exterior objects or structural portions of opponent vehicle.

As a countermeasure against this secondary contact, adopted is development of body structure by dividing into the cabin compartment zone and the crushable zone comprising the sections in front of and at the back of compartment(Fig.5). By allowing this crushable zone to absorb the impact energy, impact shocks applied to the occupants is reduced and deformation of the compartment is minimized. On the other hand, the crushable zone is so designed as to achieve maximum absorption of impact energy within the restriction of limited space availability.

For instance, to increase the reaction force during deformation of vehicle body, we reinforce the frame members. Or, to widen the ranges of breakage plasticity deformation at multiple points, we form the beads (sectional dents) for causing stress concentration so that deformation occurs at targeted spots (Fig6). To achieve optimum designing of body structures incorporating these points, computer simulations and various collision test are conducted.

Further, different means are adopted for making the vehicle cabin compartments sturdier and stronger against the crushing force. Included in this series of work are enlargement of cross-sectional areas of such major structural members as body sills, pillars, and side members, employment of high-strength materials, and use of various reinforcement pieces. Also, since the steering assembly is caused to intrude by deformation of the dash panel, this steering assembly is secured to the steering member connected to both sides of body so that effects of deformation can be reduced. Additionally, the steering assembly itself is provided with the mechanism to make it collapsible for minimizing the amount of intrusion into the compartment interior.

Another countermeasure for preventing the secondary contact to head is supported by the use of occupant restraint devices, a representative type being seat belts. As is well known, the seat belts function in the preventive work of secondary contact to heads by restricting the movement of occupants and reducing the shift distances at the time of collision. These shift distances of occupant are chiefly determined by the length of belt extension and also by the amout of belt elongation caused when the belt is rolled into the retractor tightly. Therefore, an attempt is made to restrict belt elongation by using the webbing materials with low extendibility or the clamping mechanism is provided on the outlet end of retractor for preventing excessive belt stretching. Further, increasingly adopted recently is the preloading retractor which is designed to upgrade the restraint performance (Fig.7). Through instantly detecting occurrence of collision, this preloading retractor positively winds up the slacks caused by clothes between the belt and occupant's body.

Air bags represent another new type of device becoming popular in recent years as the device for preventing the secondary contact to heads (Fig8). Presently, these air bags are considered as a supplementary restraint device for supporting the function of seat belts. In other words, the air bags are primarily aimed at preventing the hard objects from impacting the heads that cannot be sufficiently protected with seat belts alone. Generally, an air bag is composed of collision sensor, an inflator, and a bag. The sensor, upon detecting the deceleration occuring on the colliding car, sends signals to the inflator to generate the gas and instantly inflate the bag.

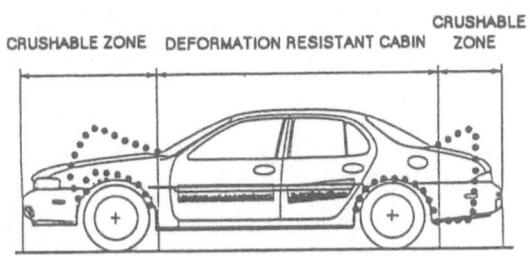

Fig.5 Crushable Zone and Cabin Compartment

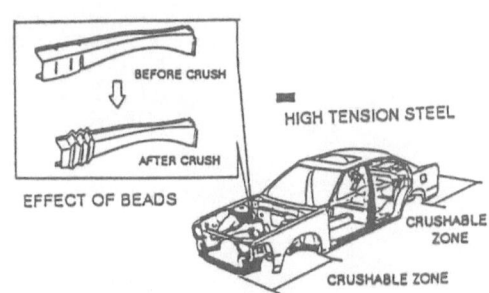

Fig.6 Example of Car Body Countermeasures

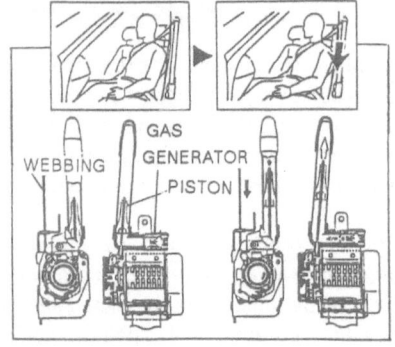

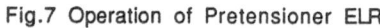

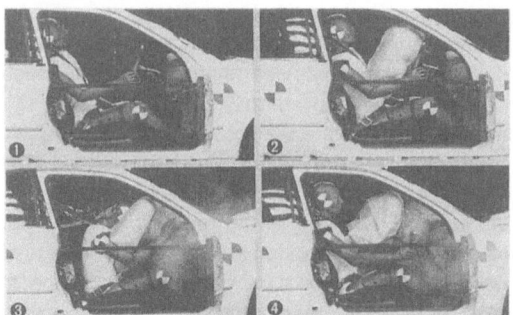

Fig.7 Operation of Pretensioner ELR   Fig.8 Operation of Air Bag

3.2 Impact Alleviation Countermeasures During Secondary Contact

Next, we like to touch upon the countermeasures to cope with head injuries adoptable in case the secondary contact is unavoidable. In the real world, various types of accidents are occuring day after day and even if different countermeasures mentioned above are applied, the secondary contact to heads resulting from extensive car body deformation is bound to occur, for instance, when the collision speed is exceptionally fast. Therefore, on the portions which are liable to be involved in the secondary contact, we apply the means of providing the structure designed for absorbing the impact energy. Major structural sections where this countermeasure is incorporated are located in front of the occupants including the steering wheel before the driver and the instrument panel before the front passenger. The seatbacks in front of rear passengers are also included in this category.

We shall explain by referring to the example of steering wheel. The shock energy absorbing medium is installed within the space provided in front of the hard structure required for maintaining the steering performance (Fig. 9). Generally, the material used for this absorbing medium is steel plate easy to be deformed, urethane pad, or other rather soft object. By permitting this energy absorbing medium to deform when the head contacts it, speed of the head is reduced and injuries by impact with hard structure of steering wheel are prevented.

Similar preventive countermeasures are also applied to the seats and the instrument panel. In addition, the sections inside the compartment where contact with the head may occur are designed to become free from sharp corners or edges by interconnecting flat and smooth surfaces. Further, switches and other components are rounded in shapes to eliminate square protrusions or installed in recesses so that contact of sharp edges with head can be minimized (Fig.10).

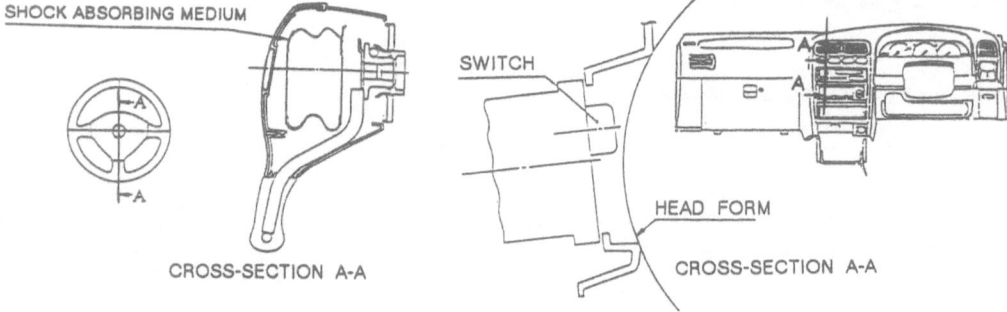

Fig.9 Countermeasure for Steering Wheel   Fig.10 Countermeasure for Instrument Panel

4. TESTING METHODS

Assessment of safety pertaining to the head injury reduction countermeasures is achieved by conducting actual vehicle collision tests, sled collision tests, and unit impact tests. The actual vehicle crash tests provide the results highly effective for use on evaluation of safety countermeasures for head injuries because this is a type of tests conducted under the conditions very closely resembling real-world car accident status. Therefore, in our vehicle development activities, adoption of this actual vehicle collision tests mean that our assessment is made on collision styles representative of the conditions existing in real world accidents. On the other hand, since entire vehicles are used for assessment by these actual collision tests, there lies a problem of "relatively extensive variations of experimental results." For the purpose of compensating for this drawback of the actual vehicle collision tests, two other additional types of tests, namely, sled impact tests and unit impact tests, are performed for further pinpointing assessment factors. This testing method with concentrated assessment factors applied to these two types of tests is able to offer a merit to allow rather easy repetition of test phenomena that are difficult to be reproduced by the acutual vehicle collision tests.

The actual vehicle collision tests are conducted by causing test cars to collide against the test barriers (Fig. 11). These cars are loaded with test dummies and after the tests, the dummies are examined as to spots of head impacts and generation of acceleration factors. At present, the HIC values calculated by the Equation 1 shown below are used for evaluating head injury levels. This HIC is mathematical function for expressing degrees of acceleration applied to the centers of gravity of heads and according to the Federal regulation of U.S.A., FMVSS, HIC=1000, is designated as the safety limit. It is reported that when HIC=1000 is exceeded, linear fractures possessing correlative relations with cerebral concussion threshhold are liable to occur.

$$\text{HIC} = [1/(t2 - t1) \int_{t1}^{t2} a\,dt]^{2.5} (t2-t1) \quad t1,t2; \text{any time during the crash}, \ t2-t1 \leqq 36\text{msec} .. \ \text{Eq. (1)}$$

a; dummy's head acceleration

The sled collision tests are conducted chiefly for evaluating safety of vehicle interior components. Test car bodies are loaded with dummies and components which affect injury levels at the time of collision and the car bodies thus loaded are set on the test-use sleds (Fig12). The test system is so designed that when the sled collided, deceleration occurs in the same manner as acutual vehicle impact. Similarly to the actual vehicle collision tests, the HIC values are used for assessment of head injury levels of dummies. Since no cars are actually crushed on these sled impact tests, advantage of limited test expenses is available.

On the unit impact tests, evaluations are made by using head impactors to strike the sections of heads possible to be impacted by the secondary contact (Fig.13). This testing method offers the merits of limited time for completing test preparations, not requiring large-scaled test facilities, minimum parts necessary for tests, and low experiment costs. Excellent reproducibility of tset phenomena is another prominent feature of this testing method. On this testing method, generated deceleration factors are generally used for achieving assessment to check avoidance of head impact to hard objects.

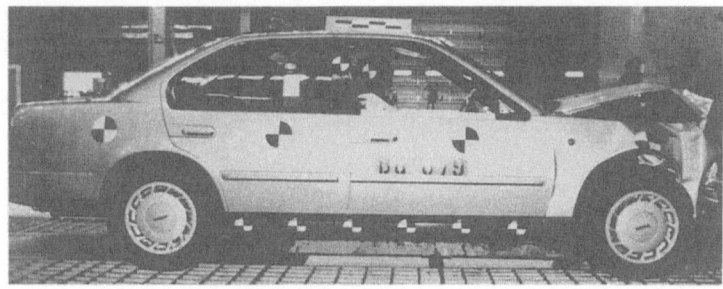

Fig.11 Vehicle Collision Test

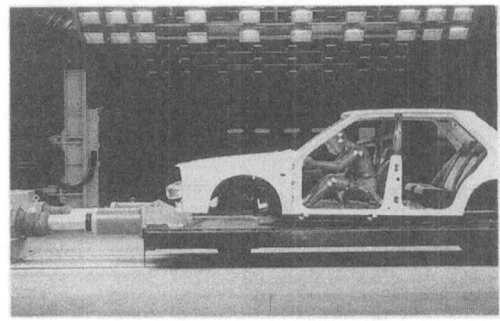

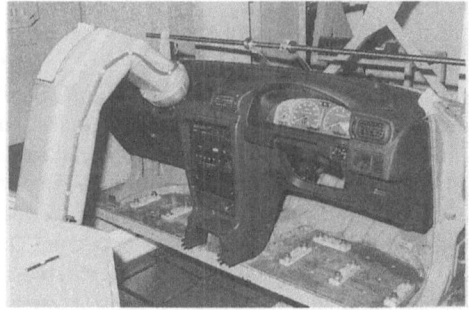

Fig.12 Sled Collision Test   Fig.13 Unit Impact Test

5. CONCLUSION

Explanations up to this point cover the outline of our head injury preventive countermeasures during car collision. Besides these countermeasures,as the safety enhancement means viewed from the vehicle side, we implement other countermeasures related to upgrading of visual fields/visibility, drive stability, and brake performance. In broad sense of words, our efforts for improvements in these areas may equally fall into the category of countermeasures for prevention of head injuries.

Countermeasures for ensuring safety on vehicles are usually processed through the courses of full analyses of real-world accidents, complete investigations of damage-inflicted portions and damage-inflicting sections/status, and incessant repetition of experiments to reproduce investigation results, thereby finally arriving at determination of assessment methods. Then, target performance for development viewed from the standpoint of human tolerance is subsequently determined and extensive structural research and studies are initiated for realizing those targets. This way, until a single countermeasure can be fully established, efforts by a number of technicians and engineers are indispensable. In the future too, by obtaining close cooperation and guidance from many specialists not only at automobile manufacturers but also in other professional fields, all of us the engineering staff are determined to continue our efforts for developing safer vehicles.

REFERRENCES
1."White Paper for Traffic Safety"(1992).Prime Minister's Office
2.Accident Investigation Data(1981-90). Ministry of Transport
3. Sato T,(1980) "Safety on Automobile". Sankaido Printing.

3—Disaster Assistance in Neurotrauma

The Organisation of Health Care in Civilian Disasters

F. SERVADEI[1], S. BADIALI[2], G. STAFFA[1], MT. NASI[1], and MT. FIANDRI[2]

[1]Division of Neurosurgery, Ospedale Bufalini, Cesena and [2]Intensive Care Unit, Ospedale Maggiore, Regione Emilia Romagna, Italy

SUMMARY

The authors studied a series of mass emergencies occurred in the Region Emilia Romagna,North Est of Italy from 1974 to 1990.The results of the interventions were compared to the different organisation of emergency medical services in the event's periods(presence of coordination centers,presence of emergency service with helicopters,presence of ambulance with Casualty doctors,establishment of a protocol for mass casualties).The conclusion is that the improvement of the everyday trauma care allowed a better response even in the case of a catastrophe.

KEY WORDS
emergency medical service-mass casualty-disaster planning

INTRODUCTION

The main characteristic of a catastrophic event is that an acute imbalance develops between the quantity of available resorses and the acute request of medical aid.The medical response to mass emergencies must aim at razionalising these available and hireable resorses.There are two main field of intervention:a)organisational, by planning criteria of emergency care and supplies of men and materials b)clinical,by identifying the therapeutical priorities.In our area we unfortunately observed a number of catastrophies (table 1);the analysis of the most impressive one (bomb at Bologna railways station in 1980) led a group of swedish traumatologists (1) to criticize the absence of a proper disaster planning system.
Since then we improved the everyday treatment of traumatic emergencies.In this paper we analyze the mass casualties to see how the improvement of trauma care in our area could have influenced the medical aid in disasters.

MATERIAL,METHODS and RESULTS

Year	Event	Dead	Involved
1974	Bomb on Italicus Train	12	48
1978	Derailment of "laguna" Train	48	117
1980	Bomb at Bologna raiways station	85	291
1984	Bomb on a 904 Train	15	193
1986	Derailment of "Brenner exp" Train	0	88
1987	Fire on ship "E.Montanari"	13	13
1989	Chain of crashes on A 13 Motorway	8	50
1990	Air crash on "Salvemini"school	12	94

Table 1:List of mass emergencies in the region Emilia Romagna

We then examine the type of medical response to the most important catastrophies in relation to the emergencies organisation available at the time of the event. In our region (4 milion people,North est of Italy)we established,starting in 1980 in Bologna,a net of coordination centers for ambulances.In 1986 and 1987 an emergency medical service with helicopters was organized in 3 bases in different regional locations.From 1988 the emergency medical service was improved with the use of Casualty doctors on the ambulances.In 1991 a mobile truck with a communication and a dispatch center became available.
In 1974,first mass emergency examined,there were no link or coordination between hospitals and voluntary services.The call for the event concerned a"sickness at the railway station" and the actual place of the disaster was identyfied only one hour later.The ambulances were therefore dispatched with considerable delay and most victims were rescued by volounteers.In 1980,bomb explosion in Bologna,it was already established a center coordinating 80% of the ambulances but no protocol was available for mass emergencies with consequent overcrowding of the hospitals.In 1984 the established protocol for mass emergencies was applied to the bomb on a train catastrophy: one hour after the explosion an advaced medical post was set up near the event location;70 minutes after the explosion 6 doctors,27 ambulance,a lorry with supply materials were on the scene.Meantime the medical and nursing staff in the regional referring hospitals was doubled according to emergency protocol.In this case the response was fast,well coordinated with a good dimensioning also of the hospital organisation.The negative aspects concerned the lack of some equipments and a partial lack of immediate information.In 1990 a military plane crushed on a school in Bologna.Four minutes later the emergency medical helicopter took off . Meantime ,4 ambulances were dispatched to the scene of accident; two of them carried a doctor from the Casualty Deparment.At 8 minutes from the event the helicopter comunicated to the coordinating center the aproximated entity of the disaster as seen from above.12 minutes after the event on the accident location was organized an advanced medical post and a triage center.The evacuation was concluded 30 minutes later.The only critical points in this event concerned the collapse of the hospital administration facing so many admissions at the same time and the collapse of the traffic in the roads near the accident scene.

DISCUSSION

A mass casualty is defined by a disaster were the local health sistem is overwhelmed completely by the entity of the event(5).
The scenario will then be different according to the accident's location (urban areas, mountains,tunnels) and the nearby available resourses.In any of these location the organisation of an advaced medical post (AMP) is most helpful in diciding treatment priorities on the scene of accident(4).A number of different scale have been published for patients' triage(2):basically there is the immediate need to identify,apart from the deaths which must be separated,patients "critical"(possible survival with non sophisticated care),"catastrophic"(non probable survival and/or need for sophisticated care)"severe"(possible survival with non sophisticated care even after 1 hour)"minor"(survival with care

even hours later).If the nearest hospitals (even increasing medical and nursing staff(6)according to a mass casualty protocol) are able to treat all the above mentioned categories of patients, the role of the AMP is of basic life support before triage as in all our mass emegencies.On the other hand,if(owing to accident location and/or lack of local resourses)there are no possibilities to treat properly the patients ,the AMP must be organized in a "cross" shape with an area for surgical procedures and an area for the intensive care , either using a tend or adapting an adjacent building (4).The end of the"cross" is the triage area   where helicopters and ambulances rescue patients.We adopted this system in 1984 for the bomb on the train:the accident location was a tunnel in the mountains not easy to reach.The presence of a medical service with helicopters is most helpful in case of mass casualty if integrated in the emergency planning(3).In the last of our mass emergencies the helicopter was useful in giving to the coordinating center an immediate information about the entity of the disaster.In conclusion, medical treatment of mass casualty in our area improved toghether with the everyday treatment of trauma patients.The first of the ten golden rules(5) in case of catastrophies ("as much as possible follow day to day routine") is ,in our experience, the most important one.

REFENCES

1)Brismar   B,Bergenwald   L:The   terrorist   bomb   explosion   in Bologna,Italy   1980:an   analysis   of   the   effects   and   injuries sustained J Trauma 22:216-220,1982
2)Champion HF:Trauma triage JWAEDM 3:1-4,1987
3)Jacobs LM,Gabrham SG,Stohler SA:The integration of a helicopter emergency medical service in a mass casualty response system Prehosp Dis Med 6:451-454,1991
4)Julien H,Fontaine P,Menage P,Lienhard A:Caracteristiques des postes medicaux avances de situation de catastrophe civile Urgences 9:293-306,1990
5)Pepe PE,Stewart RD,Copass MK:Ten golden roules for urban multiple casualty management Prehosp Dis Med 4:131-134,1989
6)Smith JS:Hospital Disaster and evacuation planning Prehosp Dis Med 5:357-362,1990

4—Chronic Subdural Hematoma

An Experimental Chronic Subdural Hematoma in Dogs – with a Brain Atrophy Model

FUMIHITO KANEKO, MASAAKI OHBAYASHI, TSUTOMU OHSHIMA, and KEIZO MATSUMOTO

Department of Neurological Surgery, School of Medicine, The University of Tokushima, Tokushima, 770 Japan

SUMMARY

A new model of chronic subdural hematoma in dogs with brain atrophy is described. In reviewing clinical cases, we considered the possibility that brain atrophy may play a role as one of the causative factors. The cisterna magna of adult mongrel dogs was punctured, and 10-15 ml of cerebrospinal fluid was drained. Subsequently, 6-hydroxydopamine (6-OHDA) 1mg/kg body weight dissolved in artificial cerebrospinal fluid containing 0.01% ascorbic acid, was injected into the cisterna magna. Marked ventricular enlargement was confirmed by computerized tomography (CT) three to four weeks later, at which time fresh autologous blood (2-3 ml) was inoculate into subdural space. Progressively enlarging hematomas were found by CT in four of the 10 dogs two to four weeks later. Gross and histological examinations of the hematomas revealed a condition closely resembling human chronic subdural hematoma. Two of the dogs showed drastic deterioration four weeks after subdural inoculation of blood. In these brain atrophy models, chronic subdural hematomas were experimentally reproduced at a high rate. The results suggest that brain atrophy may play an important role in the formation of chronic subdural hematoma.

KEY WORDS: chronic subdural hematoma, brain atrophy, 6-hydroxydopamine, experimental, dog

INTRODUCTION

It is well known that the creation of an experimental model of chronic subdural hematoma is seldom successful. In our laboratory a pathological state closely resembling human chronic subdural hematoma was experimentally produced in dogs by subdural inoculation of blood-CSF mixture with CSF drainage and intravenous administration of D-mannitol[1]. In reviewing clinical cases, another possibility was considered that brain atrophy may play a role as one of the causative factors.

MATERIALS AND METHODS

Mongrel dogs of both sexes, ranging in weight from 10 to 15 kg, were used for this study. The cisterna magna was punctured and 10-15 ml of CSF was drained. Subsequently 6-hydroxydopamine (6-OHDA) dissolved in artificial CSF containing 0.01% ascorbic acid was injected in a dose of 1 mg/kg body weight into the cisterna magna. Marked ventricular enlargement was confirmed by computed tomography (CT) three to four weeks later.

Gross and histological findings:

The ventricular system was markedly enlarged (Fig.1).

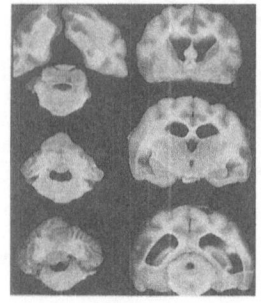

Fig.1. Coronal section of three weeks after 6-hydroxydopamine (1mg/kg) cisternal injection.

Almost no adhesion of meninges was observed. Ependymal cells were enlarged, but in the subependymal region there was no spongy appearance as has been in experimental hydrocephalus induced by cisternal injection of kaolin. Neurons in the spinal anterior horn and hippocampus showed pyknotic changes. Nuclear membranes of neurons in the vicinity of locus caeruleus showed a tendency to disappear (Fig.2).

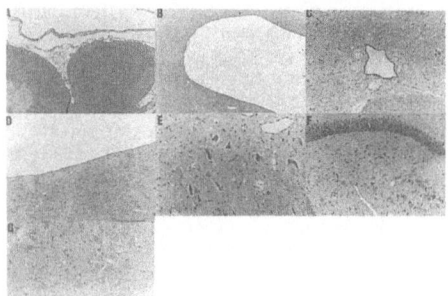

Fig.2. Histological findings of dogs three weeks after 6-hydroxydopamine cisternal injection (HE stain). A: basal cistern (x20), B: anterior horn of lateral ventricle (x10), C: central canal spinal cord (x40), D: ependymal cell lying of central canal (x100), E: spinal anterior horn (x100), F: hippocampus (x100), G: locus caeruleus (x100).

Cerebral blood flow and brain water content:

Five dogs were examined three weeks after 6-OHDA cisternal injection with five normal controls. They were anesthetized with intramuscular ketamine hydrochloride (10 mg/kg), intubated, immobilized with intravenous pancronium bromide (0.01 mg/kg), fixed in a stereotaxic frame in the prone position, ventilated with a 60% NO_2 mixture, and maintained on controlled respiration. Arterial pO_2 was 95 to 100 mm Hg and pCO_2 was 35 to 45 mm Hg. Regional cerebral blood flow (rCBF) was measured by a microspheric method. Microspheres (15+5 μm in diameter and labeled with ^{57}Co) in 1.0 ml of 10% dextran were injected into the left ventricle. The rCBF of the gray matter and the white matter decreased by 49% and 47%, respectively (Fig.3 left).

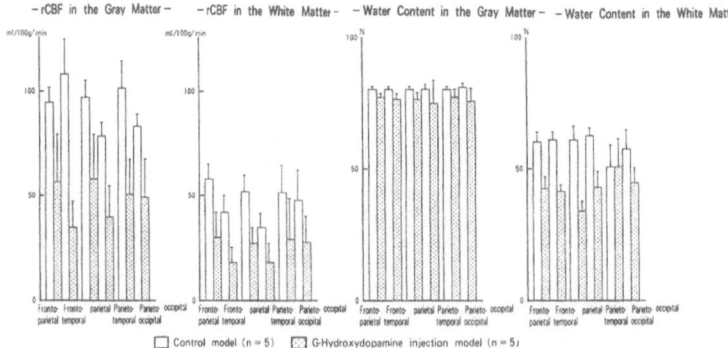

Fig.3. Regional cerebral blood flow and brain water content of the 6-hydroxydopamine injection model.

46

Water content was measured by the freeze-dry method immediately after measurement of the rCBF, the water content of the gray matter and the white matter decreased. The tendency to decrease was particularly evident in the white matter (Fig.3 right). Ventricular dilatation was attributed to brain atrophy, not to hydrocephalus.

Inoculation of flesh blood into subdural space:

Ten Dogs were used three weeks after 6-OHDA intracisternal injection. They were immobilized with intramuscular ketamine hydrochloride (10 mg/kg), intubated, anesthetized with intravenous pentobarbital sodium (10 mg/kg), and fixed in a stereotaxic frame in the prone position. Fresh autologous blood (2-3 ml) was introduced into the subdural space via a burr hole, and subsequently symptoms and CT-scan findings were observed.

RESULT

Progressively growing hematomas were found by CT in four of the 10 dogs two to four weeks later. Gross and histological examinations of the hematomas revealed the condition closely resembling human chronic subdural hematoma. Two of these dogs (cases 1 and 2) showed drastic deterioration of symptoms four weeks after subdural inoculation of blood. Before this, the ventricle had been remarkably enlarged by the 6-OHDA cisternal injection. The subdural mass showed an expanded high density area 30 days after inoculation of fresh autologous blood (Fig.4A). Midline shift was also seen. In the extracted brain and hematoma of case 1 (Fig.4B), the dura and hematoma could be carefully reflected en bloc. The photomicrograph of the neomembrane The neomembrane showed a sinusoidal channel layer and a fibrous layer (Fig.4C).

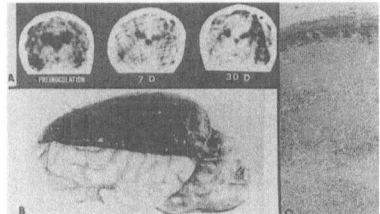

Fig.4. Case 1. A: Serial CT (D: day), B: Extracted brain and hematoma, C: Photomicrograph of the neomembrane (HE stain, x13).

In serial CT of case 2 the subdural mass showed expanded low density area 28 days after inoculation (Fig.5A) and the extracted brain showed the encapsulated hematoma (Fig.5B). The outer membrane of hematoma could be carefully reflected. The neomembrane had sinusoidal channel layer and fibrous layer (Fig.5C).

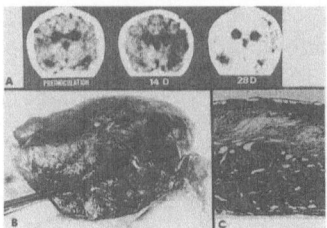

Fig.5. Case 2. A: Serial CT (D: day), B: Extracted brain and hematoma, C: Photomicrograph of the neomembrane (Azan-Mallory stain x13).

DISCUSSION

Experimental studies of chronic subdural hematoma have been sporadically attempted[2,3,4], but were not successful until 1970, when Watanabe et al.[5], first reported a form of experimental chronic subdural hematoma by inoculating a clot of blood mixed with CSF into the subdural space of dogs and monkeys. They stated that a peculiar type of fibrin was essential for inducing the capsule formation. Apfelbaum, et al.[6], pursued Watanabe's experiment, however they could not substantiate their hypothesis. Labadie and Glover[7] compared histological and biochemical aspect of subcutaneous hematoma in rats and subdural hematoma in man. They found a remarkable similarity and stated that inflammatory mechanism appeared to be essential and that CSF played no role in the process of chronic hematoma formation. Aikawa and Suzuki[8] reported spontaneous chronic subdural hematomas in mice with induced hydrocephalus by a single intraperitoneal injection of 6-aminonicotinamide. As perforation of the occipital cortex was observed in almost all experimental mice, they stated that abrupt decompression of the hydrocephalic lateral ventricle caused pulling and tearing of the bridging veins. That caused spontaneous chronic subdural hematoma. They noted that similar phenomenon has been observed in clinical hydrocephalic patient who frequently develop subdural hematoma after shunt operation.

In reviewing clinical cases, chronic subdural hematoma occurs more often in the aged than the non-aged. It suggests that brain atrophy may play a role as one of its causative factors. We had successful experimental chronic subdural hematomas in a very limited number of cases by inoculating blood mixed with CSF into dogs' subdural space and maintaining a subdural gap with D-mannitol and CSF drainage. We speculated that brain shrinkage is needed for expansion of chronic subdural hematoma[1]. And in this brain atrophy model, chronic subdural hematoma was developed in four of ten dogs by subdural inoculation of the blood. In our previous experiment, inoculation of blood-CSF mixture produced neomembrane formation but no expansion of the hematoma. This can be regarded as one of causative factors of neomembrane formation (beta factor). Fresh blood inoculation caused organization in normal dogs, but brain atrophy model. Therefore, reduction of the brain volume may be counted as one of the factor of hematoma expansion (gamma factor). In the evolution of chronic subdural hematoma succession of sequences of trigger or initiation (alpha factor), beta and gamma are supposed to be necessary.

REFERENCES

1. Ohshima T (1982) Experimental study on the evolution of chronic subdural hematoma. Neurol Med Chir (Tokyo) 22:696-706

2. Putnam TJ, Putnam IK (1927) The experimental study of pachymeningitis hemorrhagica. J Nerv Ment Dis 65:260-272

3. Gardner WJ (1932) Traumatic subdural hematoma. With particular reference to the latent interval. Arch Neurol Psychiatry 27:847-858

4. Goodell CL, Mealey J Jr (1963) Pathogenesis of chronic subdural hematoma. Experimental study. Arch Neurol 8:429-437

5. Watanabe S, Shimada H, Ishii S (1972) Production of clinical form of chronic subdural hematoma in the experimental animals. Adv Neurol Sci (Tokyo) 14:387-396

6. Apfelbaum R, Guthkelch AN, Shulman K (1974) Experimental production of subdural hematomas. J Neurosurg 40:336-346

7. Labadie EL, Glover D (1976) Pathogenesis of chronic subdural hematoma - Experimental studies -. J Neurosurg 45:382-392

8. Aikawa H, Suzuki K (1987) Experimental chronic subdural hematoma in mice.Gross morphology and light microscopic observations.J Neurosurg 67:710-716

Significance of Cholesterol Metabolites in Chronic Subdural Hematoma

KAZUYA NAGATA[1], MAGNUS AXELSON[2], INGEMAR BJOERKHEM[3], MASAO MATSUTANI[4], and KINTOMO TAKAKURA

[1]Department of Neurosurgery, New Tokyo Hospital, Nemoto, Matsudo, Chiba, 271 Japan, [2]Department of Clinical Chemistry, Karolinska Hospital, 104 01 Stockholm 60, Sweden, [3]Department of Clinical Chemistry, Huddinge University Hospital, Stockholm, Sweden, and [4]Department of Neurosurgery, The University of Tokyo, Bunkyo-ku, Tokyo, 113 Japan

SUMMARY

We have previously reported the high level of 7α-hydroxy-3-oxo-4-cholestenoic acid in chronic subdural hematoma. In order to clarify the underlying mechanism of this high concentration, the levels of possible precursors and metabolites were examined. Compared to the reported normal plasma levels, low levels of 7α-hydroxy-4-cholesten-3-one were observed while the levels of the other precursors or metabolites were similar or higher than the plasma levels. Intracranial conversion from 7α-hydroxy-4-cholesten-3-one was considered to be one possible cause of the high levels of 7α-hydroxy-3-oxo-4-cholestenoic acid. Since the former compound is less polar and more lipo-soluble than the latter, and brain tissue is abundant in lipid, the possibility of a biological detoxication mechanism is discussed. Another possible mechanism for the accumulation of 7α-hydroxy-3-oxo-4-cholestenoic acid is a concentration of this and other polar metabolites in the hematoma.

KEY WORDS: chronic subdural hematoma, cholestenoic acid, cholesterol metabolite, bile acid, 26-hydroxylase

INTRODUCTION

In order to clarify the underlying mechanisms in the capsular formation of chronic subdural hematoma (CSDH), we have analyzed the content of hematoma using biochemical techniques [1]. In these analyses, we incidentally found a cholesterol metabolite specific to CSDH. This substance was always found in the content of chronic subdural hematoma, while it was not detected in the subdural hygroma, whose pathogenesis is similar to CSDH except for the lack of capsular formation. Using several chemical techniques, we identified its chemical structure as 7α-hydroxy-3-oxo-4-cholestenoic acid [2]. We also found the concentration of this substance in CSDH to be approximately the five-fold of the normal plasma level.

As previously reported [3], 7α-hydroxy-3-oxo-4-cholestenoic acid is not believed to be a usual intermediate from cholesterol to bile acids, but in an alternative pathway to chenodeoxycholic acid. From its chemical structure, a possible model for the biosynthesis of 7α-hydroxy-3-oxo-4-cholestenoic acid is proposed as shown in Fig.1. The main purpose of this study was to clarify the underlying mechanism producing this high concentration of the substance by measuring the levels of possible precursors and metabolic products in CSDH.

MATERIALS AND METHODS

Eleven patients with CSDH were selected for this study. The hematoma contents were surgically evacuated and stored at -20°C until analysis. In order to clarify the cause of the high level of this cholestenoic acid, the levels of possible precursors, 7α-hydroxy-4-cholesten-3-one, 3β-hydroxy-5-cholestenoic acid, 3β,7α-dihydroxy-5-cholestenoic acid were measured in five patients (Fig.1). The levels of cholic acid and chenodeoxycholic acid as possible metabolic products were also examined in eleven patients.

The level of 7α-hydroxy-4-cholesten-3-one was measured with high performance liquid chromatography (HPLC) reported by Axelson et al [4]. Following the addition of ^{3}H-labelled 25-hydroxyvitamin D_3 (approximately 10,000 cpm), 1 ml of sample was diluted with 2 ml of isotonic saline. The solution was heated to 64°C for 5 min and then passed through a 1.0 x 0.8 cm column of octadecylsilane (ODS)-bonded silica (Preparative C_{18}, particle size 55-105 mm, Waters Associates Inc., Milford, MA), which was washed with 5 ml of methanol, methanol-chloroform 1:1 (v/v), methanol, and water prior to use. The column was washed with 10 ml of water (at 64°C) and 10 ml of 65% aqueous methanol (at room temperature). Prior to elution of steroids with 8 ml of hexane/chloroform (95:5, v/v), a gentle stream of nitrogen was passed through the column for 0.5 min. The eluate was taken to dryness under a stream of nitrogen and the residue was redissolved in 0.1 ml hexane. HPLC was carried out on a column (250 x 4.5 mm) of LiChrospher (Hibar, Si 100, 5 µm, Merck-Darmstadt) connected to a pump (Constametric III) and a fixed-wavelength (254 nm) detector (LDC/Milton Roy, Riviera Beach, FL). The mobile phase was hexane/isopropanol (95:5, v/v). The amount of 7α-hydroxy-4-cholesten-3-one was determined by comparing its peak area with that of known amounts of the reference compound. Since the recoveries of 7α-hydroxy-4-cholesten-3-one is known to be similar to those of 25-hydroxyvitamin D_3, ^{3}H-labelled 25-hydroxyvitamin D_3 was used to correct for losses and variations in injection volumes.

The levels of 3β-hydroxy-5-cholestenoic acid and 3β,7α-dihydroxy-5-cholestenoic acid were measured with gas-chromatography reported by Axelson et al [5]. 1 ml of sample was diluted with 3 ml of methanol and 3 ml of 80% aqueous methanol. After centrifugation at 1,500 rpm for 10 min, the supernatant was passed through a 1.0 x 0.8 cm column of octadecylsilane (ODS)-bonded silica (Preparative C_{18}, particle size 55-105 µm, Waters Associates Inc., Milford, MA), which was washed with 5 ml of methanol, methanol/chloroform 1:1 (v/v), methanol, and water prior to use. Following the wash with 10 ml of 80% aqueous methanol, the eluate was concentrated to approximately 3 ml with a rotary evaporator, and the concentrated solution mixed with 5 ml of water was again extracted on the washed column of ODS-bonded silica (flow rate about 1 ml/min). The column was washed with 5 ml each of water and 10% aqueous methanol, and steroids were eluted with 10 ml of 95% aqueous methanol. The eluate was passed through a column (6 x 0.4 cm) of TEAP-LH-20 in HCO_3^--form, packed in 95% aqueous methanol. Following a wash with 5 ml each of 95% aqueous methanol and methanol/chloroform 1:1 (v/v), unconjugated steroids with one carboxyl group were eluted with 4 ml of 0.15 M acetic acid in 95% aqueous methanol. This fraction was taken to dryness in vacuo and the residue was dissolved in methanol. Following the addition of 1 µg of triacontane as an internal standard, samples were methylated with freshly prepared diazomethane and trimethylsilylated with pyridine-hexamethyldisilazane-trimethylchlorosilane 3:2:1 (v/v/v). Gas chromatography was carried out using a Carlo Erba HRGC 5300 gas chromatograph connected to a Spectra-Physics SP 4270 integrator. An on-column injector system and a fused silica column (25 x 0.32 µm) coated with a 0.25 µm layer of cross-linked methyl silicone (Quadrex Corp., New Haven, CT) were used with a flame ionization detector. The temperature of the oven was 80°C during the injection and was then programmed

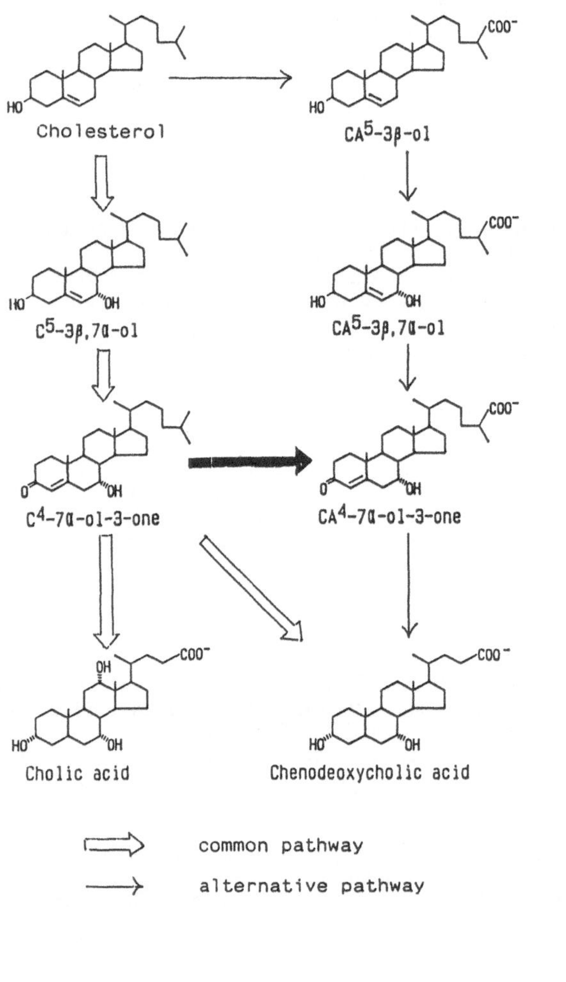

Cholesterol

$CA^5-3\beta-ol$

$C^5-3\beta,7\alpha-ol$

$CA^5-3\beta,7\alpha-ol$

$C^4-7\alpha-ol-3-one$

$CA^4-7\alpha-ol-3-one$

Cholic acid

Chenodeoxycholic acid

⟹ common pathway

⟶ alternative pathway

Fig. 1 Proposed model for the biosynthesis of 7α-hydroxy-3-oxo-4-cholestenoic acid.

from 80°C to 280°C at a rate of 25°C x min^{-1}. The amounts of cholestenoic acids were calculated by comparisons of the peak areas with those given by known amounts of the corresponding reference compounds. The internal standard, triacontane, was used to normalize the injection volumes.

The levels of cholic acid and chenodeoxycholic acid were measured with the isotope dilution mass-spectrometry technique reported by Björkhem et al [6]. Deuterium-labeled internal standards, D_5-cholic acid and D_4-chenodeoxycholic acid, were synthesized as described previously [6]. Following the addition of 1 μg each of D_5-cholic acid and D_4-chenodeoxycholic acid, 0.5 ml of sample was hydrolyzed prior to extraction. The hydrolysis was performed by refluxing at 120°C for 8 hr with KOH/ethanol (1:20 v/v). Cholic acids were extracted with diethyl ether. The ether layer was taken to dryness in vacuo, and was redissolved in a small amount of choloroform/methanol (2:1, v/v). The fractions containing bile acids were converted into trimethylsilyl ether derivative before analysis by mass spectrometry. The mass spectrometric assays was performed with an LKB 9000 instrument equipped with a multiple ion detector. A column of 1.5% SE-30 was used for gas-liquid chromatography. The multiple ion detector was focused on the ions at m/e 623 and 628 for the analysis of cholic acid, and at m/e 370 and 374 for chenodeoxycholic acid, respectively. The amounts of unlabeled cholic acid and cheno deoxycholic acid were determined with use of standard curves obtained by analyses of standard mixtures of a fixed amount of the deuterium-labeled internal standard (100, 200, 400, 800 ng) and varying amounts of the unlabeled steroid.

RESULTS

The level of 7α-hydroxy-3-oxo-4-cholestenoic acid was 658.09 ± 137.53 ng/ml in CSDH, while it was 126.27 ± 17.73 ng/ml in serum, as reported previously. The difference was statistically significant (p<0.01, Welch-t-test). The levels of 3β-hydroxy-5-cholestenoic acid and 3β,7α-dihydroxy-5-cholestenoic acid in CSDH were 84.6 ± 16.5, 71.0 ± 23.0 ng/ml, respectively. The levels of these cholestenoic acids in normal human plasma/serum has been reported by Axelson et al.[5] to be 67.2 ± 27.9, 38.9 ± 25.6 ng/ml, and were statistically not siginificant (Student-t-test). The levels of bile acids in CSDH were 976.5 ± 288.3 ng/ml in chenodeoxycholic acid, and 260.2 ± 119.3 ng/ml in cholic acid. The average levels in normal plasma, as measured by the same method, were 324 ± 128 ng/ml in chenodeoxycholic acid (p<0.05) and 116 ± 72 ng/ml in cholic acid (N.S.) [6]. It is worth noting that 7α-hydroxy-4-cholesten-3-one was not detected in any of the five cases of CSDH, while the normal plasma level is reported to be 50 ± 10 ng/ml by Bjoerkhem et al.[7] (p<0.01). All these results are summarized in Table 1.

Table-1 Obtained levels of several cholesterol metabolites in chronic subdural hematoma and the reported respective normal serum level as a comparison.

	chr subdural hematoma	normal serum	
CA^4-7a-ol-3-one	658.1 ± 137.5	126.3 ± 17.7	(p<0.01)
CA^5-3b-ol	84.6 ± 16.5	67.2 ± 27.9	(N.S.)
CA^5-3b,7a-ol	71.0 ± 23.0	38.9 ± 25.6	(N.S.)
C^4-7a-ol-3-one	not detected	50.0 ± 10.0	(p<0.01)
Cholic acid	260.2 ± 119.3	116 ± 72	(N.S.)
Chenodeoxy- cholic acid	976.5 ± 288.3	324 ± 128	(p<0.05)

DISCUSSION

These experiments showed a relatively high concentration of 7α-hydroxy-3-oxo-4-cholestenoic acid and an extremely low level of 7α-hydroxy-4-cholesten-3-one in CSDH, compared to their normal levels in serum. Since the levels of 3β-hydroxy-5-cholestenoic acid and 3β,7α-dihydroxy-5-cholestenoic acid, both of which are possible precursor of 7α-hydroxy-3-oxo-4-cholestenoic acid, in CSDH were not very different from the normal plasma level, it would be reasonable to conclude that the high level of 7α-hydroxy-3-oxo-4-cholestenoic acid may in part be caused by the conversion of 7α-hydroxy-4-cholesten-3-one. Since cholic acid and chenodeoxycholic acid levels in the hematoma were about three-fold higher than the corresponding serum levels obtained with the same methodology, it is aslo reasonable to conclude that there is some concentration of the polar bile acids as compared to plasma. The mechanism behind this concentration is unknown. The relative importance of this concentration mechanism and enzymatic conversion of 7α-hydroxy-4-cholesten-3-one into the corresponding acid is unknown.

The structural difference between the latter two compounds is the existence of 26-carboxyl moiety. 26-hydroxylase has been .reported to exist in several tissues other than the liver, including brain [8,9]. Thus, the enzymatic conversion from 7α-hydroxy-4-cholesten-3-one to 7α-hydroxy-3-oxo-4-cholestenoic acid via 7α,26-dihydroxy-4-cholesten-3-one may be theoretically possible even in the cranial cavity. Since the actual extrahepatic bile acid formation has, hitherto, not been reported, further studies will be required to demonstrate this intracranial cholestenoic acid production.

From the chemical properties of these compounds, the following hypothesis for part of the high level of 7α-hydroxy-3-oxo-4-cholestenoic acid is advanced. It is well known that brain tissue is abundant in lipid. Hence, lipo-soluble compounds may be more harmful to brain tissue than water-soluble ones. Because of the existence of 26-carboxyl moiety, 7α-hydroxy-3-oxo-4-cholestenoic acid is more polar, which means less lipo-soluble, than 7α-hydroxy-4-cholesten-3-one. Since the cerebrospinal fluid usually does not contain this lipo-soluble 7α-hydroxy-4-cholesten-3-one (unpublished data), once the compound, which is included in normal circulating blood, is exposed to the brain tissue by the intracranial hemorrhage, some detoxication mechanism mayb occur to eliminate this potentially harmful 7α-hydroxy-4-cholesten-3-one may occur in the cranial cavity. Continuos microhemorrhage is known to occur in CSDH [10], leading to accumulation of less harmful 7α-hydroxy-3-oxo-4-cholestenoic acid. It is not known with certainty if 7α-hydroxy-4-cholesten-3-one is toxic on the brain tissue. Further study on the biological activity of this compound is now under way.

Aknowledgements: The skillful technical assistance of Kristina Garmark, Birgitta Mörk, and Anita Lovgren is gratefully acknowledged.

REFERENCES

1. Nagata K, Asano T, Basugi N, Tango T, Takakura K (1988) Neurol Surg 16: 1347-1353
2. Nagata K, Takakura K, Asano T, Seyama Y, Hirota H, Shigematsu N, Shima I, Kasama T, Shimizu T (1992) Biochim Biophys Acta 1126: 229-236
3. Axelson M, Sjövall J (1990) J Steroid Biochem 36: 631-640
4. Axelson M, Aly A, Sjövall J (1988) FEBS Lett 239: 324-328
5. Axelson M, Mork B, Sjovall J (1988) J Lipid Res 29: 629-641
6. Bjorkhem I, Falk O (1983) Scand J Clin Lab Invest 43: 163-170
7. Björkhem I, Skrede S, Buchmann MS, East C, Grundy S (1987) Hepatology 7: 266-271
8. Pedersen I, Oftebro H, Bjorkhem I (1989) Biochem Int 18:615-622
9. Andersson S, Davis DL, Dahlback H, Jornvall H, Russel DW (1989) J Biol Chem 264: 8222-8229
10. Ito H, Yamamoto S, Komai T, Mizukoshi H (1976) J Neurosurg 45: 26-31

The Role of the Kallikrein-Kinin System in Chronic Subdural Hematoma

HIROSUKE FUJISAWA[1], HARUHIDE ITO[1], JUNKOH YAMASHITA[2], KENICHI SAITO[2], and SOTARO HIGASHI[2]

[1]Department of Neurosurgery, Yamaguchi University School of Medicine, Ube, Yamaguchi, 755 Japan and
[2]Department of Neurosurgery, School of Medicine, Kanazawa University, Kanazawa, 920 Japan

SUMMARY

The outer membrane of chronic subdural hematoma (CSDH) is morphologically composed of inflammatory granulation tissue. Increased permeability of new macrocapillaries, perivascular hemorrhages, migration of all inflammatory cells and interstitial edema in the outer membrane have been suggested as factors which cause hematoma enlargement. Bradykinin (BK), an end product of the kallikrein-kinin system, causes enhancement of vascular permeability, vasodilatation and migration of leukocytes. We have measured prekallikrein (PKK), high molecular weight kininogen (HMWK) and BK, which are components of the kallikrein-kinin system, in 67 hematoma sites of 57 patients. The activities of both PKK and HMWK in the hematoma were significantly lower than in plasma, and there was a significant correlation between them. The concentration of BK in the hematoma was significantly higher than in plasma. The kallikrein-kinin system is thus activated in CSDH. CSDH contains quantities of red and white blood cells, and the total protein concentration in the hematoma was higher than in plasma and similar to the fluid exudate of inflamed tissue. The kallikrein-kinin system may accelerate plasma exudation and hemorrhage from new macrocapillaries both into the membrane and also into the hematoma cavity to cause enlargement of the hematoma. The kallikrein-kinin system is related to the fibrinolytic system which is generally accepted as a main etiological factor in CSDH. We postulate that the kallikrein-kinin system and the fibrinolytic system are involved in the etiology of CSDH by stimulating each other.

KEY WORDS: chronic subdural hematoma, kallikrein-kinin system, bradykinin, fibrinolysis, etiology

INTRODUCTION

The kallikrein-kinin system basically consists of prekallikrein (PKK), high-molecular weight kininogen (HMWK) and bradykinin (BK). Prekallikrein is transformed into kallikrein, which in turn converts HMWK into BK (see Fig. 2). BK has strong biological effects such as enhancement of vascular permeability, vasodilatation and migration of leukocytes[1]. In the outer membrane of CSDH, perivascular hemorrhages, inflammatory cells migration and interstitial edema are observed, and increased permeability of macrocapillaries has been suggested to cause enlargement of the hematoma[2]. We have measured PKK, HMWK and BK in patients with CSDH and the role of the kallikrein-kinin system in the etiology of CSDH is discussed.

MATERIALS AND METHODS

Fifty-seven patients between 36 to 85 years old (mean 66.6 years) with CSDH were studied. They had received no previous treatment for CSDH. The total number of hematomas was 67 (bilateral in 10). Hematoma samples

53

(obtained through the dura) during surgery, and peripheral blood were taken before or during surgery. Hematoma samples were put into siliconized vacuum tubes containing 3.8 % sodium citrate for measurement of PKK and HMWK activity, and tubes containing aprotinin, soybean trypsin inhibitor, protamine sulfate and disodium ethylenediaminetetra-acetic acid for measurement of BK levels. The samples were then centrifuged and supernatant obtained. PKK and HMWK activity were measured by the one-stage activated partial thromboplastin time method, using Fletcher factor (PKK) deficient plasma and Fitzerald factor (HMWK) deficient plasma, respectively[3,4]. Bradykinin was measured by radioimmunoassay. Total protein, protein fraction, white blood cells (WBC), red blood cells (RBC) were also measured.

RESULTS AND DISCUSSION

PKK and HMWK activities, and BK levels

PKK and HMWK activities in the hematoma were significantly lower than in plasma (Table 1), and there was a significant correlation between PKK and HMWK activity (Fig. 1). BK levels was significantly greater in the hematoma than in plasma (Table 1). These results indicate that the kallikrein-kinin system is locally activated in CSDH. In the outer membrane of CSDH, gaps between adjacent endothelial cells of macro-capillaries have been demonstrated at the sites of vascular leakage [2]. It has been suggested that BK enhances vascular permeability by increasing the gaps between endothelial cells[5]. Thus, it is proposed that perivascular hemorrhage, inflammatory cell migration and inter-stitial edema in the outer membrane are caused by the activation of the kallikrein-kinin system.

Table 1 Prekallikrein activities, High molecular weight kininogen (HMW-kininogen) activities and Bradykinin levels. Values are Mean ± S.E.M. ***;p<0.001 by unpaired Student's t-test, *; p<0.05 by Wilcoxon signed rank test.

		Hematoma		Plasma	
Prekallikrein	(%)	54.6 ± 2.6 ***	(n=65)	79.4 ± 2.7	(n=36)
HMW-kininogen	(%)	42.4 ± 2.4 ***	(n=64)	79.2 ± 3.2	(n=48)
Bradykinin (pg/ml)		63.9 ± 12.1 *	(n=25)	36.4 ± 5.6	(n=22)

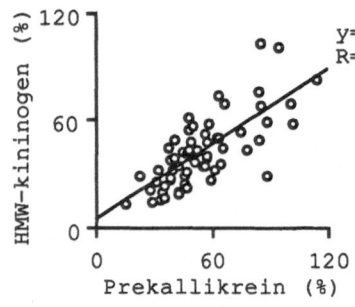

y=4.2905+0.70308x
R=0.74

Fig. 1 Correlation between prekallikrein and HMW-kininogen activity in the hematoma. p<0.001 by Spearman rank correlation test.

Protein fractions, white blood cell count and red blood cell count

The results are shown in Table 2. Total protein in the hematoma was significantly higher than in the peripheral blood and as high as in the fluid exudate of inflammed tissue. The difference in total protein concentration was a result of the difference in α2- and β-globulin. The hematoma contained a considerable amount of WBC and RBC, derived from the outer membrane. It has been reported that capillaries open from the outer membrane into the hematoma cavity[2]. Thus, it may be that the openings of the vessels into the hematoma cavity are large enough for blood cells to pass through, or that the activation of the kallikrein-kinin system causes their leakage from the outer membrane.

Table 2 Total protein, protein fraction, white blood cells (WBC) and red blood cells (RBC). Values are Mean ± S.E.M. ***;p<0.001, **;p<0.01, *;p<0.05 by Student's t-test.

	Hematoma			Peripheral blood	
T. protein (g/dl)	8.4 ± 0.4	***	(n=61)	6.3 ± 0.1	(n=39)
albumin	3.8 ± 0.1			3.9 ± 0.1	
α1-globulin	0.2 ± 0.02			0.2 ± 0.01	
α2-globulin	1.6 ± 0.3	*		0.6 ± 0.02	
β-globulin	2.2 ± 0.3	**		0.6 ± 0.02	
γ-globulin	0.8 ± 0.05			0.9 ± 0.05	
WBC (/ml)	5781 ± 1068		(n=52)	6994 ± 361	(n=48)
RBC (10^4/ml)	303 ± 18		(n=53)	383 ± 7	(n=48)

It is now generally accepted that local hyperfibrinolysis in the outer membrane is a main etiological factor of CSDH[6]. Interestingly, the kallikrein-kinin system is related to the fibrinolytic system (Fig. 2); kallikrein converts plasminogen into plasmin, plasmin can activate HMWK [7, 8] and FDP enhances the action of BK[9].

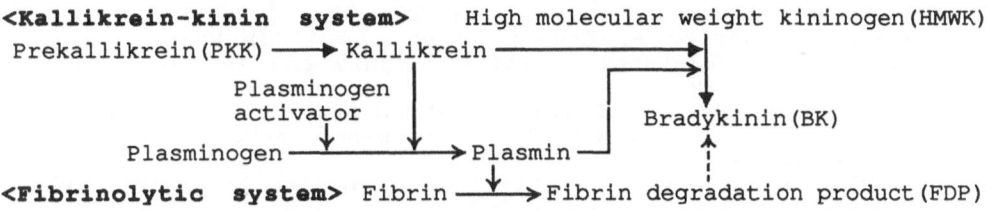

Fig. 2 Relationship between the kallikrein-kinin and the fibrinolytic system.

A diagram of the putative etiology of CSDH is shown in Fig.3. Blood extravasation, plasma exudation and migration of inflammatory cells into both the membrane and the hematoma cavity are caused by the activation of the kallilrein-kinin system (1). Although platelets aggregate and fibrin clots are formed at the opening sites of capillaries into the hematoma cavity or at the endothelial gaps, these clots may be very fragile because the hematoma contains a large amount of FDP[6] which inhibits both platelet aggregation[10] and fibrin polymerization[11]. Thus, the clots are easily broken down by increased fibrinolytic activity (2). Hemorrhage, plasma exudation and migration of inflammatory cells from the capillaries then recur, resulting in enlargement of the hematoma (3). Fibrin is produced in extravasated blood and exudates in the outer membrane and forms a matrix for the migrating fibroblasts. BK has been reported to stimulate proliferation of fibroblasts and collagen synthesis[12]. Thus, it is suggested that the kallikrein-kinin system may also play a role in the growth of the outer membrane (3).

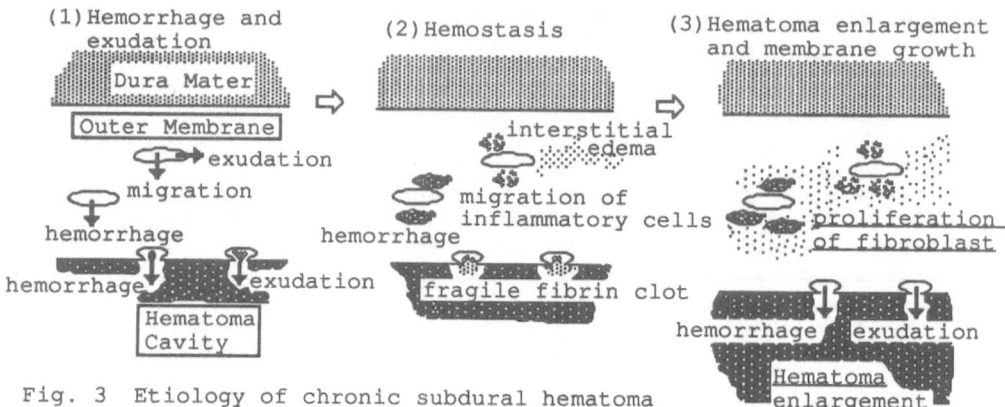

Fig. 3 Etiology of chronic subdural hematoma

REFERENCES

1. Ratnoff OD (1976) Mediators of inflammation. J Allergy Clin Immunol 58:438-446
2. Yamashima T, Yamamoto S, Friede RL (1983) The role of endothelial gap junctions in the enlargement of chronic subdural hematomas. J Neurosurg 59:298-303
3. Saito H, Goldsmith G, Waldmann R (1976) Fitzgerald factor (high molecular weight kininogen) clotting activity in human plasma in health and disease in various animal plasmas. Blood 48:941-947
4. Saito H, Poon MC, Vicic W, Goldsmith GH Jr, Menitove JE (1978) Human plasma prekallikrein (Fletcher factor) clotting activity and antigen in health and disease. J Lab Clin Med 92:84-95
5. Marceau F, Lussier A, Regoli D, et al (1983) Pharmacology of kinins: Their relevance to tissue injury and inflammation. Gen Pharmac 14:209-229
6. Ito H, Yamamoto S, Komai T, Mizukoshi H (1976) Role of hyperfibrinolysis in the etiology of chronic subdural hematoma. J Neurosurg 45:26-31
7. Back N, Steger B (1965) Activation of bovine bradykininogen by human plasmin. Life Sci 4:153-157
8. Ratnoff OD (1965) Increased vascular permeability induced by human plasmin. J Exp Med 122:905-921
9. Buluk K, Malofiejew M (1969) The pharmacological properties of fibrinogen degradation products. Br J Pharmac 35:79-89
10. Kowalski E, Kopec M, Wegrynowicz Z (1964) Influence of fibrinogen degradation products (FDP) on platelet aggregation, adhesiveness and viscous metamorphosis. Thromb Haemostas 10:406-423
11. Alkjaersig N, Fletcher AP, Sherry S (1962) Pathogenesis of the coagulation defect developing during pathological plasma proteolytic ("fibrinolytic") states. II. The significance, mechanism and consequences of defective fibrin polymerization. J Clin Invest 41:917-934
12. Goldstein RH, Wall M (1984) Activation of protein formation and cell division by bradykinin and des-Arg^9-bradykinin. J Biol Chem 259:9263-9268

Histochemical Profile of Chronic Subdural Hematoma from a Wound Healing Viewpoint

SHIN NISHIDA, MASAYOSHI MATSUMOTO, and NORIO NAKAMURA

Department of Neurosurgery, The Jikei University School of Medicine, Minato-ku, Tokyo, 105 Japan

SUMMARY

The concentration of blood coagulation factor X Ⅲ (F X Ⅲ), fibronectin, and α_2-plasmin inhibitor (α_2-PI) in chronic subdural hematoma was measured, and the localization of fibronectin and fibrin in the outer membrane was immunohistologically examined. Based on the results, the relationship between these factors and the etiology of the hematoma were investigated. Seventy-five chronic subdural hematoma patients who had had burr hole opening surgery became the subjects of the study, and hematoma fluid retrieved during their operations was analyzed. The hematoma membrane attached to the dura mater was immunohistologically examined in 20 samples. In most of the typical hematoma cases, concentration of fibronectin in the hematoma fluid was more than the normal plasma range. The value of F X Ⅲ was extremely low, and the degree of the tissue healing factor in the hematoma fluid was unfavorable, despite a normal healing process. Fibrin and fibronectin were contained in the outer membrane. The authors can assume from the results that the outer membrane was granulation tissue which recovery process was delayed. The guess was that an imbalance in the condition of factors in the healing of the tissue very much related to the etiology and natural history of the chronic subdural hematoma.

KEY WORDS: fibronectin, blood coagulation factor X Ⅲ, wound healing, chronic subdural hematoma, spontaneous recovery

INTRODUCTION

Chronic subdural hematoma occasionally demonstrates spontaneous recovery. However, in the the case of natural healing, the time it takes to heal is longer than for common injuries. There are several reports of studies of the outer membrane of the chronic subdural hematoma as one kind of granulation in the healing of the wound. However, the authors look at the entire subdural hematoma was one kind of injury. In order to do that, it is necessary to determine what role is played by factors relating to the healing of injuries in chronic subdural hematoma. The authors are interested in fibronectin and its related substances; fibronectin is important in the recovery process; F X Ⅲ is the medium forming the cross-linked bond between fibronectin and fibrin; α_2-PI relates to the recovery process and the coagulation fibrinogenolysis system. The authors studied what significance these factors had in chronic subdural hematoma. In addition to these, localization of the fibronectin and fibrin at the outer membrane were investigated.

MATERIALS AND METHODS

Our study looked at 75 cases of chronic subdural hematoma which had
undergone burr hole opening surgery. Seventeen of the cases had
bilateral chronic subdural hematoma, and three were re-stagnation
hematoma cases (all male, aged 15,68,72 years). Among the 75 were
seven cases which were considered special. Details of those are as
follows: two were acute subdural hematoma cases which were becoming
chronic, two had a history of severe head injury complicated with
traumatic subarachnoid hemorrhaging, one had complications with DIC,
another had complications with cirrhosis, and the last had
complications with renal failure. One exceptional case was judged
through diagnosis by CT-Scan examination and findings in the operation
to have right-side subdural hygroma. The hematoma fluid was
centrifuged at a rate of 3000 rpm for five minutes, then the separated
supernatant was immediately cooled to −80 degrees C, stored
temporarily, and measured. In cases of re-stagnation of hematoma and
bilateral chronic subdural hematoma, each fluid is separately assayed
as an independent hematoma fluid. The number of assayed samples,
including the special cases described above were as follows: 90 cases
of fibronectin, 86 cases of F X Ⅲ , and 85 cases of the α_2-PI. The
fibronectin, F X Ⅲ , and the α_2-PI in the peripheral blood were
measured as one part of the cases. The fibronectin and the fibrin in
the outer membrane of the chronic subdural hematoma were
immunohistologically stained. Rabbit-anti-human-fibronectin or
fibrinogen (600 fold dilution) were used as a primary antibody. This
was followed by methyl green or hematoxylin as post-staining agents.
The findings of the CT-scan of the chronic subdural hematoma were
classified into low, iso, high, and mix density, and the fibronectin
value was compared with it.

RESULTS

Of the 68 cases of chronic subdural hematoma which were typical, there
were 44 cases with a history of head injury. The fibronectin content
in the hematoma fluid was within the range of 40−1068 μ g/ml.
Considering the correlation with the injury, the value was relatively
high when the period between the head injury and the operation was
less than 8 weeks (Fig.1). This corresponds to the hematoma formation

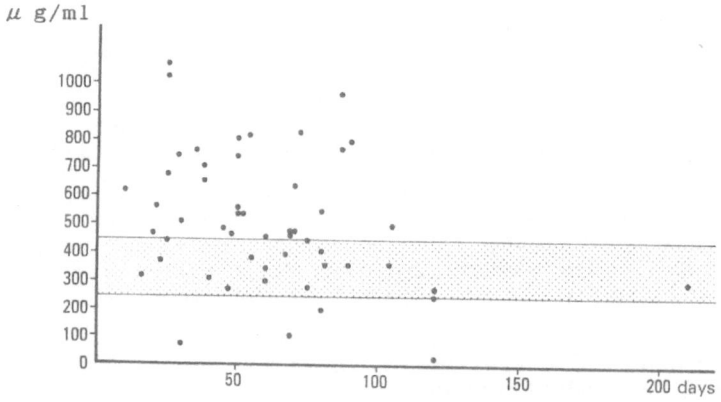

Fig.1 Fibronectin of hematoma in each day
        between the head injury and the operation

period. Also, a tendency was demonstrated that the longer the period between the head injury and the operation, the lower the value of the fibronectin. In the case of the subdural hygroma, the value was extremely low; less than 40 μ g/ml.

In all cases, the value of α_2-PI was less than the lower limit of the normal range (the normal value is 85-115%). In most of the samples, the value was less than 25%. The content of F XIII was extremely low, with the exception of one case that was out of the normal range of values for blood plasma (the normal value is 72-144%). The difference between the seven special cases and the others was found in respect only to the measured amount of fibronectin. The average value of seven cases was a low 237.1 μ g/ml. Fibronectin in the tissue sample was found at the outer membrane of the hematoma but not at the dura. Fibrin was also contained only in the outer membrane. The relationship between the density found in the CT-Scan and the density of the fibronectin, was found on average to be 310.0, 442.2, 445.5, and 609.6 μ g/ml respectively.

DISCUSSION

The significance of fibronectin

Fibronectin, whose molecular weight is about 440,000, is deposited locally along with fibrin whenever tissue is damaged. As with fibrin and collagen, fibronectin also plays an important role in forming a cross-linked bond with fibrous proteins which are necessary for tissue repair. This is how a solid "fibrin-matrix" is created. The fibroblasts proliferates there and tissue repair proceeds[1]. In this way, fibronectin and fibroblast appear together as the injury heals, and disappear as the healing process goes on. The healing process of a wound is completed experimentally in 5 weeks time [2]. However, in cases of chronic subdural hematoma, clinical symptoms show about eight weeks after the head injury. Therefore, in the case of natural healing, the process takes a long time. In fact, fibronectin in the hematoma fluid stays at a relatively high level until about eight weeks after the injury and decreases to a normal plasma range with time. Accordingly, as Nakamura and Mochizuki have pointed out, the healing of the wound may be retarded in cases of chronic subdural hematoma[3][4]. In the case of subdural hygroma, fibronectin levels are extremely low. The level of fibronectin in cerebrospinal fluid is also extremely low (i.e. the ratio of plasma to cerebrospinal fluid is about 400.) It is assumed that the cerebrospinal fluid will be concerned to the chronic subdural hematoma. Then, the question may be arise as to what significance there is in the presence of fibronectin in the outer membrane. According to pathological retrievals, the outer membrane itself is still in the damaged tissue healing process. It is assumed that the area where fibronectin exits is the delicate tissue in the early healing process before scar contraction.

The role of F XIII in the chronic subdural hematoma

The F XIII is responsible for the last stages of blood coagulation, and this function is mainly related to the healing of an injury. Currently, four kinds of the cross-linked bonds which progress with F XIII have been confirmed[5]. The gamma bond is fragile, but if even a trace is present, it may rapidly form the cross-linked bond. The fibrin inter-molecular rigid crosslinks, made up of alpha bonds, progress slowly when the level of the F XIII exceeds the normal value of 25%[6]. In addition, there must be at least 70% or more of the normal level in order that an incomplete clinical recovery does not occur. However, the bond of α_2-PI to the fibrin progresses with less than 25% of F X III, but it is common for the level of F X III in the hematoma fluid to be less than 25%. Therefore, in hematoma fluid, the fragile bonding of the fibrin molecule gamma chain proceeds rapidly. The rigid cross-links of the alpha bonds, however, have difficulty advancing in hematoma fluid. In other words, the hematoma is physically unstable as a result of the low level of F X III. This cross-linked bond which mediates the F X III is insufficient. As a result, it causes the physical fragility of the tissue over a long period of time. Accordingly, hemorrhaging may occur naturally, or as the result of a slight external force. This can cause repeated hemorrhaging from the outer membrane in the same way as the above α_2-PI deficiency condition, or in local hyper-fibrinolytic activity[7]. In chronic subdural hematoma fluid, factors relating to the healing of tissue are in a state of imbalance. It has already been reported that the fibrinogen in hematoma fluid decreases. This situation is very difficult to treat from the viewpoint of healing a wound. Aoki et al., have reported that the quality of the fibrin-matrix formation in the early stages of healing the wound is the essential condition in the restoration of tissue which follows[8]. Therefore, it is possible that chronic subdural hematoma may be the result of some interference in the first stages of the healing process of the wound. As such, this might be the reason that chronic subdural hematoma exists for a long time, and that it gets gradually larger as a result of recurrent hemorrhaging in the weak membrane.

REFERENCES

1. Ueyama M, Amano H, Hirakawa S, Urayama T (1979) The role of factor X III in fibroblast proliferation. —The cell growth dependent on α — crosslinking of fibrin— Blood & Vessel 10: 505-509
2. Kurkinen M, Vahere A, Roberts PJ, Stenman S (1980) Sequential appearance of fibronectin and collagen in experimental granulation tissue. Laboratory Investigation 43: 47-51
3. Nakamura N (1966) The relationship between head injuries and chronic subdural hematoma. Brain and Nerve (Tokyo) 18: 30-37
4. Mochizuki R (1987) The role of tissue plasminogen activator in chronic subdural hematomas. Brain & Nerve 39: 947-952
5. Matsuda M (1982) Fibronectin and its related substances —Their roles in tissue repair. Connective Tissue 13: 177-184
6. Matsuda M (1977) Wound healing and Factor X III. Acta Haem Jap 40: 995-1002
7. Saito K, Ito H, Hasegawa T, Yamamoto S (1989) Plasmin-α_2-plasmin inhibitor complex and α_2-plasmin inhibitor in chronic subdural hematoma. J Neurosurg 70: 68-72
8. Aoki N, Sakata Y, Matsuda M, Tateno K (1980) Fibrinolytic states in a patient congenital deficiency of α_2-plasmin inhibitor. Blood 55: 483-488

The Role of Platelet-Activating Factor (PAF) in the Development of Chronic Subdural Hematoma

YUTAKA HIRASHIMA[1], RYOKO KATO[1], TOMOAKI OHMORI[1], TAKESHI NAGAHORI[1], MICHIHARU NISHIJIMA[1], SHUNRO ENDO[1], AKIRA TAKAKU[1], and KEN KARASAWA[2]

[1]Department of Neurosurgery, Toyama Medical and Pharmaceutical University, Toyama-shi, Toyama, 930-01 Japan and [2]Faculty of Pharmaceutical Sciences, Teikyo University, Kanagawa, 199-01 Japan

SUMMARY

The PAF level in the plasma of patients with chronic subdural hematoma was higher than that in the plasma of healthy volunteers($p<0.01$). The PAF level in the hematoma of the old hematoma group(more than 14 days from the day symptoms appeared to the day of operation)was lower than that in the fresh hematoma group(less than 14 days)($p<0.05$). On the other hand, the PAF-acetylhydrolase activity in the hematoma of the old hematoma group was higher than that in the fresh hematoma group($p<0.05$). The PAF level in the plasma of cured patients decreased rapidly after operation, but did not decrease rapidly or turned to increase in the plasma of the recurrent hematoma and delayed cure patients. Etizolam, PAF antagonist was effective for preventing the development of hematoma. Only one patient with hypo-PAF-acetylhydrolasia showed the recurrence of subdural hematoma. The fluorescent antibody method for staining PAF demonstrated the localization of PAF around the sinusoidal vessels in the outer membrane. These findings suggest that PAF plays an important role in the development of chronic subdural hematoma.

KEY WORDS: platelet-activating factor, PAF-acetylhydrolase, Etizolam, fluorescent antibody method, chronic subdural hematoma

INTRODUCTION

The inflammatory reaction has been thought to stimulate the growth of subdural hematoma[1]. The platelet-activating factor(PAF), a highly potent mediator of inflammation, can induce the chemotaxis of inflammatory cells including eosinophils[2,3]. Eosinophile infiltration to the capsule of chronic subdural hematoma contributes to bleeding into the hematoma cavity. Because, the secretion of plasminogen-rich granules from eosinophils may initiate local hyperfibrinolysis[4]. Increasing vascular permeability, one of PAF's activities[5] may also contribute to the development of chronic subdural hematoma. In this study, the PAF and PAF-acetylhydrolase activity in the plasma and hematoma of patients and clinical courses of these patients are discussed including the effect of Etizolam, a PAF antagonist.

MATERIAL AND METHODS

Patients

We examined the PAF level and/or PAF acetylhydrolase activity in hematoma and/or plasma from a series of 28 patients with chronic subdural hematoma. These two parameters in plasma were also followed in 15 patients after surgery. Etizolam, PAF antagonist was administered orally to seven patients and the sequential changes on the brain CT were followed.

Analysis of PAF Content
Total lipids were extracted from both hematoma and plasma specimens by the method of Bligh and Dyer[6]. Extracts were applied to a silica gel cartridge(Sep-Pak cartridge, Waters). After washing with 10 ml of chloroform, 10 ml of acetone, 10 ml of an acetone and methanol mixture(1/1, v/v) and 10 ml of a chloroform and methanol mixture(7/3, v/v), the elute, with 10 ml of a chroloform, methanol and water mixture(1/2/0.8, v/v/v), was collected and extracted again by the method of Bligh and Dyer[6]. The lipid extract was subjected to TLC(Silicagel G, Merck) and developed with a solvent system consisting of chloroform, methanol and water(65/35/6, v/v/v). The area corresponding to PAF was scraped off and reextracted. PAF was quantified by a bioassay, in which the radioactivity of[^{14}C]serotonin released from rabbit platelets [7] was measured.

Measurement of PAF-acetylhydrolase Activity
The enzyme activity was measured according to the method of Miwa et al.[8].

Fluorescent Antibody Staining for PAF
Preparation of antibody Dimethylcarbamoyl-CPGPC/BSA conjugates with Freund's complete adjuvant were injected into rabbits as previously described[9]. One week after the booster injection, blood was obtained. The IgG fraction was separated from antisera by protein A-Sepharose CL-6B column chromatography.

Tissue processing All specimens were embedded in OCT compound(Tissue-Tek, Miles Pharmaceuticals) and frozen at - 20°C. Cross-sections 5 μm thick mounted on a glass slide were exposed to the primary antibody, anti-PAF IgG, for 60 min at room temperature. After washing with cold PBS, the slide was incubated for 60 min at room temperature with FITC-labeled goat anti-rabbit IgG. After washing again in cold PBS, the slide was viewed under a fluorescence microscope. As a control, sections were also processed without the primary antibody or with preimmune rabbit immunoglobulin at the same concentrations.

RESULTS AND DISCUSSION
The PAF level in patient's plasma and hematoma was 0.72 ± 0.12 pmol/ml(M $\pm$ SEM, n=25) and 0.5 ± 0.12 pmol/ml(M $\pm$ SEM, n=28), respectively. The level in plasma from the 7 healthy volunteers was 0.18 ± 0.02 pmol/ml(M $\pm$ SEM, n=7), ie., higher in the patient than the healthy volunteers(p<0.01). Patients with chronic subdural hematoma were divided into two groups, fresh and old hematoma according to the interval from the day symptoms appeared to the days of operation, being 1 to 14 days for fresh hematoma and more than 14 days for old hematoma. The PAF level in the plasma in the fresh hematoma group, 0.81 ± 0.17 pmol/ml (M $\pm$ SEM, n=11), did not differ from that in the old hematoma group, 0.74 ± 0.13 pmol/ml (M $\pm$ SEM, n=14). However, the PAF level in the hematoma in the old hematoma group, 0.17 ± 0.023 pmol/ml (M $\pm$ SEM, n=15), was much lower than that in the fresh hematoma group, 0.59 ± 0.17 pmol/ml (M $\pm$ SEM, n=13)(p<0.05)(Fig. 1A). On the other hand, the activity of PAF-acetylhydrolase in the hematoma

in the old hematoma group, 1.04 ± 0.16 nmol/min/mg (M ± SEM, n=13), was higher than that in the fresh hematoma group, 0.55 ± 0.072 nmol/min/mg (M ± SEM, n=12)(Fig. 1B)(p<0.05).

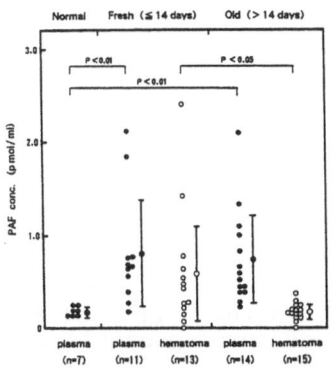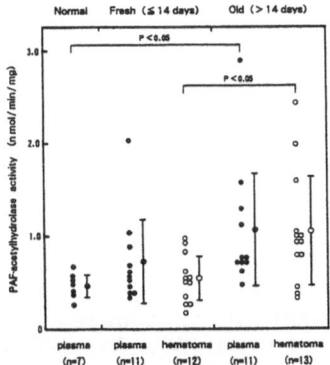

Fig. 1. PAF levels(A) and PAF-acetylhydrolase activity(B) in the plasma and hematoma in patients with chronic subdural hematoma and healthy volunteers.

On fifteen patients who had evacuation of hematoma, brain CT scanning and measurement of PAF level in plasma were performed. Seven patients were cured within 1 month(cured group), while 8 patients showed recurrence of hematoma or over 1-month delay of cure(recurrent hematoma and delayed cured group). The PAF level in the plasma of the cured group decreased rapidly after the operation, while that in the recurrent and delayed cured group did not decrease smoothly after operation or turned to increase at some point after operation(Fig. 2A,B). These findings suggest that plasma PAF plays a role in the recurrence of hematoma or the delay of cure. PAF induces the chemo-taxis of many inflammatory cells such as eosinophils[2,3] and stimu-lates degranulation[10]. The secretion of plasminogen-rich granules from eosinophils may initiate local hyperfibrinolysis and contribute to repeated bleeding into the hematoma cavity[4]. PAF has many activ-ities, including increasing vascular permeability[4]. These activi-ties of PAF may contribute to the recurrence or development of chron-ic subdural hematoma. Etizolam, a PAF antagonist, is clinically available. We administered 1 mg - 3 mg Etizolam orally, per day to 7 patients with chronic subdural hematoma. Five patients were adminis-tered Etizolam after operation, while 2 patients were treated conser-vatively with Etizolam. None of the patients showed the recurrence after administration of Etizolam(data not shown). Only one patient in this study was PAF-acetylhydrolase-negative in both plasma and hema-toma. Interestingly, his hematoma recurred and developed (data not shown). These two findings also suggest that PAF is involved in the pathogenesis of chronic subdural hematoma. Fig. 3 is a visual demon-stration of PAF localization in the capsule stained by fluorescent antibody method developed by us. PAF was stained predominantly on the hematoma cavity side of the outer membrane, surrounding the sinusoidal vessels. This histochemical demonstration also supports the possibility of the contribution of PAF to development of chronic subdural hematoma.

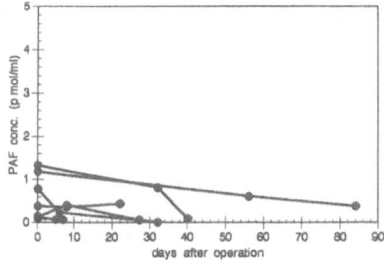 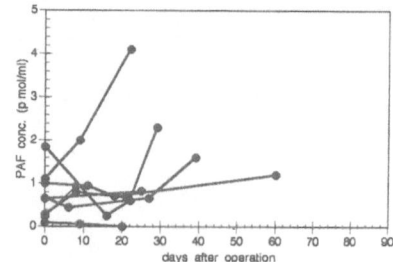

Fig. 2. Sequential changes of PAF level in the plasma after operation. Cured group(A), Recurrent and delayed cured group(B)

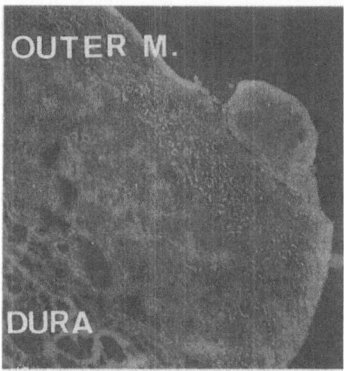

Fig. 3. PAF localization in the outer membrane

REFERENCES
1. Labadie EL, Glover D (1976) J Neurosurg 45: 382-392
2. Tamura N, Agrawal DK, Suliaman FA, Townley RG (1987) Biochem Biophys Res Commun 142: 638-644
3. Wardlaw AJ, Mogbel R, Cromwell O, Kay AB (1986) J Clin Invest 78: 1701-1706
4. Yamashima T, Kubota T, Yamamot S (1985) J Neurosurg 62: 257-260
5. Bjork J, Lindbrom L, Gerdin B, Smedegard G, Arfors K-E, Benveniste J (1983) Acta Physiol Scand 119: 305-308
6. Bligh EG, Dyer WJ (1959) Can J Biochem Physiol 37: 911-917
7. Hanahan DJ, Weintraub ST (1985) In: Glick D (ed) Methods of Biochemical Analysis. Wiley and Sons, pp 195-219
8. Miwa M, Miyake T, Yamanaka T, Sugatani J, Suzuki Y, Sakata S, Araki Y, Matsumoto M (1988) J Clin Invest 82: 1983-1991
9. Karasawa K, Satoh N, Masuda M, Setaka M, Hashimoto K, Ishibashi K, Nojima S (1991) J Biochem 110: 683-687
10. Kroegel C, Yukawa t, Dent G, Chanez P, Chung KF, Barnes PJ (1988) Immunology 64: 559-562

Significance of Platelet-Activating Factor (PAF) and PAF – Acethylhydrolase in the Pathogenesis of Chronic Subdural Hematoma

Mamoru Abe[1], Masaharu Matsuzaki[2], Takashi Inoue[1], Hirotoshi Sano[3], and Tetsuo Kanno[3]

[1]Department of Neurosurgery, Yachiyo Hospital, Anjyo, Aichi, 446 Japan, [2]SRL Research Institute, Hachioji, Tokyo, 192 Japan, and [3]Department of Neurosurgery, Fujita Health University, School of Medicine, Toyoake, Aichi, 470-11 Japan

SUMMARY

The pathogenetic mechanism of chronic subdural hematoma(CSH) has not been satisfactorily clarified until now. To make clear the mechanisms, we carried out an investigation into the levels of platelet-activating factor(PAF) and PAF-acethylhydrolase activity(PAFAH) in the plasma and hematoma of the patients with CSH(N=49, 31 males, 17 females) by the method of radioimmunoassay. Both the PAF(p<0.01) and PAFAH(p<0.05) value of the hematoma more significantly increased in comparison to the one in the plasma. Compared to the plasma PAFAH values for the people aged 30 and over, the level of PAFAH in the group of people aged between 30 and 70 was significantly lower(p<0.05) than the one in the group of people aged 70 and over of both sexes. Additionally, even compared with the plasma PAFAH values in the age matched groups of normal subjects and cerebral infraction, the one in the group of CSH was significantly lower(p<0.01), and the plasma PAF value was not significantly different. These results suggest that the plasma PAF value in CSH is high. We speculated that the high value of PAF in the hematoma plays an important role in the pathological findings of CSH, having chronic inflammation, eosinophilic infiltration and hyperfibrinolysis. And further, the cause of the pathogenesis of CSH may result in the conditions, that the PAF level of plasma is high and on the other hand, that the PAFAH levels of one is low, or the reaction of that over the one of PAF is low.

KEY WORDS: platelet-activating factor, acethylhydrolase, pathogenesis, chronic subdural hematoma

INTRODUCTION

Chronic subdural hematoma (CSH) is a popular disease in the neurosurgical field. But the pathogenetic mechanisms of CSH have not been satisfactorily clarified until now. For instance, it is said that there are particular conditions in CSH such as eosinophilic infiltration into the capsule, hyperfibrinolysis in the hematoma, which are curable by a barr hole operation, or even by natural course. Platelet-activating factor (PAF) has been known as a potent chemical mediator, which lots of cells (endothelial cells, neutrophils, eosinophils, monocytes, macropharges, fibroblasts, platelets, etc) synthesize and release into conditions such as inflammation, and vascular function etc(1-6). PAF-acethylhydrolase (PAFAH)(7) is a specific inhibitor against PAF. The production of that is said to be lung, liver, brain and kidney(7). The balance of both the PAF and PAFAH in various conditions is thought to have an important role. We measured the presence of PAF and PAFAH in the hematoma with the plasma in the patients with CSH to further clarify it's pathogenesis.

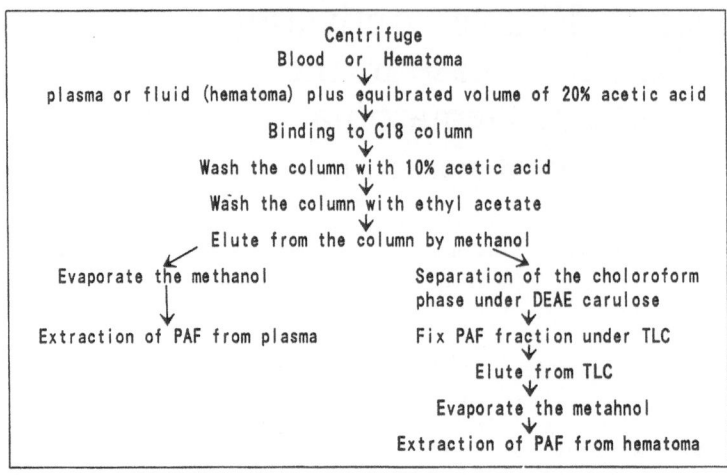

Fig.1 Procedure for extraction of PAF from blood
and hematoma.

MATERIALS AND METHODS

Forty nine patients with CSH, aged 31-91 years (31 males, 17 females),
who were diagnosed using CT image, were included in this study. The
blood samples were obtained just before the operation and the hematoma
samples were obtained during the operation. The procedure for
extraction of PAF from the blood and the hematoma was shown in Fig.1.
The PAF activity was measured by the method of radioimmunoassey (RIA)
using the PAF-RIA kit (NEN Co). The minor PAF volume measured by this
method using the PAF-RIA kit is 20 pg/0.1ml. And so, the PAF value of
less than 20 pg/0.1ml in the plasma and the hematoma was calculated as
20 pg/0.1ml. The arranged procedure of the measurement of PAFAH
activity by Stafforini et al was used. In 10 cases out of 49 cases we
measured the PAF and the PAFAH values in both the plasma and the
hematoma. And also, the data of the PAF and the PAFAH value in the
plasma in all 49 cases was studied with regards the difference across
age and gender. Further, the PAF and the PAFAH values in the plasma
of the CSH group were compared with the ones in nomral subjects and
cerebral infarction of the group. They statistically matched with
regards age.

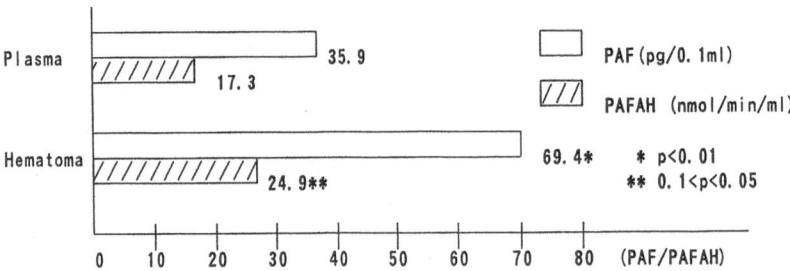

Fig.2 PAF and PAFAH values (mean) in both the plasma
and the hematoma in 10 cases.

RESULTS

The PAF and the PAFAH value in the hematoma of 10 cases were both significantly higher than the one in the plasma (Fig.2) The PAF and the PAFAH values in the plasma samples of all 49 cases were shown in Table 1. In analyzing the PAF and the PAFAH values for patients aged 30 and over, the ones in patients aged 30-50 and the ones in patients aged 60-70 were statistically lower than the ones in other age groups (Table 1). Additionally, comparing the PAFAH value in patients aged 30-50 (mean age 42.5) with CSH, to the one in the age matched group of normal subjects (mean age 40.29), the one in the group of CSH was statistically lower (Table 2). That tendency was the same even in the comparison between the PAFAH value in patients aged 30-70 with CSH (mean age 60.52) and the one in the age matched group of cerebral infarction (mean age 56.68) (Table 2). And also, the PAF values in the plasma of the CSH group would be higher as suggested in Table 2. Further, the PAFAH value in the patients aged 30-70 was significantly lower than the one in the patients aged 70 and over, in both sexes (Table 3).

Table 1. PAF and PAFAH values (mean) in the plasma samples of all 49 cases and the ones for patients aged 30 and over.

Age (n) Name	40 — 50 (n=6)	— 60 — (n=6)	70 (n=10)	— 80 — (n=18)	90 (n=9)	Total (n=49)
PAF	48. 0	59. 0	32. 9	47. 1	42. 6	43. 8
PAFAH	*17. 3	25. 3	**9. 4	31. 1	25. 9	23. 3

PAF (pg/0. 1ml) PAFAH (nmol/min/ml)   * p<0. 05
                                       ** p<0. 01

Table 2. PAF and PAFAH values (mean) in the plasma between the group of normal subjects (age 40.29) vs CSH (30-50y, age 42.5) and the one of CT (age 56.68) vs CSH (30-70y, aged 60.52).

Group Name	PAF	PAFAH
Normal subjects (Age 40. 29, n=7)	20. 5	33. 4
CSH (30-50y) (Age 42. 5, n=6)	*48. 0	**17. 4
CI (Age 50. 68, n=27)	37. 2	30. 2
CSH (30-70y) (Age 60. 52, n=22)	44. 6	***16. 5

PAF (pg/0. 1mol) PAFAH (nmol/min/ml)
*, **, *** p<0. 01
CI: cerebral infarction

Table 3. PAF and PAFAH values (mean) in the plasma for patients aged 30-70 and ones aged 70 and over, in both sexes.

Age Sex	30 - 70 (n=22)		70 - 90 - (n=27)	
Name	Males	Females	Males	Females
PAF	49. 3	37. 9	52. 7	28. 7
PAFAH	*17. 3	**13. 8	28. 0	31. 4

PAF (pg/0. 1ml)   *** p<0. 05
PAFAH (nmol/min/ml)

DISCUSSION

PAF has a lot of biological activities including an increased vascular permeability and destructiveness(8), a potent inducing factor of eosinophils, a release of a tissue-type plasminogen activator(6) from vessel walls and increased fibroblasts via tissue necrotic factor and interleukin-I(4). And also, the metabolism of PAF(PAF cycle) is related to the one of arachidonic acids. Increased PAF and PAFAH activities in the hematoma would chronically show the active PAF cycle. This may play a centrol role to induce particular findings, such as hyperfibrinolysis, eosinophilic infiltration, increased vascular permeability and bleeding, and increased membrane, in CSH. PAFAH said to be a specific inhibitor against PAF is also most important to control in the mechanism related to the PAF. Our results of increased PAF and decreased PAFAH activities in the plasma may be ascribed to the chronically active PAF cycle in CSH. The PAF activity in older males is reported to be higher than the one in older females(9). However, the PAFAH activity is not significantly different across age and sex(10). These differences in sex might contribute to the fact that the incident rate of CSH is greater in older males than in older females.

REFERENCE

1) Bussolino, F., Camussi, G., and Baglioni, C. (1988) J. Biol. Chem. 263: 11856-11861
2) Lellouch-Tubiana, A., Lefort, J., Pfister, A., Vargaftig, B.B. (1987) Int. Archs. Allergy Appl. Immun. 83: 198-205
3) Valone, F.H., Philip, R., Debs, R.J. (1988) Immunol. 64:715-718
4) Michel, L., Denizot, Y., Themar, Y., Jean-Louis, F., Pitton, C., Benveniste, J., Dubertret, L. (1988) J. Immunol. 141: 948-953
5) Mencia-huerta, J.M., Hosfound, D., Braguet, P. (1989) Clin Exp. Allergy. 19: 125-142
6) Eneis, J.J., Kluft, C. (1985) Blood 66: 86-91
7) Blank, M.L., Lee, T., Fitzgerald, V., Synder, F. (1981) J. Biol. Chem. 256: 175-178
8) Humphrey, D.M., Hanahan, D.J., Pinckard, R.N. (1982) Lab. Invest 47:227-234
9) Taylor, R., Sturm, M., Kendrew, P.J., Vandongen, R., Beilin, L.J. (1989) Clin Science 76: 195-198
10) Matsuzaki, M. (1989) SRL HOKAN 13: 51-56

Coagulation and Fibrinolysis in Chronic Subdural Hematomas

KOICHI YAMASHITA, TATSUO HAYASHI, and HIROAKI SEKINO

Division of Neurosurgery, Second Department of Surgery, St. Marianna University School of Medicine, Kawasaki, Kanagawa, 213 Japan

SUMMARY

We studied changes in the activity of coagulation and fibrinolysis in two groups of patients with chronic subdural hematoma and minor head injury in order to know the etiology of CSH. In 61 cases with CSH, coagulation and fibrinolysis in hematoma contents and in venous blood were studied. These activities were evaluated by 7 parameters, fibrinopeptide A (FPA), fibrinopeptide Bβ 15-42(FPB) in systemic blood and α2 plasmin inhibitor (A2PI), plasmin-α2 plasmin inhibitor complex (PLN-A2PIC), fibrinogen, D-dimer, antithrombin-III (AT-III) in hematoma contents. In the 27 patients with minor head injury, older than 65 years old, we measured FPA and FPB in venous blood taken within 1 week and at 3 weeks after injury, and thereafter them. From our observations, it was learned that the majority of patients with minor head injury with or without subdural fluid collection showed hyperfibrinolytic activity. Moreover, in one case, it was observed that subdural fluid collection developed into chronic subdural hematoma concurrent with gradual increase in fibrinolytic activity. Therefore, we reached a tentative conclusion. Systemic hyperfibrinolytic activity in old age people may play an important role as one of causes of chronic subdural hematoma following minor head injury.

KEY WORDS: chronic subdural hematoma, coagulation, fibrinolysis, fibrinopeptide

INTRODUCTION

The pathogenesis of chronic subdural hematoma has not been clarified yet. As an etiology of chronic subdural hematoma, a few reports showed excessive local activation of fibrinolysis played an important role [1, 2] and it was already well known that hyperfibrinolysis in the hematoma was caused by tissue type plasminogen activator released from outer membrane [3]. Furthermore, it has been recently intimated that FPB as the indicator of fibrinolytic activity is elevated in the systemic blood and remained above normal in postoperative systemic blood [4]. However it has been still unknown why fibrinolytic activity is elevated in systemic blood and remained above normal postoperatively. Systemic fibrinolysis might be affected with hyperfibrinolytic activity in the hematoma. Then we studied changes in the activities of coagulation fibrinolysis in two groups of patients with chronic subdural hematoma and minor head injury.

MATERIALS AND METHODS

Group of chronic subdural hematoma

Sixty-five patients with chronic subdural hematoma (CSH) were studied. There were 13 females and 48 males, with a mean age of 70 years. In this group, we made a burr hole and aspirated the contents of the hematoma through the dura with a sharp needle. During removal of the hematoma, care was taken to avoid contamination by peripheral blood. The contents of the hematoma were sampled for the following tests of coagulation and fibrinolysis: fibrinogen, D-dimer, antithrombin-III (AT-III), plasmin-α2 plasmin inhibitor complex (PLN-A2PIC) and α2 plasmin inhibitor (A2PI). And a blood sample was drawn from a vein at the time of surgery. Fibrinopeptide A (FPA) levels as an indicator of thrombin activity and fibrinopeptide Bβ15-42 (FPB) levels as an indicator of plasmin activity were measured in systemic blood.

Group of minor head injury
Twenty-seven patients with minor head injury whose age was more than 65 years. We measured FPA and FPB in venous blood taken within 1 week (early stage) after minor head injury. All of the patients had no abnormalities in the physical examination and laboratory data (serum glutamic oxaloacetic transaminase, glutamic pyruvic transaminase, lactate dehydrogenase, serum bilirubin, alkaline phosphatase, blood urea nitrogen, serum creatinine, red blood cell count, hematocrit, and hemoglobin concentration). At the time of admission, all of the patients were studied on CT scanner. And they were followed for more than 3 weeks (late stage) with CT scans and sampling of venous blood for measurement of FPA and FPB. Therefore, 11 out of 27 cases with minor head injury showed subdural fluid collection.

RESULTS

Group of chronic subdural hematoma
The results in the hematoma contents were as follows: No fibrinogen was detected in any samples of hematoma contents. Reversely D-dimer had a extremely high concentration, at a level of 177 $\pm$ 138 µg/ml (mean $\pm$ SD). PLN-A2PIC was highly elevated comparing with normal value of serum (p<0.01) in all 53 patients and the mean value was 6.9 $\pm$ 5.0 ug/ml. A2PI was less than normal in all 31 patients and the mean value was 4.7 $\pm$ 5.3 mg/dl. AT-III was less than normal in all 51 patients and the mean value was 19.4 $\pm$ 5.5 mg/dl. In venous blood, FPA and FPB were measured in 59 patients immediately before surgery. Both of values for FPA and FPB was markedly higher than normal value of serum (p<0.01). And the mean value of FPA was 18.2 $\pm$ 18.6 ng/ml and the mean value of FPB was 7.7 $\pm$ 4.4 ng/ml. In 3 cases followed up more than 3 months postoperatively, FPA fell to normal range immediately, whereas FPB still remained above normal, which may reflect persistence of accelerated systemic fibrinolytic activity.

Group of minor head injury
After minor head injury 11 out of 27 cases showed subdural fluid collection on CT scan. Majority of cases had also high levels of FPA and FPB. The mean value of FPA was 13.5 $\pm$ 19.0 ng/ml in the early stage and 5.6 $\pm$ 6.8 ng/ml in the late stage. The mean value of FPB was 7.0 $\pm$ 2.5 ng/ml in the early stage and 10.6 $\pm$ 12.9 ng/ml in the late stage. There were no difference between the two stages significantly. On the other hand, 16 out of 27 cases with minor head injury showed no abnormal findings on CT scan but elevated FPA and FPB were found in most of these cases. The mean value of FPA was 7.4 $\pm$ 8.1 ng/ml in the early stage and 3.6 $\pm$ 2.5 ng/ml in the late stage. The mean value of FPB was 7.4 $\pm$ 4.0 ng/ml in the early stage and 7.1 $\pm$ 3.3 ng/ml in the late stage. There is an example of followed up case after minor head injury. The patient was a 78-year-old female. At the time of minor head injury, FPA raised remarkably and fell immediately, whereas FPB was within the normal limits. Three weeks later, subdural fluid collection was observed on CT scan, and demonstrated gradual increase in volume and in density on CT scan, accordingly FPB increased. Then chronic subdural hematoma was found on CT scan 52 days after injury. FPB remained high even after operation.

DISCUSSION

It is already well known that hyperfibrinolysis in the hematoma is caused by tissue type plasminogen activator released from outer membrane [3], and that plasminogen and fibrinogen are extremely low in hematoma contents which also contain elevated FDP's. In this study, no fibrinogen was detected and D-dimer showed extremely high in any samples of hematoma. Therefore, PLN-A2PIC as an indicator of plasmin had trend toward increase. In contrast, A2PI and AT-III were present in low concentration. From these results, increased fibrinolytic activity was present in the hematomas. Our results in hematoma contents showed similar findings to other previous reports [5,6,7]. On the other hand, both FPA and FPB in venous blood were elevated at the time of surgery. Particularly, increased fibrinolytic activities were found not only in the hematoma contents but in the systemic blood. In several cases with CSH followed up postoperatively, systemic blood FPB remained above normal, which may reflect persistence of accelerated systemic fibrinolytic activity, whereas, FPA markedly fell to normal range immediately after surgery. But this does not explain why FPB, as the indicator of fibrinolytic activity, is elevated and remained above normal in postoperative systemic blood. However, from our observations, it was learned that the majority of patients with minor head injury with or without subdural fluid collection showed hyperfibrinolytic activity. Moreover, in one case, it was observed that subdural fluid collection developed into chronic subdural hematoma concurrent with gradual increase in fibrinolytic activity. Therefore, we reached a tentative conclusion. Systemic hyperfibrinolytic activity in old age people may play an important role as one of causes of chronic subdural hematoma following minor head injury. To draw any definitive conclusion from our observations, further research needs to be done.

REFERENCES

1. Ito H, Yamamoto S, Komai T, Mizukoshi H (1976) J Neurosurg 45: 26-31
2. Komai T, Ito H, Yamashima T, Yamamoto S (1977) Neurol Med Chir (Tokyo) 17: 499-505
3. Ito H, Komai T, Yamamoto S (1978) J Neurosurg 48: 197-200
4. Harada K, Orita T, Abiko S, Aoki H (1989) Neurol Med Chir (Tokyo) 29: 113-116
5. Weir B, Gordon P (1983) J Neurosurg 58: 242-245
6. Kawakami Y, Chikami M, Tamiya T, Shimamura Y (1988) Neurosurgery 25: 25-29
7. Saito K, Ito H, Hasegawa T, Yamamoto S (1989) J Neurosurg 70:68-72

Fibrinolytic Activities of the Chronic Subdural Hematoma and Efficacy of the Antifibrinolytic Agent for the Chronic Subdural Hematoma

KATSUZO FUJITA, HIDEMI NAKAMURA, KAZUMASA EHARA, and NORIHIKO TAMAKI

Department of Neurosurgery, Kobe University School of Medicine, Kobe, Hyogo, 650 Japan

(SUMMARY)

The subdural hematoma contents were collected after operation to measure the fibrinolytic activities in 31 patients with chronic subdural hematoma. Raised level of FDP, t-PA and t-PA-PAI complex was demonstrated in the hematoma. From the finding of the hyperfibrinolysis in the hematoma, the efficacy of the antifibrinolytic agent of tranexamic acid was examined in 46 subdural hematoma cases. By antifibrinolytic therapy, there were no recurrent cases of the chronic subdural hematoma after surgery. Fifteen cases of the subdural hematoma was medically treated by antifibrinolytic agent and 14 cases were cured without surgery.

(KEY WORDS)

chronic subdural hematoma, hyperfibrinolysis, antifibrinolytic agent, medical treatment

(INTRODUCTION)

Since the introduction of computed tomography (CT) and magnetic resonance image (MRI), the number of the chronic subdural hematoma (CSH) cases has been increasing in our clinic. The etiological factors for the origin and development of CSH have, however, remained unclear. The purpose of this paper is to investigate the fibrinolytic activities in the contents of CSH and the efficacy of antifibrinolytic agent for CSH.

(CLINICAL MATERIALS AND METHODS)

From April 1988 to August 1992, 46 patients with CSH were admitted to Kobe University Hospital. Thirty one patients with CSH were treated by small burr hole craniotomy with the evacuation of the hematoma. The hematoma contents were collected to measure the fibrinolytic activities in the hematoma. After operation, these 31 patients were medically treated by antifibrynolytic agent of tranexamic acid (1000 mg/ day) and carbazochrome sodium sulfonate (60 mg/day) to prevent the reaccumulation of the subdural hematoma. In contrast, the other 15 patients with CSH who were not operated on initially because of patient's refusal or old age were also medically treated by antifibrynolytic agent with careful observation. The duration of the medical treatment ranged from 1 to 2 months. Follow up CT was taken every 2 weeks after medical therapy was started.

Fibrinogen was measured by the thrombin test, and FDP (fibrin/fibrinogen degradation products), by the latex agglutination method. The enzyme-linked immunoabsorbent assay (ELISA) kit (American Diagnostica Inc) applying the double antibody sandwich assay principle was used to measure the t-PA (tissue-plasminogen activator) levels and t-PA-PAI(t-PA-plasminogen activator inhibitor) complex was measured by the capture/tag antibody technique using polystilene beads.

(RESULTS)
 Forty six patients with CSH were divided into two groups, surgical group (31 patients) and medical group (15 patients) and CSH was categolized into 2 types, early stage (Group A, 14 patients) and advanced stage (Group B, 32 patients) according to CT findings. Patient s age and sex were summarized in Table 1.
(1) Fibrinolytic activities of the hematoma
 The level of fibrinogen, FDP (fibrin/fibrinogen degradation products), PIC(-plasmin inhibitor plasmin complex), t-PA (tissue plasminogen activator), t-PA-PAI complex (t-PA-plasminogen activator inhibitor) of the hematoma and the plasma was measured in patients operated on. Fibrinogen was not detected in the hematoma , but level of FDP was exceedingly high and scaled out over 160 mg/ml in the both types of hematoma (Fig. 1). PIC was significantly higher only in group(B) (Fig. 2). T-PA and, t-PA-PAI complex were also significantly higher in both type of the hematoma, especially in group (B) (Fig. 3, 4,).
(2) Antifibrinolytic therapy for the chronic subdural hematoma
 Thirty one patients were treated by antifibrinolytic agent of tranexamic acid after evacuation of the hematoma. No cases were reoperated on because of reaccumulation of the hematoma. Other 15 patients were treated medically by antifibrinolytic agent without surgery. CSHs eventually resolved in 14 of 15 patients without surgery, and no recurrence was observed during the follow up period ranging from 4 months to 3 years. One patient in advanced stage of CSH was operated on because of no symptomatc improvement by medical therapy (Table 2).   No adverse effects by antifibrolytic therapy were observed in 46 cases.

(DISCUSSION)
 Chronic subdural hematoma may occur after minor head injury in individuals of old age associated with brain atrophy. Although various causes have been reported, exact etiology is still unknown. Inflammation of the dural membrane(10), osmotic pressure (4), trauma(9) or intermittent hemorrhage caused by local hyperfibrinolysis (5) has been advocated as its etiology. Virchow(10) reported "pachy meningitis hemorrhagica interna" in 1857. In order to explain the mechanism of the CSH, the osmotic gradient theory was proposed by Gardner(4). Weir(11), however, was unable to find significant differences in the osmotic pressure between hematoma fluid, venous blood. These findings don't support the osmotic gradient theory as the etiological factors of CSH. Later the recurrent hemorrhage from the hematoma capsule due to local hyperfibrinolysis was proposed by Ito (5). The vessels of the hematoma capsule were reported to have marked proliferative potential and fragile nature. These findings suggested high permeability and fragility of these capillaries, allowing them to bleed easily. Ito has shown high plasminogen activator levels in the vascular membrane and that plasminogen and avairable plasmin are extremely low in hematoma which also

contains elevated FDP. This suggested enhanced fibrinolytic activity, which might then be associated with further bleeding. The results of our study show findings similar to those of Ito. However, we also measured t-PA-PAI complex which may be a new molecular marker that reflects t-PA release from outer membrane. The facts that t-PA and t-PA-PAI complex were significantly higher in hematoma mean that t-PA is a main factor of hyperfibrinolysis in the chronic subdural hematoma.

Although surgical removal constitutes the essential therapeutic approach for the chronic subdural hematoma(2, 3, 6,) postoperative reaccumulation of the hematoma has been reported with the rate of 2.6 % to 20 % (2, 6, 8). In our cases, however, there were no postoperative recurrent cases after antifibrinolytic therapy was given.

Non-surgical treatment of the chronic subdural hematoma was reported by some authors(1, 7), such as steroid or mannitol therapy, but these treatments have not been widely accepted as a treatment of choice. While we employed the antifibrinolytic agent of tranexamic acid for CSH of the early stage, the observed effect of tranexamic acid appeared to be effective to prevent the progression of the hematoma or the reaccumulation of hematoma after surgery.

(References)

(1) Bender MB, Christoff N : Nonsurgical treatment of subdural hematomas. Arch Neurol 31 : 73-79, 1974
(2) Cameron MM : Chronic subdural hematoma :A review of 114 cases. J Neurol Neurosurg Psychiatry 41 : 834-839 ,1978
(3) D'Avella D, Blasi FD, Rotilio A, Pensabene V, Pandolfo N, : Intracerebral hematoma following evacuation of chronic subdural hematomas. J Neurosurg 65 : 710-712, 1986
(4) Gardner WJ : traumatic subdural hematoma with particular reference to the latent interval. Arch Neurol Psychiatry 27:841-858, 1932
(5) Ito H, Yamamoto S, Komai T, Mizukoshi H : Role of local hyper fibrinosis in the etioology of chronic subdural hematoma J Neurosurg 45 : 26-31, 1976
(6) Markwalder TM : Chronic subdural hematomas ; A review, J Neurosurg 54 : 637-645, 1981
(7) Suzuki J, Takaku A : Nonsurgical treatment of chronic subdural hematoma. J Neurosurg 33: %$ (-553, 1970
(8) Svien HJ, Gelety JE : On the surgical management of encapsu lated subdural hematoma : A comparison of the results of membra nectomy and simple evacuation. J Neurosurg 21: 172-177, 1963
(9) Trotter W : Chronicsubdural hemorrhage of traumatic origin and its relation to pachymeningitis hemorrhagica interna. Br J Surg 2 :271-291, 1914
(10) Virchow R : Das Hamatom der Dura Mater. Verhandlungen der Psysikalisch-Medizinischen Gesellschaft zu Wurzburg 7 : 134-142, 1857
(11) Weir B: Oncotic pressure of subdural fluids. J Neurosurg. 53:512-515, 1980

Table 1

Table 2

Clinical Summary of Chronic Subdural Hematoma

1. Surgical group 31 cases.
  Age 46y ～ 84y
  Sex M. 24
   F. 7
2. Medical group 15 cases.
  Age 65y ～ 80y
  Sex M. 12
   F. 3

Clinical Summary of Chronic Subdural Hematoma
Treated by Antifibrinolytic Agent

cases	sex	age	symtoms & signs	CT Type	Ope	results
1	M	66y	headache	A	(-)	cured
2	M	75y	headache	A	(-)	cured
3	M	74y	headache	A	(-)	cured
4	M	78y	asymptomatic	A	(-)	cured
5	M	65y	asymptomatic	A	(-)	cured
6	M	71y	asymptomatic	A	(-)	cured
7	M	74y	asymptomatic	A	(-)	cured
8	M	68y	headache	A	(-)	cured
9	F	67y	headache	A	(-)	cured
10	M	80y	headache	A	(-)	cured
11	M	78y	headache & hemiparesis	B	(-) (+)	cured cured
12	M	80y	headache	A	(-)	cured
13	F	75y	headache	A	(-)	cured
14	F	74y	headache	A	(-)	cured
15	M	78y	asymptomatic	A	(-)	cured

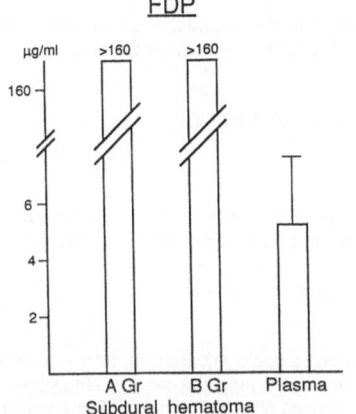

(Fig. 1) Level of FDP in the hematoma and the plasma. FDP was significantly higher in both stage of CSH.

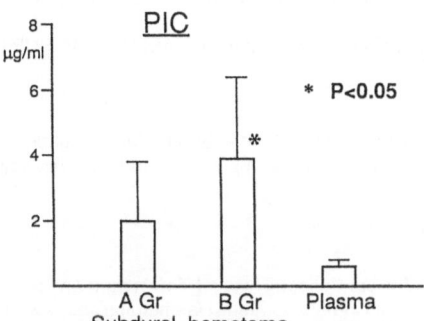

(Fig. 2) Level of PIC in the hematoma and the plasma. PIC was significantly higher in the hematoma of the advanced stage

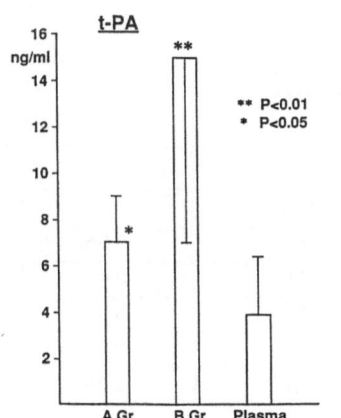

(Fig. 3) Level of t-PA in the hematoma and the plasma. T-PA was significantly high in CSH at both stages, but higher at the advanced stage of CSH.

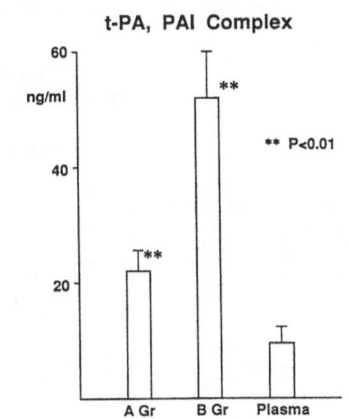

(Fig. 4) Level of t-PA-PAI complex T-PA-PAI complex was also significantly high in CSH at both stage.

Chromic Subdural Haematoma Experience with 2245 Cases

M. SAMBASIVAN

Former Director & Prof. of Neuro Surgery, Medical College, Trivandrum, Consultant Neuro Surgeon, Cosmopolitan Hospital, Trivandrum, India

Summary

Since 1966 over a period of 26 years 2245 cases of Chronic subdural haematoma were seen and treated. Male preponderance amongst the cases was seen as 5:1. The condition presented with Variegated manifestations compared pre C.T. Scan period when 900 cases were seen for 1980 after that 1345 cases were encountered. Since 1968 the cases were managed by temporal craniectomy with dura left open and subdural space communicating with subtemporalis area. This procedure has resulted in marked reduction of recurrences and membranectomy was not required. There has been an overall mortality of 0.8% only.

KEY WORDS: CHRONIC SUBDURAL HAEMATOMA SUBTEMPORALIS DRAINAGE

Introduction

As early as 1656 J.J. Wepfor reported about Chronic Subdural haematoma. Since then many reports have appeared in the literature and this condition is considered as a malady, very well treatable Neurosurgically giving gratifying results.

Case Material

Since 1966 at Medical College Hospital Trivandrum and at Cosmopolitan Hospital Trivandrum, over a period of 26 years 2245 cases of Chronic Subdural Haematoma cases were encountered. Amongst the cases of Neurotrauma this group constitutes 9%. Chronic Subdural haematomas got referred to us from all over the Kerala State which has a population of 29 million. Trivandrum, Capital city of Kerala has a population of 1.0 million. Eventhough neighbouring institutions did have neurosurgical treatment, they took up only referred cases. All trauma, and emergencies came to Medical College Hospital. This has contributed to the large number of subdural haematoma being tackled at Medical College hsopital. Table I shows the age sex incidence of the cases.

TABLE I
CHRONIC SUBDURAL HAEMATOMA

Age Sex Incidence

Age group	Male	Female	Total	%
0 - 10	38	17	55	2.5 %
11 - 20	30	19	49	2.0%
21 - 30	96	21	117	5.0%
31 - 40	382	81	463	20.0%
41 - 50	484	86	570	25.0%
51 - 60	342	63	405	18.0%
61 - 70	362	49	411	18.4%
71 -	123	52	175	8.0%
All ages	1857	388	2245	100 %

It is seen that a higher percentage of cases occured from the third decade. The male preponderance in this series. M:F - 5:1. This may be due to (1) The exposure of male population to injuries more than females, (2) Less of females seeking medical advice (3) There may be an estrogen and their derivatives potentiating capillary integrity.

This last factor needs to be evaluated in the prospective studies. As it is no such study is available. This also opens up the question of using estrogen derivatives for management or prevention of recurrence of subdurals, with the hope that it may potentiate the capillaries integrity.

Clinical presentation of cases are summarised in Table II

TABLE II
CHRONIC SUBDURAL HAEMATOMA
CLINICAL PRESENTATION

1. Fully conscious with signs of Raised I.C.T.	337	(15%)
2. Behavioural disturbance	404	(18%)
3. Seizures	269	(12%)
4. Visual disturbances	269	(12%)
5. Stroke	629	(28%)
6. Coma	337	(15%)
	2245	(100%)

Clinical story of Chronic Alcoholism was available in 14% of the cases. Anticoagulant therapy, Blood dyscrasias or coagulation defect was noted in 6% of cases.

Definite history of head injury could be obtained only in 76% of the cases. In the remaining 24% of cases they could not remember any episode of Trauma at all.

337 cases had refractory headache with periods of remissions and exacerbations. The increase in the head ache was noticed on assuming upright posture from lying position. With increase in the severity of headache, vomiting followed. So these cases were afraid to assume upright posture. They had also all the classical signs of raised intracranial tension, headache, vomiting and Papilloedema. These cases did not have any neurological deficit.

404 cases had behavioural disturbances. This consisted of garrullousness, emotional outbursts, unkempt appearances, lack of concentration, sleep disturbances maniacal and depressive states. These cases did go for psychiatric consultations and then got referred to us. In fact some of the cases were brought by relatives with the story of head injury of a minor nature 2 weeks or 2 months prior to these behavioural disturbances. Investigations proved the existence of subdural haematoma.

269 cases presented with late onset seizures. In some these were focal in nature and in others of a generalised nature. With the previous history of head injury, and Post Traumatic epilepsy as a favourite diagnosis they were investigated and were found to harbour chronic subdurals.

The next group of cases had only visual problems as blurring of vision, or double vision. They had taken ophthalmology consultation and then got referred for further investigations. Isolated sixth nerve deficit or 3rd nerve deficit or severe papilloedema resulting in visual blurring were seen.

Completed stroke like picture was seen in 629 cases. This constituted the largest single group. With previous history of Trauma, and history of stuttering weakness of one side or other even without any signs of raised intracranial tension one should suspect Chronic Subdural haematoma as a strong possibility.

Some of these case did take treatment elsewhere for transient ischaemic attacks with Dipyridamole or Aspirin. This aggravated the bleeding tendency and they came with a completed stroke like picture. Angiograms were done in these cases earlier on for diagnosis. With C.T. scan the diagnosis has been much easier and more definite.

337 cases come in Coma to the emergency department. In older age group presence of catracts bilaterally prevented the fundoscopy. Yet if there was a history of Trauma the diagnosis of C.S.D.H. was suspected. C.T. clinched the diagnosis.MRI was done as the primary diagnostic. Procedure elsewhere and the case got referred here.

TABLE III
CHRONIC SUBDURAL HAEMATOMA

UNILATERAL	-	1672	(74.4%)
BILATERAL	-	564	(25%)
INTERHEMISPHERIC	-	9	(0.5%)

It is noteworthy that 25% of the cases had bilateral subdural haematomas.

From 1966 to 1980 over a period of 14 years 900 cases were seen and treated. From 1981 to 1992, 1344 cases was seen and treated. C.T. facility available from 1981 did play a dominant role in early diagnosis and picking up more cases.

Management

From 1966 to 1968 the subdural haematomas were drained by multiple burr holes. This consisted of 51 cases. In six cases semisolid collections were released after raising a bone flap craniotomy. These cases also had membranectomy. Multiple burr hole drainage group, 11 cases had recurrences. Of these five cases needed multiple reaspiration and six cases needed Membranectomy. Overall mortality in this group was two - that is 3% and both had infective complications.

From 1968 to 1992, 2188 cases were treated by the following procedure. The subdural collection has taken through a cranicetomy 3 to 4cm in diameter subtemporally - extending it towards frontal, Parietal or Occipital region as the C.T. picture warranted. Dural opening was made in a cruciate manner and the dural edges were hitched up, the outer membrane was opened and excised at the exposed area. All the collected material evacuated including altered blood clots. Washed out the subdural space with Normal saline till the effluent was clear. The inner membrane also was opened and removed at the exposed area. Sub dural drain was put and connected to water seal drainage bottle or Romovac. Dural edges were coagulated and left open. Temporalis approximated over, so that provided a surface for absorption and wound was closed in layers.

Post operatively patients were hydrated with 5% Dextrose Saline 2000 ccs. to induce Cerebral oedema. So that it helped in obliteration of subdural space.

Drain was kept on for 24 Hr. and then removed. Patient was mobilised as early as possible with physiotherapy. In 80% of the cases the deficits started recovering within 48 Hrs. and were up and about in 4 days. Scalp sutures were removed on the 6th day and patient could go home on 7th or 8th post OP day. Post OP C.T. Scan showed good obliteration of subdural space. Complications like intercurrent infections, cardiac or pulmonary problems, contributed to mortality.

Results

Table IV shows the results. Among the 51 cases when drainage was effected by multiple burrholes, there was 20% recurrence. They had to come for further surgery - reaspiration in five cases and membranectomy in 6 cases. Six cases had craniotomy with bone flap being raised. These cases had no membranectomy at the primary sitting. All inter hemispheric haematomas were drained through burr holes, and all did well. 2179 cases had subtemporarlis marsupialisation procedure. Of these only 0.27% had a recurrence.

TABLE IV
Chronic Subdural Haematomas
Results

A. DRAINAGE THROUGH MULTIPLE BURRHOLES	-	51
B. CRANIOTOMY - Solid Subdurals	-	6
RECURRENCE	-	11 (20%)
MEMBRANECTOMY	-	6
REASPIRATIONS	-	5
MORTALITY	-	2 (3%)
C. Burrhole evacuation Inter Hemispheric Haematoma	-	9
D. Craniectomy Subtemporalis marsupialisation	-	2179
Recurrence	-	6 (0.27%)
Died	-	16 (0.7%)

Total Cases   - 2245 Mortality 0.8%

Follow up

All the survivors recovered very well and could support themselves. With an average follow up for 18 months, this was confirmed positively in 84%, 16% was lost for follow up.

Discussion

As early as 17th century with the reappraisal of Johann Jacob Wepfer on SDH this entity has become well known. Gian fortunat Hoesly reported this material in 1966. Putnam J & Cushing H. discussed the pathology of SDH and its relation to pachymeningitis haemorrhagica and it's surgical treatment as early as 1925. Complication of anti coagulant therapy including Neurological complication was noted by Silverstein. A. Among S.D.H. 12 to 38% were found to be due to ant coagulation. In the present series it has been 8% Tetsunori Yamashima and Shinjiro Yamamoto have found proliferating macrocapillaries in the capsule of SDH. They also noted mitotic activity of endothelial cells and vascular sprouts in the capsule besides increased permeability. This accounted for recurrent bleeds and enlargement of SDH.

Recurrence of SDH posed a serious problem Munro reported 14 recurrence among 314 cases (4.5%) Mc Laurin and Tutor found 9 recurrences among 34 cases (26.5%). In the present series with multiple burr holes and evacuation of SDH there has been a recurrence rate of 20%. But after employing the subtemporalis marsupilization procedure it had dropped to 0.27%

Bryce Weir and Philip Gorodon noted factors affecting Coagulation and fibrinolysis in Chronic S.D.H. Boyle 150 yrs ago suggested that Chronic rebleeding caused growth of SDH. SDH fluid does not clot on standing, and it also inhibits normal clotting process. Defective local haemostasis and chronic rebleeding contributes to growth of SDH. SDH fluid has a high concentration of Fibrin degradation products and high plasminogen activator levels in vascular outer membrane. These also contribute to further bleeding into SDH (ITO.H.) Sedimentation and level visible in C.T. scans was described by Ming Chein Kao and is an accepted feature of many S.D.H. He noted this in 5% of C.T. Scans of SDH. In this series it was seen in 19% of cases.

Present series of cases managed by Subtemporal marsupialisation appears to be an effective treatment and recurrence are very low, (0.27%). This procedure may be practiced by many, yet unknown to me. All the same this procedure of managing chronic SDH is found to be safe and effective, giving good results.

References

(1) Bryce Weir and Philip Gorodon Factors affecting Coagulation, Fibrinolysis in Chronic Subdural fluid collection. J. Neurosurgery 58 - 242 - 245 . 1983

(2) Gian Fortunat Hoessly. Chronic Subdural Haematoma. J. Neurosurgery - 24. 493 - 496. 1966

(3) ITO.H, Yamamoto.S. and Komai. T. Role of hyper fibrinolysis in the etiology of chronic subdural Haematoma. J. Neurosergery 45 26-31-1976

(4) ITO.H, Komai.T., Yamamoto.S. Fibrinolytic enzyme in the lining walls of chronic subdural Haematoma. J. Neurosurgery 48: 197-200 1978

(5) Johan Jacob Wepfer as quoted by Gian - Fortunat Hoessly.

(6) Ming Chein Kap. Sedimentation levels in Chronic Subdural haematoma visible on C.T. J. Neurosurgery 58. 246-251 1983

(7) Putnam J, Cushing.H. Chronic Subdural Haematoma, it's pathology its relation to pachymeningitis haemorrhagica and it's surgical treatment - Archives of Surgery 11 - 329 - 393 - 1925

(8) Silver-stein.A. Neurological Complication of Anti coagulation Therapy. A Neurologists' review. Arch Int. med. 139, 217-220 1979.

(9) Tetsumori Yamashima and Shinjiro Yamamoto - How do vessels proliferate in the Capsule of Chronic SDH Neurosurgery - 15.5.672 - 678 . 1984

Evaluation of Cerebral Blood Flow by SPECT in Patients with Chronic Subdural Hematomas

MASAYOSHI MATSUMOTO, SHIN NISHIDA, TOSHIAKI ABE, TAKUO HASHIMOTO, and NORIO NAKAMURA

Department of Neurosurgery, The Jikei University School of Medicine, Minato-ku, Tokyo, 105 Japan

SUMMARY

We compared neurological symptoms with CT findings and SPECT findings in 38 patients with chronic subdural hematomas(CSH).
All patients had reduction in cerebral blood flow(CBF), especially in the deep cerebral areas of the basal ganglia and thalamus ipsilateral to the hematoma. Depressed CBF in deep cerebral areas was thought to be the common pathogenesis of CSH.
Cerebral diaschisis was closely related with severe dementia or disturbance of consciousness. Crossed cerebellar diaschisis was found in cases with marked midline shift on CT scan or severe hemiplegia.
Thus, diaschisis was closely related to the development of symptom in CSH. The SPECT image demonstrated that persistence of postoperative CD indicated a high possibility of recurrence.
We reported the usefulness of SPECT and the significance of diaschisis on CSH.

KEY WORDS: chronic subdural hematomas, SPECT, CT scan, diaschisis

INTRODUCTION

We report our experience using Tc-99m hexamethylpropyleneamine oxime (HM-PAO) in patients with chronic subdural hematomas.
The aims of our research were to study cerebral perfusion changes in this disease with HM-PAO and single photon emission computed tomography(SPECT), and to compare these cerebral perfusion changes with the morphologic changes demonstrated with computed tomographic (CT) scans.

MATERIALS AND METHODS

The study group consisted of 38 patients (33 men, 5 women) who had chronic subdural hematomas documented by CT scan. The patient's mean age was 70.1 years (range 40-87 yr), these patients underwent 38 operations (6 patients underwent bilateral operation).
Neurologic findings were evaluated according to classification scheme the authors developed as a modification of Bender's classification (Table 1)(1). Dementia was evaluated using Hasegawa's dementia scale.
Using a personal computer (PC-9801VX), the hematoma was calculated as an integral sum of the CT images.
A head rotating scintillation camera (GCA901A, GE400AT) was used for SPECT. A dose of approximately 20 mCi HM-PAO was administered intravenously. Data acquisition started 5 minutes after injection of the tracer, rotation time was 30 minutues for 60 projections.

Regions of interest (ROI) were defined by frontal, temporal, and occipital lobe, central brain structure (thalamus and basal ganglia), and cerebellar hemisphere on both sides. Indices of regional isotope uptake were calculated by dividing the count rate of a region by the mean count of cerebellar hemisphere.

Five healthy volunteers underwent identical examinations: these were our control examinations. Their SPECT and CT scans were performed at the same time.

All examinations were performed before and after evacuation of a chronic subdural hematoma. The second study was done 2 or 3 weeks postoperatively, when all the patients had improved clinically.

The correlation between clinical symptoms and cerebral perfusion was examined.

RESULTS

Group Classification

The size of the hematoma was clearly correlated with the degree of impairment.

SPECT findings

Cerebral blood flow (CBF) was consistently decreased most markedly, on the affected side, independent of clinical symptoms. In case with bilateral lesions, CBF in the central brain areas of the thalamus and basal ganglia decreased more on the side with the larger hematoma (Table 3). CBF in the deep cerebral areas was proportional to the severity of the conditon. The SPECT findings did not vary significantly with the location of the hematoma.

Cerebral diaschisis (CD) was observed in thirteen patients. It was in this group of patients that severe dementia or decreased consciousness was observed.

Crossed cerebellar diaschisis (CCD) was seen in nine patients. This coincided with a marked midline shift of CT scan in these patients and was seen in patients with severe hemiplegia. Diaschisis was seen in approximately 53.3% of the patients in G.III and approximately 90.0% of the G.IV patients. These findings demonstrated that in patients with severe condition.

We observed three patients with postoperative persistent CD. The recurrence in two of these patients required reoperation.

Representative Cases

Case 2 (Group II)

A 61-year-old man was admitted with severe dementia and headache. Preoperative CT revealed CSH at left side. The SPECT images demonstrated bilaterally reduced CBF, especially in the thalamus and basal ganglia. The CBF was diffusely reduced contralateral to the hematoma, which is diagnostic for CD. Symptoms disappeared after operation. Postoperative CT scan demonstrated the successful removal of the hematoma, and SPECT images showed a recovery of the CBF (Fig. 1).

Case 12 (Group IV)

A 76-year-old man was admitted with severe right hemiplegia and stupor. Preoprative CT scan revealed CSH at right side and marked midline shift. The SPECT images showed ipsilaterally reduced CBF, mainly in the thalamus and basal ganglia. Reduced CBF in the contralateral cerebellar hemisphere was also noted. The diagnosis of CCD was made based on these observations. Symptoms disappeared after operation. Postoperative CT scan demonstrated the successful removal of the hematomas, and the SPECT images showed a recovery of the CBF (Fig. 2).

DISCUSSION

A hematoma not only increases intracranial pressure but also reduces the CBF beneath it. This contributes to the development of CSH.

According to published reports, in dementia, the ipsilateral cerebral perfusion in reduced in the frontal lobe and the thalamus. In hemiplegic patients, there is a local decrease in cerebral perfusion in the frontal and parietal lobes (2,3).

However, our study showed that cerebral perfusion decrease independently of the location of the hematoma or neurological symptoms. The basic mechanism appears to be ipsilateral decrease in CBF, mainly in deep cerebral areas like the ipsilateral thalamus and basal ganglia.

Cases with severe dementia or severe disturbance of consciousness present with a generalized reduction in CBF. This is due to callosal hypoactivity. This is turn initiates remote effects which reduce CBF in the cerebral hemispheres, including the contralateral side.

Since patients wiht CCD had severe hemiplegia or marked midline shifts on CT scan, we hypothesize that CCD is due to corticopontile and corticocerebellar tract damage as a result of central herniation caused by increased intracranial pressure.

Thus, in CSH, CD is related to disturbance of consciousness in the same way that CCD is related to severity of clinical manifestation, motor disorders (4).

In those cases with recurrence, two of the three patients with postoperative persistent CD required reoperation. We considered that careful follow-up should be done in patients with postoperatively persistent CD.

We reported the significance of diaschisis and importance of SPECT on CSH.

REFERENCES

1. Bender MB, Christoff N (1974) Nonsurgical treatment of subdural hematomas. Arch Neurol 31:73-79
2. Ikeda K, Kano A, Hayase H, Yamashima T, Ito H, Yamamoto S (1984) Relationship between symptoms of chronic subdural hematoma and hematoma volume or regional cerebral blood flow. Neurol Med Chir 24:869-875
3. Ueda M, Takahashi Y, Ohmiya N, Mikami J, Ito K, Sato H, Matsuoka T, Takeda S, Ohkawara S (1985) Single photon emission CT findings in chronic subdural hematoma. Prog Comput Tomogr 7:623-630
4. Feeney DM, Baron JC (1986) Diaschisis. STROKE 17:817-830

Table. | Clinical classfication of chronic subdural hematoma

Group	Findings
I	Neurologically intact, headache
II	Mental syndrome, disturbance of consciousness, few or no focal signs
III	Mild or moderate focal neurologic deficit, with or without disturbance of consciousness
IV	Severe focal neurologic deficit, with disturbance of consciousness
V	Coma

Table. 2 Summary in each group

Group	No. of cases (male/female)	Average age (years)	Mean hematoma volume (㎖)	Percentage of cases with diaschisis (%)
I	5(3/2)	58.8	82.8	20.0
II	7(5/2)	70.7	115.3	42.8
III	15(14/1)	74.1	126.5	53.3
IV	11(9/2)	75.8	159.7	90.0

Table. 3 Pre-and postoperative cerebral blood flow on hematoma side and non-hematoma side in each group　*F:frontal, T:temporal, O:occipital, C:central(thalamus, basal ganglia), ( ):Number of cases.

Group	Hematoma side				Non-hematoma side			
	F	T	O	C	F	T	O	C
G. I Pre-op	0.86±0.06	0.77±0.10	0.76±0.11	0.81±0.10	0.86±0.06	0.86±0.08	0.93±0.08	0.87±0.10
(5) Post-op	0.94±0.08	0.89±0.08	0.90±0.10	0.89±0.10	0.88±0.08	0.87±0.08	0.97±0.12	0.91±0.10
G. II Pre-op	0.74±0.07	0.73±0.10	0.78±0.09	0.71±0.10	0.84±0.11	0.73±0.08	0.85±0.12	0.75±0.06
(7) Post-op	0.87±0.10	0.90±0.08	0.97±0.08	0.90±0.10	0.84±0.11	0.86±0.08	0.86±0.12	0.87±0.12
G. III Pre-op	0.84±0.07	0.68±0.12	0.78±0.07	0.62±0.10	0.86±0.07	0.84±0.06	0.84±0.08	0.85±0.08
(15)Post-op	0.84±0.08	0.83±0.12	0.88±0.10	0.88±0.10	0.82±0.08	0.84±0.09	0.86±0.09	0.88±0.11
G. IV Pre-op	0.71±0.12	0.58±0.12	0.68±0.10	0.56±0.08	0.72±0.12	0.68±0.11	0.69±0.12	0.70±0.08
(11)Post-op	0.84±0.12	0.84±0.08	0.82±0.08	0.86±0.12	0.81±0.08	0.79±0.15	0.81±0.09	0.84±0.11

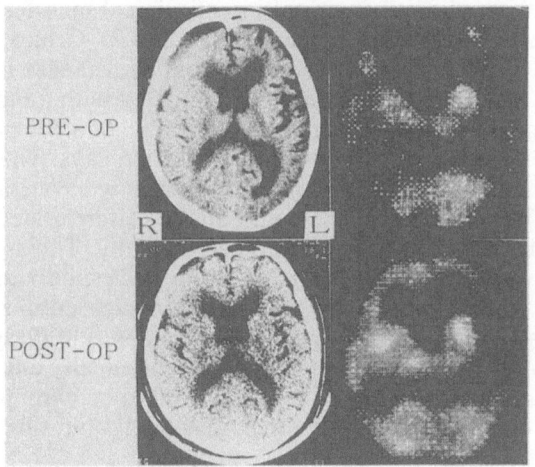

Fig. 1　CT scan and SPECT in case 2

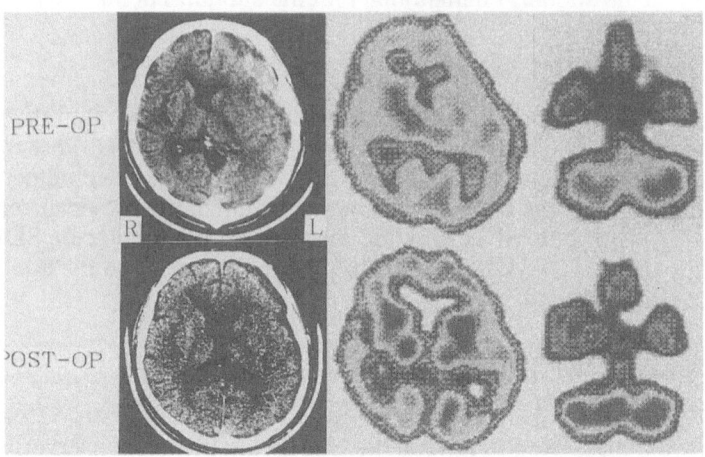

Fig. 2　CT scan and SPECT in case 12

Evolution from Acute Subdural Hematomas to Chronic Subdural Hematomas

Yoshio Taguchi, Yoshitaro Yamaguchi, Tatsuo Hayashi, and Hiroaki Sekino

Division of Neurosurgery, Second Department of Surgery, St. Marianna University School of Medicine, Kawasaki, Kanagawa, 216 Japan

SUMMARY

We analyzed 52 patients of acute subdural hematoma treated conservatively because of mild clinical symptoms and/or thin subdural hematoma to elucidate the evolution from acute subdural hematomas to chronic subdural hematomas. Based on the follow-up CT findings, these patients were classified into two groups: subdural hematomas increased in size gradually with or without deterioration of clinical manifestations(group 1) and subdural hematomas disappeared spontaneously(group 2). Group 1 included 23 patients. In most patients, CT showed the increase in size with a decrease in hematoma density 8 to 14 days after the insult. Fifteen patients were treated with a burr hole craniectomy and the evacuation of liquid hematoma content because of a deterioration of signs and symptoms. Average time elapsed to be operated was 26 days. The neomembrane similar to the outer membrane of chronic subdural hematomas was verified in 11 out of 15 operated patients. These neomembrane could not be differentiated from that of ordinary chronic subdural hematomas pathohistologically. The average age in 29 patients of group 2 was younger than that of group 1. Despite variable changes in hematoma density, subdural hematomas in group 2 decreased in size gradually or rapidly, and eventually disappeared. Average time elapsed to disappear was 25 days. When chronic subdural hematomas are defined as chronically enlarged and encapsulated subdural hematomas, a part of group 1 is considered to be chronic subdural hematomas and the evolution from acute subdural hematomas to chronic subdural hematomas can be present.

KEY WORDS: acute subdural hematoma, chronic subdural hematoma

INTRODUCTION

The cause of chronic subdural hematoma(SDH) is still unknown, but the advent of CT scans has given a clue to clarify the pathogenesis of chronic SDH. Post-traumatic subdural fluid collection has been known to contribute to the development of chronic SDH[1]. Although there has been a few reports documenting the occurrence of chronic SDH originating from acute SDH[1,2], the relationship between acute SDH and chronic SDH is not fully studied. To know this relationship, we analyzed the adult patients with acute SDH treated conservatively.

MATERIALS AND METHODS

During the 7-year period from January, 1985, to December, 1991, 52 out of 188 patients who were diagnosed to have acute SDH were treated conservatively. They were followed up intimately by using a CT scan and the surgical treatment was carried out when the patient had a deterioration of clinical manifestation. This study is partly retrospective and partly prospective. No patients with more extensive lacerations of the brain, with an epidural or intracerebral hematoma, or with an acute subdural hygroma were included in this material. Based on the follow-up CT findings, these patients were classified into two groups. Group 1 included 23 patients whose SDH increased in size gradually with or without deterioration of clinical manifestation. While, in 29 patients of group 2, SDH decreased in size in the follow-up study and eventually disappeared. The age distribution, gender and the type of injury in both groups were shown in Table 1. Both groups included highly elderly patients. Thirty five patients were more than 60 years of age. The average age of group 1 was slightly higher than that of group 2.

Table 1 Classification of patients with acute subdural hematoma treated conservatively

	Group 1	Group 2
Changes of Hematoma Volume	Increase	Decrease
No. of Patients	23	29
Age (Mean)	37-84 (65)	17-89 (60)
Gender (M:F)	13:10	15:14
Type of Injury		
Fall Down	15	6
Fall	5	4
MVA	3	12
Others		7

MVA: motor vehicle accident

ILLUSTRATIVE CASE PRESENTATION

Case 3 of group 1(Fig.1)

This 79-year-old woman fell down accidentally and hit her occipital area on the ground. She had transient loss of consciousness. On admission, she had no neurological deficit, but a CT scan showed a moderate amount of SDH on the right. In the follow-up CT scans, the SDH decreased in density gradually, but increased in size. On the day 22, she underwent a burr hole craniectomy and the evacuation of hematoma because she became to have headache and the left motor weakness. A considerable amount of brownish fluid was evacuated and both outer and inner membranes of the hematoma were identified. The pathohistological specimen showed a granulation tissue containing a rich neovascularity.

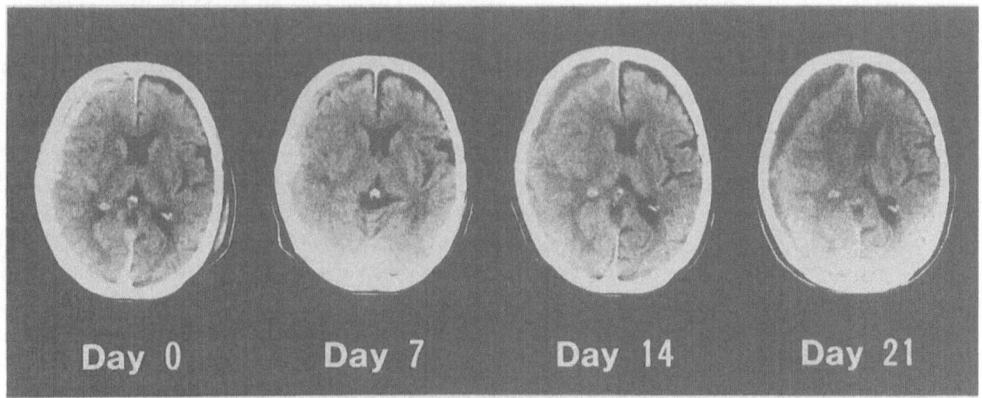

Fig. 1 Serial CT scans of case 3 in group 1 showing a decrease in hematoma density with an increase in size of hematoma.

Case 5 of group 2(Fig.2)

This 82-year-old woman had a minor head injury followed by an impaired consciousness. Glasgow coma scale score on admission was 13. A CT scan showed a thin SDH on the right. She was conservatively treated. Her consciousness level improved gradually and the SDH was shown to be decreased in size. On the day 47, the SDH disappeared completely.

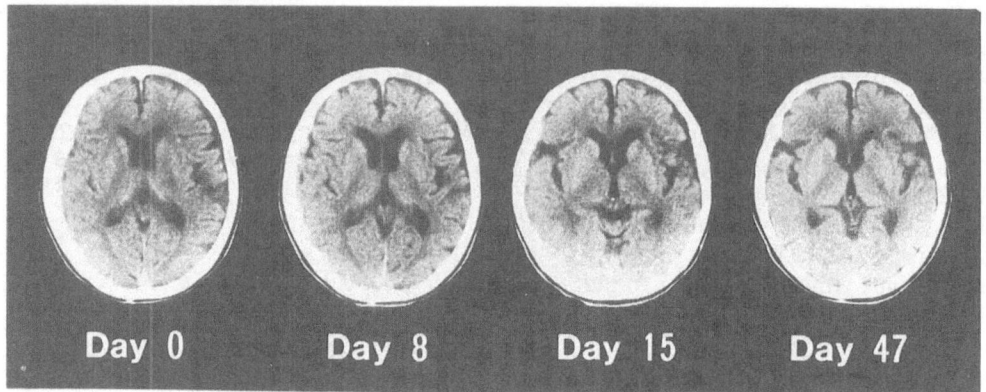

Fig. 2 Serial CT scans of case 5 in group 2 showing a gradual decrease in hematoma volume.

RESULTS

The summary of group 1 was shown in Fig.3, where the chronological changes of density and thickness of hematoma were illustrated. In seventeen out of 23 patients, CT scan revealed an increase in size accompanied with a decrease in hematoma density 8 to 14 days after the head injury. In four patients, both size and density of SDH were shown to be decreased in a subacute stage and increased in a chronic stage. Fifteen patients were treated surgically because of a clinical deterioration. Average time elapsed to be operated was 26 days. The neomembrane similar to the outer membrane of chronic SDH was verified in 11 out of 15 operated patients. In some patients, the inner membrane was confirmed macroscopically. These eleven patients underwent a surgical treatment more than 19 days after the head injury. Pathohistologically these neomembranes could not be differentiated from those of ordinary chronic SDHs. Four patients having no neomembrane were carried out a surgery within 14 days after the insult. In the patients of group 2, most SDHs disappeared gradually, though the time elapsed to disappear and the changes of hematoma density were variable. In four patients, SDH disappeared rapidly within 24 hours probably due to redistribution. No correlation was found between the time elapsed to disappear and the severity of head injury or the associated parenchymatous lesions. Most SDH thickness in initial CT scan were less than 10 mm. Comparing with the patients of group 1, the initial size of SDH in group 2 tended to be thin. However, this was not true in some patients. Therefore, we still do not know the way to predict which SDH increase in size and progress to have a clinical deterioration. The outcome was favorable both in two groups except for 2 patients with death from unrelated diseases.

DISCUSSION

SDHs are arbitrarily grouped as acute, subacute, or chronic. This is based on the interval from trauma to development of symptoms from the hematomas[3]. While, chronic SDH is clearly differentiated from acute SDH in their pathological feature.

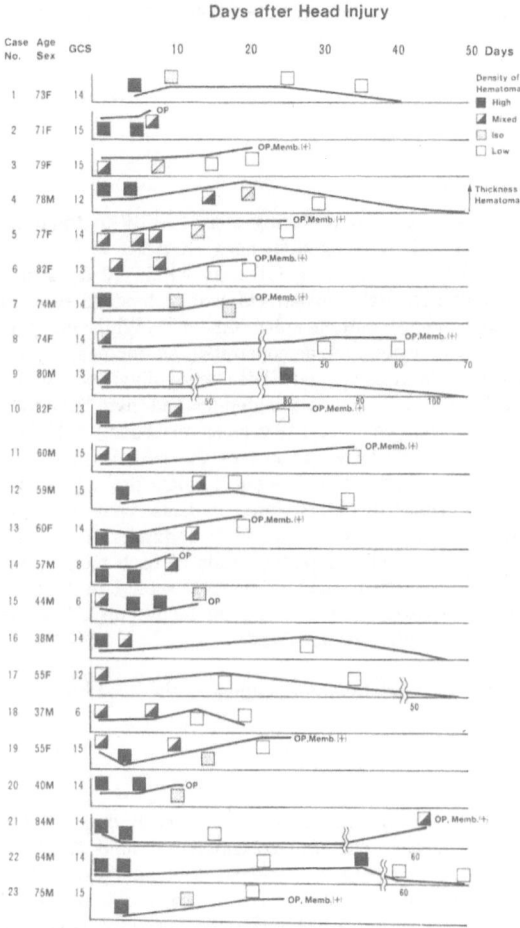

Although there has been a few report presenting chronic SDH originating from acute SDH[1,2], the relation-ship between them is still unclear. When chronic SDH was defined as chronically enlarged and encapsulated SDH, a part of group 1 was considered to be chronic SDH. We conclude that the evolution from acute SDH to chronic SDH is present especially in the elderly patients. No information to explain the mechanism of this evolution had been given in our study. However, an increase in colloid osmotic pressure caused by the breakdown of red blood cells[4] may play a major role to facilitate the cerebrospinal fluid(CSF) influx into the subdural space and to enlarge the SDH because the increase in volume was highly related to the decrease in density suggesting the destruction of red cells. Since the mixture of CSF and the blood was reported to be an important factor in the development of chronic SDH[5], the influx of CSF into the subdural space may encourage to make a neomembrane. No matter what the mechanism is, it is necessary to investigate to know the way to predict which SDH has a such evolution.

Fig. 3 Chronological changes of subdural hematomas in Group 1. Each square and solid line shows the density of hematoma and the thickness of hematoma respectively.

REFERENCES

1. Taguchi Y, Nakamura N, Sato J, Hasegawa Y (1982) Neurol Med Chir(Tokyo) 22: 276-282
2. Aoki N, Tsutsumi K (1990) Acta Neurochir(Wien) 102: 149-151
3. McKissock W, Richardson A, Bloom WH (1960) Lancet 1: 1365-1369
4. Ito H, Shimoji T, Yamamoto S, Saito K, Uehara Y (1988) Neurol Med Chir(Tokyo) 28: 650-653
5. Watanabe S, Shimada H, Ishii S (1972) J Neurosurg 37: 552-561

Chronic Subdural Hematoma Secondary to Traumatic Subdural Hygroma: Consequence or Coexistence?

CHUN KUN PARK, JANG HOI HWANG, JOON KI KANG, and CHANG RAK CHOI

Department of Neurosurgery, Kangnam St. Mary's Hospital, Catholic University Medical College, Seoul 137-040, Korea

SUMMARY

We experienced 13 patients with chronic subdural hematoma (CSDH) occurring consequently to traumatic subdural hygroma (SDHy) over a 6-year period. The patients ranged in ages from 20 to 80 years (mean 52.1 years). Twelve of them were male. All patients underwent CT scan within 10 days after head trauma, and presented small to moderate amount of subdural effusion (<20 of Hounsfield units in density) in uni- or bi-lateral frontal areas without surrounding contrast enhancement. While managed conservatively, follow-up CT scan was performed in 9 patients and demonstrated an increase in the amount of subdural effusion, but no evidence of increase in density. CSDHs were diagnosed in the same areas as SDHy without any history of further head trauma, eight unilaterally and five bilaterally, at mean interval of 53.4 days. During the interval, new symptoms had developed insidiously following a period of stabilization of the initial symptoms manifested by SDHy in most of the patients, but 4 of the 13 patients (30%) had not had any new symptom. Ten patients underwent surgical drainage of the hematoma and the membrane formation was confirmed, while the other three patients were managed conservatively followed by complete resolution of the hematoma. Our experience indicates that SDHy can be a prodromal disease of CSDH in certain situations, although the pathogenesis of each deasese has been considered to be totally different. Patients with SDHy, even small in amount, should be followed up for at least 3 months. Particularly, a patient with the SDHy getting larger in follow-up CT scans, should be carefully monitored, although their symptoms and signs are stabilized.

KEY WORDS: head trauma, chronic subdural hematoma, subdural hygroma, pathogenesis, evolution

INTRODUCTION

Post-traumatic subdural hygroma (SDHy) and chronic subdural hematoma (CSDH) each has different pathogenesis. SDHy is a term used to describe clear, watery subdural collections of fulid devoid of limiting membranes after head trauma [4], and believed to develop after arachnoid disruptions, permitting unidirectional flow of cerebrospinal fluid into the subdural space [1,3]. The pathogenesis of CSDH, especially the mechanism of increase in volume remains obscure, but it has been currently suggested that effusion and recurrent hemorrhage from the capillaries of the subdural hematoma membrane following the initial bleeding and establishment of membranes contribute to enlargement of hematomas [2,6]. Accordingly, these two diseases have been considered to be in different clinical or pathological entity. The authors have experienced 13 cases of CSDH, which developed sometime after and in the same region as SDHy had occurred without any history of further head trauma but the initial injury. In the present paper, we summarize our experience and discuss the mechanism of the development of CSDH secondary to SDHy.

MATERIALS AND METHODS

This series includes 13 consecutive cases with CSDH, all of which had been initially diagnosed as SDHy within 10 days after the initial head trauma based on their finding on brain CT scans. CT scan demonstrated small to moderate amount of subdural fluid collection in uni- or bi-lateral frontal areas.

Subdural hygroma was defined as watery subdural fluid collection (<20 of Hounsfield units in density) without surrounding contrast enhancement on CT scan. The development of CSDH had been observed by a follow-up CT or MRI scan, which was performed on the routine basis or because of the development of new symptoms and signs. In every surgical case, membrane formation had been confirmed.

RESULTS AND DISCUSSION

The 13 patients all had experienced only a single event of closed head injury throughout their clinical course based on their statements. They ranged in ages from 20 to 80 years (average, 52.1 years). Only one was female. Motor vehicle accidents were the cause of injury in 10 cases, and falls resulted in 3 cases. At the diagnosis of SDHy, Glasgow Coma Scale (GCS) score was more than 11(average, 12.8) in most of the patients, and the symptoms and signs varied from only a headache to lowered consciousness and mental confusion. The hygroma was bilateral in all cases. Evidence of concurrent brain atrophy was found on CT scan in only 5 of the 13 patients. Nine cases had a follow-up CT scan on at least one occasion to monitor the change of the hygroma, and progressive increase in the amount of the hygroma was observed in the all 9 patients before they were newly diagnosed as CSDH. After a period of some improvement and stabilization, 7 of the 13 patiens had insidiously developed new symptoms and signs manifested by mental confusion, headache and/or hemiparesis, or had aggravation of the initial symptoms requiring follow-up CT scan to demonstrate newly developed subdural hematoma. By contrast, 5 patients had a clinical course that stabilzed with the initial symptoms or without any symptom or sign, and the subdural hematoma happened to be observed on a routine follow-up CT or MRI scan. In one patient, CSDH developed alternatively in each side of the hemisphere at different intervals: the one without new symptom or sign; the other with new findings such as hemiparesis 70 days later. The hematoma developed unilaterally in 8 patients and bilaterally in 5 patients. The interval from the diagnosis of SDHy to CSDH was ranged from 10 to 114 days (average, 53.4 days), and about 80% of the patients had developed CSDH in a period of 3 months. All the hygroma had been treated conservatively. Eleven CSDH had been treated with burr hole trephination and subdural drainage, and the remaining 3 CSDH with no symptom or sign had been simply observed and followed up without any aggressive management such as the administration of hyperosmolar agents (Fig. 1). Post-treatment CT scans in all of the 13 patiens showed that complete resolution of CSDH and SDHy had occurred.

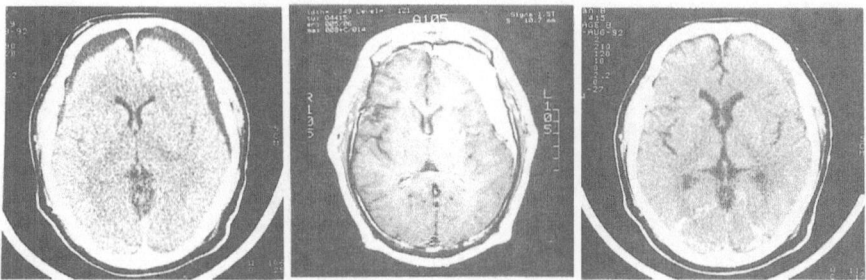

Fig. 1. A illustrative case (Age: 50; Sex: male). Left: CT scan, examined 22days after injury, demonstrating subdural hygroma in the bilateral frontal areas. Middle: Magnetic resonance image, T2-weighted, examined 3 months postinjury, showing a high-intensity subdural hematoma in the left frontal area. Right: Follow-up CT scan, examined 6 months postinjury, showing almost complete disappearance of the subdural hematoma only with conservative management.

A retrospective analysis of the 13 patients with CSDH indicates that the hematoma does not simply coexist with the subdural hygroma, but develops secondary to the initial diease, SDHy. However, the mechanism by which the hematoma is evolved from the hygroma remains unclear. Stone and his colleagues reported that the subarachnoid hemorrhages were frequently observed in the patients with

SDHy (53 of the 57 cases having lumbar puncture) and might be caused by concurrent leptomeningeal vascular trauma [5].   And it has been reported that damaged or irritated capillaries could be responsible for the delayed evolution of SDHy with arachnoid disruption [1,3].   These concurrent leptomeningeal vascular damages may not only predispose the increase of the hygroma by disturbing the cerebrospinal fluid resorption and forming secondary effusions, but also trigger a process of the events in the development of CSDH under unknown circumstances.   It is also considered that the conditions increased venous pressure such as coughing, sneezing, and of straining may play a role in initiating subdural bleedings in a patient with damaged leptomeningeal vessels as well as large amount of subdural collection.   It appears that brain atrophy is not responsible for the development of CSDH secondary to SDHy.

Our experience suggests the necessity of follow-up for at least 3 months in patients with SDHy, even in small amount and whose symptoms related with the hygroma are well stabilized.   Enlarging hygroma on follow-up CT scans could be the most important factor to foresee the development of secondary CSDH.

REFERENCES

1. Hooper R(1969) Patterns of acute head injury. Williams and Wilkins. Baltimore, pp61-63
2. Markwalder TM(1981) J Neurosurg 54:637-645
3. McConnell AA(1941) J Neurol Neurosurg Psychiatry 4:237-256
4. Naffziger HC(1924) JAMA 82:1751-1752
5. Stone JL, Lang RGR, Sugar O, Moody RA(1981) Neurosurgery 8:524-549
6. Yamashima T, Yamamoto S, Friede RL(1983) J Neurosurg 59:298-303

Development of Chronic Subdural Hematomas from Acute Thin Subdural Hematomas: Determinants of Their Evolution

Takamitsu Yamamoto, Yoichi Katayama, and Takashi Tsubokawa

Department of Neurological Surgery, Nihon University School of Medicine, Itabashi-ku, Tokyo, 173 Japan

SUMMARY

Since 1988, we have conservatively treated 90 cases of acute thin subdural hematomas (ATSDHs). These hematomas were less than 4 mm in width and disappeared spontaneously within 2 weeks in most cases. In 7 cases (7.8%), however, chronic subdural hematomas (CSDHs) developed. Craniotomy was performed in 3 cases and irrigation through a burr hole in the other 4 cases. We analyzed the characteristics of these cases of ATSDH in which CSDHs were later formed. The results indicated that (1) most of the cases were older than the remaining cases and had sustained minor head trauma; (2) cerebral atrophy was frequently evident on initial CT scans; (3) CT scans taken at 2 weeks after trauma demonstrated unresolved clots more frequently than in the other cases; (4) the development of voluminous CSDH was first identified on CT scans at as early as 3 weeks after trauma; (5) an external membrane, but not an inner membrane, was noted on surgery at approximately 3 weeks after trauma, implying that this form of CSDH may often develop quite rapidly; (6) the arachnoid membrane beneath the CSDH was frequently non-transparent and might have acted as an inner membrane; (7) the contents of the hematomas were identical to those observed in other CSDHs. These findings suggest that a large subdural space and low intracranial pressure may delay the resolution of ATSDH, and CSDHs may be rapidly formed from the unresolved clots. In addition, it appeared that CT scans taken at 2 weeks after trauma could be important for predicting subsequent development of CSDH.

KEY WORDS: chronic subdural hematoma, acute subdural hematoma, intracranial pressure, subdural space, subdural clot

INTRODUCTION

It has been demonstrated that chronic subdural hematoma (CSDH) can develop from hemorrhage occurring in the subdural space [1-7] . It is also recognized that only some cases of subdural hemorrhage develop into CSDH within several weeks or several months after head injury. Since 1988, we have conservatively treated 90 cases of acute thin subdural hematomas (ATSDHs). These hematomas were less than 4 mm in width and disappeared spontaneously within 2 weeks in most cases. In 7 cases (7.8%), however, CSDH developed [7] . The aims of this study were to clarify which factor is important in determining whether or not ATSDH progresses to CSDH and what are the essential features of this type of CSDH.

MATERIALS AND METHODS

All 7 cases of CSDH which developed from ATSDH were at first treated conservatively using regimens of diuretics, bed rest and corticosteroids, since the patients complained only of headache and nausea without definite disturbance of their consciousness at the time of admission. The 7 cases comprised 3 males and 4 females. The age distribution of the patients was as follows: 40-49 years, one case; 50-59 years, 2 cases; 60-69 years, one case; and 70-79 years, 3 cases.

RESULTS AND DISCUSSION

The causes of the head injury included one case of falling down and 6 cases of minor head injury including bruising and falling. Transient unconsciousness occurring immediately after the head injury was not observed in 6 of the 7 cases, and no patient suffered skull fracture. The initial CT scans revealed findings of a low intracranial pressure (ICP), with cerebral thrombosis, brain atrophy and subdural fluid collection in 6 of the 7 cases. All 7 cases displayed clinical signs of ICP elevation and disturbance of consciousness, while the CT scans demonstrated a definite mass effect (such as a shift of the midline structures) within 3 weeks after the head injury. The CT scan findings showed no difference from usual CSDHs which require further long-term follow-up showed for the expression of the clinical signs and CT findings (Fig-1). All cases underwent surgery within 3 weeks after head injury. Craniotomy was performed in 3 cases and irrigation through a burr hole in the other 4 cases. All cases presented a good prognosis.

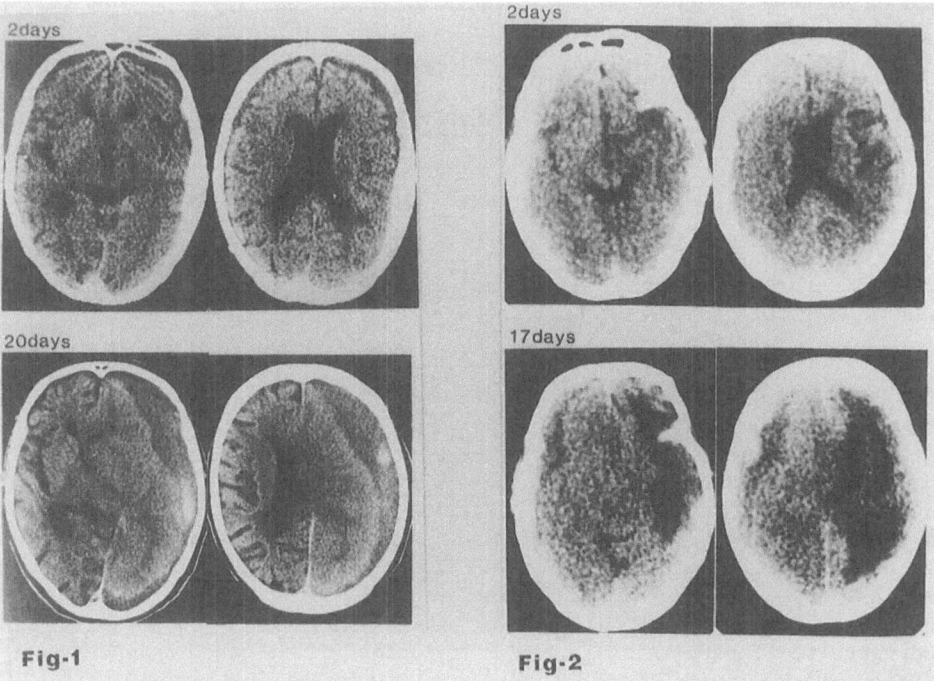

Fig-1. CT scan findings at 2 days (upper) and 20 days (lower) after head injury. The CT scan shows bilateral subdural fluid collection and a slight enlarged ventricle (upper). CSDH is containing clots (lower). Fig-2. CT scan findings two days (upper) and 17 days (lower) after head injury. CT scan shows cerebral thrombosis with acute subdural hematoma.

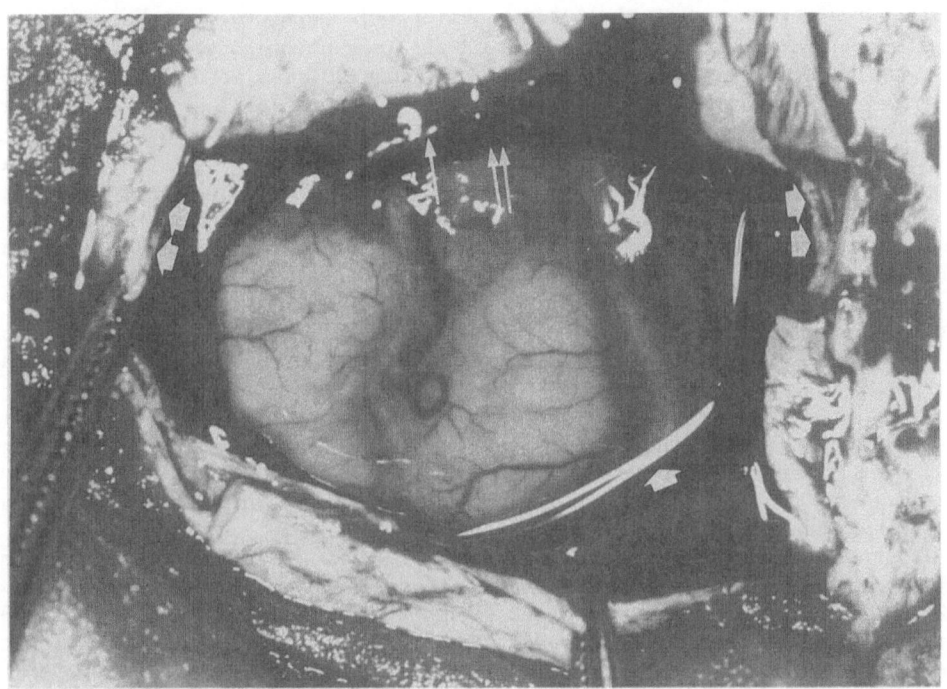

Fig-3: Operative findings of a chronic subdural hematoma which developed from an acute thin subdural hematoma. After opening the dura (➡➡), a thin fiber layer (↑) was apparent. Thick granulation tissue (↑↑) formed a membrane beneath the fibrin layer, and granulation tissue was adherent to the fibrin layer. After opening the granulation tissue, a dark red-colored liquid-type hematoma (➡) was expelled. No inner membrane of the hematoma capsule was visible over the cortex with the naked eye.

The common features of the operative findings were an external hematoma capsule, such as a fibrin layer and granulation tissue, which could be recognized beneath the dura, and a fluid-type hematoma identical to a chronic subdural hematoma which was present beneath these structures. No inner membrane of the hematoma could be identified with the naked eye (Fig-3).

Case Report: A 77-year-old female sustained minor bruising through contact with a signboard while out walking, but she suffered no initial unconsciousness. The next day she complained of headache, and a CT scan revealed a right hemispheric acute subdural hematoma and bilateral fluid collection with brain atrophy. The CT scan findings at 20 days post-injury showed CSDH, and unconsciousness also appeared (Fig-1).

A 69-year-old male who had left hemiparesis fell on the floor without without being aware of head injury; on the following day he noticed a headache. A CT scan revealed left hemispheric acute subdural hematoma and right hemispheric atrophy caused by cerebral infarction. Although he had no initial unconscious or skull fracture, he became somnolent and developed tetraparesis 17 days post-injury. Repeated CT scan on the same day showed a remarkable shift of the midline structure caused by an isodense hemispheric hematoma (Fig-2).

McKissoch, Richardson and Bloom applied the term chronic subdural hematoma to those cases which presented symptoms at more than 20 days after head injury. It has, however, been reported that between 25% and 48% of patients with CSDH have no obvious history of head injury [1,3,4,5,6] . The term chronic subdural hematoma is thus usually based on the clinical signs, radiological findings and operative findings. We experienced 7 cases of CSDH which developed from ATSDH that was definitely identified on CT scans within 2 days after head injury. These cases presented with essentially identical features on their CT scans, and there were clinical signs and pathological findings of CSDH except that no inner membrane could be identified with the naked eye. One special feature of this group was the rapid development (after an average of 16.1 days) of clinical and radiological findings of CSDH. All cases of this type, except one, had only minor head injury and CT findings with low ICP signs which included cerebral thrombosis, brain atrophy or subdural fluid collection with ATSDH. These observations suggested that the ICP is very important in determining whether ATSDH will disappear or develop into CSDH. We consider that a large subdural space and low ICP may delay the resolution of ATSDH, and CSDH may be formed rapidly from unresolved hematoma clots.

No inner membrane was identified with the naked eye in our cases. This may be a reasonable observation, since these cases displayed clinical signs from 12 to 20 days, and surgery was performed within 3 weeks post-head injury. Reports of pathological studies have indicated that an inner membrane appears during the third week [2] . The fact that a liquid-type hematoma was present beneath the external capsule raises the possibility that an inner membrane, which could not be identified with the naked eye, might already have formed or that the arachnoid membrane acted as an inner membrane at this stage.

REFERENCES
1. McKissoch, W., Richardson, A., Bloom, W.H. (1960) Subdural hematoma: A review of 389 cases. Lancet 1: 1365-1369
2. Munro, D. and Merritt, H.H. (1936) Surgical pathology of subdural hematoma, based on a study of one hundred and five cases. Archives of Neurology and Psychiatry 35: 64-78
3. Forgelholm, R. and Waltimo, O. (1975) Epidemiology of chronic subdural hematoma. Acta Neurochirurgia 32: 247-250
4. Marshall, L.F., Toole, B.M., Bowers, S.A. (1983) The national traumatic coma data bank. Part 2. Patient who talk and deteriorate; implications for treatment. Journal of Neurosurgery 59: 285-288
5. Richter, H.P., Klein, H.J., Schafer, M. (1984) Chronic subdural hematomas treated by enlarged burr-hole craniotomy and closed system drainage: retrospective study of 120 patients. Acta Neurochirurgia 71: 179-188
6. Svien, H.J., Gelety, J.E. (1964) On the surgical management of encapsulated subdural hematoma: a comparison of the results of membranectomy and a simple evacuation. Journal of Neurosurgery 21: 172-177
7. Yamamoto, T., Katayama, Y., Tsubokawa, T., Sasaki, J., Kumagawa, H. (1990) Features of chronic subdural hematoma developed from definitely identified acute subdural haematoma. Brain Injury 4: 135-145

Surgical Treatment of Chronic Subdural Hematoms in Adults

R. VAN SCHAYCK, R. KALFF, and D. SEYDA

University of Essen, Medical Center, Neurosurgical Department, 4300 Essen 1, Germany

KEY WORDS

chronic subdural hematoma - burr-hole - craniotomy - outcome - mortality

SUMMARY

One hundred and eighty patients with chronic subdural hematoma were surgically treated by burr-hole craniostomy (150) or by craniotomy (30). The age ranged from 21 to 91 years, mean 64.2 years. At presentation 61.1 % of the patients showed reduced vigilance, 3.9 % were comatose, 31.7 % had hemiparesis. Minor head trauma was detected in 49 %. At discharge the thickness of the hematoma was clearly reduced. Eightythree per cent of the patients were conscious and fully orientated, hemiparesis was diminished to 6.7 %. The outcome was not significally different for the burr-hole craniostomy and for the craniotomy, but the mortality raised from 3.1 % to 13.3 %. We conclude that burr-hole trepanation was a save and effective treatment of chronic subdural hematoma in adults and that craniotomy should be confined to recurrent unsuccessful burr-hole trepanations, multiple cavities and solid hematomas.

INTRODUCTION

The chronic subdural hematoma consists of a blood and fluid accumulation within the subdural space usually caused by minor head injury [1]. The treatment of subdural hematomas varries from non-surgical therapy [2,3] to surgical treatment including burr-hole craniostomy and craniotomy combined with closed-system subdural drainage [1]. We compared 150 patients after burr-hole craniostomy and subdural drainage with 30 patients after primary craniotomy to answer the question: What is the indication for craniotomy?

PATIENTS AND METHODS

From 1986 to 1991 180 consecutive adult patients with subdural hematoma were reviewed. The hematoma was identified in case of intraoperatively proved black fluid collection within the subdural space covered by a membrane. In all patients computerized tomography (CT) was applied to detect the subdural hematoma. Commonly, we performed one or two burr-hole trepanations in the frontal and parietal area to irrigate the subdural space with physiological saline solution via a flexible red rubber or silicone catheter. After washings were clear a subdural drainige was inserted from 1 to 7 days, mean 3 days. The cranotomy consisted of a standard frontoparietial bone flap, removal of the hematoma and membranectomy.

95

RESULTS

The age distribution of 180 patiets with chronic subdural hematoma is shown in Fig. 1. One hundred and nineteen patients were male, 61 female, mean age 64.2 years. One hundred and fifty patients underwent burr-hole craniostomy and 30 patients primary craniotomy. There was no obvious difference between the age distribution of both groups.

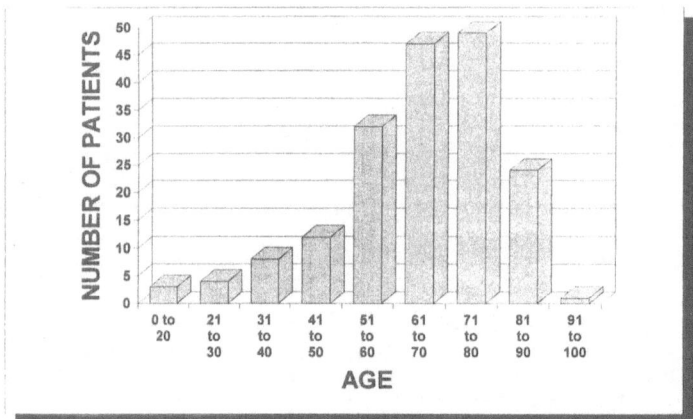

Fig. 1   Age distribution of 180 patients with chronic subdural hematoma

At presentation 110 patients i.e. 61.1 % showed an impaired state of consciousness, only 70 patients (38.9 %) were conscious. Seventy three patients (40.6 %) suffered from headache, hemiparesis was present in 57 patients (31.7 %), other abnormal neurological signs were anisocoria, facial nerve palsy, aphasia and convulsions (Table 1). The hematoma of 49 % of the patients developed from the 7th to the 98th day after minor head trauma, 51 % were spontaneous hemorrhages. For other risk factors see table 2.

Tabel 1 Symtoms at presentation

fully orientated	38.9 % (70)
somnolent	47.2 % (85)
soporose	10.0 % (18)
comatose	3.9 % (7)
headache	40.6 % (73)
hemiparesis	31.7 % (57)
anisocoria	7.2 % (13)
facial nerve palsy	6.7 % (12)
aphasia	5.0 % (9)
convulsions	1.7 % (3)

Table 2 Risk Factors

no head trauma	51.0 % (92)
minor head trauma	49.0 % (88)
abuse of alcohol	16.0 % (29)
diabetes	11.7 % (22)
anticoagulants	6.7 % (12)
thrombocytopenia	1.7 % (3)

In 160 patients (88.8 %) unilateral hematoma was detected by CT, 20 hematomas (11.2 %) occured bilateral. Thickness varied from below 10 mm to 40 mm and correlated well with the midline shift.
One hundred and twenty eight patients underwent burr-hole trepanation, 7 patients with recurrent burr-hole craniostomy. Craniotomy was performed secondly in 22 unsuccessfully treated patients due to multiple cavities. Thirty patients underwent primary craniotomy, repeated craniotomy was necessary in 5 patients. The single and recurrent burr-hole craniostomy group showed a mortality of 3.1 %, 4 patients of 128 died. The mortality raised to 13,3 % in the primary and recurrent craniotomy group, 4 patients of 30 died. The mortality rate was siginifcantly higher in the craniotomy group (p<0,01), but the outcome showed no clear difference. At discharge 150 of the 180 surgical treated patients (83.3 %) were in an essentially normal or good condition, 10 (10.7 %) were confused or somolent and hemiparesis showed a siginificant reduction (p<0,01), the mortality of the total series was 6.7 % (Table 3). A clear decrease in size and thickness of the hematoma was evident on CT (Fig. 2).

Table 3 Outcome at discharge

mortality	6.7 % (12)
fully orientated	83.3 % (150)
somnolent	10.0 % (18)
soporose	0
comatose	0
hemiparesis	6.7 % (12)
aphasia	2.8 % (5)

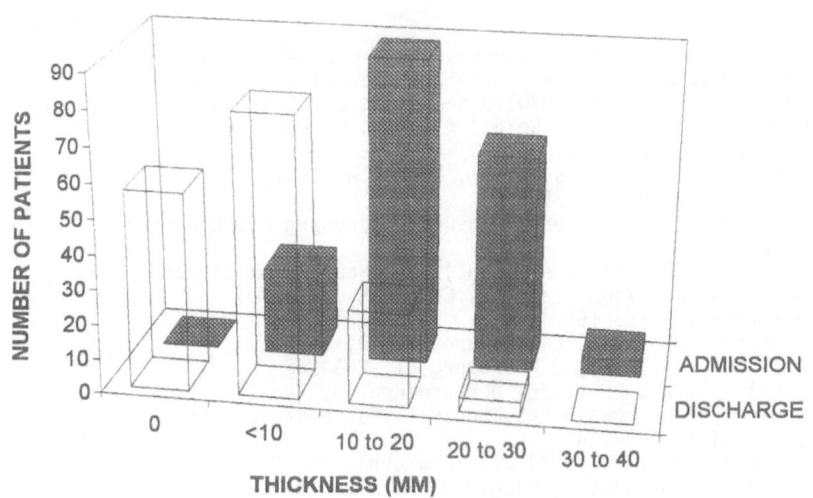

Fig. 2   Thickness of the hematoma, Admission and discharge

DISCUSSION

A subdural drainage increased the rate of successfully evacuated subdural hematomas, but might also have increased the rate of infectious complications [4]. We inserted a subdural drainage to reduce the amount of remaining subdural fluid collection postoperatively. Under the treatment with antibiotics we observed no infectious complication, even if the drainage lasted one week. Furthermore the persistence of subdural fluid collection postoperatively induced a reaccumulation of the hematoma [4,5,6,7]. However, the follow-up of our series from 6 to 18 months after discharge revealed complete reabsorption of the subdural fluid collection.

The nonsurgical treatment of chronic subdural hematomas were demonstrated as effective to some extent. But the hospitalization was needed for at least 3 weeks and deterioration of some patiens required surgical intervention [2,3]. Under surgical treatment most of our patients improved and the average stay in hospital was 14 days.

The mortality of chronic subdural hematoma treated by burr-hole ranged from 0 % to 16.6 % as reported in the recent literature [4 to 12]. In these studies 25 of 523 burr-hole treated patients died. The mortaliy of our 128 burr-hole treated patients was 3.1 % and therefore slightly lower than the reported mortality of 4.1 %. The clear increase of mortality to 13.3 % in our craniotomy group corresponded well to the literature [13,14].

We conclude that a surgical approach to chronic subdural hematomas in adults results in a good outcome and low mortality and is therefore the treatment of first choise. Most chronic subdural hematomas are satisfactorily treated by burr-hole craniostomy and subdural drainage. The craniotomy and membranectomy should be confined to recurrent uneffective burr-hole trepanations, multiple cavities and extensive solid hematomas.

REFERENCES

1. Markwalder TM (1981) J Neurosurg 54: 637-645
2. Bender MB, Christoff N (1974) Arch Neurol 31: 73-79
3. Suzuki J, Takaku A (1970) J Neurosurg 33, 548-553
4. Harders A, Eggert HR, Weigel K (1982) Neurochirurgia (Stuttg) 25: 147-152
5. Markwalder TM, Steinsiepe KF, Rohner M (1981) J Neurosurg 55, 390-396
6. Moussa A, Joshy N (1982) J Neurol Neurosurg Psychiatry 45: 1156-1158
7. Victoratos GC, Bligh AS (1981) Surg Neurol 15: 158-160
8. Dolinskas CA, Zimmermann RA, Bilaniuk LT (1979) J Trauma 19, 163-169
9. Galbraith JG (1982) Clin Neurosurg 29, 24-31
10. Robinson, RG (1984) J Neurosurg 61, 263-268
11. Camel M, Grubb RL (1986) J Neurosurg 65, 183-187
12. Firsching R, Frowein RA, Thun F (1989) Neurosurg Rev, 12 Suppl 1: 207-214
13. Kalff R, Braun W (1984) Zbl. Neurochir 45, 210-218
14. Schulz W. Saballus R, Flugel R, Harms L (1988) Zbl Neurochir 49: 280-289

Consideration of Pathophysiology of Chronic Subdural Hematoma by Measurements of Cerebral Blood Flow, Intracranial Pressure and EEG Topography

AKIRA TANAKA, MASATO KIMURA, SHIGEHIKO KUMATE, SHINYA YOSHINAGA, and MASAMICHI TOMONAGA

Department of Neurosurgery, Fukuoka University, Chikushi Hospital, Fukuoka, 818 Japan

SUMMARY

CBF reductuon was more marked in the thalamus and putamen than in the hemisphere and cortex, and CBF enhancement by Diamox was impaired in the formers and preserved in the latters. The resting and enhanced CBF was restored after surgery. ICP was within normal limits. CBF in the thalamus and putamen correlated negatively with the slow waves in the frontopolar, frontal and central regions on the side with the hematoma. CBF in the other regions and on the side without the hematoma had no correlation with any EEG quotinent. We speculate that chronic subdural hematoma displaces and distorts the central cerebral areas without significant increase of ICP, and has them dys- functioned. The other brain structures including the cortex seem to undergo a trans- neuronal suppression from the dysfunctioned thalamus with a resulting reduction of CBF.

KEY WORDS: brain distortion, cerebral blood flow, chronic subdural hematoma, diaschisis, thalamus

INTRODUCTION

Chronic subdural hematomas are slowly expanding intracranial mass lesions that can cause reversible reduction of cerebral function by compressing and displacing the brain. However, the pathophysiology of the cerebral dysfunction is still unclear. We have done the following studies to elucidate it.

PATIENTS AND METHODS

The studies were performed on 25 patients, aged 23 to 83 years (average, 69 yr), before and after evacuation of a chronic subdural hematoma. CBF was measured by a xenon-enhanced CT scan CBF analyzing system adapted to a SOMATOM DR-III while the patients inhaled 30% xenon gas for 6 minutes. CBF enhancement was tested to infuse 1g of Diamox. ICP was measured during a surgery to place a transducer-tipped catheter in the epidural space through a burr hole. EEG was recorded from 12 points on the scalp according to the 10/20 international system. Power spectral analysis was carried out between 2.0 and 29.8 Hz by the Processor. Percentage power fraction (PPF) was defined for each frequency band as delta-PPF, theta-PPF, alpha-PPF and beta-PPF. As a single parameter reflecting the degree of slowing of background EEG activity, a power ratio index (PRI) was calculated.

RESULTS

The ICP values at a time of surgery were 40-137(88.5±43.0) mmH2O in the
headache group (patients who had only headache and minimal mass effect on a CT scan)
and 54-161 (107.4±29.8) mmH2O in the neurology group (patients who had hemiparesis
and/or mental disturbance, and moderate or severe mass effect). CBF reduction of the
headache group was, on the side with the hematoma, 6.9-17.0% of normal values
and CBF was adversely elevated by 13.2% in the cortex (Fig. 1). After surgery, it was
further reduced in all regions, most markedly in the cortex. CBF reduction of the
neurology group was, on the side with the hematoma, 35.8-51.1% (Fig. 1). After
surgery, it returned to 74.4-83.1% of normal values. The postoperative increase was,
on the side with the hematoma, 23.9-52.1%, most markedly in the thalamus (p<0.01).
CBF enhancement by Diamox was, on the side with the hematoma, 54.6% in the hemisphere
, 62.8% in the cortex, 19.3% in the thalamus and 27.8% in the putamen (Fig. 2).
The preoperative mean value of PRI was 147.3±110.3% on the side with the hematoma
and 143.9±112.2% on the side without. PRI was reduced to 56.0±23.8% and to 55.1±
24.6% postoperatively. The reduction was mainly due to a decrease of delta-PPF. In a
linear regression analysis of CBF correlation with EEG quotients, CBF in the thalamus
correlated negatively with delta-PPF in the frontal and central regions (p<0.05),
theta-PPF in the frontopolar (p<0.05) and central (p<0.01) regions and PRI in
the frontal and central regions (p<0.05) on the side with the hematoma (Table 1).
CBF in the putamen also correlated negatively with delta-PPF in the frontal region
(p<0.05) and theta-PPF in the central region (p<0.05). No CBF in the other regions
and on the side without the hematoma correlated with any EEG quotinent.

DISCUSSION

CBF reduction in chronic subdural hematoma, which is more marked in the thalamus and
putamen than in the hemisphere and cortex, seems to suggest that central cerebral
areas are more responsible for clinical symptoms than the cortex. Elevation of ICP
can be the cause of CBF reduction, but it was within normal limits in this sudy.
However, Wozney et al [1] reported a patient in whom a frontal lobe hematoma caused
a central herniation without increase of ICP. After removal of the hematoma, both
clinical status, and local and cental CBF improved. The report demonstrated that a
pressure elevation exerted by a focal mass lesion is not uniform and can cause a
central herniation without significant change of ICP. This may be true for a chronic
subdural hematoma. CBF enhancement by Diamox can be an indicator of whether a CBF
reduction reflects an ischemia or is a secondary phenomenon since the ischemic brain
tissue can hardly respond to a vasodilator for CBF augmentation [2] . In our study,
CBF enhancement was preserved in the hemisphere and cortex, but impaird in the
thalamus and putamen. This result may indicate that the thalamus and putamen undergo,
ischemia by a central herniation, and the hemisphere and cortex undergo a transneural
suppression of "diaschisis" from the dysfunctioned thalamus and other upper brain
stem structures. The ischemia in the thalamus and putamen might be caused by a
distortion of the vessels like the lenticulostriate and thalamoperforating arterial
systems [3] . Focal slow wave, particularly monorythmic delta wave, is known to
appears in the frontal region as the brain displacement and distortion proceed on EEG
in chronic subdural hematoma and it is speculated to originate from the thalamus [4, 5]
. In this study, delta wave was dominant in all regions, particularly in the front
opolar and frontal regions. CBF in the thalamus and putamen correlated negatively

with the delta- and/or theta-PPF in the frontopolar, frontal and central regions. Only CBF in the thalamus had a correlation with PRI in the frontal and central regions. CBF in the other regions and on the side without the hematoma had no correlation with any EEG quotient. The results of EEG studies seem to substantiate that a dysfunctioning of the thalamus is a core of pathophysiology of chronic subdural hematoma.

REFERENCES

1. Wozney P, Yonas H, Latchaw RE, Gur D, Good W (1985) Central herniation revealed by focal decrease in blood flow without elevation of intracranial pressure: A case report. Neurosurgery 17: 641-644
2. Yamashita T, Kashiwagi S, Nakano S, Takasago T, Abiko S, Shiroyama Y, Hayashi M, Ito H (1991) The effect of EC-IC bypass surgery on resting cerebral blood flow and cerebrovascular reserve capacity studied with stable Xe-CT and acetazolamide. Neuroradiology 33: 217-222
3. Tanaka A, Yoshinaga S, Kimura M (1990) Xenon-enhanced computed tomographic measurement of cerebral blood flow in patients with chronic subdural hematomas. Neurosurgery 27: 554-561
4. Kusumoto K, Kobayashi E, Yamamoto K, Mihara T, Asakura T (1981) Computed tomography and electroencephalogram in chronic subdural hematoma: A review of 50 cases. Rinshou Nouha (Tokyo) 23: 720-726
5. Shima F, Maeyama R, Takeno Y, Nagatomi H, Nishimura K, Matsuoka S (1973) The electroencephalogram in subdural hematoma: With reference to cerebral angiography and other clinical findings. Brain Nerve (Tokyo) 25: 321-328

Table 1

Correlation Significance in the Linear Regression Analysis between the Hemispheric Mean Values of EEG Quotients and CBF in the Hemisphere, Cortex, Thalamus and Putamen on the side with the hematoma

	Frontopolar	Frontal	Central	Temporal	Occipital	Frontal-Midline	Parietal-Midline
Detla-PPF							
vs. H. CBF	ns	ns	ns	ns	ns	ns	ns
vs. C. CBF	ns	ns	ns	ns	ns	ns	ns
vs. T. CBF	ns	$p<0.05$	$p<0.05$	ns	ns	ns	ns
vs. P. CBF	ns	$p<0.05$	ns	ns	ns	ns	ns
Theta-PPF							
vs. H. CBF	ns	ns	ns	ns	ns	ns	ns
vs. C. CBF	ns	ns	ns	ns	ns	ns	ns
vs. T. CBF	$p<0.05$	ns	$p<0.01$	ns	ns	ns	ns
vs. P. CBF	ns	ns	$p<0.05$	ns	ns	ns	ns
PRI							
vs. H. CBF	ns	ns	ns	ns	ns	ns	ns
vs. C. CBF	ns	ns	ns	ns	ns	ns	ns
vs. T. CBF	ns	$p<0.05$	$p<0.05$	ns	ns	ns	ns
vs. P. CBF	ns	ns	ns	ns	ns	ns	ns

CBF, cerebral blood flow; PPF, percentage power fraction; PRI, power ratio index; H., hemispheric; C., cortical; T., thalamic; P., putaminal; ns, statistically not significant.

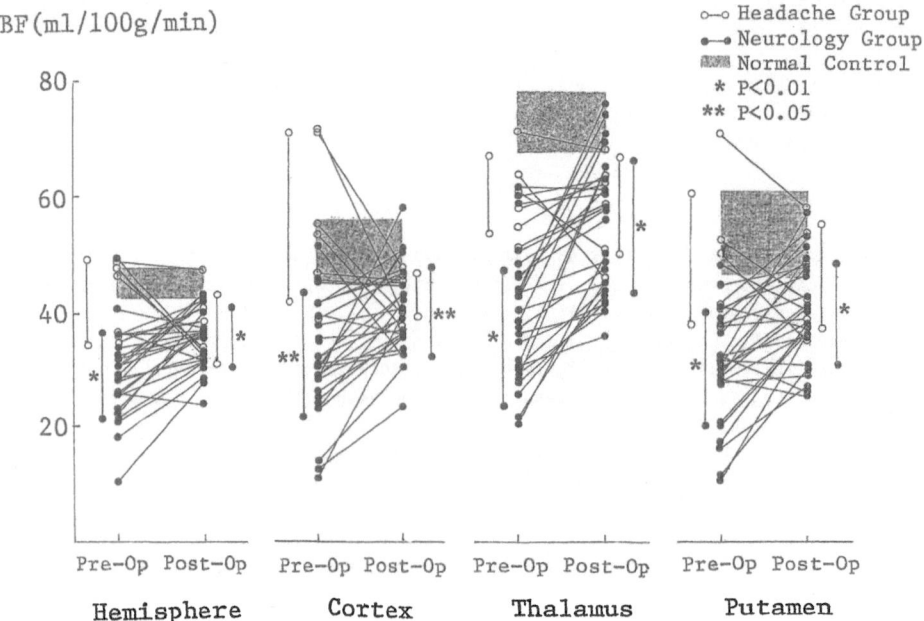

Fig. 1 CBF changes before and after surgery in chronic subdural hematoma

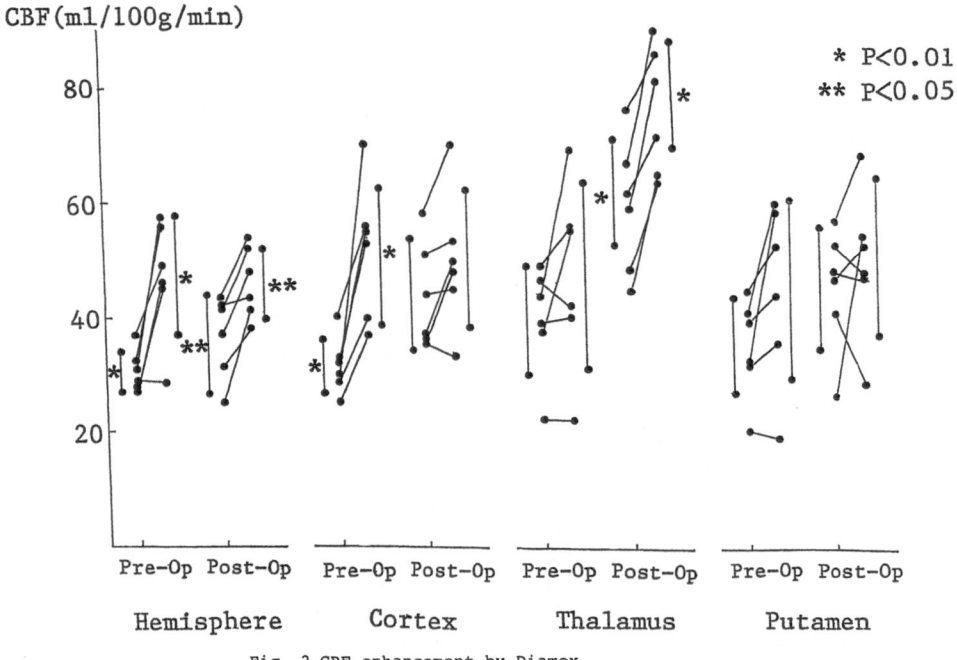

Fig. 2 CBF enhancement by Diamox

Analysis of Intracerebral Stress Distribution and Its Effect on Regional Blood Flow in Chronic Subdural Hematoma

SEIJI HAMANO[1], TATSUYA NAGASHIMA[2], KAZUMASA EHARA[2], SHIGEKIYO FUJITA[1], NORIHIKO TAMAKI[2], and YUKIO TADA[3]

[1]Department of Neurosurgery, Brain and Heart Center at Himeji Himeji, Hyogo, 670 Japan, [2]Department of Neurosurgery, Kobe University School of Medicine, Kobe, Hyogo, 650 Japan, and [3]Department of Faculty of Engineering, Kobe University, Kobe, Hyogo, 657 Japan

SUMMARY

Deformation of brain and intracerebral stress distribution in cases with chronic subdural hematoma were computer simulated by finite element method(FEM).The deformation of the brain by chronic subdural hematoma was well represented by the simulation.The stress concentrated in the area just beneath the hematoma and around the falx cerebri.The area of stress concentration coincides with the area of decreased regional cerebral blood flow measured by SPECT.

KEY WORDS: finite element method(FEM),computer simulation, stress distribution chronic subdural hematoma, regional cerebral blood flow(r-CBF)

INTRODUCTION

Various sensors made it possible to measure intracranial pressure, but it is immposible to directly measure intracerebral stress.To simulate to brain deformation and the stress distribution in cases with chronic subdrural hematoma, finite element method(FEM) was applied in this study.

MATERIALS AND METHODS

From the slices of CT and MRI, four finite element models of cerebral section were made.The number of nodes were 125, 100, 78, 64,respectively, and the number of triangular elements were 182, 156, 116, 102,respectively.The brain was assumed to be a viscoelastic material in this simulation.The program of the simulation was made to calculate with the models made by less than four different materials.The mechanical properties(Young's modulus, coefficient of viscosity, Poison raio)were quoted from literatures.[1,2,3,4,5,6,] The Young's modulus of the dura was determined 10 times larger than that of the brain.

Using these models, simulation of left temporal compression and left frontal compression by chronic subdural hematoma were performed.To calculate these simulations, the main computer of the total information center at Kobe University was used. Then the results were computer simulated by a NEC ACOS 1000 computer.

RESULTS

1)Models of Temporal Compression by Chronic Subdural Hematoma

The similated brain deformation was similar to the CT findings. The deviation of the frontal part of the midline is more apparent than that of the posterior part.

Intracerebral stress distribution visualized by contour mapping showed that the stress concentrate just beneath the subdural hematoma and around the falx cerebri.The stress concentraion means that the brain is compressed to the falx.On the other hand, the stress diminished markedly in the contralateral hemisphere.The falx and the ventricles appeared to be a buffer zone.

Comparing the area of stress concentraion with the regional cerebral blood flow, it coincidesd with the area of decreased regional cerebral blood flow measured by SPECT.

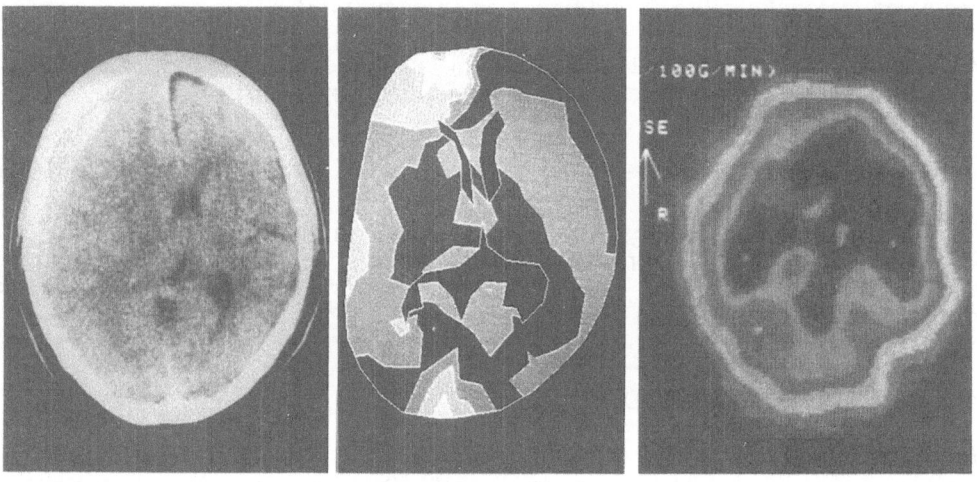

Figure 1	Figure 2	Figure 3
CT of a left temporal	Simulated principal stress	r-CBF of the patient
chronic subdural	distribution in a temporal	in Figure 1
hematoma	compression	

2)Models of Frontal Compression by Chronic Subdural Hematoma

Using the same finite element model, a simulation of left frontal compression by chronic subdural hematoma was performed.Similar to the CT findings,the deformation of the frontal lobe and that of ventricles were more obvious than that of the posterior part.

The stress concentrated not only just beneath the hematoma, but also in the frontal part of the falx cerebri.The difference from the simulation of temporal compression was that the stress markedly concentrated anterior part of the brain and the falx cerebri.The stress diminished markedly in the contralateral hemisphere and the occipital lobe.

Comparing the stress distribution with the r-CBF by SPECT,the area of stress concentration coincides with the decreased r-CBF.

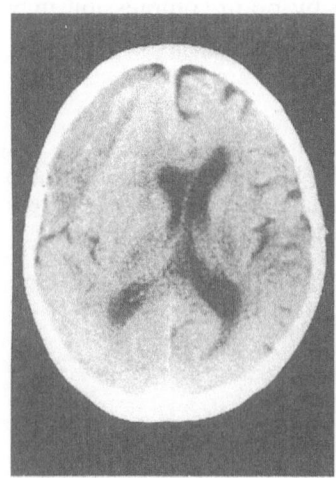 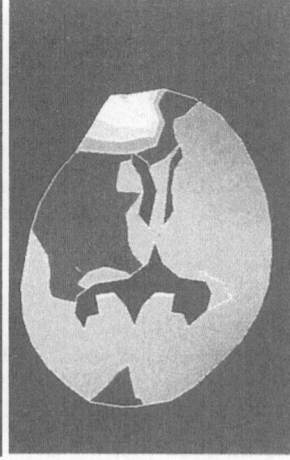 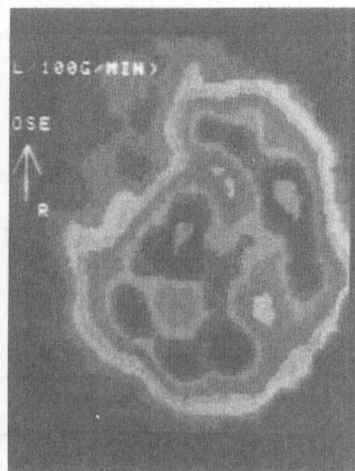

Figure 4	Figure 5	Figure 6
CT of a left frontal	Simulated principal stress	r-CBF of the patient
chronic subdural	in a case of fromtal	in Figure 4
hematoma	compression	

3)a Model of Coronal Section Compressed by Chronic Subdural Hematoma

A model of coronal section compressed by parietal chronic subdural hematoma was made by a section of MRI.

The simulated deviation of the midline and the deformation of the ventricles were not so much as those of the MRI.

The stress distribution was, concentrated beneath the hematoma and around the falx cerebri.The stress beyond the falx and the ventricles was markedly decreased.The diminished stress is speculated from the clearly visualized sulci of the contralateral parietal lobe in the MRI.

DISCUSSION

The finite element method(FEM) is used to smiulate deformation and stress distribution of continuum by deviding it in many subdivisions.The viscoelastic model, that we used was more suitable to simulate mechanical behavior of the living brain than applying elastic models.However, the results of the simulation may depend on the boundary and loading conditions.Therefore, we must be careful to interprete the results.

To date, many studies are reported as the properties about animal and human brain[1,2,3,4,5,6,7,8,9].Formerly the modulus were measured with the non-living brain.[4,7,8,9,10,11] But recent study , on the material properties of living brain [1,2,3] showed elastic property depends on vascular tone in living condition.The elastic modulus of the brain is increased by the bypertension and decreased by hypotension.On the contrary, our study showed that the stress concentration in the brain decreases f-CBF.The decreased cerebral blood flow by brain compression may cause the clinical symptoms of chronic subdural hematoma.

CONCLUSION

Simulations of cerebral compression by chronic subdural hematoma were made with viscoelastic model by FEM.The finite element analysis of intracergrl stress distribution revealed that the intracerebral stress concentration decreases r-CBF.

REFERENCES

1.Aoyagi T,Masuzawa H,Sano K,Kihira M,Kobayasi S:Compliance of the brain:Brain and Nerve 32:47-56,1980
2.Alfonso S. and Walsh,E.G.:Pressure relaxation of the intracranial system in vivo. American Journal of Physiology,225:513-517,1973
3.Alfonso,S.and Walsh,E.G.:Experimental indentification of the subarachnoid and subpial compartment by intracranial pressure measurement.:J.Neurosurg.,40:609-616,1974.
4.Galford,J.and McElhaney,J:A Viscoelastic study of scalp,brain adn dura.:J.Biomechanics 3:211-221,1970
5.Nagashima T,Tamaki N,Matsumoto S,Seguchi Y:Biomechanics and a theoretical model of hydrocepahlus.Application of the finite element method.:Intracranial Pressure 4,Springer-Verlag,Berlin-Heidelberg-New York,Tokyo,:441-446,1986
6.Nagashima T.,Tamaki N,Matsumoto S,B.Horwitz,Seguchi Y:Biomechanics of Hydrocephalus:A new theoretical model:Neurosugery 21:898-904,1987
7.Walsh E.K. and Alfonso S:Elastic behavior of brain tissue in vivo.:American Journal of Phisiology,230:1058-1062,1976
8.Brock M,Hartung C:Glossary of difinitions,standards and deviations.:Intracranial Pressure:Springer-Verlag,Berlin-Heidelberg-New York,:372-375,1972
9.Dodgson,M.C.H.:Colloidal structure of brain,Biorheology,1:21-30,1962
10.Falkenstein,G.:Dynamic mechanical properties of human brain tissue.ASME Oaoer Bi,69-BHF 13,1968
11.Estes M.S.and McElhaney J.H.:Response of brain tissue to compressive loading.Fourth ASME Biomechanics Conference,June,ASME Paper No.69-BHF 13

Chronological Change in Biomechanical Indices of Chronic Subdural Hematoma During and After Closed Drainage – When Should Fluid Drainage Cease?

A. WACHI, O. TSUJI, K. BANDOH, Y. ABE, and K. SATO

Department of Neurosurgery, Juntendo University, Bunkyo-ku, Tokyo, 113 Japan

SUMMARY

Patients with chronic subdural hematoma (ages 33 - 83) were investigated to elucidate the biomechanical status of the hematoma and to determine the time for termination of external hematoma drainage. After trepanation, initial pressure within hematoma was first recorded, followed by pressure-volume measurement. In conclusion, mean initial intrahematoma pressure of 27 mmHg, remarkably higher than in previous reports, was found. Pressure buffering capacity within hematoma after successive drainage of hematoma demonstrated that there were two groups of patients, one in which there was a decrease in PVI and the other with slow increase in PVI. Usually, fluid outflow ceased within few days after surgery in former group, while CSF continuously drains in latter group. External drainage may therefore be terminated when there is normalization of intrahematoma pressure-volume status or fluid outflow disappears.

KEY WORDS: chronic subdural hematoma, pressure volume index

INTRODUCTION

Several surgical procedures for chronic subdural hematoma have been established. Among them, irrigation of hematoma with burr hole and closed drainage are favorable method for patients (1,2), especially for aged or high risk patients. One reason why drainage is effective on chronic subdural hematoma may be clarified by reaccumulation of fluid within the hematoma cavity after irrigation. We determined the classification of hematoma in 2 groups and established the drainage protocol based on biomechanical status of hematoma.

STUDY POPULATION AND METHODS

28 cases including 23 males and 5 female of chronic subdural hematoma were listed on this study. Age distribution of these cases is between 33 and 83, and mean age is 61 years. 24 cases had unilateral hematoma (left 14 and right 24), rest of 4 cases had bilateral hematoma. Pressure monitoring within hematoma was carried out with conventional pressure transducer or fiber-optic pressure monitoring catheter. Pressure within hematoma initially was recorded and subsequently, Pressure-Volume Index (PVI) as indicator of pressure-volume relationship was measured by bolus withdrawal test (3). After measurement of PVI, a drainage tube

was inserted into the cavity, and the fluid was closely drained for several days after surgery. Pressure to drain were at levels of 2-7 mmHg. Pressure, PVI, and accumulated fluid volume were daily monitored. Head CT scan was performed preoperatively, 3 day and 7 day after surgery.

RESULTS

Postoperatively, there were 2 types of hematoma in this study according to accumulation of drained fluid. Communicating type of hematoma indicates that CSF continuously outflows from drainage tube even several days after surgery. Non-Communicating hematoma, on the other hand indicates that fluid outflow ceased until few days after surgery. Communicating type had 5 males and 2 females, and Non-Communicating type had 18 males and 3 females. There were no difference in age, initial pressure within hematoma, and initial PVI. Duration of drainage for Communicating type is 4.3±1.9 days, while 2.1±0.3 day for Non-Communicating type. Cerebral sulci on lesion side shown by CT scan appeared until 7 days after drainage on Communicating type, but is not remarkable on Non-Communicating type. Initial PVI of Communicating type was 7.5±3.4 ml (mean and SD) and it gradually increased until postoperative day 5 and reached to 17±6 ml at that time, while initial PVI of Non-Communicating type was 6.8±4.4 ml and this value rapidly decreased 3±2 ml for 3 days.

DISCUSSION

Surgical treatments of chronic subdural hematoma, especially to drain or not to drain were discussed in the literatures. Wakai et al reported the possibility of reaccumulation of fluid within hematoma cavity and insisted that closed drainage system may reduce rate of fluid reaccumulation, but the system is not necessary after postoperative day 1 since no reduction of cavity was recognized in their study. Markwalder (1) reported that one problem of surgical treatment without hematoma drainage was due to subdural CSF accumulation after surgery, and this fluid accumulation often becomes pressurized afterwards and clinically it makes patients worse. Although these can be the reasons why they emphasized the efficacy of burr hole surgery and continuous drainage with closed system, when a drainage tube stays in the cavity for long period, it may cause severe intracranial infection. Thus, it is important to consider the timing of drain removal.
Membrane located inner side of chronic subdural hematoma is usually well vasculalized and sometimes it is clearly visible on enhanced CT scan, and the hematoma can be isolated from intracranial subarachnoid space by this membrane and its existence may also distinguish subdural hematoma from non hematomatous subdural fluid collection.
Our results indicates that any chronic subdural hematomas are closed within the intracranial cavity preoperatively because the pressure within hematoma is considerably high, and pressure buffering capacity (PVI) is very low. PVI is considered an indicator of pressure buffering capacity and Shapiro (4) reported that PVI of infant is smaller that of adult since the volume of cranial cavity in infant is smaller than that in adult. Therefore,

it was reasonable that PVI within closed hematoma should be very small. But, after surgery, in case of Communicating Hematoma, CSF becomes freely to move through the inner membrane and gradually accumulates within the hematoma cavity. This concept is not inconsistent with Wakai and Markwaler's opinions, and this continuous CSF outflow may be explained by membrane tearing or immature membrane formation. Because values of our biomechanical indices (pressure and pressure buffering capacity) within the cavity are gradually closed to these of normal intracranial environment, the cavity may become a part of subarachnoid space, thus, no longer drain should be necessary. While in case of Non-Communicating type of hematoma which may have a well developed membrane, this membrane prevents CSF from flowing into the cavity even after surgery and as well as no drain of fluid, low PVI and normalized cavity pressure may indicate that drain should be removed at that point.

In conclusion, continuous CSF outflow and increased PVI may occur when hematoma cavity freely communicates with normal subarachnoid space possibly due to immaturity in formation, or tearing, of inner hematoma membrane. Fluid drainage should be removed when no fluid drains (Non-Communicating Hematoma) or when CSF continuously outflows, and PVI is improved (Communicating Hematoma).

REFERENCE

1. Markwalder TM, Seiler RW: Chronic Subdural Hematomas: To Drain of Not to Drain?
Neurosurgery 16: 185-188, 1985

2. Wakai S, Hashimoto K, Watanabe N, Inoh S, Ochiai C, Nagai M: Efficacy of Closed-System Drainage in Treating Chronic Subdural Hematoma: A Prospective Comparative Study.
Neurosurgery 26: 771-773, 1990

3. Marmarou A, Shulman K, LaMorgese J: Compartmental analysis of compliance and outflow resistance of the cerebrospinal fluid system.
J Neurosurg 43: 523-534, 1975

4. Shapiro K, Marmarou A, Shulman K: Characterization of clinical CSF dynamics and neural compliance using the pressure-volume index. I. The normal pressure-volume index.
Ann Neurol 7: 508-514, 1980

Evolution of Surgical Treatment of Chronic Subdural Hematomas

ALEXANDER POTAPOV, LEONID LIKHTERMAN, ALEXANDER KRAVCHUK, and
HÍKMAT EL-KADI
The Burdenko Neurosurgical Institute of the Russian Academy of Medical Sciences, Moscow, Russia

SUMMARY

We analyzed results of the surgical treatment of chronic subdural hematomas (CSH) in 148 patients. It's estimated that removal of hematoma through the burr hole with further closed external drainage is the most adequate method for CSH treatment, especially in the elderly patients. Craniotomy with membranectomy is recommended only in cases of vast dense clots in the hematoma cavity, rarely- in cases with its calcification and also in patients with the real recurrence and insufficiency of the drainage operations.

KEY WORDS:chronic subdural hematomas, surgical treatment,outcome.

INTRODUCTION

The use of CT and MRI, new knowledge of the CSH pathogenesis caused the evolution of the surgical tactics in this pathology (1,2,3). We report the results of CSH treatment by craniotomy with membranectomy and closed external drainage.

MATERIALS AND METHODS

We reviewed our experience in 148 patients with CSH ranging from 1 to 85 years (the mean age - 43,3;males-131,females-17). The most frequent causes of CSH are head injury-68%, vascular pathology-7%,iatrogenic factors-5%;the unknown etiology -20%).Bilateral CSH were diagnosed in 23 cases.From 1970 to 1984 the basic method for surgical treatment of CSH was craniotomy and membranectomy (70 patients;mean age -37;group1). From 1985 the CSH evacuation through the burr hole with further closed external drainage was used (78 patients;mean age -49,7; group II).
The integral indicator of severity of CSH patients state on admission to the Institute was clinical phase of desease,that was defined as a unity of the neurological and somatic symptoms. The following phases were distinguished in the CSH clinical courses.
1.Compensation. Hypertensive and focal symptoms are absent. II.Subcompesation.Mild focal symtoms,moderate headache. III.Moderate decompensation.Moderate stunning.Focal symptoms are variable, prolapse symptoms and irritation symptoms as well as separate secondary brain stem symptoms are observed. IY.Severe decompensation. Consciousness is disturbed from deep stunning to coma. Severe hypertensive,focal and dislocation symptoms, disturbances of vital functions. 2/3 of CSH patients (100 patients -68%) were admitted in a state of moderate and severe compensation,1/3 (47 patients -32%) in a phase of clinical subcompensation.

RESULTS AND DISCUSSION

Patients status in both groups before operation is presented in Table1
As seen from Table 1,the status of patients in group II was more sever
than in Group I. These patients were older (mean age-49,7 years and 37
years respectively).

Table 1. Phasic distribution of patients with CSH the group I and
group II

Clinical phases	Group I		Group II.	
	No of pa-tients	%	No of pa-·tients	%
Subcompensation	28	40	19	24
Moderate decompensation	24	34	29	37
Severe decompensation	18	26	30	39
Total	70	100	78	100

Frequency and character of complications in both CSH groups are
presented in Table 2.

Table 2. Complications and mortality in respect to different operative
interventions in chronic subdural hematomas

Operative intervention	Craniotomy and membranectomy	Burr-hole and closed system drainage
No of cases	69 (70%)	78
Complication		
epidural hematoma	11 (16%)	—
re-accumlation of subdural hematoma	6 (9%)	4 (5%)
infection	3 (4,3%)	1 (1,3%)
others	3 (5,7%)	2 (2,7%)
total	24 (35%)	7 (9%)
Mortality	2 (2,9%)	2 (2,6%)

As seen from Table 2, in closed external drainage the number of all
complications is almost four times less than in craniotomy with
membranectomy (9% and 35% respectively). It's also important that the
character of complications changed due to disappearance or sharp
decrease of postoperative complications,recurrence of epidural and
subdural hematomas.
Thus,the evacuation of the hematoma content through the burr hole with
it's washing by the saline solution and further applied closed
external drainage system is safer. This method gives us a number of
benefits:the drainage is conducted step by step(thus decreasing the
occurrence of postoperative hematomas); creates better condition for
gradual cerebral decomression,diminishes the infection risk; allow to
make simultaneous drainage of bilateral hematomas, to conduct some
manipulations under local anesthesia. Etiology of the disease, age of
the patients, clinical phase, brain conditions and craniocerebral

relations together with a number of the factors determine the volume of the evacuated liquid after washing out CSH and the drainage duration. Several studies (4,5,6) showed the increase of the fiber disintegration products in the hematoma cavity causing the local hyperfibrinolisis and provoking repeated hemorrhages from the vessels of the external membrane. The evacuation of the CSH content and it's washing out from CSH cavity by the saline solution disrupt,the self-supporting cycle of microhemorrages from the pathologic newly-formed capillaries. Dynamic CT and MRI showed total disappearance
of CSH after drainage. Our findings show,that the process of brain reexpansion takes from 1 to 3 months after operation (depending on the age of the patient, age of the hematoma, the clinical phase and craniocerebral complications).That is why the liquid remnants in the hematoma cavity after its washing by the saline solution and drainage of its content without clinical deterioration,can't be an indication for the second operation and/or the prolonged stay in the hospital. We consider that further optimization of the CSH treatment demands studying pathogenic mechanisms of the CSH formation.

REFERENCES

1.Tabbador K, Shulman K(1977) Diffinitive treatment of chronic subdural hematoma by twist-drill craniostomy and closed-system drainage. J.Neurosurgery,46,220-226.
2.Markwalder Th.-M.,Reulen H.J.(1986) Influence of Neomembraneous Organization, Cortical expansion and Subdural Pressure on the Post-operative Course of Chronic Subdural Haematoma - an Analysis of 201 cases. Acta Neurochirurgica,79,100-106.
3. Rychlicki F,Recchioni M.A.,Burchiani M.,Marcolini P., Messoria A., Papo J. Percutaneus Twist-Drill Craniotomy for Treatment of Chronic Subdural Haematoma

4. Labadie E.L.,Glover D. (1975) Local alterations of hemostatic-fibrinolitic mechanisms in reforming subdural hematomas. Neurology,25,669-675.
5. Ito H, Yamamoto S, Komai T, Mizukoshi H (1976) Role of local hyperfibrinolisis in the etiology of chronic subdural hematoma. J.Neurosurgery,45,26-31.
6. Ito H, Saito K, Yamamoto S, Hasegawa T (1988) Tissue-type plasminogen activator in the chronic subdural hematoma.Surg.Neurol.30: 175-179.

Chronic Subdural Hematoma in Adults as Compared with Aged Group

Hiroshi Takahashi and Shozo Nakazawa
Department of Neurosurgery, Nippon Medical School, Bunkyo-ku, Tokyo, 113 Japan

SUMMARY

Recently, 150 patients with chronic subdural hematoma, including 50 who were over 70 years old, were surgically treated. The clinical features and prognosis of these aged patients were analyzed. In the aged group (over 70 years old), dementia and urinary incontinence were seen in 50% and 24% of the patients, respectively. These rates were significantly different from those in the adult group (under 69 years old). Headache occurred in only 2% of the patients in the aged group, but in 58% of the patients in the adult group, a significantly difference. After surgery, the recovery of dementia was good (87%) in the group with dementia after chronic subdural hematoma (15 cases), but very poor in the group with dementia before chronic subdural hematoma (10 cases). In the aged group, bilateral hematoma occurred, more frequently, and CT scan showed mixed density hematoma more often than in the adult group. This type of hematoma sometimes causes apoplectic onset of chronic subdural hematoma. This study suggests that exact diagnosis is important when faced with aged patients with unusual dementia.

KEY WORDS: chronic subduarl hematoma, aged, dementia, headache,

INTRODUCTION

With regard to brain disease in the aged, there are few symptoms of intracranial hypertension, but the incidence of psychological symptom is high. Accordingly, there is a real risk of misunderstanding the patient's condition as senile psychotic or mental disturbance or even a cerebrovascular disease. Therefore, it is very important to focus discussion on aged patients who show dementia at the time of chronic subdural hematoma (CSDH). In the present study, we carried out clinical investigations on adult patients with CSDH as compared with aged group, and various interesting findings were obtained.

MATERIALS AND METHODS

During a recent five-year period, 150 patients with CSDH were surgically treated at the Department of Neurosurgery, Nippon Medical School and its associated hospitals. Those patients included 50 aged cases of 70 or more years, with a mean age of 76.2 years (Aged Group). The remaining 100 patients were less than 70 years of age, and their mean age was 57.3 years (Adult Group). By performing comparative studies on these two patient groups, we investigated the characteristics and outcome of the disease state of CSDH in the aged patients as compared with adult cases.

RESULTS

1. Sex

The 50 patients in the Aged Group consisted of 35 (70%) males and 15 (30%) females, with the 100 patients in the Adult Group included 72 (72%) male and 28 (28%) female patients. Thus, both groups contained a preponderance of male patients.

2. Trauma

Trauma had been experienced by 88% of the Aged Group patients who showed symptoms of dementia, and by 92% of the Aged Group patients without symptoms of dementia. In the Adult Group, the comparable percentages were 92% and 90%. Thus, almost no difference were found between the two patient groups in regard to the presence or absence of trauma.

3. Symptoms

As shown in Fig. 1, symptoms of dementia were seen in 50% of the Aged Group patients, which was clearly higher than the 35% of the Adult Group patients showing dementia (p<0.05). Urinary incontinence was seen in 24% of the Aged Group patients, which was again clearly higher than the 11% seen in the Adult Group patients (p<0.05). However, headache-which is thought to be indicative of intracranial hypertension- was experienced by 58% of the Adult Group patients, but by only 2% of the Aged Group patients. Thus, the incidence of headache was significantly higher in the Adult Group than the Aged Group (p<0.05). In addition, hemiparesis, which must be distinguished from cerebral infarction in elderly patients, was observed in 40% of the Aged patients and 52% of the Aged Group patients, the difference between the groups for this symptom was not statiscally significant.

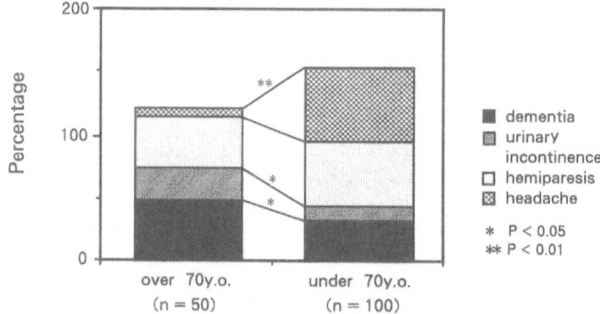

Fig. 1   Symptoms of chronic subdural hematoma in Aged and Adult Groups.

4. Outcome

We divided the Aged Group into two subgroups, depending on whether or not the patient had experienced dementia-like symptoms even prior to the development of CSDH. Fifteen of the aged patients had not shown any particular clear symptoms of dementia before the CSDH, while 10 patients had. Fig.2 presents the data on the rates of

114

postoperative recovery of these two aged patient subgroups from the symptoms of dementia and hemiparesis. It is seen that the aged patients who manifested dementia only after the development of CSDH showed a comparatively high, 87% rate of recovery from the dementia symptoms after the surgery. In contrast, the postoperative recovery rate was a low 30% for the aged patients who had manifested dementia symptoms even prior to the CSDH and which had become more severe after the development of CSDH. The difference between these two recovery rates was statistically significant (p<0.05). The rates of recovery from the symtom of hemiparesis were high values of 93% and 09% for these two subgroups of aged patients.

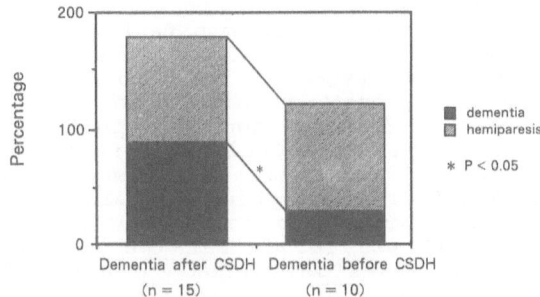

Fig. 2   Recovery of symtoms after operation in Aged and Adult Groups of chronic subdural hematoma.

5. Type of Hematoma

As shown in Fig.3, the analysis of hematoma revealed that the apoplectic type, which is accompanied by sudden manifestation of severe disturbance of consciousness and hemiparesis, was present in only 1% of the Adult Group, compared with a high 6% of the Aged Group. This difference was statistically significant (p<0.05). In addition, the incidence of bilateral hematoma was only 10% in the Adult Group, compared with a high incidence of 32% in the Aged Group (P<0.01). Finally, the hematoma showed a mixed density on the CT scan in 8% of the Adult Group, but in a significantly higher 20% in the Aged Group (P<0.05). Also, a CT scan often revealed bilateral CSDH of mixed density, with niveau formation. Thus, these three types of hematoma were surmised to be characteristic of CSDH in elderly patients 70 years of age or more.

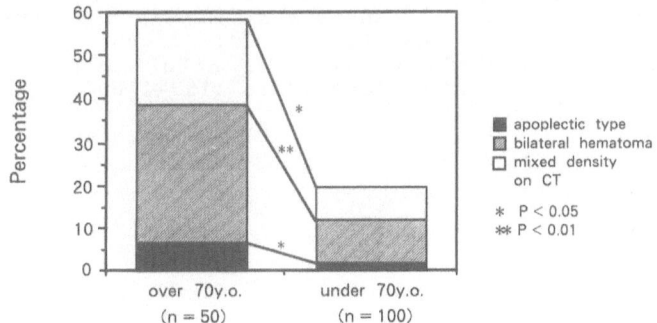

Fig.3   Significant clinical findings in Aged and Adult Groups of chronic subdural hematoma.

DISCUSSION

Regarding the distribution of CSDH by sex and age, it has been reported that CSDH is generally more common in males, and in the 30-60 year-old age bracket [1]. In the present study, the patients in the Adult Group showed a tendency to be almost the same as the general population. It was especially noteworthy that, even in the Aged Group of patients aged 70 years or more, males still predominant as same as in the Adult Group. In addition, regarding the involvement of an earlier trauma to the head, as well, there was no great difference between the Aged Group and the Adult Group. On the other hand, as characteristic feartures of CSDH in the elderly patients, it has been reported that intracranial hypertension does not readily manifest, whereas there are many cases that manifest psychotic symptoms [1]. Our present study provided similar findings. Moreover, we demonstrated that dementia is more likely to be a chief complaint in the elderly patients and that urinary incontinence is present as a complication at a high rate in the aged patients.

Analysis of the outcome of these CSDH patients after surgical removal of the hematoma yielded interesting findings. First, after the surgery, the hemiparesis that had been seen in the patients prior to the surgery was greatly improved in both the Aged Group and the Adult Group. In contrast, it was found that the degree of recovery from the symptoms of dementia was influenced to a considerable extent by the nature of their manifestation prior to the operation for the CSDH. In the present study, we elucidated the characteristic features of hematomas in aged patients. That is, we demonstrated that the Aged Group patients showed significantly greater incidences of hematomas that were bilateral and of mixed density on CT scans, as well as the apoplectic type, which is known to progress to sudden aggravation of symptoms. It has been explained that the reason for the greater incidence of mixed-density subdural hematoma on CT scans in aged patients is due to new hemorrhage into subdural space or subdural hygroma that already exists in the aged brain [2]. In addition, another paper reported that niveau formation was much more commonly observed in elderly patinets [3]. The results of our present study support the findings of these earlier reports.

In summary, it is necessary to take into sufficient account the various findings of CSDH documented in the present study, and it is hoped that clinicians will carry out careful diagnosis and treatment of these cases.

REFERENCES

1. Fogelholm R (1975) J Neurosurg 42: 43-46
2. Miyazaki S, Ohmori H, Kanazawa Y, Munekata K, Fukushima H, Kamata K (1980) Neurol Med Chir (Tokyo) 20: 875-881
3. Fujioka S, Matsukado Y, Kaku M, Sakurama N, Nonaka N, Miura G (1981) Neurol Med Chir (Tokyo) 21: 1153-1160

Development and Treatment of Chronic Subdural Hematoma

HIROMICHI MIYAZAKI, NAOMI ISHIYAMA, KIYOTAKA TAMURA, and
HIROSHI KAGAMI

Department of Neurosurgery, Hiratsuka City Hospital, Hiratsuka, Kanagawa, 254 Japan

SUMMARY

One hundred eleven adult patients with chronic subdural hematoma (SDH)
were reviewed. In 28% of the cases it was observed that traumatic subdural fluid collection (SFC) developed into chronic SDH in successive
computed tomographic (CT) scans after the initial head injury. In 43%
of the cases which had not been followed up after their head injury,
it was assumed that there was also traumatic SFC initially which later
developed into chronic SDH, considering the similarity in temporal
course with the former group. It was proposed that traumatic SFC played an important role in the development of chronic SDH. As for treatment, 99 cases were operated upon; 31 patients underwent craniotomy
and evacuation with membranectomy and later 68 patients had burr-hole
and continuous drainage (simple drainage). Both methods produced comparable good results, clinically and radiographically. The advantages
of simple drainage, i.e., gradual decompression and simplicity of the
procedure make this method a first operative procedure. A theoretical
basis supporting simple drainage is discussed.

KEY WORDS: subdural hematoma, head injury, subdural fluid collection,
drainage

INTRODUCTION

Recently, traumatic SFC has been noted to be a preexisting state of
chronic SDH[1,2]. Our first aim in this study was to estimate how
often chronic SDH developed from traumatic SFC. Although the operative
procedure for chronic SDH has been modified in the past, the consensus
regarding the optimal method has not been established. Our second aim
was to evaluate the efficacy of simple drainage of chronic SDH,
comparing it with other conventional methods.

MATERIALS AND METHODS

A consecutive series of 111 adult patients with chronic SDH between
April 1984 and July 1992 was reviewed. The ages ranged from 32 to 93
years (mean, 69 years). Eighty were male and 31 were female. Twenty-
two patients had bilateral chronic SDH. In all the cases, the course
until the diagnosis of chronic SDH was made was reviewed. Some
patients had been followed since the initial head injury because of
the presence of traumatic SFC on the early CT scans. A traumatic SFC

117

was diagnosed when a crescentic area with CSF (cerebrospinal fluid)-like density, mainly situated on the frontal lobe was found and the change in size and density on successive CT scans was observed. On the other hand, a chronic SDH was diagnosed when the lesion was apparently of higher density than CSF regardless of clinical symptoms. Ninety-nine cases were treated surgically and 12 cases which remained asymptomatic were followed up without treatment. Thirty-one cases (33 SDHs) were treated by evacuation of SDH by craniotomy and irrigation of subdural space with partial membranectomy. Of these, 24 cases were operated under general anesthesia. From March 1988, 68 cases (84 SDHs) underwent burr-hole craniostomy with continuous drainage (simple drainage) under local anesthesia. After making a cruciform incision in the dura and a small incision in the external neomembrane, a ventricular catheter was immediately inserted about 3 cm into the hematoma cavity, brought out from a separate wound and connected to a Jackson-Pratt bulb without suction and placed just below head level. The patient was kept supine until the flow of lique-fied hematoma ceased and the drain was removed, with a mean duration of 2 days. The operative results of these two methods were compared with respect to clinical improvement, resolution of SDH on CT scan, motality, morbidity, complications, and recurrence. Perioperative neurological status was assessed according to Markwalder's classif-cation[3]:Grade 0: normal, Grade 1: alert and orientated; mild symptoms such as headache; absent or mild neurological deficit, Grade2 : drowsy or disorientated with variable neurological deficit, Grade 3: stuporous but responding appropriately to noxious stimuli; severe focal signs, Grade 4: comatose with absent motor response to painful stimuli; decerebrate or decorticate posturing.

RESULTS

According to the course until the diagnosis of chronic SDH was made, the cases were grouped as follows: In 31 cases (Group I : mean age 66 years), it was observed that traumatic SFC developed into chronic SDH on successive CT scans after the initial head injury. Head injury in this group varied in severity from minor trauma to cerebral contusion. In 48 cases (Group II : mean age 69 years) with a history of head injury, mostly minor trauma, but had not been followed up afterwards, the first CT scan showed chronic SDH. The clinical courses from the time of injury to diagnosis of chronic SDH in Group I and II were compared and were apparently similar (Fig. 1) . In three cases (Group III : mean age 71 years), acute SDH treated conservatively developed into chronic SDH. The remaining 27 cases(Group IV: mean age 68 years) had no history of head injury. Two cases with a recurrent hematoma after the first operation from another hospital were excluded.
    The results of evaluation of the two operative procedures(craniotomy vs. simple drainage) are shown in Table 1. The patients are comparable with respect to age, sex, and mean preoperative neurological grade. Mean postoperative neurological grades at 1 week were 0.52 and 0.43, the difference being statistically insignificant and indicates similar rapid improvement in both series. Finally, morbid patients (Grade 1 or 2) were 3 and 1 respectively, excluding initially morbid patients (dementia, etc.). One patient died from cardiac failure 16 days after

the simple drainage, who was an 88-year old female and was comatose preoperatively. No complication occured in either series. Only one patient required a reoperation after simple drainage, due to poor drainage and residual hematoma, as revealed on CT scan after 2 days. A second simple drainage was performed and another intact neomembrane was found. Reaccumulation of hematoma which needed a second operation was not seen in either series. Normal CT scan was obtained within 2 months in 51% and 45% cases of respective series, and cases which showed normal CT scan after 3 months were 36% and 30%, respectively. These imply that the rate of resolution of postoperative subdural collection and reexpansion of the brain is similar in the two methods.

Fig. 1 Relationship between the interval from head injury to diagnosis of chronic SDH and % cases in Group I (open bar) and Group II (shaded bar).

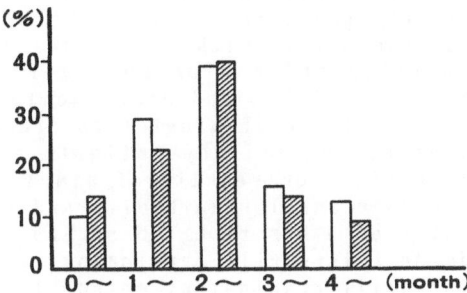

Table 1 Comparative results of two operative procedures.

	cases	mean age(ys)	male/ female	mean neurological grade preop. /postop.1 week		%normal CT scan postop.2 months
craniotomy	31	65	23/8	1.52 /	0.52	45%
drainage	68	69	51/17	1.46 /	0.43	51%

DISCUSSION

The development of chronic SDH are presently explained in terms of formation of a subdural neomembrane, defective hemostasis (hyper-fibrinolysis) and chronic rebleeding[4]. Production of the neomembrane is considered to be triggered by subdural bleeding resulting from various causes, such as injury, coagulation disorder, intracranial hypotension, and infectious diseases[4]. Head injury has long been considered as the most important etiologic factor. Recently, traumatic SFC is noted as a preexisting state of chronic SDH[1,2]. It is esti-mated that nearly 50% of traumatic SFC transform to chronic SDH[2]. On the other hand, it is not clear how often chronic SDH results from traumatic SFC. In the present study, 28% of the chronic SDH had been followed up from the state of SFC. The other 43% of the cases with a history of head injury also seemed to develop from traumatic SFC, because their temporary course from trauma to diagnosis of chronic SDH was quite similar to that of the former group. Although 27% of the patients had no history of head injury, preexistence of traumatic SFC resulting from slight head injury cannot be ruled out, as there were no other etiologic factors. Another study of ours proved that even slight injury could cause traumatic SFC, especially in the elderly[5]. We therefore concluded that most cases of chronic SDH developed from traumatic SFC and other causes are probably rare. It is postulated that traumatic SFC is CSF mixed with varying amounts of blood resulting from arachnoid tear caused by injury, and that persistence of SFC for more than 3 weeks results in the formation of a neomembrane[1]. Transformation from acute SDH to chronic SDH has been reported[3] and was also observed in our study(3%). The mechanism of this transformation is thought to be essentially similar to that of SFC. While various surgical techniques have been proposed for chronic SDH, the present study convinced us that simple drainage is one of the optimal operations. Both of our methods, the conventional method (evacuation by craniotomy with partial membranectomy) and simple drainage (burrhole craniostomy with continuous drainage), showed comparable results clinically and radiographically. It has been shown that complete evacuation of SDH and membranectomy are not necessarily required. It took only 10 to 15 minutes to drain a unilateral chronic SDH by simple drainage, and all the patients could be treated safely under local anesthesia. Our results of simple drainage with no complications or recurrence and low morbidity and mortality rates are superior to the results of other reported series treated by burr-hole evacuation[6] or bedside twist-drill craniostomy with continuous drainage[7]. Although twist-drill craniostomy method is basically similar which avoids rapid decompression of the brain[8], we believe that simple drainage is a more familiar and reliable method which can be performed under most circumstances. The only exception may be a rare existence of a true loculated SDH. Chronic SDH has a natural healing ability, which leads to spotaneous resolusion not rarely encountered (11% of all our cases) [2,8]. Whereas neomembrane is formed as a reparative tissue to absorb SDH, it produces tissue plasminogen activator in excess which causes increased fibrinolytic activity in the SDH producing a large amount of plasmin and fibrinogen degradation products (FDP)[9]. Hyperfibrinolysis and impaired hemostasis destabilizes normal clotting and causes repeated microhemorrhages from the neomembrane. This unbalance betweew absorption and rebleeding brings about expansion of SDH. Simple drainage is effective enough to reduce the fibrinolytic factors and make absorption dominant leading to resolution of SDH.

REFERENCES

1. Yamada H, Watanabe T, Murata S, Shibui S, Nihei H, Kohno T, Itoh T (1980) Surg Neurol 13: 441-448
2. Ohno K, Suzuki R, Masaoka H, Matsushima Y, Inaba Y, Monma S (1987) J Neurol Neurosurg Psychiatry 50: 1694-1697
3. Markwalder TM, Steinsiepe KF, Rohner M, Reichenbach W, Markwalder H (1981) J Neurosurg 55: 390-396
4. Giuffre R (1987) Rivista di Neurologia 57: 298-304
5. Miyazaki H, Ishiyama N, Nakamura A (1991) Neurotraumatology 14: 239 (abstract in Japanese)
6. Robinson RG (1984) J Neurosurg 61: 263-268
7. Camel M, Grubb RL (1986) J Neurosurg 65: 183-187
8. Tabaddor K, Shulman K (1977) J Neurosurg 46: 220-226
9. Ito H, Komai T, Yamamoto S (1978) J Neurosurg 48: 197-2009

Chronic Subdural Hematoma Associated with Middle Cranial Fossa Arachnoid Cyst. Is Cyst Peritoneal Shunt Treatment of Choice?

JUZO ABE, YOSHIO TAGUCHI and HIROAKI SEKINO[1]

[1]Division of Neurosurgery, Second Department of Surgery, St. Marianna University School of Medicine, Kawasaki, Kanagawa, 213 Japan

SUMMARY

We reviewed operative results of 9 patients with chronic subdural hematoma accompanied with arachnoid cyst and also 9patients with arachnoid cyst. We also reviewed incidence and age distribution of patients with arachnoid cyst founded by CTscan out of 14998 patients in our university hospital between 1979 and 1986.As for surgical treatment of arachnoid cyst with cyst-peritoneal shunt is considered good treatment of choice. Considering possible disappearance of arachnoid cyst, some of them may not need operation, if they are followed closely. Unsupported vessels on the surface of arachnoid cysts are most likely course of chronic subdural hematoma.

KEY WORDS: chronic subdural hematoma, middle fossa arachnoid cyst, cyst peritoneal shunt

INTRODUCTION

Combination of middle fossa arachnoid cyst(MFAC) and ipsilateral chronic subdural hematoma(CSDH) are well known. Treatment strategy in this situation has been controversial as well as in arachnoid cyst, no matter what it is symptomatic or incidental. We reviewed operative results of 9 patients with chronic subdural hematoma accompanied with arachnoid cyst and also 9 patients with arachnoid cyst.

MATERIALS AND METHODS

For the past 9 years (January,1983-December,1991), we experienced 181 cases of chronic subdural hematoma out of all patient who came to our university hospital. Their average age was 63.9 years. Nine of them was accompanied with middle fossa arachnoid cyst, with average age of 28.3 years. On the other hand, 33 cases of arachnoid cyst (24 in middle fossa, 8 in posterior fossa, 1 in cerebello-pontine angle) were diagnosed by CT scan out of all patients in our university hospital between 1979 and 1991. Twenty cases of middle fossa arachnoid cyst were found on CT scan out of 14998 patients in our university hospital between 1979 and 1986(Table 1). All patients with MFAC

Table 1 Incidence of middle cranial fossa arachnoid cyst

Age Distribution	0- 9	10-19	20-29	30-39	40-49	50-59	60-69	70-79	80-89	90-99	TOTAL
No. of cranial CT scan	1806	1348	1194	1474	1859	2301	2232	1996	647	41	14998
No. of MFAC	2	8	5	3	2	0	0	0	0	0	20

MFAC=middle fossa arachnoid cyst

was younger than 50 years of age, whereas 49% of 14998 patients were older than 50 years of age.

RESULTS

Nine patients with middle fossa arachnoid cyst were treated surgical-ly(Table 2). Five of them are accompanied with chronic subdural hematoma, and in 4 of them, arachnoid cyst were found incidentally following minor head injury. Craniotomy, membranectomy of arachnoid cyst and cyst peritoneal shunt(C-P shunt) were performed. In 4 pa-tients, C-P shunt was removed after disappearance of arachnoid cyst. In 8 patients arachnoid cyst remains disappeared even after removal of C-P shunt. In one patients, whose C-P shunt was removed because of low pressure headache, arachnoid cyst was slightly enlarged thereaf-ter. No other complication was noted. Four out of 9 patients with chronic subdural hematoma underwent burr hole and irrigation of chronic subdural hematoma(Table 3). In two of such patients, arach-noid cyst became smaller and disappeared during follow up period.

Table 2 Surgical result of cyst-peritoneal shunt for middle fossa arachnoid cysts

Case No.	Age(yrs)	Sex	Type of head injury	Signs and symptom	CSDH	Shunt removal	Compilation	Outcome of MFACs
1 K.A.	10	F	HI type 2	headache	lt.CSDH	9 month later	low ICP headache	slightly enlargement after removal of shunt
2 H.Y.	24	F	HI type 1	headache	lt.CSDH	-	-	
3 T.K.	25	M	HI type 1	headache	rt.CSDH	-	-	disappeared
4 S.S.	33	M	HI type 1	headache	lt.CSDH	-	-	disappeared
5 Y.M	24	F	HI type 1	headache	lt.CSDH	-	-	disappeared
6 A.S.	8	M	HI type 1	headache	-	9 months later	-	disappeared
7 T.I	17	M	HI type 1	no symptom	-	7 months later	-	disappeared
8 T.K.	28	F	HI type 1	no symptom	-	-	-	disappeared
9 K.H.	41	M	HI type 2	no symptom	-	13 months later	-	disappeared

HI type 1=head injury without loss of consciousness ; HI type 2=head injury with loss off consciousness; CSDH =chronic subdural hematoma ; MFAC=middle fossa arachnoid cyst ; ICP=intra cranial pressure ; - =none

Table 3 Surgical result of patients with middle fossa arachnoid cyst accompanied by chronic subdurall hematoma

Case No.	Age(yrs)	sex	Type of head injury	Duration between head injury and operation	Signs and symptoms	Surgical procedures	GOS	Post operative change of MCFACs
1 K.A.	10	F	HI type 2	29 days	headache	C-P shunt menbrenectomy	GR	disappeared
2 H.Y.	24	F	HI type 1	5 months	headache	C-P shunt menbrenectomy	GR	disappeared
3 T.K.	25	M	HI type 1	2 months	headache	C-P shunt menbrenectomy	GR	no change
4 S.S.	33	M	HI type 1	4 month	headache	C-P shunt menbrenectomy	GR	disappeared
5 T.K.	25	M	HI type 1	28 days	headache	C-P shunt menbrenectomy	GR	decreased in size
10 M.T.	15	M	HI type 1	61 days	headache rt.hemiparesis	burr hole irrigation	GR	disappeared
11 A.K.	18	F	HI type 2	61 days	headache	burr hole irrigation	GR	disappears
12 Y.T.	25	M	HI type 1	2 months	headache	burr hole irrigation	GR	disappears
13 T.K.	62	M	HI type 1	1 months	headache rt.hemiparesis	burr hole irrigation	GR	no change

HI type 1=head injury without loss of consciousness ; HI type 2=head injury with loss of consciousness; C-P shunt=cyst peritoneal shut

CASE REPORT

Case 13   25-year-old   man
While he has follow up for incidental arachnoid cyst, he suffered
from traffic accident, hit from behind. Two month later chronic
subdural hematoma was found, and he underwent burr hole and irrigation of CSDH. During followedup period arachnoid cyst became smaller
and one year after operation, it disappeared. Fig. 1

Fig. 1

A
September 1987

B
September 1989

C
December   1990

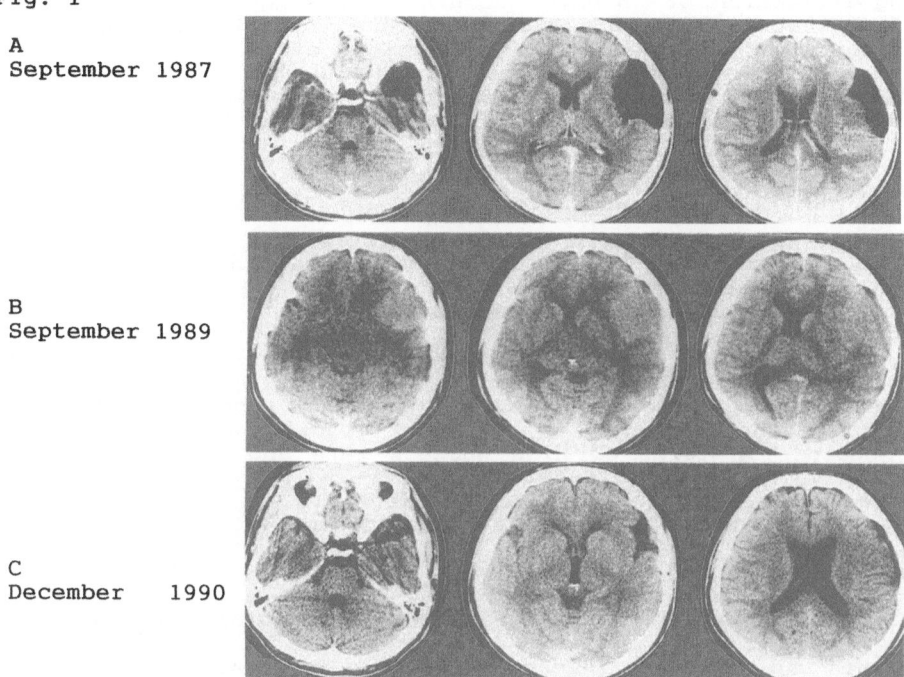

DISCUSSION

Many paper reported arachnoid cysts accompanied with chronic subdural
hematoma[1][2]. Our review showed average years of patients with
chronic subdural hematoma is 63.9 years, whereas patients with arachnoid cyst accompanied with chronic subdural hematoma is apparently
younger as average years of 28.3 years. Incidence of chronic subdural
hematoma accompanied with arachnoid cyst was high as 37.5%. Previous
paper also reported as about 20%[1][3]. Therefore it dose not look
like incidental that these two diseases occurred together. As a cause
of chronic subdural hematoma in patients with arachnoid cyst, we
consider small vessels, confirmed at the time of operation, which
goes through about 5 mm holes of septum between hematoma cavity and
arachnoid cyst, are significant. These small vessels are probably
responsible as source of bleeding at the time of head injury, changing to chronic subdural hematoma later. Treatment strategy has been
controversial including incidental arachnoid cyst. As treatment of
choice, cyst peritoneal shunt, membranectomy of arachnoid cyst making
communication to basal cistern, are reported as about 70% of success
rate[4][5][6][7]. Our method of craniotomy, membranectomy of outer

membrane and C-P shunt resulted disappearance of arachnoid cysts in all patients before removal of C-P shunt. Even if we consider one patients as non successful case, because arachnoid cyst slightly enlarged after removal of C-P shunt, still it makes 89% of disappearance rate. Furthermore with low complication rate, we recommended our method as treatment of choice. Before 1988, it was our policy that all arachnoid cysts, including incidental ones, should be operated with craniotomy, because they had potential risk of bleeding. But with experiences of two patients whose arachnoid cyst disappeared following irrigation of chronic subdural hematoma, and also looking at the fact that no arachnoid cysts was found in patients older than 50 years in this study, we postulate that some of arachnoid cysts may disappear with time. With these back ground, we now think operation is not always necessary for arachnoid cyst, and some of them can be followed safely especially in Japan, where CT scan is easily available.

CONCLUSION

Average years of patients with arachnoid cyst accompanied with chronic subdural hematoma was 28.3 years, much younger than patients with chronic subdural hematoma.
All chronic subdural hematomas accompanied with arachnoid cysts were found following minor head injury.
Unsupported vessels on the surface of arachnoid cysts are most likely course of chronic subdural hematoma.
As for surgical treatment of arachnoid cyst, resection of outer membrane of arachnoid cyst with C-P shunt is considered good treatment of choice, in terms of high success rate and low complication rate.
Considering possible disappearance of arachnoid cyst, some of them may not need operation, if they are followed closely.

REFERENCES

1. Aicardi J, Bauman F (1975) Supratentorial cerebral cysts in

   infants and children. J Neurol Neurosurg Psychiatry 38: 57-68
2. LaCour F, Trevor R, Carey M (1978) Arachnoid cyst and associated subdural hematoma. Arch Neurol 35: 84-89
3. Robinson RG (1955) Intracranial collection of fluid with local bulging of the skull. J Neurosurg 12: 345-353
4. Dyck P, Gruskin P (1977) Supratentorial arachnoid cysts in adults. Arch Neurol 34: 276-279
5. Menzes AH, Bell WE, Perret GE (1980) Arachnoid cysts in children. Arch Neurol 37: 168-172
6. Kaplan BJ, Mickle JP, Parkhurst R (1984) Cystoperitoneal shunting for congenital arachnoid cysts. Child's Brain 11: 304-311
7. Stein SC (1981) Intracranial developmental cysts in children. Treatment by cystoperitoneal shunting. Neurosurgery 8: 647-650

The Relationship Between Cephalic Index and Chronic Subdural Hematoma

MASAZUMI SATO, NOBUMASA KUWANA, YASUHIRO KOJIMA, NOBUMASA TANAKA, and SYUTARO OCHIAI

Department of Neurosurgery, Yokohama Minami-Kyosai Hospital, Yokohama, Kanagawa, 236 Japan

SUMMARY

A low cephalic index, also called 'dolichocephaly' has been observed in patients with chronic subdural hematomas. So we paid close attention to the cephalic index in head trauma patients and evaluated its relationship with chronic subdural hematoma. Sixty-five patients with chronic subdural hematomas who were treated between January, 1983, and December,1987, and 65 patients aged 40 years or older who were treated for head trauma which caused no intracranial hematoma, randomly sampled, as a control group, a total of 130 patients were studied for cephalic index on plain craniogram. The mean cephalic index was smaller in the chronic subdural hematoma group than in the control group for both males(79.0 vs 82.0) and females(80.8 vs 82.9). The percentage of males with dolichocephaly was significantly higher in the chronic subdural hematoma group(15.1% or 8/53 cases)than in the control group (1.9% or 1/53 cases)($p = 0.014$). The smaller the cephalic index, the greater the rotatory moment in the cranial axial direction. This moment may generate angular acceleration and cause a traction of the bridging vein. Thus, resulting in the onset of chronic subdural hematoma. On the other hand, the same endocrine environment may be related to the development of both dolichocephaly and chronic subdural hematoma. Particular attention should be given to chronic subdural hematoma after head trauma in adults with dolichocephaly on plain craniogram.

KEY WORDS: cephalic index, chronic subdural hematoma, dolichocephaly, head trauma

INTRODUCTION

We had an opportunity to treat two impressive chronic subdural hematoma patients with so-called 'hyperdolichocephaly'. Both had extremely long cranial lengths and small cephalic indices (one of these cases is shown in Fig. 1). The similarities of these two cases prompted us to pay close attention to the cephalic index in head trauma and evaluate its relationship with chronic subdural hematoma.

MATERIALS AND METHODS

Between January 1983 and December 1987, we treated 65 chronic subdural hematoma patients, 53 males and 12 females. Sixty-five randomly selected patients aged 40 years or older, 53 males and 12 females, were also treated for head trauma in the same period. This second group had no intracranial hematoma in the subsequent clinical follow-up and they served as a control group. The cephalic index (breadth× 100/ length) was determined on plain craniograms obtained from these 130 patients.

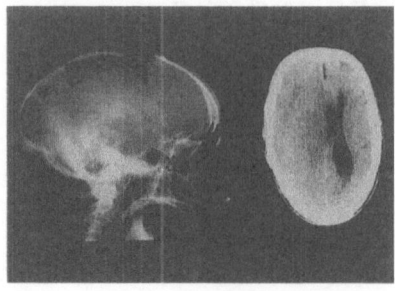

Fig. 1 A chronic subdural hematoma in a 69-years-old man with "hyperdolichocephaly"

Table 1 Mean cephalic index of each group

| | Cephalic Index (mean±standard deviation) | |
	CSDH (mean 66.4y)	Control (mean 64.3y)
Male	79.0±4.22 (n=53)	82.0±3.56 (n=53)
Female	80.8±4.75 (n=12)	82.9±2.76 (n=12)

The breadth was defined as the maximum diameter of the cranium on anteroposterior view and the length as the distance between glabella and inion. Of the 65 patients with chronic subdural hematoma, 54 patients (45 males and 9 females) had a known history of head trauma, while the history of head trauma remained ambiguous in the remaining 11 patients. However, it was thought that these 11 patients also had some trauma which served as a trigger, because other contributing factors such as craniotomy, shunting procedure, other intracranial lesion, hemorrhagic diathesis and anticoagulant therapy were not included [5. 9] Although almost all of these patients lived in the eastern part of Kanagawa Prefecture, their origins unknown. The meanage of the patients with chronic subdural hematoma was 66.4 years, andthose in the control group was 64.3 years.

RESULTS

The mean cephalic index was smaller in the chronic subdural hematoma group than in the control group for both males(79.0 vs 82.0) and females (80.8 vs 82.9) as shown in Table 1. The percentage of males with dolichocephaly was higher in the chronic subdural hematoma group (15.1% or 8／53 cases)than in the control group (1.9% or 1／53 cases) as shown in Table 2 and Fig. 2. The difference between the two percentages was statistically significant(p = 0.014). Among the patients with known history of head trauma, dolichocephaly was observed in 7 out of the 45 males (15.6%), this figure was also significantly higher than the control group (p = 0.015).

Table 2 Distribution of cephalic index in each group

| No. of Cases | Male | | | Female | |
	CSDH	CSDH with HI	Control	CSDH	Control
Dolichocephaly	8 (15.1%)	7 (15.6%)	1 (1.9%)	1 (8.3%)	0 (0 %)
Normocephaly	42 (79.2%)	35 (77.8%)	41 (77.4%)	8 (66.7%)	10 (83.3%)
Brachycephaly	3 (5.7%)	3 (6.7%)	11 (20.8%)	3 (25.0%)	2 (16.7%)
Total	53	45	53	12	12

Abbreviation. CSDH, chronic subdural hematoma; HI, head injury

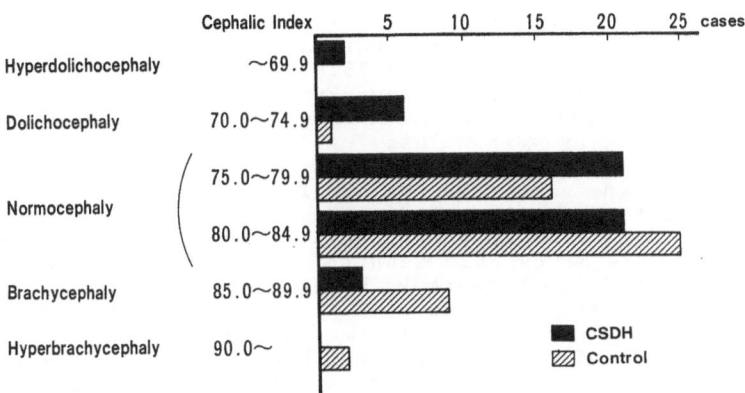

Fig. 2 Graph illustraring the distribution of cephalic index in each group

DISCUSSION

Individual differences in cephalic index can be explained by various factors. In infancy and early childhood, it is mainly determined by the timing of closure of sagittal and coronal sutures. In adolescent males, it decreases due to the development of arcus superciliaris and protuberantia occipitalis externa under the influence of androgen and growth hormone. Both androgen and growth hormone may precipitate chronic subdural hematoma, the former by inducing aggressive behaviors and the latter by stimulating the synthesis of collagen [2]. It is therefore likely that such endocrine environment is related to the development of both dolichocephaly and chronic subdural hematoma. This may explain why chronic subdural hematoma is more prevalent in males than in females.

Dynamically, rotatory moment is likely to be produced by excentric external force upon injury of the head, like a football hitting the ground. Suppose that the cross section of the cranium is an ellipse with a shorter radius "a" and a longer radius 1, as shown in Fig. 3. If the stress produced upon impact of this ellipse with a plane at a given point $P(x_1, y_1)$ is defined as F, moment M is given by the following equilibrium.

$$M = C\ x_1 y_1 (1 / a^2 - 1)\ F$$

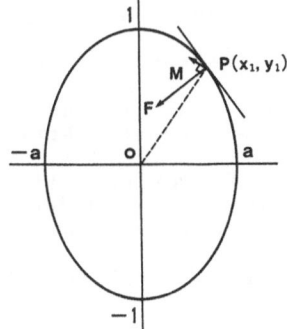

Fig. 3 If the stress at a point P is defined as F, moment M is given by the equilibrium above.

Table. 3 Moment at the same stress on various shape of cranium

Cephalic Index(a)	Moment(M)
70.0	1.04 Cx_1y_1F
75.0	0.79 Cx_1y_1F
80.0	0.56 Cx_1y_1F
85.0	0.38 Cx_1y_1F
90.0	0.23 Cx_1y_1F

"M" increases as "a" decreases.　　In other words, the smaller the cephalic index, the greater the moment in the cranial axial direction. In the case whose cephalic index is 75.0, the moment is about twice as much as in the case of 85.0, as shown in Table 3. This moment may generate angular acceleration in the cranial axial direction and cause a tension of the bridging vein.　Thus, resulting in the onset of chronic subdural hematoma.　Dynamically, other traumatic lesions such as acute subdural hematoma may also occur by similar mechanisms, but this issue will be dealt with in further studies.

In general, Japanese have shorter cranial lengths than Caucasians, but reported incidences of chronic subdural hematoma are higher in Japan (5.0-5.3 ／ 100,000 inhabitants in Miyagi Prefecture between 1983 and 1986 [8]) than in Western countries (1.72 ／ 100,000 inhabitants in Helsinki between 1967 and 1973 [1]).　Since various factors are involved in the onset of chronic subdural hematoma, a simple comparison can not be made between different races with different life styles.

The cephalic index also differs from one region to another in Japan: in general, it is longer in northern Japan than in western Japan [4] . In addition, the tendency has been to become shorter over the last several decades [6] , with younger Japanese having lower cephalic indices than older generations.　Thus in this study, the two groups of Japanese were in the same age group and from the same geographical area so that individual differrences could be focused on.

Although there have been various studies to explain the etiology of chronic subdural hematoma, no author, to our knowledge, has dealt with the implication of anthropological measurements such as the cephalic index.　Based on this study, doctors treating adult patients with dolichocephaly on plain craniogram, that have head trauma should take care the possibility of chronic subdural henatoma.

REFFERENCES

1. Fogelholm R, Heiskanen O, Waltimo O (1975) Chronic subdural hematoma in adult; Influence of patient's age on symptoms, signs, and thickness of hematoma. J Neurosurg 42: 43-46
2. Ganong WF (1987) Review of medical physiology, 13th ed. Lange Medical Publ. pp373-397
3. Miklashevskaya NN (1968) Sex distinction in the cephalic growth of children and adolescents of different races. Proc 8th Intern Cong Anthrop Ethn Sc 1-8
4. Miyamoto H (1924) An anthropological study of the human skelton in modern Japanese. J. Anthrop. Soc. Nippon 39: 307-450
5. Nakamura N (1966) The relationship between head injuies and chronic subdural hematoma. Brain and Nerve 18: 702-709
6. Nakashima T (1986) Brachycephalization in the head form of school girls in North Kyushu. J UOEH 8: 411-414
7. Sato M, kuwana N, Kojima Y, Tanaka N (1992) Cephalic index in the case of chronic subdural hematomas; A preliminary report. Neurol Surg 20: 153-155
8. Suzuki S, Niizuma H, Sakurai Y, Yoshimoto T, Suzuki J (1988) Recent tendency of the occurrence of 716 cases of chronic subdural hematoma in Miyagi prefecture. Proceeding of 11th conference of Japanese society of neurotraumatology: 24-27
9. Yamamoto S (1979) Chronic subdural hematoma. Neurol Med Chir 19: 401-409

Analysis of MR Findings on Initial Stage of Chronic Subdural Hematoma – Evaluation of Proton Density Image

YUKIHIRO MATSUMOTO[1], KAZUO MORINAGA[1], MIKIYA UEDA[1], SHUJI OKAWARA[1], and YOSHIO TAKAHASHI[2]

[1]Okawara Neurosurgical Hospital, Muroran, 050 Japan, and [2]Hokkaido Children's Hospital and Medical Center, Otaru, 047-02 Japan

SUMMARY

Among 42 patients with chronic subdural hematoma after head trauma over a period of 2 year, 9 patients could be performed serial MR scan on a 0.2 Tesla permanent magnetic system. In process of changing from subdural fluid collection to chronic subdural hematoma,the findings of proton density image (spin echo 2000/38), T_1-weighted image (spin echo 500/25), and CT were compared.

As a result, the initial changes of MR findings were as follows : First, the increased signal of subdural fluid collection was observed on proton density image, which made the borderline between subdural fluid collection and subarachnoid space. The borderline on proton density image was detected from 7 to 32 days (mean 17.9 days) after head trauma, which was earlier than T_1-weighted image (from 17 to 56 days, mean 36.4 days) in each case.

It is considered that the above-mentioned borderline on proton density image is the earliest change on MR findings of chronic subdural hematoma, and possibly this borderline suggest the formation of inner membrane of chronic subdural hematoma.

Key words : chronic subdural hematoma, subdural fluid collection, MRI, proton density image

INTRODUCTION

Recently, reports of MR findings of chronic subdural hematoma gradually increase, but there have been few studies of MR findings on the initial stage of chronic subdural hematoma[1]. The purpose of this study is to evaluate MR findings on initial of chronic subdural hematoma, especially according to comparison of proton density image and T_1-weighted image.

MATERIALS AND METHODS

Among 42 consecutive patients with chronic subdural hematoma after head trauma over a period of 2 years, 9 patients could be performed serial MR and CT scan. There were 7 men and 2 women ranging in age from 59 to 88 years. MR was performed with a 0.2 Tesla permanent magnetic system (Hitachi MRP-20). The pulse sequences were used proton density image (spin-echo technique TR/TE = 2000/38) and T_1-weighted image (spin-echo technique TR/TE = 500/25). All patients were performed serial MR and CT scan from 3 to 9 times In the process of changing from subdural fluid collection to chronic subdural hematoma, proton density image, T_1-weighted image and CT findings were compared.

ILLUSTRATIVE CASE

〈Case 1〉 70-year-old man (Fig. 1, 2)

On 22 days after head trauma, CT showed bilateral subdural fluid collection. On T_1-weighted image, subdural fluid collection showed low signal intensity. But on proton density image, the signal intensity of subdural fluid

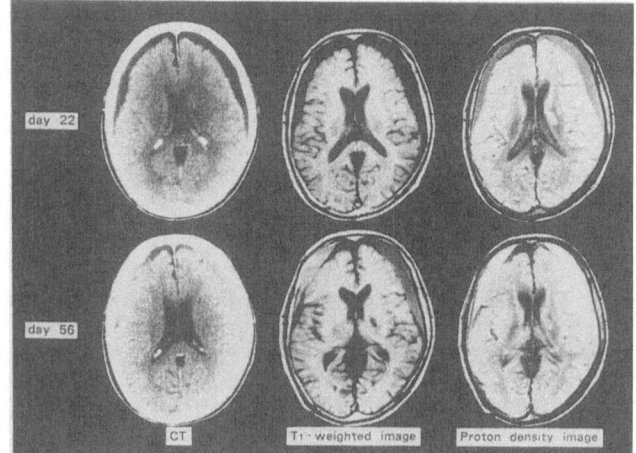

Fig. 1　Case 1　70 y.o M

collection demonstrated slightly higher than that of subarachnoid space, and the borderline due to difference of the signal between subdural fluid collection and sub-arachnoid space at left frontal region was observed (Fig. 2 arrows).

On proton density image 56 days later, the high signal of subdural fluid collection became more evident. In addition, the signal inten-

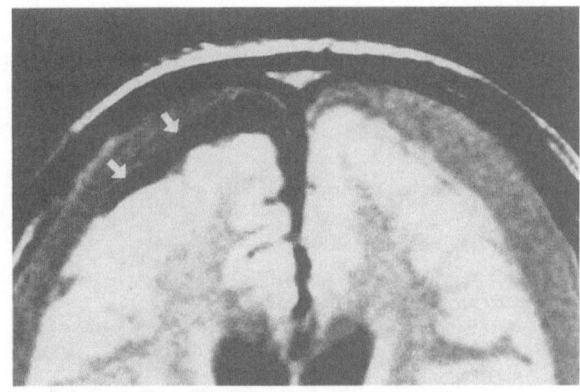

Fig. 2　Magnified image of proton density image（day 22）

sity of subdural fluid collection on T_1-weighted image changed high signal and it made the borderline between subdural fluid collection and subarachnoid space. CT on the same day was allowed a diagnosis of chronic subdural hematoma.

Retrospectively, the borderline between subdural fluid collection (high signal) and subarachnoid space (low signal) on proton density image was observed earlier than that of T_1-weighted image.

RESULTS

As a result of this study, the initial changes of MR findings in process from head trauma to chronic subdural hematoma were as follows : First, subdural fluid collection appeared after head trauma, and the increased signal of subdural fluid collection was observed on proton density image, which made the borderline between subdural fluid collection and subarachnoid space. Subsequently, T_1-weighted image also demonstrated the

Tabel 1　Period from head trauma to appearance of the borderline between subdural fluid collection and subarachnoid space

Case	Age/Sex	Proton density image	T_1-weighted image
1	70/M	22 days	56 days
2	70/M	13	27
3	67/M	11	19
4	72/M	32	46
5	59/M	17	30
6	65/M	24	38
7	74/M	21	56
8	75/F	7	17
9	88/F	14	40
		Mean 17.9 days	Mean 36.4 days

high signal of subdural fluid collection and the borderline.

In all 9 patients, the period from head trauma to appearance of the borderline between subdural fluid collection and subarachnoid space were summarized in Table 1. The borderline on proton density

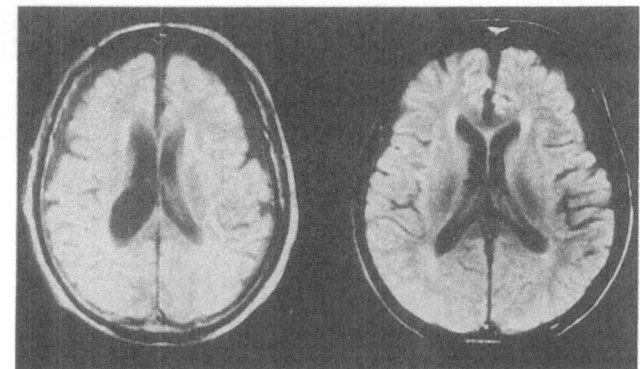

Fig. 3   Subdural fluid collection in cases with cerebral atrophy. The borderline between subdural fluid collection and subarachnoid space were not observed on proton density image.

image was detected from 7 to 32 days (mean 17.9 days) after head trauma,which was earlier than T_1-weighted image (from 17 to 56 days, mean 36.4 days) in each case.

Those findings were not observed in cases with cerebral atrophy (Fig. 3).

It is considered that the increased signal of subdural fluid collection and the borderline on proton density image are the earliest changes on MR findings of chronic subdural hematoma, and possibly this borderline suggest the formation of inner membrane of chronic subdural hematoma.

CONCLUSION

1) The increase of signal intensity of subdural fluid collection and the borderline between subdural fluid collection and subarachnoid space were observed on proton density image earlier than T_1-weighted image.

2) Proton density image is useful for assessment on initial stage of chronic subdural hematoma.

REFERENCES

1) Tsuchiya N, Muraki M, Ninchoji T, et al : Magnetic resonance imaging in chronic subdural hematoma of early stages. CT Kenkyu 12 : 505 − 512, 1990

Chronic Subdural Hematomas: Pathophysiological Studies with MR Imaging and SEP

MAKIO KAMINOGO, AKIO ICHIKURA, AKIRA OCHI, MASANARI ONIZUKA, and JIRO MOROKI

Department of Neurosurgery, Yamaguchi Central Hospital, Hofu, Yamaguchi, 747 Japan

SUMMARY

Comparative evaluations of the MR findings, clinical symptoms, and hematoma fluid contents of 19 chronic subdural hematomas(CSHs) in 16 patients were performed to clarify the etiology of the development of CSH. CSHs were classified into four groups according to the MR findings. Hematomas showed iso-or hypointense on T1-weighted(T1-W) images and proton density-Weighted(D-W) images and hypointense on T2-weighted(T2-W) images in 6 CSHs (group A). They were hyperintense on T1-W and D-W images and hypointense on T2-W images in group B (10 CSHs) and hyperintense on T1-W, D-W, and T2-W images in 2 CSHs (group C). In the remaining CSH (group D), the hematoma showed mildly hypointense on T1-W images, isointense on D-W images, and hyperintense on T2-W images (group D). The intervals between the onset of symptoms and MR examinations were less than 5 days in 5 of 6 CSHs of group A, 4-16 days in all but one CSHs of group B (the exceptional one being an incidental case), 22 and 32 days in group C, and 46 days in group D. RBC counts, Hb , and the Hct of the hematoma fluid were also the highest in group A and the lowest in group D. This finding indicates that large amount of rebleeding took place as neurological symptoms developed and that rebleeding into a hematoma cavity was also responsible for the enlargement of CSH. The central conduction times (CCTs) of somatosensory evoked potentials(SEPs) were examined, because not only the motor pathway but also the sensory pathway should be affected by the extraaxial mass. CCTs were examined in 8 of 14 CSHs with motor weakness, however no case showed an abnormality of the sensory pathway. This suggests that the motor function was more vulnerable to extraaxial compression than the sensory pathway. Further studies are indicated for the evaluation of these mechanisms.

KEY WORDS: chronic subdural hematoma, magnetic resonance imaging, hematoma fluid, somatosensory evoked potential, central conduction time

INTRODUCTION

The characteristic findings of magnetic resonance imaging(MRI) in chronic subdural hematoma(CSH) have been reported as hyperintense on both T1 and T2 weighted(T1-W and T2-W) MRI[1, 2]. However, this seems inconsistent with the pathogenetic consideration of CSH that recurrent bleeding from the hematoma capsule is important in the etiology of the CSH[3]. In this study, the MR findings, clinical symptoms, and the content of the hematoma fluid were comparatively evaluated to clarify the etiology of the development of CSH.

Motor weakness is one of the most frequent symptoms in CSHs, however, sensory deficit is not so often reported. The motor pathway seems to be predominantly affected by the extraaxial mass. However, the degree to which the sensory pathway is also affected is not yet clear. Since the central conduction time(CCT) of somatosensory evoked potential(SEP) is reported to be a sensitive indicator of the functional integrity of the sensory pathway[4], it was also examined in order to evaluate the effect of CSH on the somatosensory system.

MATERIALS AND METHODS

19 CSHs in 16 patients (ages 41 to 96 years old) were reviewed retrospectively. In general, imaging was carried out on a 1.5-T GE imager (Signa) using spin-echo(SE) sequences with 300-500 / 20-30 (TR/TE) and 2000-2200/30-90/2. All hematomas were evacuated within a day after the MR examinations using a one burr hole evacuation and irrigation with saline through the catheter placed in the cavity. The indication for surgery was the presence of severe headache, motor weakness, or altered consciousness in all but one incidental case. The diagnosis of CSH was confirmed by the presence of outer and inner capsule membranes. SEPs were recorded from the sensory cortex and the second cervical spine through median nerve simulation(2Hz, 128 times). The CCT was obtained as a time interval between the first negative peak from the second cervical spine (N14) and the initial negative potential from the somatosensory cortex (N20). Since the CCT in the control groups were 5.6± 0.4 msec, a CCT longer than 6.5 msec (>mean+2sd) was defined as abnormal.

RESULTS

Preoperative symptoms, of altered consciousness, headache, and motor weakness were observed in the sixth, twelfth, and, fourteenth CSHs respectively. One incidental CSH was operated on because of the presence of a midline shift (about 1cm) on CT scan and MRI. A history of head injuries preceding the development of symptoms were reported in 12 CSHs of 11 patients. The injuries were minor in all cases. The mean intervals between the head injuries and the onset of symptoms was 63.6 ± 34.0 days.

Hematomas showed mixed signal intensities in some instances, however, CSHs could be classified into four groups according to the main signal intensities on T1-W, proton density-weighted(D-W), and T2-W images(Table 1). The recurrence of symptoms and reaccumulation of hematoma fluid occurred in 2 CSHs, one was from group A and the other was in group D.

Table 1. MR findings of CSHs

Group	Number of cases	signal intensity T1 - W	signal intensity D - W	signal intensity T2 - W
A	6	L or I	L or I	L
B	10	H	H	L
C	2	H	H	H
D	1	L	I	H

L: hypo-signal intensity   I: iso-signal intensity
H: hyper-signal intensity

The interval between the onset of symptoms and MR studies were less than 5 days in 5 CSHs of group A, between 4 and 16 days in 9CSHs of group B (the one incidental case was excluded), 22 and 32 days in group C, and 46 days in group D. RBC counts, Hb content, and the Hct value of the hematoma fluid were the highest in group A and the lowest in group D (Table 2).

Table 2. Analysis of hematoma fluid and intervals between onset of symptoms and MR studies

Group	Mean intervals (days)	Hematoma fluid RBC (x 104)	Hematoma fluid Hb (g / dl)	Hematoma fluid Hct (%)
A	5.0 ± 5.7	448 ± 87	14.2 ± 3.2	48.2 ± 10.1
B*	9.0 ± 3.9	397 ± 84	12.0 ± 2.4	43.8 ± 8.8
C	28.5 ± 4.9	281± 89	8.3 ± 2.0	29.2 ± 8.6
D	46	12	0.5	1.2

mean intervals: between onset of symptoms and MR studies(mean±sd)
*: one incidental case was excluded from the calculation of mean interval.

As the parenchymal changes with CSH, the flattening cortical gyri underlying the hematoma was always observed. However, changes of signal intensity indicating brain edema could not be detected in any of the cases. The CCT were examined in 8 of 14 patients with motor weakness. However, no pathological prolongation of the CCT on the lesion side was detected.

DISCUSSION

In this study, it was demonstrated that CSHs showed a greater variety of kinds of signal intensity on MRI than previously reported [1, 2]. In our series, MRI indicated that the fluid contained in the hematoma cavity was much fresher than we expected. It was verified by the examination of hematoma fluid obtained during surgery. According to the reported

MRI study on the various stages of hematoma[5], the MR findings of group A, B, C, and D were considered to be acute, subacute, chronic, and very chronic stage of subdural hematomas. Since the intervals between the onset of symptoms and MR examinations were identical with the ages of the hematomas, rebleeding into a hematoma cavity was thought to be responsible for the enlargement of CSH and the development of symptoms. These findings were also confirmed by examination of the hematoma fluid.

The burr hole evacuation and irrigation of the hematoma cavity with saline is generally accepted today as the rational approach to CSH. In our series, recurrence was observed in 2 CSHs, however, there were no specific MR findings to predict the recurrence of these hematomas.

Not only the motor pathway but also the sensory pathway should be affected by the extraaxial mass, however, only motor weakness is commonly observed. Since sensory deficit might be masked by altered consciousness or dementia developed due to CSHs, CCT which are a very sensitive indicator of the neuronal integrity of the sensory pathways were examined in patients with paresis. The results of this investigation revealed no prolongation of CCT in patients with motor weakness. This indicates that motor function is more vulnerable to the extraaxial mass than the sensory function. Since brain edema was not detected with MRI in the hemispheric white matter even in cases with paresis, functional suppression of cortical neurons, failure of blood supply to the cerebral cortex, or compression of the motor pathway at the cerebral peduncle might be important in the development of paresis. We need further studies to clarify this problem.

REFERENCES

1. Sipponen JT, Sepponen RE, Sivula A (1984) Chronic subdural hematoma: demonstration by magnetic resonance. Radiology 150 : 79-85
2. Hosoda K, Tamaki N, Masumura M, Matsumoto S, Maeda F (1987) Magnetic resonance images of chronic subdural hematomas. J Neurosurg 67 : 677-683
3. Ito H, Yamamoto S, Komai T, Mizukoshi H (1967) Role of local hyperfibrinolysis in the etiology of chronic subdural hematoma. J Neurosurg 45 : 26-31
4. Hume AL, Cant BR (1978) Conduction time in central somatosensory pathways in man. Electroenceph clin Neurophysiol 45 : 361-375
5. Fobben ES, Grossman RI, Atlas S, Hackney DB, Golberg HI, Zimmerman RA, Bilaniuk LT (1988) MR characteristics of subdural hematomas and hygromas at 1.5T. AJR 153 : 589-595

Antifibrinolytic Therapy of Chronic Subdural Hematomas

SHUHEI MIYAZAKI, YOICHI KATAYAMA, TAKASHI TSUBOKAWA, ATSUO YOSHINO, and SEIGOU KOYAMA

Department of Neurological Surgery, Nihon University School of Medicine, Itabashi-ku, Tokyo, 173 Japan

SUMMARY

We treated 182 cases of chronic subdural hematoma (CSH) by burr hole evacuation with subsequent drainage since 1987. In these cases, 36 cases showed unchanged volume of CSHs or further enlargement after initial surgery. We repeated surgical therapy in 20 of these cases which were treated before 1989 (group I). Only a medical therapy with careful observation was employed in the remaining 16 cases treated after 1989 (group II). No significant difference was noted between these 2 groups. The medical therapy in the group II patients consisted of administrations of tranexamic acid (750mg/day, P.O.) and carbazochrome sodium sulfonate (30-60mg/day, P.O.). Tranexamic acid was not administered in the group I patients. CSHs eventually resolved in all of the group I patients after one or more surgical interventions. Complete hematoma resorbence with clinical restoration was, however, also obtained in all of the group II patients with medical therapy alone. No recurrence was observed during the follow-up period ranging from 1 month to 2 years. These results indicate that recurent CSHs can be successfully treated by antifibrinolytic therapy alone and hyperfibrinolysis within CSHs plays a significant role in the enlargement of CSHs.

KEY WORDS: subdural hematoma, fibrinolysis, tranexamic acid, antifibrinolytic therapy

INTRODUCTION

The most common treatment of chronic subdural hematoma (CSH) is evacuation and irrigation of hematoma using burr holes. Such treatment is usually sufficient to achieve a complete neurological restoration and hematoma resorbence [1]. However, recurrence of hematoma sometimes occurs after the evacuation [1], which frequently requires more invasive treatments.
Repeated hemorrhages are currently thought to be the most important mechanism underlying enlargement of CSHs [2, 3]; when the hemorrhages exceed the capability of resorption mechanism, CSH enlarges. It has been proposed that hyperfibrinolysis within CSHs interferes with the hemostasis and facilitates the vascular permeability, resulting in the enlargement of the hematoma [2, 3]. We tested a hypothesis that hyperfibrinolysis plays a significant role in the enlargement by testing the effect of tranexamic acid, an antifibrinolytic agent.

MATERIALS AND METHODS

TABLE 1 Age (year: mean + SD) at the
beginning of the treatments, and hematoma thickness
and density of the patients in 2 groups are shown.
Hematoma thickness(cm: mean + SD) were evaluated on
CT just before the beginning of each treatment.
Hematoma densities were also evaluated at that time
and frequency distribution of hematoma densities was
shown as the number of the patients. No significant
difference in age and hematoma thickness on CT was
noted between these 2 groups. (p<0.39, p<0.26,
respectively)

	group I	group II
Age	66.9 ± 12.5	70.7 ± 12.8
Hematoma Thickness	1.9 ± 0.7	1.7 ± 0.4
Hematoma Density		
HighDensity	5	4
Iso Density	2	2
Low Density	10	9
Mixed Density	2	2

Since 1987, we treated 182 cases of CSHs by evacuation using burr
holes with subsequent drainage. Their ages at the time of the initial
treatment ranged from 35 years to 92 years. Initial symptoms of these
patients consisted of headache (46%), motor dysfunction (31%),
disturbance of consciousness (11%), dementia (6%) and others (6%).
Among these cases, 36 cases demonstrated unchanged volume of CSHs or
even further enlargement after initial surgery. CT scans showed CSHs
of varying density and thickness of more than 1 cm. We repeated
surgical therapy in 20 of these cases which were treated before 1989
(group I). The additional treatments consisted of evacuation of
hematoma using burr holes with subsequent drainage in 5 cases,
evacuation with craniotomy in 5 cases and subdural-peritoneal shunt
(S-P shunt) in 12 cases. In contrast, only a medical therapy with
careful observation was employed in the remaining 16 cases treated
after 1989 (group II). No significant difference in age and hematoma
thickness on CT was noted between these 2 groups (Table 1). Hematoma
densities on CT of the patients in these 2 groups were also shown on
Table 1. The medical therapy in the group II patients consisted of
administrations of tranexamic acid (750mg/day, P.O.) and carbazochrome
sodium sulfonate (30-60mg/day, P.O.). To avoid an increased risk of
obstructive cerebrovascular disease, pentoxifylline (300mg/day, P.O.)
was additionally given in some patients. Tranexamic acid was not
administered in the group I patients.

RESULTS

CSHs eventually resolved in all of the group I patients after one or
more surgical interventions. Complete hematoma resorbence with
clinical restoration was, however, also obtained in all of the group
II patients with medical therapy alone. The duration of the medical
treatments ranged from 1 to 6 months. No recurrence was observed
during the follow-up period ranging from 1 month to 2 years.
Furthermore, no adverse effect of the medical treatment was observed
in this study.

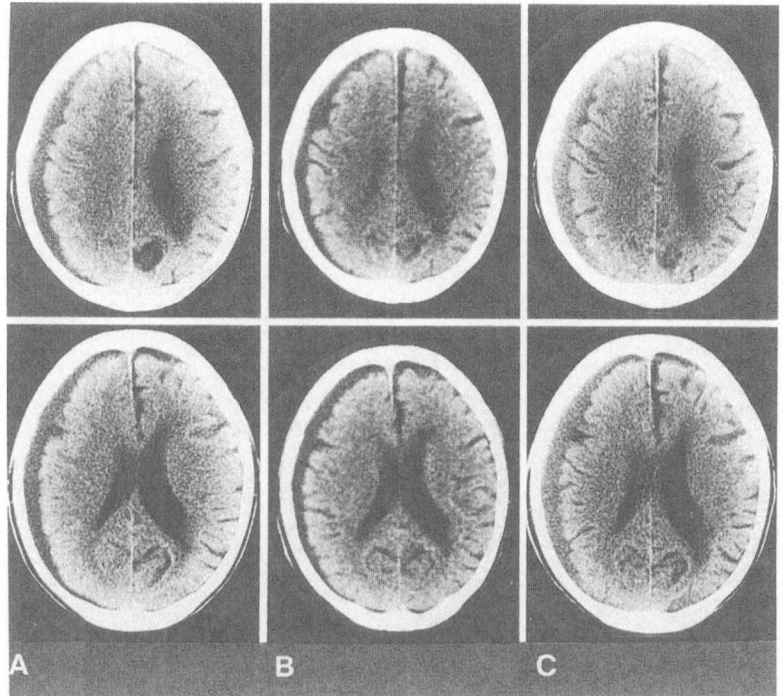

Fig. 1 CT of the reported case before and after an initial surgical treatment. A: CT just before the surgical treatment. B,C: CT of the case at 1 month and 2 months after the surgical treatment, respectively.

CASE REPORT

The patient is a 92-year old man who was referred to our hospital because of a minor head injury. He had only a small wound on the right parietal scalp without any neurological deficit.   It was noted, however, that his gait became disturbed gradually during the follow up period of a month.   CT scan revealed a CSH on the right cerebral convexity (Fig. 1A).   Evacuation of the hematoma was performed under local anesthesia using burr holes.   He showed good recovery with decrease of hematoma size shown by CT, postoperatively (Fig. 1B). About 2 months after the surgical treatment, he had gait disturbance again.   A repeated CT revealed a recurrence of the CSH (Fig. 1C, 2A). Administrations of tranexamic acid (750mg/day, P.O.) and carbazochrome sodium sulfonate (30-60mg/day, P.O.) were started and his gait restored well by 2 weeks later.   Decrease of the hematoma size and density on CT followed the clinical recovery (Fig. 2B).   Disappearance of the hematoma was obtained with antifibrinolytic therapy about 6 months after the beginning of the medical therapy (Fig. 2C).

DISCUSSION

There has been only few discussions regarding medical treatments of CSH[4,5], in contrast to surgical treatments.   Effectiveness of such treatments has been obscure, since the therapeutic assessment was made

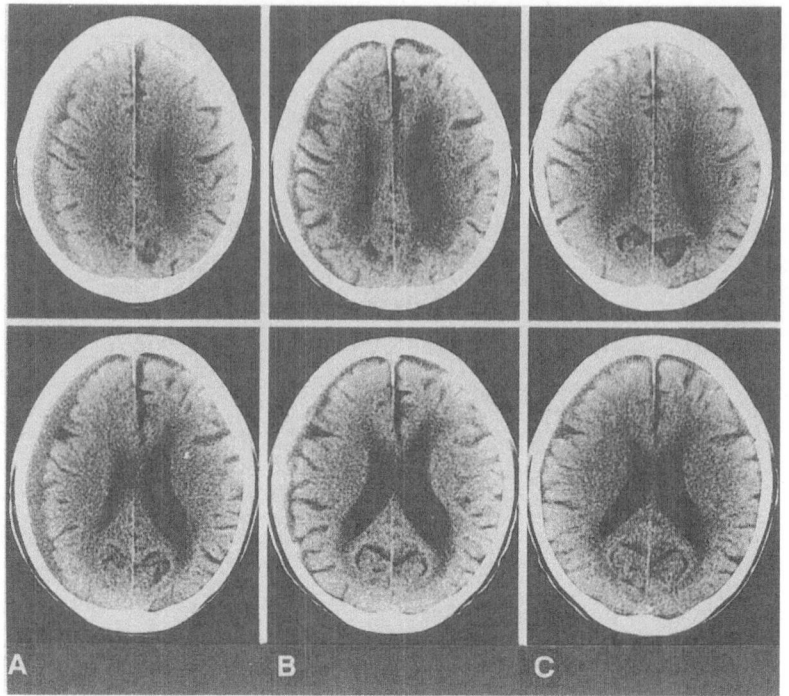

Fig. 2   CT of the reported case before, during and after the medical treatment;   A, CT just before the medical treatment;   B, CT at 3 months after the begining of the medical treatment;   C, CT at 6 months after the begining of the medical treatment.

by clinical observation and angiography[4,5].   Our results indicate that recurrent CSHs can be successfully treated by medical therapy with tranexamic acid alone in many cases.   It is well-known that tranexamic acid is an antifibrinolytic drug which exhibits powerful antifibrinolytic action in central nervous system [6].   Therefore, hyperfibrinolysis presumably within CSHs plays a significant role in the enlargement of CSHs.   While we employed medical therapy only after initial surgical intervention, the observed effect of tranexamic acid appeared to be worthy of further investigation in CSHs in general.

REFERENCES

1.   Markwalder T-M, Steinsiepe KF, Rohner M, Reichenbach W, Markwalder H   (1981) J Neurosurg 55:   390-396
2.   Ito H, Yamamoto S, Komai T, Mizukoshi H (1976) J Neurosurg 45:   26-31
3.   Ito H, Komai T, Yamamoto S (1978) J Neurosurg 48: 197-200
4.   Suzuki J, Takaku A (1970) J Neurosurg 33:   548-553
5.   Bender MB, Christoff N (1974) Arch Neurol 31:   73-79
6.   Tovi D (1973) Acta Neurol Scandinav 49:   163-175

The Treatment of Chronic Subdural Hematoma by Burr-Hole Craniostomy with or without Irrigation and Closed-System Drainage

ATSUSHI TAJIMA, SHIZUO HATASHITA, and HIDEO UENO

Department of Neurosurgery, Juntendo University Urayasu Hospital, Urayasu, Chiba, 272-01 Japan

SUMMARY

We studied to ascertain the efficacy of irrigation of hematoma through burr holes and closed-system drainage for the treatment of chronic subdural hematoma(CSDH). Twenty-two patients were treated by burr-holes irrigation and drainage(Group A) and 24 patients by a burr hole and drainage(Group B). A closed-system drainage was placed within the hematoma cavity for 1 to 2 days. Computerized tomography scans were obtained before and after surgery to assess the maximum thickness of hematoma, residual cavity and accumulation of air. Twenty-one(95%) patients in Group A and 21(88%) in Group B had a functional recovery. Only one patient in each group suffered a recurrence. The reduction rate of the hematoma cavity was 45.4% in Group A and 52.1% in Group B. In contrast, accumulation of air in the subdural space after surgery was present in 13(59%) patients in Group A and in only 3(13%) in Group B($p<0.01$). One patient in Group A developed symptomatic subdural tension pneumocephalus. These findings indicate that the irrigation of hematoma through burr holes results in an accumulation of air into the subdural space and produces a tension pneumocephalus. We conclude that the irrigation of hematoma is unnecessary for the treatment of CSDH.

KEY WORDS: head injury, chronic subdural hematoma, surgery, tension pneumocephalus

INTRODUCTION

For the treatment of chronic subdural hematoma(CSDH), irrigation of the hematoma through burr holes has been advocated as the most common operation. Some authors reported that the twist-drill or burr-hole craniostomy and closed-system drainage achieved an excellent outcome[1,2]. Since then, these procedures have been accepted as the initial choice of treatment for CSDH.

In contrast, it still remains unknown whether irrigation of the hematoma should be used as an effective procedure in addition to closed-system drainage. We studied to ascertain the efficacy of irrigation through burr holes and closed-system drainage for the treatment of CSDH.

MATERIALS AND METHODS

Forty-six patients with CSDH were treated from August 1989 through July 1992 in our department. Twenty-two patients were treated by irrigation of the hematoma through burr holes combined with closed-system drainage(Group A), and 24 patients by burr hole and closed-system drainage(Group B). The drainage system was placed within the hematoma cavity for 1 to 2 days. Computerized tomography(CT) scans were obtained before surgery and around 12 days after surgery.

The maximum thickness of the hematoma cavity before surgery and the residual cavity were measured on CT slices. The reduction rate was calculated by dividing thickness of the hematoma minus the residual cavity by the thickness of the hematoma before surgery. In addition, the accumulation of air in the subdural space was investigated after surgery. When the space filled with air was larger than the residual cavity the accumulation of air was assessed as positive.
The neurological outcome was determined according to the Glasgow Outcome Scale 2 to 6 months after surgery.

RESULTS

The clinical data of patients with CSDH treated by burr holes with or without irrigation of the hematoma and closed-system drainage are summarized in Table 1. The average age was 63.3 ± 14.6 years(mean$\pm$SD) in Group A and 75.2 ± 15.5 years in Group B. There were no significant differences between the two groups for sex, Glasgow Coma Scale before surgery, or location and density of the hematoma on CT scans.
Twenty-one patients(95%) in Group A and 21 patients(88%) in Group B had a functional recovery. Only one patient in each group suffered a recurrence. These two patients required second operations because neurological symptoms reappeared and the hematoma cavity increased after surgery. The recurrence rate was 4.5% in Group A and 4.1% in Group B.

The hematoma cavity decreased after surgery in both groups and neurological signs quickly improved. The maximum thickness of the hematoma before surgery was 25.1 ± 7.9mm and 26.5 ± 11.3mm in Group A and B, respectively, whereas the residual cavity was 13.7 ± 6.4mm and 12.7 ± 8.3mm (Fig 1). The reduction rate of the hematoma cavity was 45.4% in Group A and 52.1% in Group B. There was no significant difference in the reduction rate between the two groups.

Accumulation of air in the subdural space after surgery was present in 13 patients(59%) in Group A, but only in 3 patients(13%) in Group B(Chi-square test, P<0.01). However, neurological signs did not deteriorate in these patients with accumulation of air in either group. Only one patient treated by burr-hole irrigation of the hematoma and drainage developed a subdural tension pneumocephalus. His neurological signs deteriorated and he underwent second operation.

142

Table 1. Clinical summary of patients with CSDH treated by burr holes with and without irrigation of the hematoma and closed-system drainage.

Variables		with irrigation (Group A)	without irrigation (Group B)
Total (No of Pt)		22	24
Age	(yr)	63.3 ± 14.6	75.2 ± 15.5
Sex	(NO of Pt)		
	Male	19	21
	Female	3	3
Location (No of Pt)			
	Bilateral	5	9
	Left	10	11
	Right	7	4
Density (No of Pt)			
	High	2	8
	Iso	12	7
	Low	3	5
	Mixed	5	4
GCS before surgery		14.0 ± 1.5	13.5 ± 2.0
GOS (No of Pt)			
functional recovery		21 (95 %)	21 (88 %)
Recurrence (No of Pt)		1 (4.5 %)	1 (4.1 %)

Means are expressed $\pm$ standard deviation of the mean.
GCS : Glasgow Coma Scale, GOS : Glasgow Outcome Scale
No : Nomber, Pt : patient

DISCUSSION

In the present study, twenty-one(88%) of the patients treated by burr hole and closed-system drainage made a functional recovery and one patient(4.1%) had a recurrence. The outcome in patients with this procedure was similar to that patients by irrigation through burr holes and drainage. In addition, there was no significant difference in the reduction rate of the hematoma between patients treated by irrigation through burr holes and by closed-system drainage alone. These findings demonstrate that patients with CSDH are satisfactorily managed by burr hole and closed-system drainage, even though they are not subjected to irrigation of the hematoma. This supports the idea that slow continuous drainage of the hematoma is an optimal procedure in the treatment with CSDH[1,2].

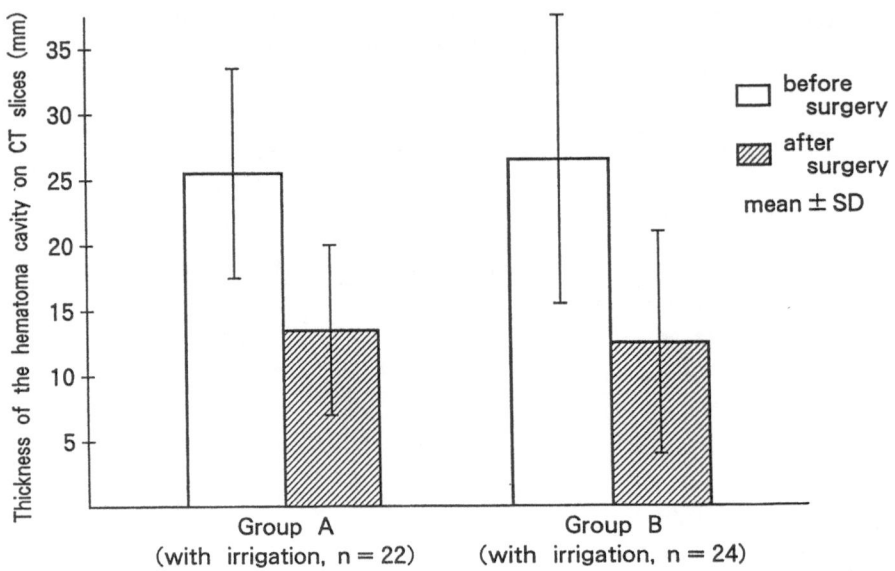

Fig. 1 The maximum thickness of the hematoma cavity before and after surgery. The reduction rate in Group A dose not significantly differ from that in Group B.

On the other hand, we found that the rate of air accumulation in the subdural space after surgery was significantly higher in patients treated by burr—holes irrigation than in those by closed—system drainage alone. One patient who was treated by irrigation of the hematoma through burr holes and drainage developed a subdural tension pneumocephalus. Bremer and Nguyen have reported that symptomatic subdural tension pneumocephalus occasionally develops after the evacuation of subdural hematoma through burr holes[3]. These findings demonstrate that the irrigation or evacuation of subdural hematoma through burr hole results in an accumulation of air in the subdural space and produces a subdural tension pneumocephalus. We conclude that the irrigation of hematoma is unnecessary for the treatment of CSDH.

REFERENCES

1. Tabaddor K, Shulman K (1977) Definitive treatment of chronic subdural hematoma by twist—drill craniostomy and closed—system drainage. J Neurosurg 46: 220–226
2. Markwalder TM, Steinsitpe KF, Rohner M, Reichenbach W, Markwalder H (1981) The course of chronic subdural hematomas after burr—hole craniostomy and closed—system drainage. J Neurosurg 55: 390–396
3. Bremer AM, Nguyen TQ (1982) Tension pneumocephalus after surgical treatment of chronic subdural hematoma. Neurosurgery 11: 284–287

Analysis of 150 Cases with Chronic Subdural Hematoma in Adult on the Factors Related to Functional Outcome

YOSHITAKA OKIMURA, JUNICHI ONO, HIROHIDE KARASUDANI, KATSUMI ISOBE, and AKIRA YAMAURA

Department of Neurosurgery, Chiba University, Chiba, 260 Japan

SUMMARY

One hundred and fifty cases with chronic subdural hematoma (CSDH) in adult were retrospectively analyzed in order to elucidate the factors responsible for long-term functional outcome. The mean age was 63 years. All the patients underwent burr hole and irrigation surgery with external drainage of a short duration. The follow-up periods ranged from 6 months to 7 years. The outcome was evaluated by Karnofsky scale. Seven cases (4.6%) had recurrence of CSDH and 11 (7.3%) had intracranial complications, such as epidural hematoma (3.3%) and intracerebral hematoma (1.3%). Four cases (2.7%) had systemic complications. These complications were significantly responsible for poor outcome. In addition, brain atrophy, which was defined as ventricular dilatation and/or subdural effusion on the follow-up CT, was the other factor responsible for poor outcome in the patients of CSDH without complications. Therefore, the poor outcome may be related to brain atrophy and potential cerebral ischemia in those patients.

KEY WORDS: chronic subdural hematoma, CT scan, long-term functional outcome, complications, brain atrophy

INTRODUCTION

Chronic subdural hematoma (CSDH) is generally accepted as a benign disease, but the information has been limited on the subject in regard to the long-term functional recovery of the patients. This retrospective study was, therefore, designed to analyze the factors related to the long-term functional outcome.

CLINICAL MATERIALS and METHODS

One hundred and fifty cases with CSDH were surgically treated in our hospital, from 1983 to 1990. There were 116 males and 34 females, whose age ranged from 29 years to 86 years and averaged 63 years. All the patients underwent burr hole and irrigation surgery with external drainage of a short duration. The follow-up periods ranged from 6 months to 7 years. Analyzed here were complications, age, interval from trauma to operation, and preoperative and follow-up CT findings.

At the long-term follow-up, the detailed clinical data were available in 61 cases and CT was checked in only 32 cases. The outcome was evaluated by Karnofsky scale: a good outcome was defined as 100% on the scale and a poor outcome as 90% or less.

RESULTS

Complications
Out of 150 cases, 7 cases (4.6%) had recurrence of CSDH and 11 (7.3%) had intracranial complications. The incidence of postoperative epidural hematoma and intracerebral hematoma was 3.3% and 1.3%, respectively. Four cases (2.7%) had systemic complications.

Outcome Related to Complications (Table 1)
In 61 cases which had detailed follow-up data on outcome, 11 (18.0%) had complications. Nine of the 11 cases (81.8%) had poor outcome. On the other hand, 26 (52.0%) had poor outcome in the 50 cases without complications. The difference was statistically significant (p<0.05).

Table 1 The relationship between outcome and complications

Outcome		Good	Poor
	(+)	2/11 cases (18.2%)	9/11 cases (81.8%)*
Complications			
	(−)	24/50 cases (48.0%)	26/50 cases (52.0%)*

*: p<0.05

Age in the 2 Outcome Groups (Table 2)
In the 50 cases without complications, the mean age was 62.1 years in the good outcome group and 65.3 years in the poor outcome group, but this difference was statistically insignificant.

Interval from Trauma to Operation in the 2 Outcome Groups (Table 2)
There was no statistically significant relationship between the interval and the outcome.

Table 2 The relationship between outcome and prognostic factors

Outcome		Good	Poor
Age		62.1±10.1	65.3±10.1
Interval	~2 weeks	1 case	2 cases
from trauma	~1 month	3 cases	2 cases
to operation	~2 months	8 cases	10 cases
	~3 months	7 cases	5 cases
	3 months~	5 cases	5 cases
	unknown	1 case	1 case

Preoperative CT Findings in the 2 Outcome Groups (Table 3)
The midline shift was 14 mm and 13 mm on the preoperative CT in the patients with good outcome and with poor outcome, respectively. The

difference was statistically insignificant. Furthermore, the difference of the hematoma density did not affect the functional outcome.

Table 3   The relationship outcome and preoperative CT findings

Outcome		Good	Poor
Midline shift		14±5mm	13±5mm
Hematoma density	high	7 cases	10 cases
	iso	6 cases	5 cases
	low	7 cases	6 cases
	mixed	4 cases	5 cases

Follow-up CT Findings in the 2 Outcome Groups (Table 4)
In 32 cases with CT follow-up, which had no complications, 15 (46.9%) had good outcome. While the mean age was statistically insignificant between the 2 groups, bifrontal index, which indicates the size of lateral ventricle, was 0.28 and 0.35 in the patients with good outcome and with poor outcome, respectively. The difference was statistically significant (p<0.05). Eleven of the 32 cases (34.4%) had subdural effusion on the follow-up CT and 9 of the 11 (81.8%) had poor outcome, whereas only 8 of 21 cases (38.1%) without subdural effusion had poor outcome. This difference was statistically significant (p<0.05).

Table 4   The relationship between outcome and follow-up CT findings

Outcome		Good	Poor
bifrontal index		0.28±0.02*	0.35±0.02*
subdural effusion	(+)	2/11 cases (18.2%)	9/11 cases (81.8%)*
	(−)	13/21 cases (61.9%)	8/21 cases (38.1%)*

*: p<0.05

DISCUSSION

CSDH is generally accepted as a benign disease, but it has been reported that the postoperative intracranial complications were not uncommon. The causes of postoperative intracranial complications were documented in detail and various surgical techniques or postoperative managements were described in the literature [1],[2],[3],[4]. In addition, our results indicated that complications were most responsible for poor outcome.
Glasgow Outcome Scale (GOS) is widely accepted to evaluate the outcome but it is less useful than Karnofsky scale in regard to fine evaluation of long-term functional recovery, such as mental state or ability to work. It is noteworthy that about 80% must have good

recovery using GOS, whereas only 48% had 100% on Karnofsky scale in our patients without complications. Minimal symptoms, such as mild headache or mild memory disturbance, are occasional problems for the patients with CSDH.

It has been generally accepted that aging was one of the factors responsible for poor outcome in the patients with CSDH. Our results, however, indicated that aging was not related to poor outcome in the patients without complications. It was also documented that the mass effect on preoperative CT was one of the poor prognostic factors. On the contrary, adverse data have been reported recently. In our study, no statistically significant relationship could be found between the midline shift and the functional outcome. In addition, it has been not definitely reported that the functional outcome might be affected by the hematoma density on preoperative CT. Conclusively, it is quite difficult to predict the functional outcome in the patients with CSDH, based on preoperative CT findings.

Brain atrophy has been generally accepted as one of the factors promoting CSDH [5], but no statistical analysis has been conducted in literature, in regard to the relationship between brain atrophy and long-term outcome. In our study, brain atrophy, which was defined as ventricular dilatation and/or subdural effusion on the follow-up CT, was one of the poor prognostic factors in the patients of CSDH without complications. Therefore, the poor outcome may be related to brain atrophy and potential cerebral ischemia in those patients.

REFERENCES

1. Robinson RG: Chronic subdural hematoma: surgical management in 133 patients. J Neurosurg 61:263-268, 1984
2. Camel M, Grubb RL Jr: Treatment of chronic subdural hematoma by twist-drill craniostomy with continuous catheter drainage.
J Neurosurg 65:183-187, 1986
3. D'Avella, Blasi FD, Rottio A, Pensabene V, Pandolfo N: Intracerebral hematoma following evacuation of chronic subdural hematoma. J Neurosurg 65:710-712, 1986
4. Aoki N: Percutaneus subdural tapping for the treatment of chronic subdural hematoma in adults. Neirol Res 9:19-23, 1987
5. Markwalder TM: Chronic subdural hematoma: a review. J Neurosurg 54: 637-645, 1981

Postoperative Morphological Recovery of Deformed Brain in Cases with Chronic Subdural Hematoma: The Difference Between a Burr Hole Closed Drainage and a Burr Hole Irrigation

CHIAKI KUDOH, KAZUAKI SUGIURA, KENTA KUNIMOTO, and HIDEO TAKIZAWA

Department of Neurosurgery, Tokyo Rohsai Hospital, Ohta-ku, Tokyo, 143 Japan

SUMMARY

This study was planned to evaluate morphologically whether a burr hole closed drainage (BD) is superior to a burr hole irrigation (BI) for a smoother re-expansion in cases with chronic subdural hematoma (CSDH). 107 cases with CSDH were treated either by BI or BD. The post-operative changes in clinical symptoms and CT findings in both groups were compared. Post-operative changes in clinical symptoms were not different significantly between the two surgical methods. The re-expansion of brain took a biphasic pattern in the BI group. In contrast, in the BD group, the course of re-expansion was not biphasic but more straight. We consider that BD is superior to BI by allowing steadier and slower re-expansion of the compressed brain.

KEY WORDS: chronic subdural hematoma, subdural drainage, intracranial pressure, rheology

INTRODUCTION

A burr hole closed drainage (BD) operation has been introduced to bring about cure in cases with chronic subdural hematoma (CSDH) [1] and to prevent the complication such as an intracerebral hemorrhage that are caused by too rapid re-expansion of the compressed brain after a burr hole irrigation (BI) [2]. This study was planned to evaluate morphologically whether BD is superior to BI for a smoother re-expansion.

MATERIALS AND METHODS

107 cases with CSDH were selected for this study, 78 males and 29 females, and mean age was 69.8 y/o ranging from 28 to 91 y/o. The patients were treated either by BI (51 cases, 38 males & 13 females) or BD (56 cases, 40 males & 16 females). The post operative changes in clinical symptoms and CT findings in both groups were compared. Edinburgh 2 Coma Scale was used for evaluation of the level of consciousness. The maximum thickness of the hematoma cavity and the maximum shift of the midline structure were measured by CT scan

preoperatively and 1,4,7 and 14 days after the operation in both groups. Subdural pressure was measured by tapping the subdural space with a needle connected to a pressure transducer in each case.

RESULTS

Post-operative changes in clinical symptoms were not different significantly between the two surgical methods (TABLE 1). 6 patients experienced reaccumulation of the hematoma after the operation (three patients in BI, the other three in BD). Re-expansion of brain took a biphasic pattern in the BI group; a rapid phase of recovery induced soon after the operation was followed by a slower recovery. In contrast, in the BD group, the course of re-expansion was not biphasic but more straight (Fig.1 & 2). Mean subdural pressure was 148 ± 18 mmH$_2$O. There were no clear correlations between the course of re-expansion, subdural pressure and the outcome.

Discussion

A little attention has been paid to the mechanical properties of brain in chronic subdural hematoma [3,4,5].
The brain has visco-elastic properties. When a visco-elastic material is subjected to load, the material is rapidly deformed to some extent and is followed by a slowly progressive deformation known as "creep" until the final equilibrium is reached [6]. It is known that the phase of "creep" takes exponential curve and it takes longer time to be completed when the viscosity of brain is playing a more dominant part than elasticity [7].
The patterns of recovery of brain after the evacuation of subdural hematoma either BI or BD were very similar to that of "creep" recovery (Fig.3 & 4). We consider that the delayed recovery of brain was same to the phenomenon of "creep" and BD would make the recovery of "creep" to be steadier.
This study suggests that BD is a simple and efficient method, and is superior to BI by allowing steadier and slower re-expansion of the compressed brain.

REFERENCES

1. Kamran T, Kenneth S (1977) Definitive treatment of chronic subdural hematoma by twist-drill craniostomy and closed-system drainage. J Neurosurg 46:220-226.
2. Medesti LM, Hodge CJ, Barnwell ML (1982) Intracerebral hematoma after evacuation of chronic extracerebral fluid colloctions. Neurosurg 10:689-693.
3. Galford JE, McElhaney JH (1970) A visco-elastic study of scalp,

brain and dura. J Biomechanics 31:211-221.

4. Ommaya AK (1968) Mechanical properties of tissues of the nervous system. J Biomechanics 1:127-138.

5. Weinstein JD, Langfitt TW, Bruno L, Zaren HA, Jackson JLF (1968) Experimental study of patterns of brain distortion and ischemia produced by an intracranial mass. J Neurosurg 28:513-521.

6. Mow V, Holmes MH, Lai WM (1984) Fluid transport and mechanical properties of articular cartilage. A review. J Biomechanics 17:377-394.

7. Takizawa H, Sugiura K, Baba M (1991) Biphasic recovery of deformed brain observed in cases with chronic subdural hematoma after operation. J J Tom 39:645-649

TABLE 1 : Pre- & postoperative condition without complication after irrigation & closed system drainage

preoperative E₂CS	irrigation				closed system drainage			
	No. of cases	GOS			No. of cases	GOS		
		GR	MD	SD~D		GR	MD	SD~D
1	18	17	1	0	21	20	1	0
2	20	19	1	0	19	17	2	0
3	6	4	2	0	5	4	1	0
4	3	2	1	0	5	3	2	0
5	1	0	1	0	3	2	1	0
6 ~ 10	0	0	0	0	0	0	0	0
Total	48	42	6	0	53	46	7	0

E₂CS ; Edinburgh 2 Coma Scale
GOS ; Glasgow Outcome Scale

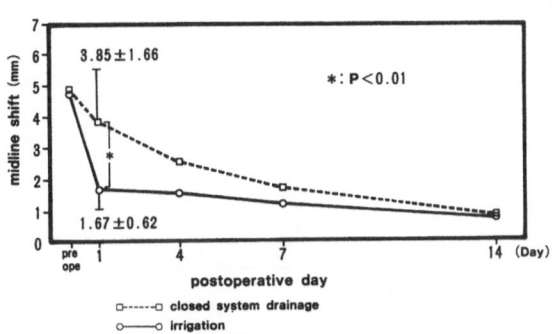

Fig. 1 : Recovery of midline shift after irrigation & closed system drainage

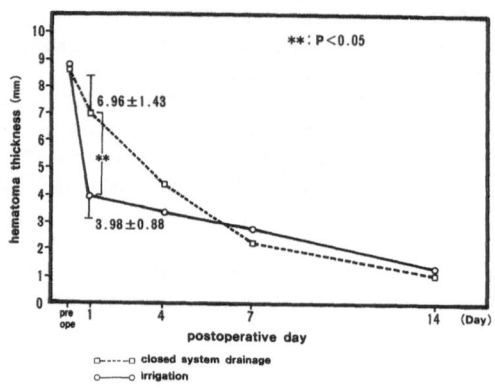

**Fig. 2 : Recovery of hematoma thickness after irrigation &
closed system drainage**

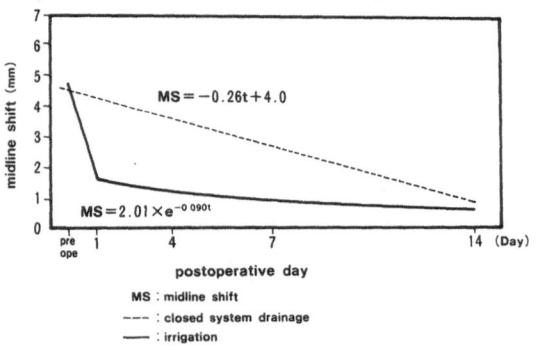

**Fig. 3 : Pre- & postoperative changes in midline shift ;
comparison between irrigation & closed system drainage**

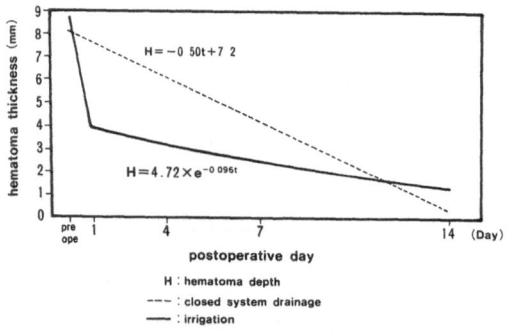

**Fig. 4 : Pre- & postoperative changes in hematoma thickness ;
comparison between irrigation & closed system drainage**

Clinical Study on Recurrent Chronic Subdural Hematoma

T. MIKI, Y. IKEDA, K. SAITO, Y. TAKEDA, and H. ITO

Department of Neurosurgery, Tokyo Medical College, Shinjuku-ku, Tokyo, 160 Japan

SUMMARY

The procedure of irrigation and external drainage was done in 131 patients with chronic subdural hematoma (CSDH), 12 of whom (9.2%) had a relapse. Recurrent hemorrhage occurred because first, stiffening of the brain with aging inhibited expansion after surgery and second, surgery performed relatively early in the course of CSDH suppressed the blood coagulation process. Relapse occurred an average of 16.8 days after surgery, but appropriate treatment resulted in a good outcome for patients.

KEY WORDS: chronic subdural hematoma, computerized tomography, rebleeding, post-operative complication

INTRODUCTION

Although irrigation via burr holes is the general approach to treat chronic subdural hematoma (CSDH), recurrence is not a rare clinical event. The clinical profiles of cases in which CSDH recurred after surgery were carefully analysed.

CLINICAL MATERIAL AND METHODS

In this study, the practice followed for a surgical approach to CSDH was irrigation via two burr holes and external drainage for a few days. Subjects consisted of 12 CSDH cases encountered in the past 10 years with postoperative recurrence requiring repeat surgery (Table 1, 2). Clinical and CT scan findings were evaluated by comparing findings from the 12 cases with 80 controls consisting of cases in which CSDH had not recurred - encountered during the same 10-year period (Table 3).

RESULTS

Postoperatively, CSDH recurred in 9.2% of the 131 CSDH cases encountered in the same 10-year period. The age of these patients ranged from 47 to 83 years and averaged 72.8 years; the average age of the controls was 64.6 years. They presented a variety of past histories: hypertension in four cases, heavy drinking in three, liver cirrhosis in one, and hemorrhagic diathesis in two. Past history of head trauma was as high as 83.3%, occurring in 10 of the 12 recurrent cases. There were no characteristic symptoms in the recurrent cases. The sides of hematoma in recurrent cases were five right-side, six left-side and one bilateral. Average hematoma volume was 118.8 ml in the recurrent cases, which was relatively greater than in the controls, for which this volume was 97.4 ml. CT scan revealed that the density of recurrent hematomas was low in 23.1%, isodense in 7.7%, high in 23.1%, and mixed in 46.2%. In the control group, density was low in 40.4%, isodense in 30.3%, high in 17.2%, and mixed in 12.1%. Thus, the patient group had lower rates of low and iso-density and higher rates of high and mixed density. Furthermore CT

Table 1 Summary of Recurrent Cases (I)

Case No.	Age	Sex	Past History	History of Head Trauma	Brain Atrophy on CT scan	Headache	Hemiparesis	Disturbance of Consciousness	Dementia
1.	69	M	hypertension	+	+		+		
2.	47	M	heavy drinking	+	–	+	+	+(GCS13)	
3.	81	M	dementia	+	+				+
4.	75	M	liver cirrhosis	?	+		+	+(GCS13)	
5.	83	M	dementia	+	+				+
6.	77	M	hypertension	+	+	+	+	+(GCS14)	
7.	55	F	hypertension	+	–	+			
8.	83	M	hypertension	+	+		+		
9.	82	M	hemorrhagic diathesis	+	+	+	+	+(GCS10)	
10.	69	M	hemorrhagic diathesis	+	+		+	+(GCS14)	
11.	79	M	heavy drinking	+	+				
12.	74	M	–	?	–	+	+		

scan showed that brain atrophy was as high as 75% in recurrent cases. The clinical course averaged 19.0 days from the time of trauma to symptom onset, 12.8 days from symptom onset to initial surgery, 16.8 days from initial surgery to recurrence (reappearance of symptoms or restagnation of hematoma), and 6.8 days from recurrence to second surgery. The average period between the time of trauma to initial surgery was 32.2 ±16.7 days in recurrent cases, which was significantly shorter than in the controls - an average of 67.0 days (P < 0.01). The data suggested that immature timing of operation had a tendency to lead postoperative reaccumulation of the

Table 2 Summary of Recurrent Cases (II)

Case No.	Side	Location	Volume (ml)	Density of CT scan	Interval (days) Trauma ->1st. ope	Density of CT scan	Clinical Symptom	Glasgow Outcome Scale
1.	L	F.T.P.	150	Mixed	21 days	Mixed	Headache	GR
2.	L	F.	175	Mixed	11	Mixed	Headache	GR
3.	L	F.T.P.	112	Low	51	Low	Dist. of Consciousness	MD
4.	L	F.P.	157	Mixed	?	Mixed	Hemiparesis	GR
5.	R	F.P.	90	Low		Mixed	–	GR
	L	F.	45	Low	47			
6.	R	F.T.P.	100	Mixed	65	Low	Dementia	GR
7.	R	F.P.	70	Mixed	21	Mixed	–	GR
8.	R	F.P.	166	High	24	High	Dist. of Consciousness	MD
9.	R	F.P.	85	Mixed	26	High	–	MD
10.	R	F.P.	110	High	25	Low	Hemiparesis	Dead(DIC)
11.	L	F.T.P.	90	High	23	Low	Hemiparesis	GR
12.	L	F.	120	Iso	?	Low	Headache	GR

F: Frontal region T: Temporal region P : Parietal region GR: Good Recovery
MD: Moderate Disabled DIC: Disseminated Intravascular Coagulation

154

Table 3 Baseline Characteristics in Recurrent Cases

Characteristics	Recurrent cases(n=12)		Controlled cases(n=80)		Significance
	No.	Percent	No.	Percent	
Age	72.8±10.9(yrs)		64.6±18.9(yrs)		N.S.
History of trauma	10	83.3%	59	73.8%	N.S.
Brain atrophy on CT	9	75%	51	63.8%	N.S.
Hematoma					
Volume	118.8±33.5ml		97.4±36.9ml		P<0.05
Density of CT					
Mixed-D	6	40.2%	12	12.1%	P<0.01
High-D	3	23.1%	17	17.2%	P<0.05
Iso-D	1	7.7%	30	30.3%	P<0.05
Low-D	3	23.1%	40	40.4%	P<0.05
Interval					
Trauma →1st. Ope.	32.2±16.7days		67.0±26.7days		P<0.01
Onset of symptom →1st. Ope.	12.8±7.5 days		7.4±5.2 days		P<0.05

hematoma (Fig. 1). Prognosis was good in all but one case with disseminated intravascular coagulation, in which the complication proved fatal.

DISCUSSION

The procedure of hematoma irrigation using burr holes and external drainage is widely adopted in the treatment of chronic subdural hematoma (CSDH). However, postoperative relapses are not rare, ranging from 3.1-36.8% (average: around 10%) in some reports [1-3] and 9.2% in our previous cases. Aritake et al. [4] reported that 50% of postoperative recurrent hematomas could be attributed to poor technique, such as insufficient hematoma irrigation or incomplete drainage. It is thus important that this simple operation be performed carefully. As the purpose of this study was to investigate the real cause of recurrent hematoma, cases apparently resulting from poor technique were excluded.

Hematoma recurrence is caused by first, insufficient brain expansion after trephination and second, incomplete hemostasis in the space left by the hematoma and recurrent hemorrhage from surgery. Action of these factors is complex. In the former case (insufficient brain expansion), postoperative cerebral distention is inhibited by 1) aging (cerebral atrophy and decreased cerebral elasticity); 2) intracranial hypotension; 3) large hematomas (severe mass effect); 4) thick hematoma capsules; 5) postoperative tension pneumocephalus; and 6) other factors. In the latter case (incomplete hemostasis and recurrent hemorrhage), systemic hemorrhagic diathesis is associated with hepatic failure or induced by drugs and then incomplete hemostasis and absorption of hematoma are related to insufficient brain expansion. In such cases, hemorrhaging cannot be stopped and absorbed by conventional therapies, such as removal and irrigation of hematoma. In order to control bleeding from the hematoma capsule with conventional procedures it is necessary to have capsule maturation, an irrigation-induced decrease of fibrin and fibrinogen degradation products (FDP) in the space left by the hematoma, and clot removal [5].

In the patients with recurrent hematoma in this study, the mean duration between trauma and the initial operation, 32.2 days, was significantly shorter than in the control group. This fact suggests that surgery performed before the capsule is mature suppresses the hemostatic process of the capsule, resulting in recurrent hematoma. Hematomas with high or mixed density were frequently observed in the CTs

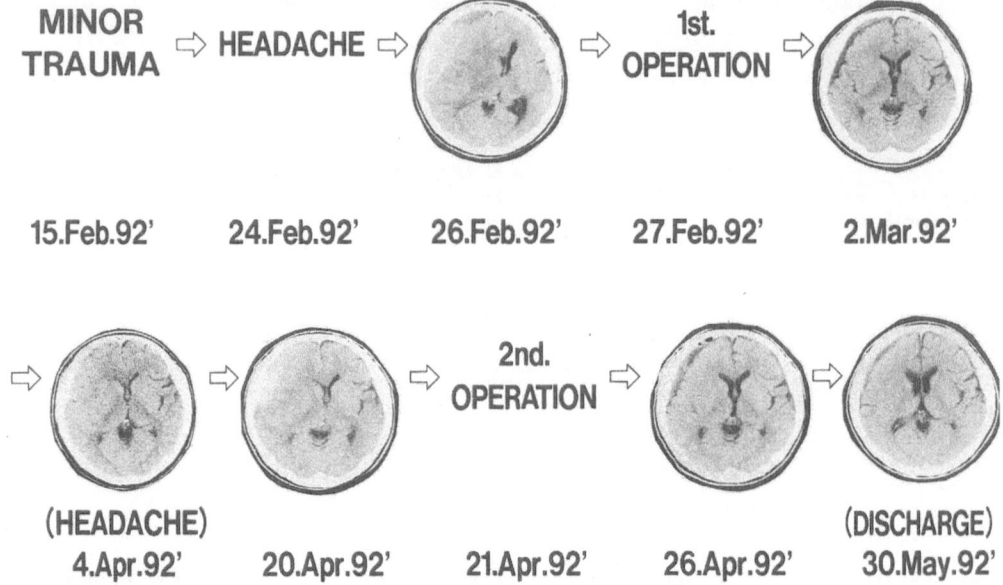

Fig. 1 Clinical Course and Serial CT Scans in Case No. 2 with Recurrent Hematoma

of patients with recurrent hemorrhage in this study, as others [6] have reported. This finding revealed that hemorrhage continued from the capsules and that capsules were being formed.

CONCLUSION

Postoperative CSDH was more apt to recur in the elderly, when initial hematoma was larger, in cases of high and mixed density on CT scan, in cases of earlier surgery from trauma, and in those complicated with hemorrhagic diathesis. The results of this study suggested that immature timing of the operation and aging (brain atrophy and hard elasticity of brain tissue) were a particularly important causative factors of recurrence. Recurrence was an average of 16.8 days after surgery. Timely management of recurrent CSDH leads to good prognosis.

REFERENCES

1. Bremer AM, Nguyen TQ (1982) Tension pneumocephalus after surgical treatment of chronic subdural hematoma. Neurosurgery 11:284-287
2. Svien HJ, Gelety JE (1963) On the surgical management of encapsulated subdural hematoma. A comparison of the results of membranectomy and simple evaluation. J Neurosurg 21:172-177
3. Weir B, Gordon P (1983) Factors affecting coagulation: Fibrinolysis in chronic subdural fluid collections. J Neurosurg 58:242-245
4. Aritake K, Miyagawa Y, Sano K (1988) Recurrent chronic subdural hematoma: Its causes and management. Neurotraumatology 11:46-50
5. Ito H, Saito K, Fujisawa H, Onishi H, Yamamoto S (1988) Role of tissue-plasminogen activator in chronic subdural hematoma. Neurotraumatology 11:78-82
6. Seki K, Kaneko S, Oowada K (1988) Study of postoperative rebleeding cases of chronic subdural hematoma. Neurotraumatology 11:142-147

Zero Postoperative Recurrence Rates in Chronic Subdural Hematoma

Masaaki Yamamoto[1], Minoru Jimbo[1], Mitsunobu Ide[1], Noriko Tanaka[1], Yutaka Umebara[1], Shinji Hagiwara[1], Eiji Takeyama[2], and Hirohisa Imanaga[3]

[1]Department of Neurosurgery, Tokyo Women's Medical College Dai-ni Hospital, Arakawa-ku, Tokyo, 116 Japan, [2]Department of Neurosurgery, Toda Chuo Hospital, Toda, Saitama, Japan, and [3]Department of Neurosurgery, Shiseikai Dai-ni Hospital, Setagaya-ku, Tokyo, Japan

SUMMARY

Although various surgical techniques and modifications thereof have been reported for chronic subdural hematoma (SDH), zero postoperative recurrence rates have yet to be accomplished. We experienced no postoperative recurrences among 251 adult cases with symptomatic chronic SDHs treated in our facilities from 1981 to 1991. The subjects include 41 cases with bilateral hematomas but none with subdural effusion. There were 189 males and 62 females. The patients ranged from 31 to 99 years old, with a mean age of 66 years. Four patients died within three months of surgery due to unrelated disorders. Full recovery within four postoperative weeks was achieved in 199 cases and significant improvement was shown in 32 cases in which, however, minimal symptoms persisted for three months or more. In the remaining 16 cases, only slight improvement was observed during the follow-up period. Although computed tomographic scan showed transient postoperative reaccumulation of hematoma in five patients, all were asymptomatic and no further procedures were required. In the interest of reducing postoperative recurrence rates, we have outlined our criteria for selecting cases appropriate for surgery and discussed our surgical technique, which entails complete removal of the hematoma through a single burr hole and subsequent drainage. In particular, we advocate meticulous application of surgical procedures designed to avoid the inflow of fresh blood into the hematoma cavity during, or after, skin closure.

KEY WORDS : chronic subdural hematoma, surgery, recurrence

INTRODUCTION

Chronic subdural hematomas (SDHs) are common lesions with virtually permanent cure being achieved by evacuation of the content via burr hole opening, with or without a drainage system [1-6]. Nevertheless, recurrence rates of 2-3%, or more, in cases with chronic SDH following successful surgical treatment, necessitating another procedure, have been reported [1-8]. We have, however, experienced no postoperative recurrences since 1981. In this paper, our criteria for selecting appropriate candidates for surgery are outlined and the application of meticulous surgical techniques designed to avoid the inflow of fresh blood into the hematoma cavity, particularly during, or after, skin closure is discussed. These measures can be considered essential for reducing postoperative recurrence rates.

MATERIALS

We reviewed 251 case histories from adults with symptomatic chronic SDH treated by evacuation of the hematoma via burr hole opening in our facility and in two affiliated clinics from 1981 to 1991. The more than 50 referrals with chronic SDH who were conservatively treated during this study period were excluded. There were 189 males and 62 females. The patients ranged from 31 to 99 years old, with a mean age of 66 years. One hundred and thirty-three patients (53%) were 70 or more years old. The subjects included 41 patients (16%) with bilateral hematomas, 36 of whom were known to have bilateral hematomas on admission and were thus operated on in one stage. The five remaining patients underwent a second procedure 2 to 4 weeks later, at which point chronic SDH had developed on the contralateral side.

CLINICAL HISTORY AND FINDINGS

In all 251 patients, the most frequent symptoms were motor problems (64%), followed by headache (25%), mental changes (16%) and disturbances of consciousness (13%). In the elderly group (70 years of age or more), mental changes were more frequent (22% vs. 10%) and headache was less frequent (11% vs. 41%) than in the younger group. Clinical findings at the time of surgery were retrospectively graded according to the scale reported by Markwalder et al. [4]. The majority of patients were Grade I (57%), followed by Grade II (30%), Grade III (12%) and Grade IV (1%). No Grade 0 patients were surgically treated during this study period.

In the 163 patients (65%) who had a history of head trauma, intervals between the trauma and symptom onset ranged from 3 to 39 weeks, with an average of 8.7 weeks. Among these 163 patients, this interval was 12 weeks or less in 129 patients (79%) and more than six months in only two. In the remaining 88 cases, neither the patients nor their relatives could recall a history of head trauma.

Five patients were known to be chronic alcoholics, four had hepatic disorders, two were on anticoagulant therapy for heart disease, one had idiopathic thrombocytopenic purpura and one had disseminated intravascular coagulopathy (DIC). Thirty patients had a history of cerebrovascular disease, five of whom had been demented since the ictus.

OPERATIVE AND POSTOPERATIVE MANAGEMENT

All patients, except nine in whom general anesthesia was required because of mental problems or delirious state, were operated on under local anesthesia with mild sedation using intravenously administered diazepam and pentazocine. A single burr hole was made at the site of maximum hematoma thickness, usually in the fronto-temporal region. After electro-cauterization of the surface, a cruciform incision was made in the dura mater and the external membrane of the hematoma. This results in four small dural flaps which adhered to the external membrane. No attempt was made to separate the two layers and the flaps were cauterized. This procedure, which results in dural flap shrinkage, carries the advantage of providing sufficient space for subsequent procedures. After evacuation of the hematoma, the cavity was irrigated with 500-1,000 ml of 37 °C saline and then a silicon catheter with multiple holes, which was connected to a closed drainage system, was placed in the cavity. Installation of the drainage system seemed, however, to be technically difficult because of immediate collapse of the cavity following evacuation of the hematoma and, therefore, could not be done in six patients. During these procedures, meticulous surgical techniques were applied to avoid injury to either the outer or inner membranes. Sampling of these membranes for histological studies was thus not warranted. The small bone defect was tightly packed with absorbable gelatin sterile sponge (Gelfoam®) to avoid the inflow of fresh blood into the hematoma cavity during, or shortly after, skin closure.

The patient was kept supine, with the drainage bag placed at bed level or 10 cm higher, for 2 to 4 postoperative days at which time the drainage system was removed. All patients were given prophylactic antibiotics but none received steroid or diuretic therapy. Patients were followed for three months or more and were examined by means of computed tomographic (CT) scan at 1, 2, 4 and 12 weeks following surgery.

RESULTS

Full recovery within four postoperative weeks was achieved in 199 cases and significant improvement was shown in 32 cases in which, however, minimal symptoms persisted for three months or more. In the remaining 16 cases, only slight improvement was observed during the follow-up period. Four patients died within three months of surgery due to unrelated disorders: Two of myocardial infarction, one of DIC and one of malignancy. No complications, such as intracranial hemorrhage or infection, were experienced. Although CT scan showed transient postoperative reaccumulation of hematoma in five patients, all were asymptomatic and no further procedures were required.

Among 143 patients with clinical grade I, 133 patients (93%) showed good recovery, as did 53 (70%) of 76 patients with clinical grade II. In contrast, only 13 (43%) of 30 patients with clinical grade III showed good recovery. In particular, mental problems persisted in elderly cases.

DISCUSSION

Although chronic SDH has been managed by both medical and surgical means, surgical evacuation is widely accepted as the treatment of choice [1-6]. In an attempt to prevent recurrent SDH after surgery, various surgical techniques, each with several modifications, have been described. Nevertheless, zero postoperative recurrence rates have yet to be accomplished and there has been considerable debate as to which procedure is best.

Our surgical technique entails complete removal of the hematoma content through a single burr hole and subsequent drainage, which is the standard procedure used in most facilities [1,4]. However, the unique modification of our procedure is that the burr hole is completely packed with absorbable gelatin sterile sponge following removal of the hematoma content and placement of a drainage device. This may be considered to be disadvantageous for promoting drainage of the content into the subgalear space as recommended by Chee [7]. This has not, however, been a problem in our experience. On the contrary, our technique carries the significant advantage of avoiding the inflow of fresh blood into the hematoma cavity, particularly during, and after, skin closure. At the beginning of the 1980s when we started our technique, there was only limited knowledge about the fibrinolytic activity which had been suggested by some authors to play an important role in the persistence and expansion of chronic SDH [9,10]. We speculated as to the possibility that the inflow of fresh blood into the cavity during, or shortly after, surgery could promote fibrinolytic activities, despite the lack of an adequate theory to explain it.

The mechanisms underlying the persistence and expansion of chronic SDH have recently been elucidated in relation to recurrent small hemorrhages from fragile blood vessels in the outer membrane, perhaps promoted by fibrinolytic enzymes, such as tissue-type plasminogen activator [11-18]. Ito et al. reported that residual clot can promote fibrionolytic activities, thereby leading to reaccumulation of hematoma [13]. Therefore, they suggested that it is theoretically possible to prevent recurrence by minimizing the inflow of blood from the dura and the subgalear tissue into the hematoma cavity during surgery [8]. Our experiences with surgically-treated hematomas supports their theory.

ACKNOWLEDGMENT

The authors would like to thank Bierta E. Barfod, M.D., University of Washington School of Medicine, for her assistance in the preparation of this manuscript.

REFERENCES

1. Weir BKA (1983) Can J Neurol Sci 10:22-26
2. Aoki N (1984) Neurosurgery 14:545-548
3. Richter HP, Klein HJ, Schaefer M (1984) Acta Neurochirurgica 71:179-188
4. Markwalder TM, Seiler RW (1985) Neurosurgery 16:185-188
5. Iwadate Y, Ishige N, Hosoi Y (1989) Neurol Med Chir (Tokyo) 29:117-121
6. Wakai S, Hashimoto K, Watanabe N, Inoh S, Ochiai C, Nagai M (1990) Neurosurgery 26:771-773
7. Chee CP (1988) Neurosurgery 22:780-782
8. Ito H, Saito K, Fujisawa H, Onishi H, Yamashita J, Shimoji T (1989) Kanazawa-daigaku Igakkai Zasshi 98:622-630
9. Ito H, Komai T, Yamamoto S (1975) Neurol Med Chir (Tokyo) 15:51-55
10. Ito H, Komai T, Yamamoto S (1978) J Neurosurg 48:197-200
11. Weir B, Philip G (1983) J Neurosurg 58:242-245
12. Ito H, Yamamoto S, Saito K, Ikeda K, Hisada K (1987) J Neurosurg 66:862-864
13. Ito H, Saito K, Yamamoto S, Hasegawa T (1988) Surg Neurol 30:175-179
14. Yatsuzuka H (1988) No To Shinkei (Brain and Nerve, Tokyo) 40:963-969
15. Saito K, Ito H, Hasegawa T, Yamamoto S (1989) J Neurosurg 70:68-72
16. Kawakami Y, Chikama M, Tamiya T, Shimamura Y (1989) Neurosurgery 25:25-29
17. Fujisawa H, Ito H, Saito K, Ikeda K, Nitta H, Yamashita J (1991) Surg Neurol 35: 441-445
18. Nishida S (1992) No To Shinkei (Brain and Nerve, Tokyo) 44:565-570

5—Neuroimaging in Central Nervous System Injury

MRI Analysis of Cerebral Contusions: Significance of Intraparenchymal Fluid-Blood Interface

Yoichi Katayama, Kosaku Kinoshita, and Takashi Tsubokawa

Department of Neurological Surgery, Nihon University School of Medicine, Tokyo, 173 Japan

SUMMARY

Fluid-blood interfaces within the cerebral parenchyma can be demonstrated on CT scans in cases with traumatic intracerebral hematomas without formation of an intraparenchymal fluid cavity. MRI suggested that the fluid-blood levels observed in 'CT scans represent layering of red blood cells within the area of contusion necrosis which may be producing voluminous edema fluid. The more extensive the brain tissue damage, the more often are fluid-blood levels formed. A poorer outcome can thus be suggested by the occurrence of intraparenchymal fluid-blood interfaces.

KEY WORDS: CT - MRI - hemorrhage - traumatic intracerebral hematoma - cerebral contusion - edema

INTRODUCTION

Intraparenchymal fluid-blood interfaces associated with cerebral contusions are not an uncommon finding in computed tomography (CT) scans [6,7]. Little is known about the detailed mechanism and significance of formation of fluid-blood levels within the cerebral parenchyma [6,10]. The present study examined clinical features of cases with such intraparenchymal fluid-blood interfaces and analyzed their characteristics in magnetic resonance imaging (MRI).

MATERIALS AND METHODS

During the last 2 years, we have experienced 40 cases with cerebral contusions complicated by intracerebral high density lesions. CT scans taken within 36 hours after trauma in these cases were reviewed retrospectively. These cases often demonstrated multiple high density lesions. A total of 70 high density lesions occurring in these cases were separately analyzed. MRI was carried out in some of these cases within 72 hours employing a 1.5-Tesla system (Gyroscan S15) or a 0.5-Tesla system (Magnetom M21). The Glasgow coma scale (GCS)[12] on admission (3-12 hours after trauma) and Glasgow outcome scale (GOS) [3,13] evaluated 6 months later were taken as measures of the severity of trauma. The size of high density lesions was expressed as the maximum diameter in cm, and the extent of edema was evaluated from the maximum width of the low density area surrounding the high density lesions on CT scans. When the width of the low density area was larger than one half of the diameter of the high density lesion, the edema was considered as extensive.

163

RESULTS

High density lesions which demonstrated fluid-blood levels were exclusively associated with contusions. Cases with high density lesions which demonstrated a fluid-blood interface were more frequently scored at 7 or less on the GCS and were more frequently associated with a poorer outcome as evaluated by the GOS (D, VS or SD), as compared with cases which did not (P<0.01, Fig. 1). Extensive contusion edema developed more frequently in high density lesions with a fluid-blood interface (33%) than in those without a fluid-blood interface (4%, P<0.01). CT scans revealed a progressive increase in edema surrounding high density lesions and an increase in the volume of the affected brain areas, although the high density lesions themselves remained unchanged. MRI indicated that large amounts of edema fluid extended along the white matter fibers. MRI in most cases suggested, however, that the fluid-blood interface was formed within contusion necrosis rather than contusion edema. When a fluid-blood interface was observed, the diameter of the high density lesions was more frequently larger than 4 cm than when a fluid-blood interface was not observed (P<0.01, Fig. 1).

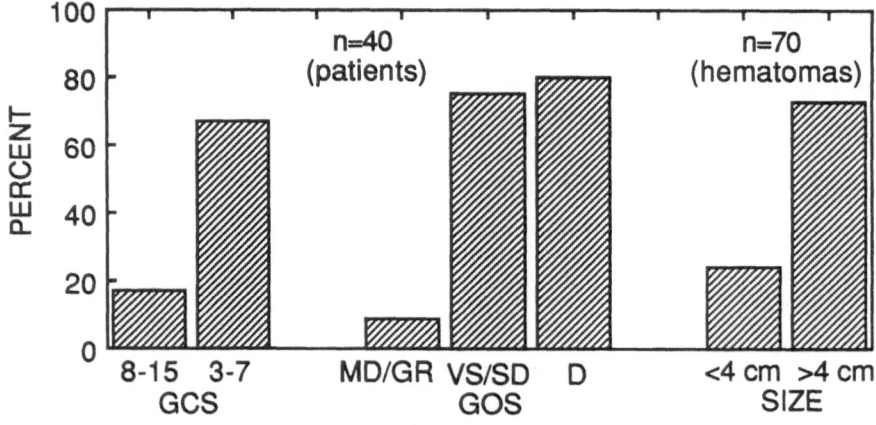

Fig. 1 Number of cases (percent) with a fluid-blood interface.

Surgical evacuation of the large high density lesions was carried out within 24 hours after trauma in 5 cases demonstrating a fluid-blood interface on CT and MRI. There was no case in which an intraparenchymal fluid cavity was observed. Thus, no blood layering within a cavity was identified at surgery.

DISCUSSION

An intracerebral fluid-blood interface may be observed in other lesions [6]. The occurrence of fluid-blood levels has been reported to be correlated with the early development of perifocal low density areas on CT scans, suggesting that the fluid-blood level may represent blood sediment in the fluid related to perifocal low density areas [2,8]. The perifocal low density areas may be induced by several factors, such as edema [4], contusion necrosis, ischemia, cerebrospinal fluid [11], and serum [5,8], or plasma [1,10] separated from clots. In contrast, it appears that intraparenchymal fluid-blood interfaces can be formed without a fluid cavity, at least in cases with traumatic intracerebral high density lesions. Similar findings have been described in cases with intracerebral hematomas secondary to coagulation defects [1, 10], in which no plasma-blood interface was identified at autopsy. It has been suggested that this might be related to the brain fixation process or perphaps to evolution of the hematoma prior to death [10]. In the present study, however, no intraparenchymal fluid cavity was identified at surgery, indicating that a fluid cavity did not exist in any event.

Fluid-blood interfaces were observed more frequently in cases with intracerebral high density lesions of traumatic origin than in those of other etiologies. Among intracerebral hematomas of various etiologies, the traumatic intracerebral high density lesion is unique because of the associated contusions [9]. In cerebral contusions, a well-demarcated area of contusion necrosis, composed of cellular disintegration and homogenation, develops within 12 to 48 hours [9]. Within the contusion necrosis, hemorrhage undergoes enlargement within the initial 6 hours after trauma [7], and red blood cells diffusely permeate the softened tissue but usually do not expand into the surrounding normal tissue [9]. The fluid-blood levels observed within the central area of contusion may represent layering of red blood cells permeating into the area of contusion necrosis. MRI finding supported this inference.

The present study also revealed that extensive edema was often observed in association with intraparenchymal fluid-blood levels. Cerebral contusions are frequently accompanied by an increased cerebrovascular permeability which results in extracellular edema [7]. In the present study, MRI demonstrated that edema fluid extended along the white matter fibers, which is consistent with extracellular edema. It has been found that the rate of CSF formation in similar cases is often elevated, suggesting that enormous amounts of extracellular edema fluid were being formed within the contused brain tissue [7]. The intraparenchymal fluid-blood levels may represent layering of red blood cells which are floating within the area of contusion necrosis producing voluminous edema fluid.

It was found that the more extensive the brain tissue damage, as evaluated from the GCS, GOS and hematoma size, the more frequently were intraparenchymal fluid-blood levels formed. More extensive contusion necrosis and edema in cases with intraparenchymal fluid-blood levels may underly this relationship. Intraparenchymal fluid-blood interfaces thus indicate a severer injury and predict a poorer outcome. In summary, a fluid-blood interface observed in CT scans appears to be indicative of the presence of contusion necrosis which is larger in size than the high density lesions and which may be producing edema fluid.

REFERENCES

1. Dolinskas CA, Bilaniuk LT, Zimmerman RA, Kuhl DE (1977) Computed tomography of intracerebral hematomas. I. Transmission CT observations on hematoma resolution. AJR 129:681-688
2. Isono M, Shindo K, Ito M, Hori S, Suzuki J (1989) CT findings of hypertensive intracerebral hematomas: Considerations of the formation of hematomas. CT Kenkyu 11:557-562 (in Japanese)
3. Giannotta SL, Weiner JM, Karnaze D (1987) Prognosis and outcome in severe head injury. In: Cooper PR (ed.) Head Injury, 2nd ed., Williams & Wilkins, Baltimore, pp.464-487
4. Kamimura K, Goto K, Ishii K, Isu T, Okudera T (1978) CT diagnosis. Shinkei Kenkyu No Shinpo 22:200-218 (in Japanese)
5. Katada K (1985) CT diagnosis of intracerebral hemorrhage. Gazoshindan 5:527-530 (in Japanese)
6. Katayama Y, Tsubokawa T, Kinoshita K, Himi K (1992) Intraparenchymal blood-fluid levels in traumatic intracerebral hematomas. Neuroradiology in press.

7. Katayama Y, Tsubokawa T, Miyazaki S, Kawamata T, Yoshino A (1990) Oedema fluid formation within contused brain tissue as a cause of medically uncontrollable elevation of intracranial pressure in head trauma patients. Acta Neurochir suppl. 51:308-310

8. Kazner E, Lanksch W, Grumme T, Kretzschmar K (1980) Diagnosis and differential diagnosis of spontaneous ICH with CT scan. In: Pia HW, Langmaid C, Zierski J (eds.), Spontaneous Intracerebral Hematomas: Advances in Diagnosis and Therapy, Springer, Berlin, pp.178-190

9. Lindenberg R, Freytag E (1957) Morphology of cortical contusions. AMA Arch Path 63:23-42

10. Livioni JP, McGahan JP (1983) Intracranial fluid-blood levels in the anticoagulated patient. Neuroradiology 25: 335-337

11. Scott WR, New PFJ, Davis KR, Schnur IA (1974) Computerized axial tomography of intracerebral and intraventricular hemorrhage. Radiology 112:73-80

12. Teasdale G, Murray G, Parker L, Jennett B (1979) Adding up the Glasgow Coma Score. Acta Neurochir suppl. 28:13-16

13. Teasdale G, Jennett B (1976) Assessment and prognosis of coma after head injury. Acta Neurochir 34:45-55

Assessment of Brainstem Distortion Associated with Supretentorial Lesions by Magnetic Resonance Imaging

Suguru Inao[1], Hiroji Kuchiwaki[1], Hidemi Kanaiwa[1], Kenichiro Sugita[1], and Masahiro Furuse[2]

[1]Department of Neurosurgery, Nagoya University School of Medicine, Showa-ku, Nagoya, 466 Japan, and
[2]Department of Neurosurgery, Nakatsugawa Municipal General Hospital, Nakatsugawa, 508 Japan

SUMMARY

Quantitative measurements of brainstem distortion and neural dysfunction were obtained in 25 cases of chronic subdural hematoma. The horizontal and rotational brainstem displacements were measured on axial and coronal magnetic resonance (MR) images in all patients pre-operatively, and brainstem auditory evoked responses (BAERs) were obtained in 11 cases. Logarithmic relationships were noted on both horizontal and rotational displacements of the brainstem and cerebrum. The type of shift changed in the rostro-caudal direction, and the difference in magnitude of distortion between cerebrum and brainstem results in midbrain kinking. The prolongation of BAER latencies and central conduction times correlated with septum shift. The results of peak-V latency indicated that brainstem rotation in the coronal plane reflects upper brainstem dysfunction most closely. This study presents objective measurements of brainstem displacement as noted on MRI, and clarifies the relationships between anatomic and physiologic changes in the brainstem that are associated with supratentorial lesions. These results suggest the importance of brainstem distortion itself affecting on brainstem dysfunction with or without transtentorial herniation.

KEY WORDS: chronic subdural hematoma, brainstem distortion, Magnetic resonance imaging, Brainstem auditory evoked response

INTRODUCTION

Recent developments in neuroradiological imaging techniques are allowing better understanding of the correlation between neural dysfunction and anatomical changes. Computed Tomography (CT) demonstrated horizontal displacement of the brainstem associated with an acute unilateral cerebral mass relates closely to depressed consciousness[1,2]. Although brainstem distortion itself is implicated in the mechanism of depressed consciousness, transtentorial herniation does not consistently correlate with the clinical status of the patient[1,3]. Using magnetic resonance imaging (MRI), we measured various parameters of brainstem distortion associated with cerebral hemispheric displacement secondary to a unilateral supratentorial mass.

MATERIAL AND METHODS

Twenty-five patients with unilateral chronic subdural hematoma (age range 39-87, mean 66.4±3.5 years) were analyzed for this study. Both axial and coronal T1-weighted MR images were obtained in all patients pre-operatively using a Shimazu SMT 150, 1.5 tesla MRI system. The maximum hematoma thickness was measured on the coronal image. The shift from the midline sagittal plane of the septum pellucidum, pineal body, vertical intercollicular sulcus, interpeduncular fossa, and the floor of the fourth ventricle were measured on axial images. Rotational displacements were measured as angles between the midline sagittal plane and the following lines: on axial images, a line connecting the septum pellucidum and pineal body, and another line connecting the midpoint of the prepontine cistern and the floor of the fourth ventricle; on coronal images, a line through the plane of the third ventricle, and another line connecting the intercollicular sulcus and midpoint of the pontomedullary junction. In 11 cases, brainstem auditory evoked responses (BAER's) were performed pre-operatively. The latency of each peak (from I to V) and central conduction time were compared with normal subjects. Statistical analysis was performed using one sample normal tests for the comparisons between normal subjects and the patient group.

RESULTS

MRI findings

Logarithmic relationships were noted between both septum (cerebral) and interpeduncular fossa (brainstem) shifts, and hematoma thickness with fair correlations (septum r= 0.64, interpeduncular r=0.57). Shifts of the pineal body and other brainstem structures were also logarithmically related to septum shift, but with better regression coefficients (pineal r=0.96, interpeduncular r=0.73, and intercollicular r=0.74). Brainstem displacement was not evident until the septum (cerebral) shift was about 3-5 mm. With septum shifts between 5 mm and 10 mm, a marked shift of the brainstem was noted, reaching a plateau in displacement even beyond 10 mm of septum shift. In the axial plane, rotations of septum-pineal (central cerebrum) line and prepontine-fourth ventricle (brainstem) line are logarithmicaly related to septum shift. In the coronal plane, rotational movements of the third ventricle (cerebrum) line and intercollicular sulcus - pontomedurally junction (brainstem) line are shown to be logarithmically related to septum shift. The difference in magnitude of rotation in this plane between the cerebrum and brainstem at higher levels of cerebral shifts results in midbrain kinking.

BAER data

Latencies of the second through fifth peaks of BAER's, labeled sequentially from I to V, appeared significantly prolonged when averaged from all patients (n=11). However, in patients with less than 8 mm of septum shift (n=6), average peak latencies were not significantly changed from controls. Central conduction times measured as the interpeak latencies between I and V, and between III and V were also similarly prolonged in all patients. However, in patients with less than 8 mm septum shift, the average III to V interpeak latency was prolonged but the average I to V interpeak latency was not significantly changed. Prolongation of peak-V latency appears to correlate best with angulation of the intercollicular-pontomedullary line (coronal brainstem rotation) (r=0.78). It does not seem to relate as well to septum shift (r=0.47), or third ventricular angulation (r=0.54).

DISCUSSION

Brainstem deformity was classified into two[4,5] or three types[6] in pathological materials; lateral (or horizontal) displacement, downward (or caudal) displacement, and rotation in the axial plane. Sunderland[6] reported that these types of displacements changed as transtentorial herniation progressed. CT scans have shown that the brainstem begins to rotate and shift in the initial phase of actual herniation[7,8]. Fisher[3] and Roper[1] reported that the mechanism of depressed consciousness in patients with a supratentorial mass was due to direct brainstem distortion rather than transtentorial herniation. Quantitative MRI data in the present study show that the brainstem as well as the cerebrum shifts and rotates in a logarithmic manner, with segmental displacement observed in the neuro-axis rostro-caudally. The coronal image presents the best view to observe midbrain deformity. We obtained BAERs in order to compare these with brainstem deformity. Tsubokawa et al.[9] report that in acute severe head injury patients BAERs provide more reliable information about brainstem function than the neurological signs or CT findings. Our results show that brainstem deformity measured by MRI correlates well with brainstem dysfunction as assessed by BAERs. The prolongation of BAER latencies and central conduction times correlated with septum shift. All peak latencies, except peak-I, and central conduction times were prolonged in the severe septum shift group indicating midbrain as well as pontine involvement; while in the mild shift group prolongation of only the III-V central conduction time suggests only midbrain dysfunction. The results of peak-V latency indicated that brainstem rotation in the coronal plane reflects upper brainstem (midbrain) dysfunction most closely, which is in agreement with experimental data[10].

REFERENCE

1) Ropper AH: Lateral displacement of the brain and level of consciousness in patients with an acute hemispheral mass. N Engl J Med 314:953-958, 1986
2) Ross DA, Olsen WL, Ross AM, et al: Brain shift, level of consciousness, and restoration of consciousness in patients with acute intracranial hematoma. J Neurosurg 71:498-502, 1989
3) Fisher CM: Acute brain herniation--a revised concept, in Semin Neurol 4, 1984, pp 417-21.

4) Howell DA: Upper brain-stem compression and foraminal impaction with intracranial space-occupying lesions and swelling. Brain 82: 525 -550, 1959

5) Johnson RT, Yates PO: Brain stem haemorrhages in expanding supratentorial conditions. Acta radiol 46:250-256, 1956

6) Sunderland S: The tentorial notch and complications produced by herniations of the brain through that aperture. Br J Surg 45:422-438, 1958

7) Osborn AG: Diagnosis of descending transtentorial herniation by cranial computed tomography. Radiology 123:93-96, 1977

8) Storving J: Descending tentorial herniation: Findings on computed tomography. Neuroradiology 14:101-105, 1977

9) Tsubokawa T, Nishimoto H, Yamamoto T, et al: Assessment of brainstem damage by the auditory brainstem response in acute severe head injury. J Neurol Neurosurg Psychiatry 43:1005-1011, 1980

10) Nagao S, Roccaforte P, Moody R: Acute intracranial hypertension and auditory brain-stem responses. Part 2: The effects of brain-stem movement on the auditory brain-stem responses due to transtentorial herniation. J Neurosurg 51:846-851, 1979

Significance of Magnetic Resonance Imaging (MRI) in Diffuse Axonal Injury

HIROYUKI YOKOTA[1], YASUHIRO YAMAMOTO[1], TOSHIBUMI OTSUKA[1], SHIRO KOBAYASHI[2], and SHOZO NAKAZAWA[2]

[1]Department of Emergency and Critical Care Medicine, and [2]Department of Neurosurgery, Nippon Medical School, Bunkyo-ku, Tokyo, 113 Japan

SUMMARY

Advantages of magnetic resonance imaging(MRI) to computerized tomography(CT) on diagnosis of diffuse axonal injury(DAI) were discussed. Twenty-three patients diagnosed as DAI defined by the criteria of Gennarelli were studied with CT and MRI. Lesions were demonstrated as high intensity area on MRI of T2 weighted imaging in all patients. These lesions were located only in cerebral white matter in the cases of mild DAI, whereas in the severe DAI located in a basal ganglia, corpus callosum,dorsal part of the brain stem as well as the cerebral white matter. As for the finding of CT, these parencymal lesions were not visualized in mild or moderate DAI.

Our series suggested that MRI is superior to CT on the diagnosis of DAI and provides some informations to evaluate the severity of DAI.

INTRODUCTION

The evaluation of patients with head injuries was significantly improved by the introducion of computerized tomography(CT). Unfortunately, CT fails to demonstrate lesions like non-hemorrhagic contusions or those located in the posterior fossa and in the frontal and temporal lobes because of artifacts from nearby high density of bony structures. Based on a phenonemon of the radiofrequency-induced excitation and relaxation of nuclei ordered in a magneitc field, MRI is thought to be superior to CT for visualizing these lesions. However, the usefullness of MRI in acute head injury has not fully explored[1,2]. In this presentation we describe the usefullness of MRI in acute head injury especially in diffuseaxonal injury(DAI) established by Gennarelli[3,4].

MATERIALS AND METHOD

Over the past two years, 249 head injuried patients were underwent studies of MRI within 3 days of injury. Of these, 23 patients were diagnosed as DAI according the criteria establised by Gennarelli. CT was carried out in all patients within 3 hours following the first MRI study.MRI was performed on HITACHI MRP-20,or TOSHIBA MRT-50 using 0.2 or 0.5Tesla magnietc strength. Imaging were obtained in continuous 10mm slices in transaxial palin using spin echo sequence as T2 weighted imaging.A patient monitoring system was devised to assist observation by doctors or nurses. The blood pressure, heart rate and electro-cardiogram were recorded automatically at 1 minute interval. If the patients was consused,diazepam equal to 10-20 mg was administered in-travenously for sedation.

Their ages ranged from 7 years to 62 years with a mean of 29.0 years. Of these, 7 patients were classified to mild DAI, 9 and 7 were classified to moderate and severe DAI by the criteria proposed by Gennarelli.

CASE REPORT
CASE 1
A 16-years old man struck his head in a motorcycle accident and was admitted our hospital without consciousness. CT performed 3 hours after injury did not demonstrate any lesions in cerebral parencyma(Fig 1-A). MRI performed a day after the injury demonstrated lesions on the temporal and frontal white matters as the high intensity areas on T2 weighted imaging.

He was diagnosed as mild DAI by the critera established by Gennarelli His conscousness became clear and he has remained asymptomatic thereafter.

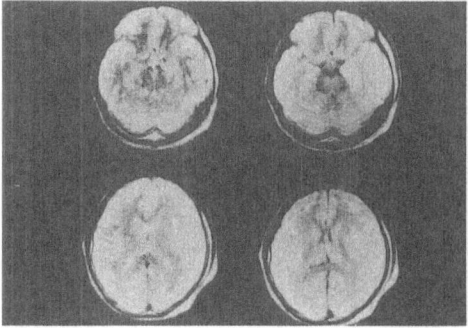

Fig.1-A

CASE 2
A 16-years old female struck her head in a automoble accident and was admitted our hospital on 8 points of Glasgow coma scale. CT performed on admission showed the subarachnoid hemorrhage(Fig.2-A), and MRI performed just after CT, demonstrated the lesion located the sub-ependymal layer on the trigone of the left lateral ventricle,
We couldmake the diagnosis as moderate DAI according to the clinical symptom. Her conscousness became gradually improving and she was disch aged without any neurological deficit 4 weeks after injury.

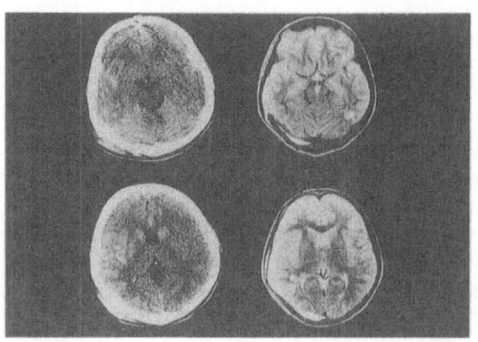

Fig.2-A

MRI performed 3 months after injury revealed the same lesion on T2 weighted imaging. We suposed that the lesion which was demonstrated on MRI but on CT was non-hemorrhagic contusion.

CASE 3

A 7-years old girl was a pedestrain who was struch over her head in an automobile accident and was admitted to our hospital with decerebrate posturing. CT performed 2 hours after injury revealed a hemorrage in the midbrain and trigone of the left lateral ventricle(Fig.3-A). MRI taken 3 days after the injury demonstrate the lesion in the dorasal part of the brainstem and the splenium of corpus callosum which was not shown on CT. We could make the diagnosis as the severe DAI and could detect the lesions which were anable to demonsterate by CT(Fig.3-B). The patients made no significant recovery and remained in a severe disability 1 month after injury.

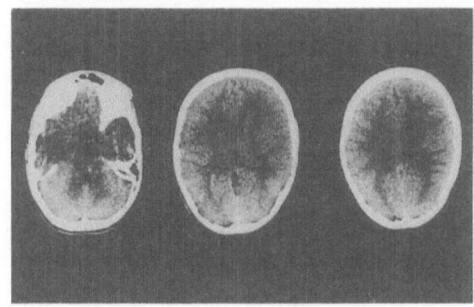

Fig.3-A

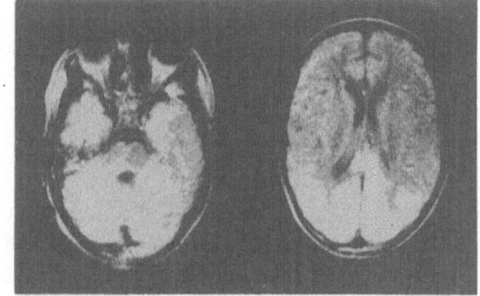

Fig.3-B

RESULT AND CONCLUSION

table 1   The number of parenchymal lesions on MRI in DAI

	mild (n = 7)	moderate (n = 9)	severe (n = 7)	total (n = 23)
hemorrhage	2	2	8	12
non-hemorrhagic contusion	5	9	7	21
focal edema	0	1	0	1
total	7	12	15	34

MRI . magnetic resonance imaging. DAI diffuse axonal injury

Using MRI, we could detect some lesions in all of the patients diagnosed as DAI. The lesions which were detected on MRI but not on CT, in mild DAI were located only in the cerebral white matter. In the moderate DAI, the lesions were located in subependymal layer, corpus callosum,basalganglia as well as the cerebral white matter which were thought to be non-hemonrrhageic contusion not to be able to demonstrate by CT. These lesions which are not demonstrated on CT but are demonstrated on MRI are considered non-hemorrhagic contusions[4], because the intensity of these lesions is not changed for more than 4 weeks onserial MRI. Lesions of severe DAI were revealed both on CT[5]. and on MRI in the cerebral white matter,basal ganglia,corpus callosum, subependymal layer and brainstem.Severe DAI has has been known to have characteristic findings of hemorrhage in these areas. In contrast, the lesion of mild and moderate DAI have been thought to be difficult to detect on CT. MRI is able to demonstrate these lesions as high intensity area on T2 weighted imaging in mild or moderate DAI as well as in the severe DAI(table.1).

table 2   Location of parenchymal lesions on MRI and CT in DAI

	mild (n = 7)	moderate (n = 9)	severe (n = 7)
white matter	5 (1)	6 (1)	4 (3)
basal ganglia	2 (1)	1 (1)	5 (3)
corpus callosum	0 (0)	1 (0)	2 (1)
subependymal	0 (0)	2 (0)	2 (0)
brain stem	0 (0)	1 (0)	2 (1)

MRI magnetic resonance imaging, CT computerized tomography. DAI diffuse axonal injury. ( ) represents the number of patients of CT findings

And MRI is also useful to evaluate the severity of DAI. The main lesions in mild DAI are located in cerebral white matter, and the lesion in severe DAI are located in all of theseareas. In severe DAI, the number of lesions which was demonstrated on MRI were much more than that demonstrated on CT(table.2).

Our study suggest the following. MRI is cleary more sensitive than CT in detecting the lesions of diffuse axonal injury. And MRI is useful to evaluate the severity of diffuse axonal injury and may be able to predict the prognosis of these patients[6]. The introduction of MRI may improve the outcome of diffuse axomal injury.

We conclud that MRI is considered to be superior to CT in the evaluation of diffuse axonal injury.

REFERENCES
1. Levin HS, Amparo E, Eisenberg H : Magneic resonance imagingand computerized tomography in relation to the neurobehavioral sequelae of mild and moderate injuries. J Neurosurg. 66:706-713,1987
2. Wilberger JE, Deeb Z, Rothfus W: Magnetic resonace imaging in acses of severe head injury. Neurosurgery,20:571-576,1987
3. Gennarelli TA : Emergency department management of head injuries. Emerg.Med.Clin.No.Amer.,2:749-760,1984
4. Gennarelli TA, Spieman GM, Langfit TW : Influence of the tpye of intracranial lesion on outcome from severe head injury. J.Neurosurg. 56:26-32,1982
5. Kobayasi s, Nakazawa S : Diffuse brain injur—Treatment and outcome. Neurosurgeons,6:27-32,1987
6. Yokota H, Kurokawa A, Otsusa T,Kobayashiu S, Nakazawa S : Significance of magentic resonance imaging in acute head injury. J Trauma 31:351-357,1991

MRI in Surgically Treated Cases of Post-Traumatic Cervical Myelopathy and Radiculopathy

TETSUYA MORIMOTO, TOSHISUKE SAKAKI, SHIGERU TSUNODA, TORU HOSHIDA, SHOICHIRO KAWAGUCHI, and TAKAO OHASHI

Department of Neurosurgery, Nara Medical University, Kashihara, 634 Japan

SUMMARY

The purpose of this study is to find the characteristic in MRI in surgical cases of cervical myelopathy and radiculopathy. From neurological findings, these cases were classified in three groups, radiculopathy group, radiculomyelopathy group, and myelopathy group. To study the dynamic change of CSF space, MRI in sagittal plane was done in both neutral position and extension position. Intramedullary lesions were recognized as high intensity area in T2WI in 8 cases with myelopathy group. These findings can be seen mainly at C3/4 level followed by C5/6.
From the configulation of cord compression, MRI findings were classified into three categolies, localized type, stenotic type, and bamboo type. In 8 myelopathy cases, 6 cases showed stenotic type with one or multiple level pincer effect. In dynamic study, CSF space became narrower and pincer effect was enhanced in extension position. These changes were more severe in myelopathy cases than radiculopathy cases. One of the mechanism of spinal cord injury is supposed to be hyperextension neck motion with pincer effect to the cord.

KEY WORDS: traumatic cervical injury, hyperextension injury, MRI, dynamic study, intramedullary lesion

INTRODUCTION

MRI shows not only extramedullary lesion but also intramedullary lesion. Dynamic study of the cord and CSF space seems to be important because of hyperextension or hyperflexion injury may be the cause of spinal cord injury. MRI provides non-invasive image of the cord in various position of the neck. We reviewed MRI findings in cases of post-traumatic cervical myelopathy and radiculopathy treated surgically.

MATERIALS AND METHODS

There are 22 cases (age:40-80, mean:56.8y.o., 15 males and 7 females). From neurological findings, these cases were classified in three groups. 1)Radiculopathy group includes 10 cases who shows radicular sign (Table 2. case 13-22). 2)Radiculomyelopathy group includes 4 cases who shows both radicular sign and long tract sign (Table 1. case

Table 1 Summary of Myelopathy and Radiculomyelopathy cases

CASE No.	AGE	SEX	Dynamic study Neut.→ Ext.	Pincer effect	Intramedullary High Intensity (T2WI)	Trauma to op.(wks)	Procedures
1	43	M	St	$C_{4/5}$	$C_{4/5} \sim C_5$	5	Lami.→Ant.
2	63	M	St → Ba	$C_{3/4}$	$C_{3/4} \sim C_6$	36	Lami.
3	69	M	Lo → Ba	$C_{3/4}$	$C_{3/4}$	21	Lami.
4	80	M	Lo	$C_{3/4}$	$C_{3/4} \sim C_4$	4	Lami.
5	71	M	St → Ba	$C_{4/5}$	$C_{4/5}$	20	Lami.
6	40	M	St	$C_{3/4}$	$C_{3/4}$	4	Lami.+Ant.
7	71	F	Ba → Ba	$C_{5/6}$	$C_{5/6}$	12	Lami.
8	45	F	St → St	$C_{5/6}$	$C_{5/6}$	4	Ant.
9	46	M	Lo	$C_{4/5}$	$C_{4/5}$	6	Ant.→Lami.
10	52	F	St → Ba	$C_{5/6}$	None	13	Lami.+Ant.
11	42	M	Lo → Lo	$C_{3/4}$	$C_{3/4}$	8	Lami.
12	59	M	Ba → Ba	$C_{3/4}$	None	11	Lami.+Ant.

St: Stenotic type Neut.: Neutral position Lami.: Laminectomy or
Lo: Localized type Ext.: Extension position Laminoplasty
Ba: Bamboo type Ant.: Anterior fusion

Table 2 Summary of Radiculopathy cases

CASE No.	AGE	SEX	Dynamic study Neut.→ Ext.	Pincer effect	Intramedullary High Intensity (T2WI)	Trauma to op.(wks)	Procedures
13	48	M	Lo → Lo	$C_{6/7}$	—	3	Ant.
14	60	M	Lo → Lo	$C_{5/6}$	—	4	Ant.
15	58	M	Lo → Ba	$C_{5/6}$	—	3	Ant.
16	42	M	St → St	$C_{5/6}$	—	12	Lami.
17	76	M	St → Ba	$C_{6/7}$	—	3	Ant.
18	63	M	Ba → Ba	$C_{4/5}$	—	5	Ant.
19	55	F	Ba → Ba	$C_{4/5}$	—	4	Ant.
20	51	F	Ba → Ba	$C_{4/5}$	—	11	Lami.
21	67	F	Lo → Lo	$C_{3/4}$	—	16	Ant.
22	48	F	Lo → Lo	$C_{3/4}$	—	8	Ant.

St: Stenotic type Neut.: Neutral position Lami.: Laminectomy or
Lo: Localized type Ext.: Extension position Laminoplasty
Ba: Bamboo type Ant.: Anterior fusion

9-12). 3)Myelopathy group includes 8 cases who shows long tract sign
(Table 1. case 1-8). The resimen of treatment in the initial stage was
as follows. Patients were fixed on the bed after roentogenological
evaluation with head CT, skull X-ray, cervical X-ray, and cervical CT.
After 2 weeks bed rest, MRI of spine was performed in all cases. In 2
cases (Table 1. case 1,4), MRI(TOSHIBA 50A 0.5T) was done in the earlier stage (case 1 on 2nd day after trauma, case 4 on 3rd day after
trauma) because of the deterioration of neurological status. Routine
medical resimen was glycerol infusion and glucocorticoid administration.
MRI was done in T1WI and T2WI in both axial and sagittal plane 2 weeks
after trauma. If neurological status was stable at this moment, MRI in
sagittal plane was done in both neutral and extension position to
study the dynamic change of cerebrospinal fluid (CSF) space. Isobist
or Metrizamide CT myelography as well as routine myelography was done
in all cases with neck collar on, to avoid inappropriate neck motion.

RESULTS

From the MRI findings, these 22 cases were classified into three
groups, stenotic type, localized type and bamboo type from the configulation of cord compression. Stenonic type indicates diffuse obliteration of CSF space from both anterior and posterior. Localized type
indicates one or two level obliteration of CSF space. Bamboo type indicates multi-level obliteration of CSF space at interspace between
vertebral body. In myelopathy group, there are 5 stenotic type, 2 localized type and 1 bamboo type. In radiculomyelopaty group, 2 localized type, 1 stenotic type and 1 bamboo type. In radiculopathy group,
5 localized type, 3 bamboo type and 2 stenotic type are observed. In
extension position, spinal cord squeezing became more severe with so
called "pincer effect". This level is indicated in table 1. Dynamic
study was done in 18 cases. In 6 cases, MRI configuration became bamboo type from stenotic or localized type.
Post-operative MRI findings was reviewed in every cases. In all 8
cases of myelopathy, intramedullary high intensity area could be detected after surgical decompression. But, in four cases of 8 myelopathy, pre-operative MRI cannot demonstrate these abnormality because of
too narrow spinal cord. The level of the detected high intensity area
are mainly at the level of C3/4 in 4 cases, and C5/6 in 3 cases. In 2
cases, high intensity area could be seen in multiple levels. In 2 of 4
radiculomyelopathy cases, intramedullary high intensity area was recognized, while in radiculopathy cases, no high intensity area could be
seen. An illustrative case is demonstrated in figure 1 and 2.

DISCUSSION

In our series, there are 8 cases in myelopathy group who showed intramedullary high intensity area on MRI. The location of the high intensity area can be most commonly seen at C3/4 and C5/6 followed by C4/5.
In 5 cases of 8 myelopathy, dynamic MRI was performed to analyze the
dynamic compression of the spinal cord on neck extension. Site of the
intramedullary lesion correlates well to the site of dynamic compression of the cord. Dynamic study also revealed multiple pincer effet
producing bamboo type cord compression, which may initially localized
or stenotic type of cord configulation in neutral position. It may be

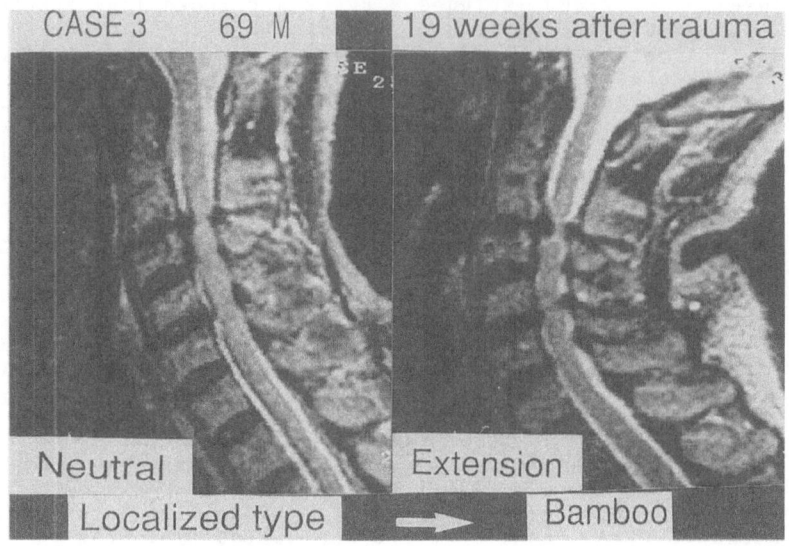

Fig.1 Preoperative MRI in sagittal plane in case 3.
Congenital fusion of C2 and C3 is noted. In extension
position, pincer effect is prominent at C3/4 level and
configulation of CSF space becomes bamboo type.

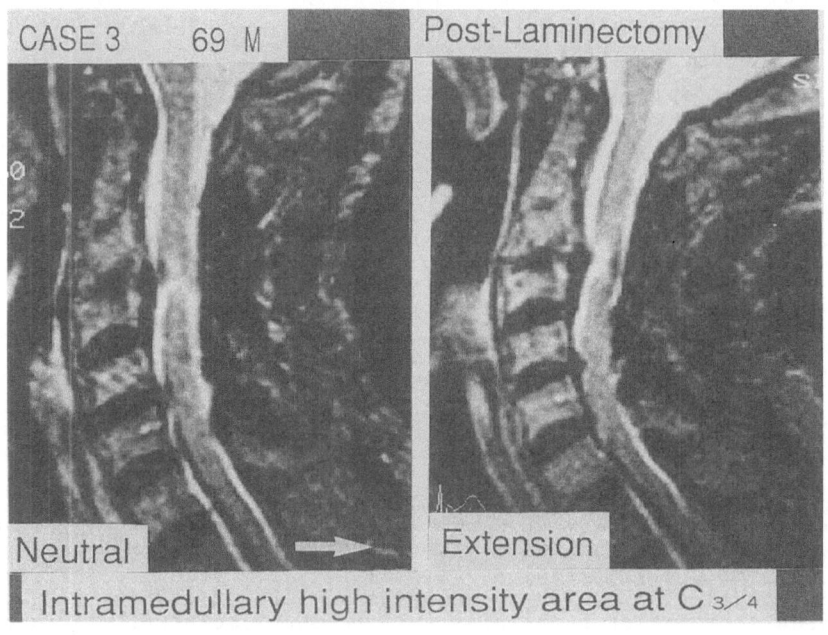

Fig.2 Postoperative MRI. Intramedullary high intensity
area is clearly demonstrated at C3/4 level.

speculated that patient of stenotic type with severe pincer effect in extension position is prone to the spinal cord injury. In acute traumatic central cord syndrome, spondylosis and canal stenosis may be one of the important factor for the development of cord injury[1]. Flanders[2] studied correlation of MR imaging findings with degree of neurologic deficit. They found no correlation between preexisting stenosis or spondylosis and severity of clinical injury.

There are some reports on MRI-pathological correlation in acute traumatic central cord syndrome. Primary findings was diffuse disruption of axons, especially within the lateral columns of the cervical cord [1]. Edema in the cord was suggested by the findings of focal high signal on the gradient refocussed echo images. Martin[3] reported a case whose MRI is very similar to histopathlogical features..T2-weighted MRI showed a central hyperintense area at C3-4. Histopathology disclosed severe axonal swelling and edema in the dorsolatral fasciculi and also recent necrosis in the right anterior horn. Common findings in our series was high intensity area on T2WI. Although immediate surgical decompression of the spinal canal remains controversial, diskectomy and laminectomy are the choice for cervical spinal cord injuries in acute and subacute stage[4]. Our surgical timing is still later than their report. For evaluation of possible improvement by surgical decompression, MRI with dynamic study is helpful in the later stage.

REFERENCES

1. Quencer RM, Bunge RP, Egnor M, Green BA, Puckett W, Naidich TP, Post MJD, Norenberg M(1992) Acute traumatic central cord syndrome: MRI-pathological correlations. Neuroradiology 34:85-94
2. Flanders AE, Schaefer DM, Doan HT, Mishkin MM, Gonzalez CF, Northrup BE(1990) Acute cervical spine trauma: correlation of MR imaging findings with degree of neurologic deficit. Neuroradiolgy 177:25-33
3. Martin D, Schoenen J, Lenelle J, Reznik M, Moonen G(1992) MRI-pathological correlations in acute traumatic central cord syndrome: case report. Neuroradiology 34:262-266
4. Mirvis SE, Geisler FH, Jelinek JJ, Joslyn JN, Gellad F(1988) Acute cervical spine trauma: evaluation with 1.5-T MR imaging. Neuroradiology 166:807-816

Diffuse Axonal Injury Caused by Traffic Accident – Long Term Serial CT Findings and Medicolegal Problem

CHIKAYUKI OCHIAI[1], TSUNEO OHNO[2], and MASAKATSU NAGAI[1]

[1]Department of Neurosurgery, Dokkyo University School of Medicine, Mibu-machi, Tochigi, 321-02 Japan, and
[2]Automobile Insurance Rating Association of Japan, Chiyoda-ku, Tokyo, 101 Japan

SUMMARY

The aim of the present study was to clarify the chronological change of CT findings in the patient with diffuse axonal injury (DAI). We utilized the clinical data of 20 DAI cases who had been subjected to Automobile Insurance Rating Association of Japan (AIRAJ) and of six DAI cases of our own hospital. Duration of follow-up, from the accident to the final CT, was up to 40 months in the AIRAJ cases and four months in our cases.

Compared with the initial CT taken on the day of accident, a most common finding on follow-up CT was a dilatation of the ventricular system, which occurred within a few weeks following the insult. Planimetry at the level of the foramen Monro showed size of the lateral ventricle became 1.4-3.8 times larger than the original one.

In 17 out of 20 AIRAJ cases, because of a difficulty for drawing a correct diagnosis solely from CT findings without seeing the patient him- or herself, DAI had been overlooked until the reevaluation was claimed. The importance to recognize DAI as a clinical entity was emphasized from a medicolegal point of view, especially in the insurance business.

KEY WORDS: diffuse axonal injury, ventricular dilatation, computed tomography, planimetry, medicolegal problem

INTRODUCTION

Patients who have survived in a disabled state after diffuse axonal injury (DAI) are usually transferred to a rehabilitation facility without staying a long term in the initial neurosurgical department. Thus, a serial long-term follow-up of computed tomography (CT) findings in the patient with DAI is very difficult. In order to overcome this difficulty we have planned to utilize the clinical data of the Automobile Insurance Rating Association of Japan (AIRAJ), a major activity of which is to set a fair rating for the automobile insurance. In the AIRAJ, for evaluating the permanent impairment of an individual suffered from a traffic accident, his or her clinical data, including CTs, are serially collected from every hospital to which he or she has been referred.

MATERIALS AND METHODS

Between 1989 and 1991, 20 cases of DAI were subjected to the AIRAJ in order to evaluate their impairment. There were 16 males and four females, aged 10 to 69 years. They had sustained a road accident while riding a motor bike in 10 cases, while walking in seven, and while driving a car in three. Immediately after the insult they had developed coma or semicoma, duration of which varied from three days to two months. Findings on the initial CT taken on the day of the accident was negative in seven cases. Remaining 13 cases showed high density areas in dorsolateral aspect of the upper brainstem in seven, in the corpus callosum in five, thick or thin subarachnoid hemorrhage in five, and subependymal bleeding in four. Duration of the follow-up period, from the accident to the final CT, was up to 40 months. In each case dilatation of the lateral ventricle was a common finding on the follow-up CTs[1] (Fig. 1).

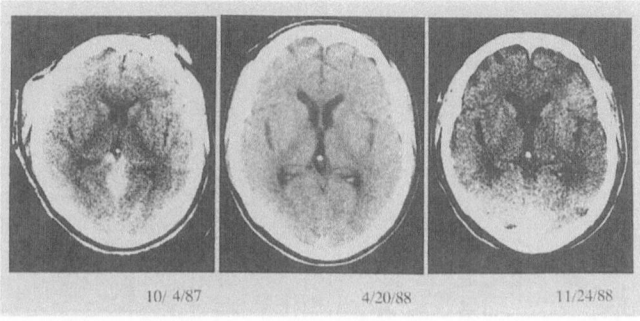

Fig. 1 Serially collected tomography scans of a representative case with DAI (40-year-old male). Left: On the day of accident. Center: Six months later. Right: 13 months later. Each scan was gathered from three different hospitals. Follow-up CTs show no abnormality other than the mild ventricular dilatation.

In order to compare the ventricular size on CT, the value of B/A was calculated in each case (fig. 2). A and B were measured by planimetry. Degree of the ventricular enlargement was expressed by the ratio of (the value of B/A on the follow-up CT)/(the value of B/A on the initial CT).

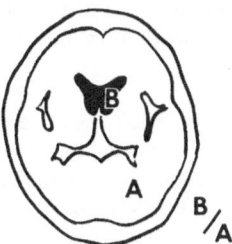

Fig. 2 Measurement of the ventricular size. Ventricular size was expressed by B/A. A and B indicate the area of the whole brain and the lateral ventricles, respectively, at the level of the foramen Monro.

181

The same analysis was carried out among the our own six cases, who survived moderate or severe DAI[2] caused by traffic accident in these three years. Male to female ratio was 4:2. The age ranged from nine to 52 years. Four out of the six cases had an episode of respiratory distress such as Cheyne-Stokes respiration immediately or shortly after the injury. Duration of follow-up period was at most four months.

RESULTS

Time course of the ventricular size in the 20 cases subjected to the AIRAJ is shown in Fig. 3. In each case, size of the lateral ventricle became 1.4-3.8 times larger while compared the final CT with the initial one. It was suggested that enlargement of the ventricular system took place within a half year after the injury.

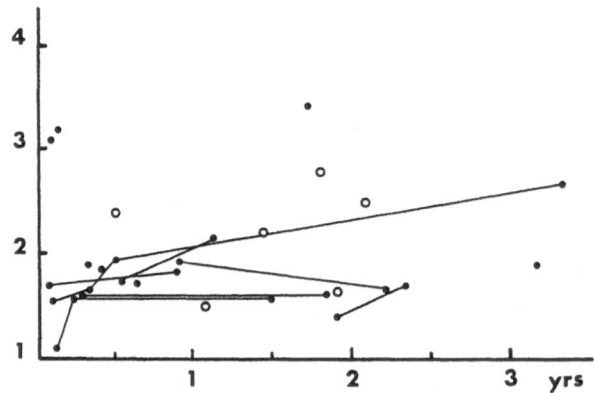

Fig. 3. Chronological change of the ventricular size. Degree of the ventricular enlargement was plotted according to the duration of follow-up period. The same cases were indicated by lines. However, the line connecting the initial CT and the first follow-up CT was omitted in each case. Closed and open circles indicate coma and semicoma, respectively, which developed after the insult.

Results of our six cases are shown in Fig. 4. Ventricular enlargement was also noticeable. It could occur even within a few weeks after the insult. Among these six cases, the fact whether a patient suffered from respiratory distress after the injury or not was not related to the occurrence of ventriculomegaly.

Serial follow-up CTs (three or more than three times) were available in seven cases in Fig. 3 and four cases in Fig. 4. Chronological course of these 10 cases strongly suggested that the lateral ventricle would remain in a similar size once the enlargement took place within a few weeks following the injury.

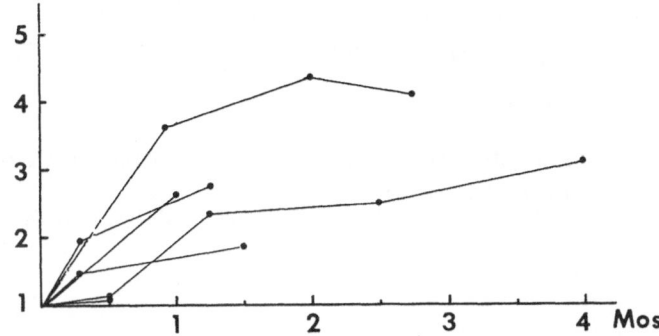

Fig. 4 Chronological change of the ventricular size of the
six cases admitted to our hospital. Degree of the ventricular
enlargement was plotted according to the duration of follow-up
period. The same cases were indicated by lines.

DISCUSSION

The lack of an apparent finding other than ventricular dilatation on
follow-up CT is a big problem for the DAI patient who is to receive the
benefit from an automobile insurance. Because, in the insurance
business, evaluation of the patient's impairment, therefore the amount
of compensation to be paid, is often decided by CT findings without
seeing the patient him- or herself. In fact, in the present series,
reassessment was necessary in 17 out of the 20 cases.

Long tract degeneration of Wallerian type throughout the cerebral
hemisphere resulted from axonal tearing has been widely accepted as the
pathogenesis of ventriculomegaly[3]. Time course of the ventricular
enlargement clarified in the present study well supports this theory.

In a chronic stage of DAI, a possible finding on CT is a ventricular
dilatation. It should be differentiated from normal pressure
hydrocephalus since shunting procedure is not effective for DAI.

REFERENCES

1. Cordobés F, Lobato RD, Rivas J, Cabrera A, Sarabia M, Castro S,
    Cisneros C, Torres ID, Lamas E (1986) Acta Neurochir 81: 27-35
2. Gennarelli TA (1987) Head injury. 2nd ed. Williams & Wilkins.
    Baltimore, pp 108-124
3. Graham DI, Adams JH, Path FRC, Gennarelli TA (1987) Head injury.
    2nd ed. Williams & Wilkins. Baltimore, pp 72-88

Comparison of MRI and X-ray CT Scan Findings in Patients with Serious Neurological Deficits Due to Head Injury

YOSHIKAZU OKADA[1], TAKESHI SHIMA[1], MASAHIRO NISHIDA[1], KANJI YAMANE[1], SHINJI OKITA[1], and AKIRA YOSHIDA[2]

[1]Department of Neurosurgery, and [2]Department of Critical Care Medicine, Chugoku Rousai Hospital, Kure, 737-01 Japan

SUMMARY

Thirty-six closed-head injury (CHI) patients who showed serious neurological deficits without causative X-ray CT findings were examined by MRI(1.5 tesla).

Intracranial hemorrhagic lesions such as epidural hematoma(EDH), subdural hematoma(SDH) and traumatic subarachnoid hemorrhage(SAH) were more easily and precisely visualized by X-ray CT scan in comparison to MRI. In contrast, MRI was superior to X-ray CT scan in detecting deep brain lesions extending from the brainstem to subcortical white matter, which were characteristics in diffuse axonal injury (DAI). The clinical outcome of 20 DAI patients was closely related to clinical grading of the patient, and seemed to be relevant to the degree of extension of lesions.

KEY WORDS: Closed-head injury, X-CT scan, MRI, diffuse axonal injury

INTRODUCTION

Recent neuroimaging studies have been reported MRI is more sensitive to visualize the lesions in patients with CHI than X-ray CT scan [1]. The purpose of this study was (1)to assess the capability of MRI and X-ray CT scan to detect intracranial lesions in patients with CHI, (2)to investigate the relationships between the findings by both neuroimagings modalities and clinical features.

MATERIALS AND METHODS

Thirty-six patients, 21 males and 15 females aged from 4 to 82 year-old, who met the criteria of this study were selected from consecutive admissions to the Chugoku Rousai Hospital for CHI. The criteria for the patients were the following: The patients presented with serious neurological deficits and disturbance of consciousness without causative intracranial lesions detected by X-ray CT scan on admission. They had undergone X-ray CT scanning within 3 hours after head injury and MRI within 72 hours. The level of consciousness was evaluated following Glasgow Coma Scale(GCS) scores and neurological examinations were carried out on the day of admission. X-ray CT scans were obtained on a Toshiba TCT-70A without contrast enhancement. MRI was performed on a Picker International using 1.5 tesla magnetic field strength. Neuro-imagings were obtained in contiguous 10 mm slices in the transaxial planes. Follow-up examinations of CT scan were performed at 1-2 weeks, 1-2 months and 3-6 months, and those of MRI were obtained at 1-3 months. Clinical outcome was estimated by Glasgow Outcome Scale (GOS) at the 6 months after head injury.

RESULTS

Clinical features and outcomes: Mean value of GCS scores on admission was 7.8, GCS score of 23 patients were less than 7, and those of the remaining 13 patients were more than 8. All patients presented with serious neurological deficits and/or disturbance of consciousness. Favorable clinical outcome (good recovery and moderate disability) and poor outcome (severe disability, persistent vegetative state and dead) were 26 and 10 patients, and their mean value of GCS scores on admission were 8.3 and 6.1, respectively.

Detection and localization of lesions by X-ray CT scan and MRI: Table 1 presents the X-ray CT scan and MRI findings in the acute period of head injury. X-ray CT scan did not show any lesions in eight patients, and MRI demonstrated no lesions in two patients. Acute EDH and SDH could be observed easily by both neuroimaging modalities. Brain contusion and/or intraparenchymal small lesions were more frequently detected by MRI. Especially, deep brain lesions which were characteristics in DAI could be evidently visualized by MRI in contrast to X-ray CT. Additionally traumatic internal carotid arterial occlusion was diagnosed in two cases by MRI. On the contrary, X-ray CT scan was more sensitive than MRI to visualize thin and/or localized SAH.

DAI: Twenty patients were diagnosed as DAI, whose findings of neuroimagings are summarized in table 2. And DAI was categorized as mild, moderate and severe following Gennarelli's criteria [2]. The mild, moderate and severe DAI were composed of five, six and nine patients, respectively. Few patients showed serious brain swelling by both neuroimagings. By X-ray CT scan in the acute period, five of 11 mild or moderate DAI demonstrated SAH in the Sylvian fissure, interhemispheric cistern and dorsolateral quadrant of the rostral brainstem, while four patients did not present evident findings. Even in severe DAI patients, small deep brain lesions could be seen in only two of nine patients by X-ray CT scan, and in five patients mild SAH and/or thin SDH were observed. By MRI, all mild or moderate DAI patients demonstrated evident lesions extending from the pons to basal ganglia. Furthermore, in severe DAI patients MRI revealed more diffusely extended deep brain lesions from the pons to subcortical white matter in comparison to those in patients with mild or moderate DAI.

The relationships between grading of DAI and GOS at 6 months after head injury are shown in table 3. There could be seen a close relationship between clinical grading of DAI and outcome. Namely, mild and moderate DAI had favorable outcome except one persistent vegetative state patient, and most of severe DAI patients had poor outcomes. Follow-up neuroimagings clarified disappearance of hyperintense lesions at the brainstem in nine patients. And all severe and half of moderate DAI patients demonstrated more rapid and progressive brain atrophy.

DISCUSSION

This study has shown that MRI is inferior to X-ray CT scan in visualizing traumatic SAH in patients with CHI, on the contrary in detecting parenchymal and extraparenchymal lesions MRI is superior to X-ray CT scan. Especially the deep brain lesions, extending from the brain stem to subcortical white matter presenting characteristics of DAI, would be more evidently observed by MRI in comparison to X-ray CT scan. These findings reconfirmed the previous results [3].

DAI has attracted special interest recently, which was an entity delivered by postmortal findings in patients with serious brain damages due to shearing injury. This neuropathological findings has been introduced one of clinical entities of patients presenting coma immediately after injury [1,2,3]. From this study, we would like to suggest that the meaning of MRI findings in DAI patients should be confirmed, because disappearance of hyperintense lesions in the deep brain could be observed in many DAI patients. Further, the extension of deep brain lesions and the following rapid and severe brain atrophy seemed to be closely related to clinical outcome with some exceptional cases. These observations may indicate that MRI is the most sensitive neuro-imaging modality to detect the deep brain lesions, but is not able to visualize all brain damages of CHI. Therefore, in future it is necessary to clarify the pathological meanings of MRI lesions and their relations with the delayed morphological changes and neuropsychological sequelae.

CONCLUSION

X-ray CT scan is very effective for detecting the intracranial hemorrhagic lesions in the acute period of closed-head injury, but MRI would be recommended for documenting deep brain lesions and for evaluating the clinical outcomes.

REFERENCES

1. Teasdale E and Headley DM(1990): Radiodiagnosis of brain injury: Handbook of Clinical Neurology 57. Elsevier Science Publishers. Amsterdam, pp 143-179
2. Gennarelli TA(1980): Emergency Medicine Clinics of North America 2: 749-760
3. Hadley DM, Teasdale GM, et al (1988): Clinical Radiology 39: 131-139

Table 1:
Comparison of X-ray and MRI findings in 36 head injured patients

	X-ray CT	MRI
EDH	(1)	(1)
SDH	(9)	(8)
Contusion (+hematoma)	(9)	(14)
DAI	(2)	(20)
TICAO	(0)	(2)
No lesion	(8)	(2)

EDH: epidural hematoma, SDH: subdural hematoma, DAI: diffuse axonal injury, TICAO: traumatic internal carotid artery, occlusion, ( ): number

Table 3:
Relationsahip between grading of DAI and Glasgow Outcome Scale (GOS)

grading of DAI	GOS				
	GR	MD	SD	PV	D
mild	(5)				
moderate	(4)	(1)		(1)	
severe		(3)	(1)	(2)	(3)

GR: good recovery, MD: moderate disability
SD: severe disability, PV: persistent vegetative state, D: dead, ( ): number

Table 2: Sites of lesions detected by X-ray CT and MRI in 20 DAI patients

No.	Age	Grading of DAI	X-ray CT	MRI
1	16	Mild	SAH	BG. & W.M.
2	36	Mild	–	pons
3	11	Mild	SAH	B.S.
4	7	Mild	SDH & contusion(FL)	SDH, B.G. & C.C
5	7	Mild	SAH	B.S
6	16	Moderate	V.H.	B.G. & C.C
7	82	Moderate	SAH	B.S.
8	4	Moderate	–	C.C., pons & B.G.
9	23	Moderate	–	C.C. & W.M.
10	20	Moderate	–	B.G. & B.S.
11	57	Moderate	EDH & SAH	EDH & C.C.
12	21	Severe	contusion(FL)	pons & W.M.
13	82	Severe	B.G. & SAH	B.G., C.C & W.M.
14	32	Severe	–	B.S. & cerebellum
15	20	Severe	SAH	C.C. & W.M.
16	42	Severe	SAH	B.G., C.C. & W.M.
17	44	Severe	EDH & contusion(MB)	EDH, C.C., B.S. & W.M.
18	21	Severe	–	B.G. & W.M.
19	76	Severe	SDH	SDH, B.S., C.C. & W.M.
20	22	Severe	SAH	B.G. & W.M.

EDH: epidural hematoma, SDH: subdural hematoma, SAH: subarachnoid hemorrhage, V.H.: ventricular hemorrhage, B.G.: basal ganglia, B.S.: brain stem, C.C.: corpus callosum, W.M.: white matter, FL: flontal lobe

The Clinical Study of Severe Diffuse Axonal Injury – A Prognostic Point of View from MRI Study in the Acute Stage

MASAO TOMINAGA[1], TETSUYA MORIMOTO[1], TOSHISUKE SAKAKI[1], TAKAHIDE SHIMOMURA[2], HIROYUKI HASHIMOTO[3], and SHIGEO TAKAI[4]

[1]Department of Neurosurgery, Nara Medical University, Kashihara, 634 Japan, [2]Seikeikai Hospital, Sakai, 591 Japan, [3]Okanami Hospital, Ueno, 518 Japan, and [4]Takai Hospital, Tenri, 632 Japan

SUMMARY

We studied the relationship between the final outcome and MRI(T2WI) findings which were evaluated within 48 hours after injury. Twenty-five patients were transfered within 6 hours after injury and underwent MRI following CT in the same day or next day of the admission. All patients were comatose more than 24 hours after injury. Brain stem symptoms were positive in the acute stage. The final outcomes were evaluated at 6 months.
Ten patients died and six were persistent vegetative state, and MRI of these patients demonstrated the high intensity in the corpus callosum, bilateral basal ganglias and mid brain. Six patients were severely disabled and three were moderately disabled. In the MRI findings of these patients, high intensity areas were localized in the unilateral basal ganglia and corpus callosum. But the mid brain was seldom involved in spite of the demonstration of brain stem symptoms in the acute stage.
In patients that high intensity areas(T2WI) were localized in the unilateral basal ganglia and corpus callosum, the prognosis was not always poor in spite of the severe state in the acute stage.

KEY WORDS: diffuse axonal injury, MRI, acute stage, final outcome

INTRODUCTION

Diffuse axonal injury is a clinical-pathological complex in which temporary or permanent damage to axons occurs after trauma. It forms a continuous spectrum of severity from minimal to severe that is associated with greater and greater disturbance of brain function and greater numbers of damaged axons. Diffuse axonal injury was classified in 1984 by Gennarelli. Since then, although the prognosis of its worst form is well known to take the poorest clinical course, it is still very difficult to speculate the final outcome of these patients in the early stage of their admission. MRI is expected to demonstrate such brain damages as those identified by neuropathological study.

MATERIALS AND METHODS

Twenty-five patients were transfered within 6 hours after injury and underwent MRI following CT in the same day or next day of the admission. All patients were injured in traffic accidents. These patients ranged in age from 17 to 65 years. Fifteen were male. All patients were comatose(GCS score=3-7) more than 24 hours after injury and underwent intubation or tracheotomy to keep the air way. Brain stem symptoms were positive in the acute stage. The final outcomes were evaluated at 6 months.

RESULTS AND DISCUSSION

Ten patients died and six were persistent vegetative stage. Six patients were severely disabled and three were moderately disabled (Table 1).
The relationship between the final outcome and MRI findings was summarized in Table 2. MRI of died or vegetative cases demonstrated the high intensity in the corpus callosum, bilateral basal ganglias and mid brain(Fig.1). In the MRI findings of severely or moderately disabled cases, high intensity areas were localized in the unilateral basal ganglia and corpus callosum. But the mid brain was seldom involved in spite of the demonstration of brain stem symptoms in the acute stage(Fig.2). In two patients, that one was severe and other was moderate disability, we didn't find any abnormal area in the MRI of acute stages.
Since Gennarelli classified diffuse brain injury clinically[1], the prognosis of its worst form(severe diffuse axonal injury) is well known to take the poorest clinical course. But it is still very difficult to speculate the final outcome of these patients in the early stage of their admission. Jenkins, et al.[2], reported that MRI(T2WI) was more available than CT on the brain of diffuse axonal injury. In our series, we could demonstrate such brain damages as those identified by neuropathological study in the acute stage.
Our conclusions are as follows.
1)In 25 patients with severe diffuse axonal injury, we studied the relationship between the final outcome and MRI findings within 48 hours after injury.
2)MRI was available to speculate the final outcome of these patients in the acute stage.
3)In patients that high intensity areas(T2WI) were localized in the unilateral basal ganglia and corpus callosum, the prognosis was not always poor in spite of the severe state in the acute stage.

REFERENCES

1.Jenkins A, Teasdale G, Hadley MDM, Rowan JO(1986) Brain lesions detected by magnetic resonance imaging in mild and severe head injuries. Lancet 2:445-446
2.Gennarelli TA(1984) Emergency department management of head injuries. Emergency Medicine Clinics of North America 2:749-760

Table 1 Final outcome of severe diffuse axonal injury

No.of cases	Final outcome
10	Death
6	Vegetative state
6	Severe disability
3	Moderate disability

Total 25

Table 2 Relationship between the final outcome and MRI findings

Final outcome	Locations(HIA)			
	cc	ubg	bbg	mb
Death	10	1	9	10
Vegetative state	5	0	6	5
Severe disability	4	4	1	1
Moderate disability	2	2	0	0

<in two patients:no abnormal area>

cc:corpus callosum,ubg:unilateral basal ganglia,
bbg:bilateral basal ganglia,mb:mid brain,
HIA:high intensity area

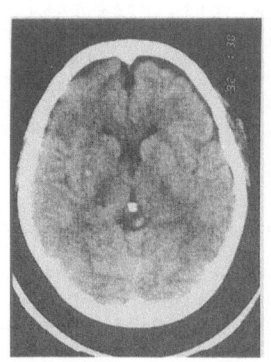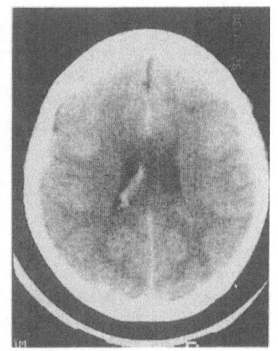

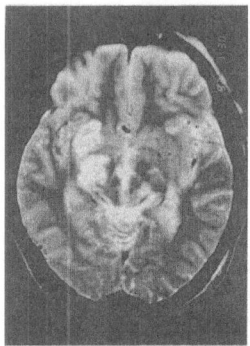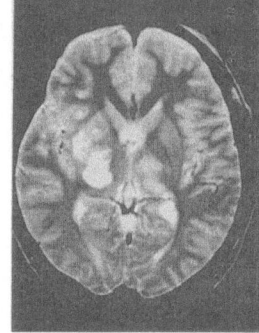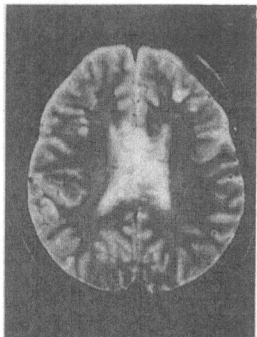

Fig.1:28-year-old man. GCS score on his admission was 4.
He was persistent vegetative state. CT scan showed very
slight lesion in the unilateral basal ganglia and intraventricular hemorrhage. But MRI demonstrated the high
intensity in the bilateral basal ganglias, mid brain and
corpus callosum.

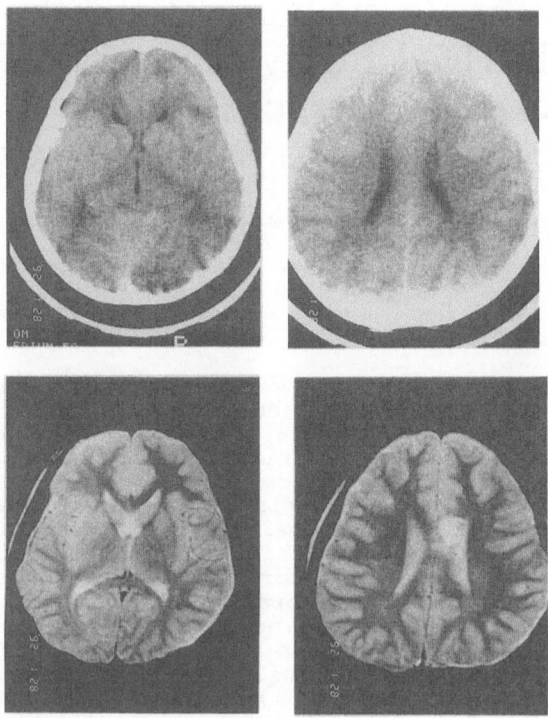

Fig.2:17-year-old woman. GCS score on her admission was 7. She was moderately disabled. CT scan showed diffuse brain swelling, but didn't show any abnormal density area. In the MRI findings, high intensity area localized in the unilateral corpus callosum. No abnormal areas were in the basal ganglia and mid brain.

Prediction of the Reversibility of the Brain Stem Dysfunction in Head Injury Patients: MRI and Auditory Brain Stem Response Study

AKIRA MATSUMURA[1], IWANE MITSUI[2], SATOSHI AYUZAWA[1], SADAYUKI TAKEUCHI[2], and TADAO NOSE[1]

[1]Department of Neurosurgery, Institute of Clinical Medicine, University of Tsukuba, Tsukuba, Ibaraki, 305 Japan, and [2]Moriya Daiichi General Hospital, Kitasoma, Ibaraki, 302-01 Japan

SUMMARY

16 cases of head injury patients were examined by magnetic resonance imaging (MRI) and auditory brain stem response (ABR) simultaneously in acute stage in order to investigate the possibility of the prediction for long term outcome. Among 13 primary brain injury patients, brain stem injury was seen on MRI in 9 cases (69%) and ABR abnormality was seen in 6 cases (46%). MRI and ABR findings were equal in 8 cases (75%). In 6 cases, only MRI could show positive brain stem findings while ABR remained normal. MRI was more sensitive in detecting primary brain stem damage. Abnormal ABR findings and normal MRI was seen only in secondary brain damage cases. In primary brain injury cases, unilateral MRI abnormality in the brain stem and normal ABR were the signs for good recovery even if the consciousness disturbance persisted for a long period. Contrary to this group, bilateral brain stem damage on MRI and/or absent ABR were the signs for poor recovery. From these findings, it was concluded that MRI is thus useful in predicting the prognosis of primary brain damage in the acute stage based on the degree of the brain stem damage.

KEYWORDS: Head injury, brain stem, magnetic resonance imaging, auditory brain stem response, clinical outcome

INTRODUCTION

Since the advent of MRI, the diagnosis of the head injury has changed significantly. Particulary brain stem injury and diffuse axonal injury are more accurately diagnosed by MRI than computed tomography(CT) (1,2,3,4,5). We have taken MRI in head injury patients in acute stage under cardiopulmonary support and monitoring if neccesary(6) and found that there is high incidence of brain stem injury in acute stage only demonstrated by T2 weighted images. We undertook therefore a prospective study to investigate how the MRI and ABR findings in brain stem injury correlates in order to find out whether the findings in acute stage can predict the long term outcome.

MATERIAL AND METHODS

Sixteen consecutive head injury patients with consciousness disturbance were investigated by MRI and ABR as soon as possible after admission. Multiple injury patients were also included in this study. MRI was obtained by 0.2 Tesla permanent MRI system (Hitachi Medico Co.Ltd., Tokyo, Japan). Full MR compatible cardiorespiratory monitoring and support were given as needed(6). ABR was performed in intensive care unit in acute stage by Neuropack mini-4 (Nihon Koden Co.Ltd., Tokyo, Japan) with auditory stimulation by 90-105dB click sound using 40dB white noise masking in the contralateral side to the stimulation. MRI and ABR were also repeated in the chronic stage and these findings were compared with initial Glasgow coma scale (GCS), Glasgow outcome scale (GOS) and the duration of the consciousness disturbance in cases with consciousness recovery.

RESULTS

The cases are summarized on Tab.1. There were GCS more than 9 in 4 cases and under 8 in 9 cases. Glasgow outcome scale (GOS) better than moderate disability (good prognosis group) was obtained in 8 patients and GOS worse than severly disabled (poor prognosis group) in 5 patients. Mean GCS of the patients with positive findings on MRI group was 9 ± 3.1 and MRI negative group was 6.5 ± 0.9. Lower GCS did not correlated with positive brain stem findings on MRI.

The MRI findings (Tab.2) and the ABR findings (Tab.3) were compared with the GOS. In good recovery group, 87.5% of the patients were negative or showed only focal/ unilateral findings on MRI. In poor recovery group, 75% of the patients showed diffuse and/or bilateral findings on MRI. The duration of the consciousness disturbance in good recovery did not differ among the degree of the MRI findings. GCS in good prognosis group was 7.3 ± 2.1 and in poor prognosis group, GCS was 9.6 ± 3.4, higher than the good prognosis group.

As shown on Tab.3, ABR correlated well with the prognosis in almost cases and improvement or deterioration were observed along its clinical course in some cases (indicated with *and**), which followed the clinical course.

Comparing the MRI and ABR findings, the both examinations were equal in 7 cases (54%) and only MRI positive in 6 cases(46%). MRI was more sensitive in detecting the brain stem damage. There was no case in which only ABR was abnormal in primary brain injury group. In secondary brain injury, ABR were abnormal in all cases and MRI was positive in only 1 case out of 3.

Tab.1 Summary of the cases

Age : 7 - 66 years old (mean 34.6)
Male:Female = 9 : 7

Type of injury

		No.cases
Diffuse axonal injury (DAI)	:	7
Acute subdural hematoma (SDH)	:	1
SDH + contusion	:	2
Epidural hematoma +contusion	:	1
Posterior fossa epidural hematoma	:	1
Primary brain stem injury+DAI	:	1
(Secondary brain injury	:	3)

Tab.2 Relationship of MRI findings and GOS in PBI

MRI	negative	focal or unilateral	diffuse or bilateral
GOS			
good #	4/8 (35 days)	3/8 (50 days)	1/8 (30 days)
poor	0/5	0/5	5/5

( ) : duration of consciousness disturbance
#: statistically significant difference (p<0.01: χ^2test) from poor group
PBI: primary brain injury cases

Tab.3 Relationship of ABR and GOS in PBI

	normal ABR	delayed ABR	no response
GOS			
good #	6/8 (41 days)	1/8* (45 days)	1/8*
poor	1/5**	0/5	4/5

( ): duration of consciousness disturbance
* : ABR improved afterwards
** : ABR deteriorated afterwards
#: statistically significant difference (p< 0.05 : χ^2test) from poor group
PBI: primary brain injury cases

ILLUSTRATIVE CASE

Case1: 17 year old girl, traffic accident. Initial GCS was 8. CT scan showed subarachnoidal hemorrhage in the right quadrigeminal cistern and right frontal contusion (Fig.1 upper row). MRI showed high intensity changes in the right dorsal midbrain and bilateral frontal contusions (Fig.1 lower row). ABR remained normal. The patient unconscious for 1 months after the accident and began to respond verebally thereafter. The patient made a gradual recovery.and she returned to the school 6 months after the accident.

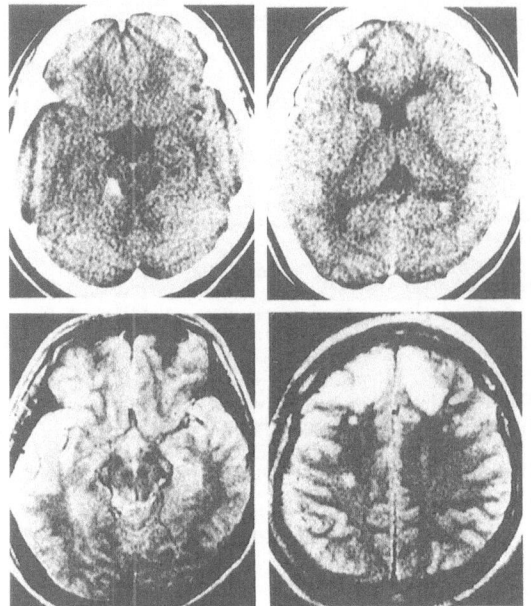

Fig.1: CT scan demonstrating SAH and the right frontal contusional hematoma (upper row). MRI showed high intensity changes in the right dorsal midbrain and bifrontal contusions (lower row)

Case2: 27 year old man, traffic accident. Initial GCS was 5 and soon after arrival, he became apnea with fixed pupils. CT scan (Fig.2 left) showed epidural hematoma in the right posterior fossa. After emergent evacuation of the hematoma, MRI was performed under barbiturate therapy. MRI demonstrated right cerebellar and bitemporal contusions and high intensity area in the right pons (Fig.2 right). Initial ABR showed only I and II waves, but after 2 weeks, almost normal ABR could be obtained. The patient remained unconscious and traechostomy was perofrmed due to the prolonged coma. However after 1 month, the patient began to improve and 4 months after the accident, the patient was discharged. He returned to normal daily life with slight unsteadiness by walking.

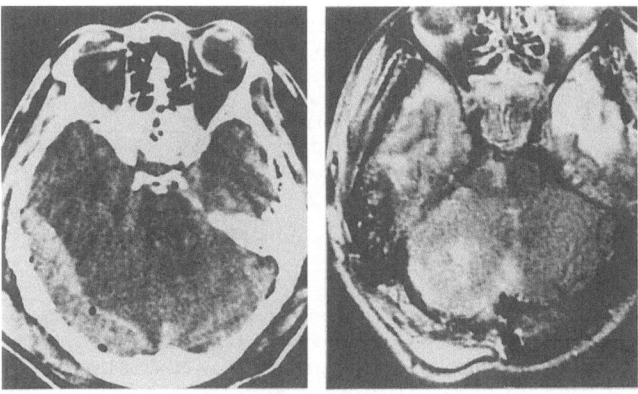

Fig.2: CT scan (left) showing the epidural hematoma in the right posterior fossa, MRI(right) demonstrating right cerebellar and bitemporal contusions and high intensity change in the right pons.

DISCUSSION

With the recent advances in MRI technique, the diagnosis of brain injury has been considerably changed. Especially in cases with DAI or brain stem injury, MRI is superior to CT scan in detecting the lesion(1,2,3,4,5). To diagnose the brain stem injury accurately, we have performed MRI examintaions in acute stage of the injury, either pre- or post-operatively. The findings seen on T2-weighted imaging as high intensity tend to disappear after weeks or months(1,5), so that the MRI in chronic stage may fail to demonstrate such findings.With the use of MRI compatible cardiopulmonary support, MRI could be performed safely in acute stage(6). The another important role of the MRI in acute stage is whether one can predict the outcome based on the MRI findings. From that point of view, if the MRI findings in the brain stem is negative or if there is a focal or unilateral findings in the brain stem, the recovery of the consciousness can be expected. In such cases, ABR were normal in the majority of the cases. The recovery from the consciousness disturbance is poor in diffuse and/or bilateral brain stem findings on MRI. In such cases, ABR showed no response. ABR was more resistive to the brain stem injury than MRI, so that the abnormal ABR findings were the definite sign for poor prognosis. MRI could demonstrate the brain stem injury more accurate than ABR and the extent and te localization was useful information in evaluating the clinical features. We used ABR for confirming the normal response in which MRI showed positive findings in the brain stem and if ABR remained normal, we could be reliable for the recovery of the patients.

The duration of the consciousness disturbance did not correlate to the degree of the brain stem injury seen on MRI in good prognosis group. The duration of the consciousness disturbance may have been influenced by the the contusions and shearing injuries seen above the level of the brain stem. Our study was focused on the brain stem injury, but multi-located various brain injury has been included in this study, so that the duration of the recovery from consciousness disturbance should be evaluated comprehensively. In conclusion, brain stem injury affect the quality of the recovery in primary brain injury, but the time course is affected by associated brain injuries.

REFERENCES

1) Ebisu T, Yamaki T, Kobori N, Tenjin H, Kuboyama T, Naruse S, Horikawa Y, Tanaka C, Higuchi T, Hirakawa K(1989) Surg Neurol 31: 261-267
2) Jenkins A, Teasdale G, Hadley MDM, Macpherson P, Rowan JO (1986) Lancet 2:445-446
3) Gentry LR, Thompson B, Godersky JC (1988) AJNR 9: 1129-1138
4) Ishige N, Pitts LH, Berry I, Carlson SG, Nishimura MC, Moseley ME, Weinstein PR (1987) J Cereb Blood Flow Metabol 7: 759-767
5) Levin HS, Amparo E, Eisenberg H, Williams DH, High Jr WM, McArdle CB, Weiner RL (1987) J Neurosurg 66: 706-713
6) Matsumura A, Meguro K, Mizutani T, Tsurushima H, Satoh N, Tsunoda T, Matsumaru Y, Nakata Y, Wada M, Kikuchi Y, Ebashi T, Nose T (1989) JJMRM 8: 268-274

Neuroimaging of Cerebral Metabolism in Severe Diffuse Brain Injury in Chronic Stage: Part 2. MR Spectroscopy and Spectroscopic Imaging

Seiichi Furuya[1], Shoji Naruse[1,2], Tarumi Yamaki[2], Yoshiharu Horikawa[2], Toshihiko Ebisu[2], Satosi Ueda[2], Chuzo Tanaka[3], Tosihiro Higuchi[3], Masahiro Umeda[3]

[1]Department of Radiology, [2]Neurosurgery, Kyoto Prefectural University of Medicine, Kamigyo-ku, Kyoto, 602 Japan, and [3]Department of Neurosurgery, Meiji College Oriental Medicine, Funai, Kyoto, 629-03 Japan

SUMMARY

We have developed the ^{31}P– and ^{1}H–magnetic resonance spectroscopic imaging (MRSI) and applied them to severe diffuse brain injury(SDBI) in the chronic stage. The three patients are all young male and had the so called diffuse axonal injury (DAI) by the traffic accident. The DAI was judged by neurological symptoms, computed tomography (CT) and magnetic resonance imaging (MRI). ^{31}P– and ^{1}H–MRSI were performed 2 to 16 months after injury. The decrease of phosphocreatine (PCr) was observed by ^{31}P–MRSI and the decrease of NAA by ^{1}H–MRSI in the wide area of the brain. The decrease of NAA reflects the neuronal damage and consequently indicates the functional deterioration. Therefore, it is suggested that the amount of NAA could be the indicator of neuronal function and ^{1}H–MRSI is useful for the examination of the neurological condition in SDBI.

KEY WORDS : diffuse brain injury(DBI), cerebral metabolism, ^{1}H–magnetic resonance spectroscopic imaging(^{1}H–MRSI), ^{31}P–magnetic resonance spectroscopic imaging(^{31}P–MRSI), N–acetyl aspartate(NAA)

INTRODUCTION

The ^{31}P– or ^{1}H–MRS are the unique methods for the analysis of the brain metabolism by non–invasive. It is possible to detect the metabolites in the living brain in situ by which other modalities can never do. Previous measurements of MRS were performed by using the single–voxel method which could obtained the localized spectrum from single, relatively large area (voxel). We have developed the magnetic resonance spectroscopic imaging (MRSI) method to obtain spectra from multiple, small voxels simultaneously. This method has additional advantage that distribution of each metabolite can be visualized by creating the metabolite mapping using obtained spectra. We have applied this method to various kinds of brain diseases such as brain tumors, cerebro–vascular accident, senile dementia, infectious diseases, degeneration diseases and pediatric diseases and are obtaining important information. Therefore, in this study, we applied the MRSI method to the SDBI and examined the usefulness of this method in the evaluation of this kind of disease.

METHOD and MATERIAL

The system used was Magnetom H15(Siemens) worked on a 1.5 Tesla magnet. Both ^{31}P–MRS and ^{1}H–MRS were measured by 3D–chemical shift imaging (CSI) methods. The 3D–CSI method offers multi–voxel MRS and the spectroscopic imaging (SI) which displays the distribution of the metabolite in the brain. The ^{31}P–MRS was obtained by applying 2 directional 8x8 phase encodings on 25x25cm FOV. The 4cm thickness slice was selected. One voxel size is about 3x3x4cm. Repetition time(TR) and echo time(TE) was 3000msec and 2msec respectively and 12 accumulation were performed. The ^{1}H-CSI was obtained by applying 2 directional 16x16 phase encodings on 18x18 cm FOV. In the FOV, a 8x8x2 cm volume of the interest (VOI) were selected by Spin echo method with water and fat suppression. Consequently 256 voxels with 1x1x2cm in size were obtained simultaneously. TR/TE was 3000/135 msec and 3 times accumulation were performed. After applying 2 dimensional Fourier Transformation of acquired data, the baseline and the phase were corrected automatically in all voxels. The spectroscopic imaging was made by using the curve-fitted spectra with interpolating to 256 square matrix.

The subjects were 3 patients with SDBI in the chronic stage. They were all young male aged 17, 19 and 25 years. They sustained a head injury in a traffic accident. The neurological condition on admission had been deep coma in all. The CT scans obtained on admission revealed neither marked mass lesions nor signs of increased intracranial pressure, but demonstrated intraventricular and subarachnoid hemorrhages as well as small subcortical hemorrhages. All patients had been treated conservatively and their neurological condition had improved gradually. The ^{31}P- and ^{1}H-MRSI studies were performed 2 to 16 month later after the injury on the same day.

The MRSI data were compared with other 162 cases examined in our MR unit.

RESULTS

^{31}P- and ^{1}H-MRSI which we developed offer high resolutional spectrum in each voxel and spectroscopic images which clearly demonstrate the distribution of metabolites. Detectable metabolites related to the cell membrane metabolism, the energy metabolism and amino-acid metabolism. ^{31}P-MRSI could detect the two groups of metabolites. One related to the metabolism of cell membrane consisting of phosphomonoesters(PME) and phosphodiesters (PDE). The other related to the energy metabolism, consisting of inorganic phosphate(Pi), phosphocreatine(PCr) and ATPs. ^{1}H-MRSI could detect the choline(Cho), phosphocreatine/creatine(PCr/Cr), N-acetyl aspartate(NAA), lactate(Lac) and other aminoacids.

In the ^{31}P-MRSI of normal volunteer, peaks of PME, Pi, PDE, PCr, gamma-ATP, alpha-ATP and beta-ATP were observed clearly in each voxels. And the SI of each metabolite could demonstrated the distribution in the brain roughly. On the ^{1}H-MRSI of the volunteer, the peaks of Cho, Cr and NAA were clearly observed in each voxels. The NAA peak was as about twice high as Cho and Cr peaks. Lactate was observed in the normal brain.

In the patients of SDBI in the chronic stage, the decrease of PCr is observed in wide area of the brain by ^{31}P-MRSI. By ^{1}H-MRSI, the NAA peak is relatively decreasing in all voxels. The spectroscopic imaging did not show any significant difference compared with the normal SI, because the decreasing of those metabolite were observed in all voxels.

DISCUSSION

Recently, ^{31}P- and ^{1}H-MRS have become to be measured on the clinical MRI/S system, and there are some reports concerning the application of MRS to some cerebral diseases. However, many of them were performed by using the single-voxel method, which has the limitation that only single area could be observed. On the other hand, the MRSI method has an advantage that spectra could be measured from multiple-voxels simultaneously and also the distribution of metabolite could be visualized by the metabolite mapping. We have developed the MRSI system both for ^{31}P- and ^{1}H nuclei and applied them to various kind of diseases. There are few reports of the application of ^{31}P– or ^{1}H–MRSI method individually to brain disorders, much less of double nuclei MRSI study simultaneously. Therefore, this is the first report which deals the ^{31}P– and ^{1}H– double nuclei MRSI studies.

In cases of SDBI at chronic stage, the decrease of PCr was observed by ^{31}P–MRSI and the decrease of NAA by ^{1}H–MRSI on wide area of the brain. The decrease of PCr and ATP in an acute stage of cerebral infarction and brain contusion were observed previously and those findings were easily attributed to the impairment of energy metabolism in acute stage. However, the decrease of PCr observed in this study is not clearly understood. At least, it is suggested that in the SDBI at chronic stage, there is some disturbance in the high energy metabolism, probably the decrease of reserver function of high energy compound in the brain tissue. But, exact elucidation is left as further problems.

The decrease of NAA observed on ^{1}H–MRSI in SDBI at chronic stage gives us a useful information for judging the viability of nerve cell. Because, NAA exists predominantly in the neuronal cell and there are many data, including our MRSI studies, that NAA decrease in a pathological condition which deteriorate the brain function such as brain tumor, hypoxic brain damage, Alzheimer's disease and so on. The decrease of NAA would not necessarily attributed to the neuronal loss. Because, we have observed the recovery of decreased NAA drastically in a case of MELAS syndrome after the appropriate treatments, preceded the neurological function. Therefore, the changes of NAA would become the indicator of neuronal function. We could not observed the recovery of NAA on cases of SDBI presented, because all were in chronic stage. However, ^{1}H–MRSI method would give us a clue to evaluate the recovery of function and/or the effectiveness of therapies in a case of brain injury especially at an acute and subacute stage. Therefore, ^{1}H–MRSI is very useful not only to examine the pathophysiology but also to evaluate the recovery of neuronal function in severe head injury.

Fig. 1 The spectrum of the ^{31}P–MRSI in the normal brain. PME, Pi, PDE, PCr and ATPs are detected.

Fig. 2 The spectrum of the ^{31}P–MRSI in the SDBI in the chronic stage. PCr peak is relatively decreasing.

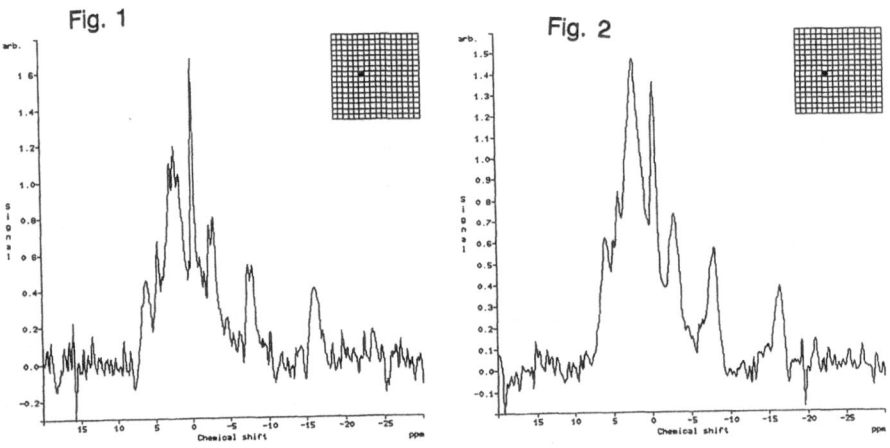

Fig. 3 The spectrum of the ¹H–MRSI in the normal brain. Cho, Cr and NAA are detected.
Fig. 4 The spectrum of the ¹H–MRSI in the SDBI in the chronic stage. NAA peak is relatively decreasing.

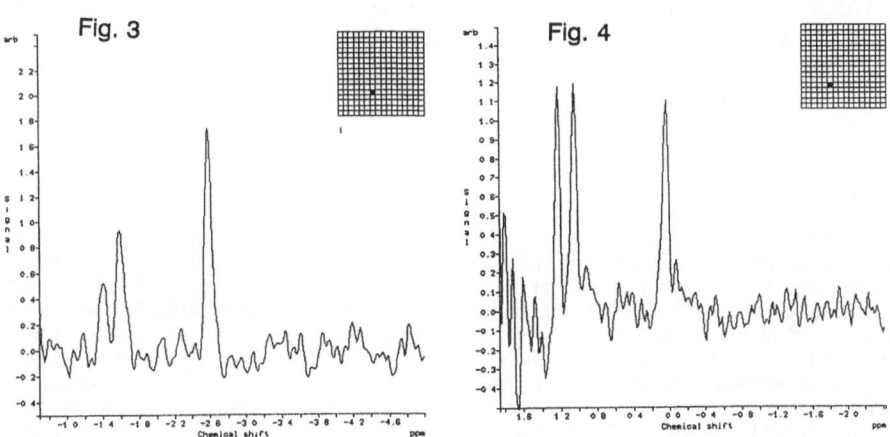

REFFERENCES
1)R.J. Ordidge, A. Connely, J.A.B. Lohman : Image–selected in vivo spectroscopy(ISIS). A new technique for spatially selective NMR spectroscopy. J.Magn. Reson. 66:283–294, 1986.
2)H. Bruhn, J. Frahn, M.L. Gyngell et al.: Noninvasive differentiation of tumors with use of localized H–1 MR spectroscopy in vivo :initial experience in patients with cerebral tumors. Radiology 172 : 541–548, 1989
3)P.R. Luyten, J.A. Hollander : Observation of metabolites in human brain by MR spectroscopy. Radiology 161:795–798, 1986.
4)P.A. Bottomley, T.B. Foster, R.D. Darrow : Depth–Resolved Surface–Coil Spectroscopy (DRESS) for in vivo 1H, 31P and 13C NMR. J. Magn. Reson. 59:338– 342, 1984
5)P.R. Luyten, A.J.H. Marien, W.Heindel et al. : Metabolic imaging of patients with intracranial tumors : H–1 MR spectroscopic imaging and PET. Radiology 176:791–799, 1990
6)S. Furuya, S. Naruse, M.Ide et al. : 1H–CSI Study of Brain Tumors. Society of Magnetic Resonance in Medicine tenth Anual Sientific Meeting Abstruct 36, 1991
7)T. Takaya, S. Naruse, S. Furuya et al. : Usefulness of 1H–CSI in Application to Pediatric Brain Disorders. Society of Magnetic Resonance in Medicine el eventh Anual Sientific Meeting Abstruct 233, 1992
8)S. Furuya, S. Naruse, M.Ide et al. : Evaluation of Clinical Usefulness of 1H–CSI Based on 125 Successful Cases. Society of Magnetic Resonance in Medicine eleventh Anual Sientific Meeting Abstruct 641, 1992
9)M. Ide, S.Naruse, S. Furuya et al. : Some Investigations of Senile Dementia of Altzheimer Type (SDAT) by 1H–CSI. Society of Magnetic Resonance in Medicine· eleventh Anual Sientific Meeting Abstruct 1930, 1992

Cerebral Hemodynamics and Metabolism in Severe Diffuse Brain Injury in Chronic Stage: Positron Emission Tomography

TARUMI YAMAKI[1], MASAHITO FUJIMOTO[2], YOSHIO OHMORI[1], YOSHIO IMAHORI[1], EIJI YOSHINO[1], TOSHIHIKO EBISU[1], and SATOSHI UEDA[1]

[1]Department of Neurosurgery, Kyoto Prefectural University of Medicine, Kamigyo-ku, Kyoto, 602 Japan, and
[2]Department of Neurosurgery, Saiseikai Shiga Hospital, Kurita, Shiga, 520-30 Japan

SUMMARY

The authors measured the cerebral hemodynamics and metabolism in patients with severe diffuse brain injury (SDBI) in the chronic stage using positron emission tomography (PET). In this study, regional cerebral blood flow (rCBF), oxygen extraction fraction (rOEF), cerebral blood volume (rCBV), cerebral metabolic rate for oxygen (rCMRO$_2$), cerebral metabolic rate for glucose (rCMRGlu), and cerebral metabolic rate were measured in three patients with SDBI in the chronic stage. The patients were all male, and aged 17, 19 and 25 years. The Glasgow Coma Scale score on admission was 3,4 and 3, respectively. In all patients, the cause of injury had been a traffic accident, computed tomography and magnetic resonance imaging revealed findings of so-called diffuse axonal injury (DAI), and the clinical course was also typical of that of DAI. The PET studies were performed 2 to 16 months after injury. The clinical condition of the patients at that time was vegetative state in two and severely disabled in one. PET revealed misery perfusion and low metabolism in two and matched low perfusion and low metabolism in one. It is interesting that any slight difference in clinical state was correlated with a slight difference in PET findings in every patients. The authors stress the usefulness of PET study in the investigation of SDBI in the chronic stage and in the assessment of its prognosis.

KEY WORDS: diffuse brain injury, diffuse axonal injury, cerebral blood flow and cerebral metabolism, positron emission tomography, chronic stage

INTRODUCTION

Although there have been several investigation of the cerebral hemodynamics and metabolism in patients with severe diffuse brain injury (SDBI) in the acute stage using several methods [1-6], there are few studies of those in the chronic stage even though the patient condition is very poor [7-9]. We therefore used positron emission tomography (PET), one of the most useful methods of examining cerebral hemodynamics and metabolism, to measure regional cerebral blood flow (rCBF), oxygen extraction fraction (rOEF), cerebral blood volume (rCBV), cerebral metabolic rate for oxygen (rCMRO$_2$), cerebral metabolic rate for glucose (rCMRGlu), and metabolic rate in three patients with SDBI in the chronic stage. In this paper, we report the results of this study and discuss the physiological status of patients with SDBI in the chronic stage.

CLINICAL MATERIALS AND METHODS

The three patients with SDBI in chronic state shared numerous clinical features. They were all young male who had sustained a head injury in a traffic accident. The neurological condition on admission had been deep coma in all. The CT scans obtained on admission had revealed neither marked mass lesions nor signs of increased intracranial pressure, but had demonstrated intraventricular and subarachnoid hemorrhages as well as small subcortical hemorrhages. All patients had been treated conservatively, and their neurological condition had improved gradually.

The PET studies were performed 2 to 16 months after injury. A Headtome 3 (SET 120W; Shimadzu Co. Japan) was used in the studies. The spatial resolution is 8.6 mm. The rCBF value was measured with C^{15}O$_2$ gas, and rOEF value with ^{15}O$_2$ gas by continuous inhalation method. The rCBV value was measured with C^{15}O gas by bolus inhalation method. The rCMRO$_2$ value was measured using inhalation of ^{15}O$_2$ gas in combination with data obtained from the preceding rCBF and rCBV studies [10,11]. The rCMRGlu value was measured using fluorodeoxyglucose (18FDG) method [12]. The metabolic rate was calculated by dividing the rCMRO$_2$ value by the rCMRGlu value. These parameters were measured in the bilateral frontal, temporal, occipital and parietal gray matter, and the bilateral white matter of the centrum semiovale. Each circular region of interest (ROI) in the gray matter included 47 pixels and was 16mm in diameter, and that in the white matter included 29 pixels and was 12mm in diameter. Each studied region in the brain included several (3-13) ROI which had been determined based on CT images obtained just before the PET study.

The same regions in 20 healthy adult volunteers (control group) were investigated by the same method (Table 1).

Case Presentations and Results of the PET study

Case 1
This 25-year-old male had sustained a head injury when the car he was driving collided with another car. He was transported to Saiseikai Shiga Hospital immediately. On admission, Glasgow Coma Scale (GCS) was 4. The CT scan disclosed a small pneumocephalus in the frontal subarachnoid space due to penetrating fracture of the frontal sinus and a small hemorrhage in the genu portion of the corpus callosum. No sign of increased intracranial pressure was seen (Fig.1A). Two months after the injury, his clinical condition assessed by the Glasgow Outcome Scale was vegetative state. The magnetic resonance imaging (MRI) revealed multiple low-intensity spots in the corpus callosum on T2-weighted image (Fig.1B). The PET study revealed decreased of rCBF, rCMRO$_2$ and rCMRGlu values (Fig.2, Table 2). The metabolic rate was 0.45.

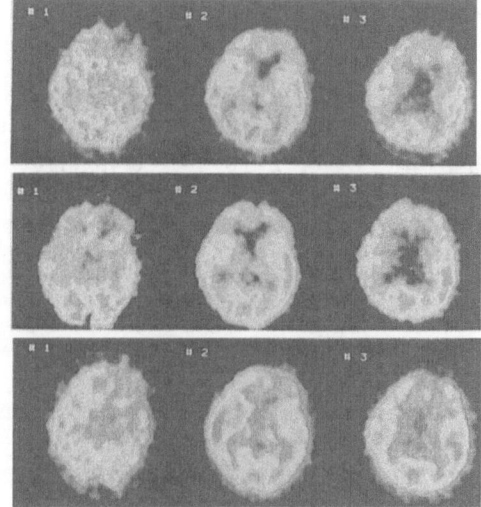

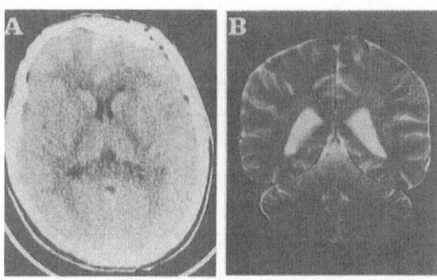

"**Fig. 1**" CT on admission (A), and MRI on 2 months after the injury (B) of Case 1.

"**Fig.2**" PET imagings of CBF (upper), CMRO2 (center) and CMRGLu (lower) of Case 1.

Case 2
This 19-year-old male sustained a head injury when his car collided with a telegraph pole. His GCS score on admission was 3, and the CT scan revealed a small hemorrhagic lesion in the right cerebellar peduncle, lateral and third ventricles, and left frontal subcortical white matter. Neither large hemorrhage nor any sign of increased intracranial pressure was noted. He was treated conservatively, and his clinical state improved gradually. The MRI and PET studies were performed 16 months after admission. At that time, his clinical status was severely disabled. T1-weighted MR images revealed mild brain atrophy and low-intensity areas in the right cerebellar peduncle and left basal ganglia. The PET study revealed markedly decreased rCBF value, increased rOEF value, decreased rCMRO$_2$ and rCMRGlu values (Table 3). The metabolic rate was 0.55.

Case 3
This 17-year-old male sustained a head injury when riding a motorbike. On admission, his GCS score was 3, and CT revealed subarachnoid hemorrhage in the suprachiasmal cistern and supracerebellar subarachnoid space. Intraventricular hemorrhage in the lateral ventricle was also noted, but no other

hemorrhagic lesion was seen. The MRI and PET studyies were performed two months after injury, followed by conservative treatment. His clinical state at that time was vegetative state. Moderate brain atrophy and a small low-intensity lesion were clearly demonstrated on the T1-weighted MR image. The PET study revealed decreased rCBF value, increased rOEF value, decreased rCMRO$_2$ value, and markedly decreased rCMRGlu value (Table 3). The metabolic rate was 0.5.

Table 1. The values of the rCBF, rOEF, rCMRO2, rCBV and rCMRGLu in the normal volunteers.

	rCBF (ml/100g/min)	rOEF	rCMRO2 (ml/100g/min)	rCBV (ml/100g)	rCMRGLu (mg/100g/min)
Gray matter	43±7	0.42±0.08	3.3±0.5	4.3±0.5	7.0±0.8
White matter	25±4	0.44±0.06	2.0±0.3	2.8±0.7	4.9±0.8

Table 2. Results of hemodynamic and metabolic studies using PET of Case 1.

	rCBF	rOEF	rCMRO2	rCBV	rCMRGLu
Rt-frontal	24±4	0.34±0.07	1.6±0.3	3.1±0.8	4.3±0.4
Lt-frontal	25±5	0.42±0.10	1.9±0,4	3.7±0.9	4.1±0.4
Rt-temporal	29±5	0.33±0.06	2.0±0.3	4.5±0.9	5.1±0.5
Lt-temporal	27±5	0.42±0.08	2.3±0.4	4.1±0.8	4.1±0.5
Rt-occipital	26±4	0.37±0.07	1.9±0.4	3.9±0.9	4.9±0.4
Lt-occipital	30±5	0.42±0.10	2.6±0.6	4.1±0.8	5.0±0.5
Rt-parietal	29±6	0.46±0.10	2.3±0.4	3.8±0.8	4.7±0.6
Lt-parietal	25±6	0.42±0.08	2.2±0.5	3.8±0.9	4.5±0.4
Average	27±5	0.40±0.08	2.1±0.4	3.9±0.9	4.6±0.5
Rt-white matter	14±2	0.35±0.07	1.1±0.2	2.5±0.6	3.1±0.4
Lt-white matter	14±3	0.50±0.10	1.2±0.3	2.3±0.6	3.2±0.4
Average	14±3	0.43±0.09	1.2±0.3	2.4±0.6	3.2±0.4

Table 3. Results of hemodynamic and metabolic studies using PET of Case 2 and 3. The values are showed as the average values.

	rCBF	rOEF	rCMRO2	rCBV	rCMRGLu
Case 2					
Gray matter	29±5	0.52±0.07	2.8±0.4	4.5±0.9	5.0±0.5
White matter	16±3	0.59±0.1	1.7±0.3	2.9±0.7	3.6±0.6
Case 3					
Gray matter	26±4	0.54±0.06	2.4±0.3	4.1±0.9	4.7±0.5

Discussion

Diffuse brain injury, especially diffuse axonal injury is one of the most difficult pathological states to treat, perhaps because the cerebral hemodynamics and metabolism in this disorder are not yet well understood. Evaluation of this disorder has consisted of morphological study from the pathological, anatomical diagnostic, or clinical perspective view [13]. However, the cerebral hemodynamics and metabolism in this disorder have rarely been investigated, since most patients die soon after injury and the clinical condition of those who survive is not amenable to evaluate, and because of the limited availability of appropriate methods of simultaneously evaluating cerebral hemodynamics and metabolism. While the PET study is an excellent method for this purpose, there have been few studies of head injury [7-9,14-16], and most of these were of patients with focal injury rather than with diffuse brain injury. The three patients in the present study presented the clinical course and diagnostic imaging findings typical of DAI.

In these cases, values of the parameters of the PET were resemble in some points but different another points. In Case 1, the values of rCBF, rCMRO2 and rCMRGLu were markedly decreased and value of rOEF was slightly decreased. These findings are consistent with matched low perfusion and low metabolism. In Case 2 and 3, the values of rCBF, rCMRO2 and rCMRGLu were decreased. Regional OEF, however, was increased. In these patients, the PET findings indicated a state of misery perfusion and decreased metabolism. The values of the PET parameters measured in the gray matter of each region as well as in the bilateral white matter were almost the same in all cases, indicating that the state of the CBF and metabolic insufficiency was due to diffuse brain injury and not to focal brain injury. In contrast, our previous PET study of brain contusions [16], we observed marked variation in the values of PET parameters, since brain contusion is a typical focal brain injury. The metabolic rate was within normal limits in all cases in the present study, indicating that the cerebral glucose metabolism was not in a state of anaerobic glycolysis in spite of the marked depressed metabolic state.

Recently, we reported a clinical evaluation of patients with so called DAI [17], in which we found that the outcome of younger patients with DAI was better than that of older patients. We plan to examine the chronological change in PET findings and clinical state in the present young patients and anticipate that this study will be helpful in clarifying the physical state in SDBI and the development of an appropriate treatment.

References

1. Yoshino E, Yamaki T, Higuchi T, Horikawa Y, Hirakawa K (1985) J Neurosurg 63: 830-839
2. Marshall LF (1990) Curr Opin Neurol Neurosurg 3: 4-9
3. Shigemori M, Moriyama T, Harada K, Kikuchi N, Tokutomi T, Kuramoto S (1990) Acta Neurochir (Wien) 107: 5-10
4. Tenjin H, Yamaki T, Nakagawa Y, Kuboyama T, Ebisu T, Kobori N, Ueda S, Mizukawa N (1990) Acta Neurochir (Wien) 104: 121-125
5. Cruz J, Miner ME, Allen SJ, Alves WM, Genarelli TA (1991). Neurosurgery 29: 743-749
6. Marion DW, Bouma GJ (1991) Neurosurgery 29: 869-873
7. Rao N, Turski PA, Polcyn RE, Nickels RJ, Matthews CG, Flynn MM (1984) Arch Phys Med Rehabil 64: 780-785
8. Langfitt TW, Obrist WD, Alavi A, Grossman RI, Zimmerman R, Jaggi J, Uzzell B, Reivich M, Patton DR (1986). J Neurosurg 64: 760-767
9. Starkstein SE, Mayberg HS, Berthir ML, Fedoroff P, Price TR, Dannals RF, Wagner HN, Leiguarda R, Robinson RG (1990) Ann Neurol 27: 652-659
10. Jones T, Chesler DA, Ter-Pogossian MM (1976) Br J Radiol 49: 339-343
11. Frackowiak RSJ, Lenzi GL, Jone T (1980) J Comput Assist Tomogr 4: 727-736
12. Hutchins GD, Holden JE, Koeppe RA, Halama JR, Gatley SJ, Nickles RJ (1984) J Cereb Blood Flow Metabol 4: 35-40
13. Adams JH, Genarrelli TA, Maxwell WL (1991) J Neurol Neurosurg Psychiatry 54: 481-483
14. Jamieson D, Alavi A, Jolles P, Chawluk J, M. Reivich M (1988) Radiol Clin North Am 26: 1075-1088
15. Humayun MS, Presty SK, Lafrance ND, Holcomb HH, Lotas H, Long DM, Wagner HN, Gordon B (1989) Nuclear Medicine Communications 10: 335-344
16. Tenjin H, Ueda S, Mizukawa N, Imahori Y, Hino A, Yamaki T, Kuboyama T, Ebisu T, Hirakawa K, Yamashita M, Nakahashi H (1990) Neurosurgery 26: 971-979
17. Nakagawa Y, Yamaki T, Murakami N, Iwamoto Y, Yamamoto K, Fujimoto M, Ueda S (1991) Neurotraumatology 14: 127-131

Effects of Decompressive Craniectomy on Regional Cerebral Blood Flow in Severe Head Trauma Patients Assessed by HMPAO SPECT

Iwao Yamakami, Akira Yamaura, Hisayuki Murai, and Katumi Isobe
Department of Neurosurgery, Chiba University School of Medicine Chuo-ku, Chiba, 260 Japan

SUMMARY

Using single photon emission computerized tomography (SPECT) with ^{99m}Tc-Hexamethylpropyleneamine oxime (HMPAO), we investigated the effect of decompressive craniectomy (DC) on regional cerebral blood flow (rCBF) in the patient with severe head trauma (SHT). SPECT studies were repeated three times in six SHT patients who underwent unilateral large DC 2–14 h after trauma; within 24 h after DC, 1 week, and then 1 month after DC. In the first 24 h of DC, SPECT uniformly found 1) PERFUSION DEFECT associated with brain contusion, and 2) HYPERPERFUSION area in the decompressed brain. The simultaneous X–CT observed mild/moderate swelling of the decompressed brain. One week after DC, SPECT found that HYPERPERFUSION area in the decompressed brain not only enlarged but also increased the severity. X–CT showed marked swelling of the decompressed brain. One month after DC, SPECT observed no HYPERPERFUSION areas in the decompressed brain. PERFUSION DEFECT associated with contusion was found to ameliorate. X–CT found no swelling of the decompressed brain. The chronology of HYPERPERFUSION area in the decompressed brain corresponded to the chronological change in the brain swelling after DC. In the SHT patient, DC significantly affects regional CBF and increases a focal CBF of the decompressed brain in the acute posttraumatic period.

KEY WORDS: brain swelling, cerebral blood flow, decompressive craniectomy, head trauma

INTRODUCTION

Decompressive craniectomy (DC) is often a useful surgical strategy in head trauma patients. Although the clinical value is still controversial [1,2,3], several effects on the pathophysiology of traumatized brain have been suggested; DC may increase the volume–compensation capacity of traumatized brain [4], and may enhance the brain swelling [5]. Its effects on cerebral blood flow (CBF) may be related to the clinical value. However, no clinical studies have investigated its effects on CBF in head trauma patients.

To clarify its effects on CBF in SHT patients, we repeated studies of rCBF in the posttraumatic one–month period. As a method to investigate rCBF, we used SPECT with HMPAO. The method is non–invasive, suitable for rCBF study in emergency situiations such as head trauma, although it does not provide absolute CBF values [6,7].

MATERIALS AND METHOD

The present study comprised 6 patients with SHT who remained comatose (≤ 8 in Glasgow coma scale: GCS score) for more than 72 h. They underwent unilateral large DC [2] 2-14 h after trauma. Hyperosmolar agents (mannitol and glycerol) were administered intravenously to manage an increased intracranial pressure, however neither barbiturates nor artificial hyperventilation was not used.

In the posttraumatic one-month period, each patient underwent HMPAO-SPECT studies three times; within 24 h after DC, 1 week, and then 1 month after DC [7].

Details in the technique of SPECT study have been published elsewhere [6,7]. In brief, five minutes after an intravenous administration of 740 MBq HMPAO, SPECT scanning was started using a single-head rotating gamma camera (Shimazu SNC-510R, Shimazu, Japan). Transaxial perfusion images parallel to the orbitomeatal line were compared with the axial images of X-ray computerized tomography (X-CT) performed simultaneously with each SPECT study.

RESULTS

In the first 24 h of DC, SPECT studies uniformly showed 1) PERFUSION DEFECT associated with brain contusion, and 2) mild and small HYPER-PERFUSION area in the decompressed brain. The simultaneously performed X-CT showed mild/moderate swelling of the decompressed brain.

One week after DC, SPECT observed that HYPERPERFUSION area in the decompressed brain not only enlarged but also increased the severity. PERFUSION DEFECT associated with contusion was also observed. X-CT showed marked swelling of the decompressed brain.

One month after DC, no HYPERPERFUSION area in the decompressed brain was observed on SPECT. PERFUSION DEFECT associated with contusion ameliorated. X-CT found that the swelling of decompressed brain dissolved.

Table 1 summarizes the relation of HYPERPERFUSION area to brain swelling in the postoperative one-month period. Within 24 h of DC, HYPERPERFUSION area was mild and small, and brain swelling was mild. One week after DC, HYPERPERFUSION area was severe and large, and brain swelling was also severe. One month after DC, no HYPERPERFUSION area was found on SPECT, and brain swelling disappeared on X-CT.

Table 1. Chronology of HYPERPERFUSION area and brain swelling in the decompressed brain

	HYPERPERFUSION area on SPECT	brain swelling on X-CT
< 24 h after DC[1]	mild and small	mild
1 week after DC	severe and large	severe
1 month after DC	none	none

DC[1]: decompressive craniectomy

DISCUSSION

Following DC in the SHT patient, SPECT studies demonstrated that HYPERPERFUSION area occurs in the decompressed brain. Since no HYPERPERFUSION area develops in SHT patients without DC (unpublished data, Yamakami), the present result suggests that DC may increase a focal CBF in the decompressed brain. The focal CBF increase in the decompressed brain may be induced by the combination of vasoparalysis in the traumatized brain [8,9] and increased transmural hydrostatic pressure gradient across brain vessels (or cerebral perfusion pressure) caused by DC [10]. Increasing CBF, DC may protect traumatized brain from an ischemic secondary neural damage.

The present result also demonstrated that the chronology of HYPERPER-FUSION area closely corresponds with the chronology of brain swelling in the decompressed brain. Since the brain swelling in the early posttraumatic period is related more to vascular congestion than to an increase in brain water content [11], the focal CBF increase induced by DC may be related to enhanced brain swelling after DC.

In conclusion, decompressive craniectomy significantly affects regional CBF in patients with severe head trauma and increases the focal CBF of the decompressed brain in the acute posttraumatic period.

REFERENCES

1. Ransohoff J, Benjamin MV, Gage EL Jr, Epstein F (1971) Hemicrani-ectomy in the management of acute subdural hematoma. J Neurosurg 34:70-76
2. Yamaura A, Uemura K, Makino H (1979) Large decompressive craniectomy in management of severe cerebral contusion: A review of 207 cases. Neurol Med Chir (Tokyo) 19:717-728
3. Gaab MR, Rittierodt M, Lorentz M, Heissler HE (1990) Traumatic brain swelling and operative decompression: A prospective investigation. Acta Neurochirurgica Suppl 51:326-328
4. Hase U, Reulen HS, Meinig G, Schurmann K (1978) The influence of the decompressive operation on the intracranial pressure and the pressure-volume relation in patients with severe head injuries. Acta Neurochir 45:1-13
5. Cooper PR, Hagler H, Clark WK, Barnett P (1979) Enhancement of experimental cerebral edema after decompressive craniectomy: Implications for the management of severe head injuries. Neurosurgery 4:296-300
6. Yamakami I, Yamaura A, Isobe K (in press) Types of traumatic brain injury and regional cerebral blood flow assessed by ^{99m}Tc-HMPAO SPECT. Neurol Med Chir (Tokyo)
7. Yamakami I, Yamaura A, Isobe K (submitted) Effects of decompressive craniectomy on regional cerebral blood flow in severe head trauma patients. Neurol Med Chir (Tokyo)
8. Enevoldsen EM, Jensen FT (1978) Autoregulation and CO2 responses of cerebral blood flow in patients with acute severe head injury. J Neurosurg 48:689-703
9. Messeter K, Nordstrom DH, Sundbarg G, Algotsson L, Ryding E (1986) Cerebral hemodynamics in patients with acute head trauma. J Neurosurg 64:231-237
10. Hatashita S, Hoff JT (1987) The effect of craniectomy on the biomechanics of normal brain. J Neurosurg 67:573-578
11. Miller JD (1979) in comments. Neurosurgery 4:300

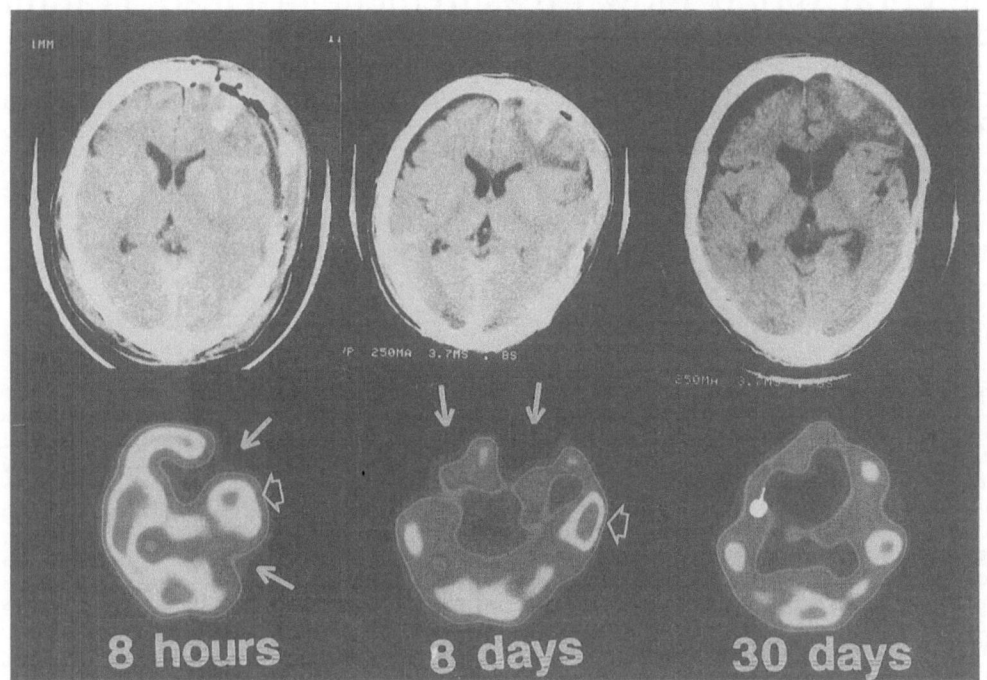

Fig. 1. X–CT (upper row) and SPECT (lower row) in the posttraumatic
one–month period of the case 2. A 49–year–old man underwent left DC
2 h after trauma for managing left acute subdural hematoma with
contusion. Eight hours after DC, SPECT showed 1) PERFUSION DEFECT
(arrows) in the left fronto–temporal lobes associated with brain
contusion, and 2) mild and small HYPERPERFUSION area (open arrow) in
the decompressed temporal lobe (lower left). Mild swelling of the
decompressed brain was observed by X–CT (upper left). Eight days after
DC, SPECT showed that HYPERPERFUSION area (open arrow) in the decompressed temporo–parietal lobe not only enlarged but also increased the
severity. PERFUSION DEFECT (arrows) associated with contusion was also
observed (lower middle). X–CT showed marked swelling of the decompressed brain (upper middle). Thirty days after DC, SPECT showed no
HYPERPERFUSION area in the decompressed temporal lobe (lower right).
The swelling of the decompressed brain also dissolved (upper right).

Cerebral Blood Flow Measurement in Head Trauma Patients

Ichiro Sunada[1], Yoshinori Akano[1], Shigeru Yamamoto[1], and Akira Hakuba[2]

[1]Department of Neurosurgery, Yamamoto Daisan Hospital, Nishinari, Osaka, 557 Japan, and [2]Department of Neurosurgery, Osaka City University, Abeno, Osaka, 545 Japan

SUMMARY

Cerebral blood flow (CBF) measurements were obtained in 40 patients with head trauma by single photon emission CT using 99m-Tc-exametazime (HMPAO) and N-isopropyl-p-(123I)iodo-amphetamine (IMP). Measurement of CBF by using HMPAO in the acute phase enabled immediate detection of brain lesions which could not be detected by CT scan performed immediately after the trauma had occurred. It, however, did not correlate the outcome of patients. In the subacute and chronic phase, it demonstrated insufficiency of cerebral blood flow which could not be detected by CT scan or MRI, but it also did not correlate the outcome. As for measurement of CBF by using IMP, early images indicated perfusion abnormalities similar to those suggested by HMPAO. The patients whose delayed images showed reduced areas of ligand accumulation defect took more favorable courses than the patients who showed no reductions in the area of ligand accumulation defect. When measured by using 99m-DTPA-human serum albumin (HSA-D), blood volume in the injured area showed increases in subacute phase, and decreases in chronic phase.
HMPAO was effective in judging the patient's condition in the acute phase, but date obtained on later occasions must carefully be analyzed. Comparisons between early and delayed images obtained by using 123I-IMP served as an effective means of prognosis.

KEY WORDS: head trauma, cerebral blood flow, cerebral blood volume, single photon emission CT

INTRODUCTION

It is difficult during the early stage of head trauma to predict its probable course by simply relying on the information from CT scans taken immediately after the trauma has occurred. This is because contusion or hematoma may later develop even if CT scan at this early stage reveals no abnormality. In the subacute of chronic phase, the patient may show clinical symptoms which cannot be explained by the results of CT scan. With the hopes of predicting the course of head trauma during its acute phase or to determining the pathological status during its subacute and chronic phases, we measured cerebral blood flow by using a single photon emission CT (SPECT) and studied head trauma in terms of blood circulation in the brain.

MATERIALS AND METHODS

We studied 40 patients who had received scores of 14 to 4 (mean 12) points on the Glasgow Coma Scale. They included 25 patients (mean age of 45 years) who were in the acute phase (within 2 days), 15 of the 25

patients being within 2 hours after the trauma had occurred. Ten patients (mean age of 51 years) were in the subacute phase (within 3 to 10 days), and the remaining 5 patients (mean age of 56 years) were in the chronic phase (1 year after the onset of trauma).
We used a SPECT (HEADTOME SET-070, SHIMADZU CORPORATION) designed exclusively for head examinations. As the radioisotope ligand, 99m-Tc-exametazime (HMPAO) was used for all patients, and N-isoproply-p-(123-I)iodo-amphetamine (IMP) was also used for 15 patients. Six patients were also subject to the cerebral blood volume measurement using 99m-Tc-DTPA-human serum albumin (HSA-D).

RESULTS

Measurements using HMPAO demonstrated local decreases in cerebral blood flow in 18 out of the 25 patients in the acute phase (Table 1). Subsequent CT scan and magnetic resonance imaging (MRI) revealed contusions in the low perfusion areas in all these 18 patients. However, the contused areas visualized by CT scan and MRI were smaller than the low perfusion areas indicated by SPECT. Five patients had extensive areas of low perfusion. Four of them showed consciousness disturbance or severe hemiparesis, and two of these patients died. However, in the remaining patient, the condition took a favorable course. Thus, in the acute phase, it was not completely possible to predict the course of a head trauma based on the degree perfusion had been lowered as indicated by HMPAO. In the 10 patients in the subacute phase, the relationship between the degree of perfusion abnormality and the subsequent course tended to be less noticeable (Table 2). In the 5 patients in the chronic phase, SPECT using HMPAO detected perfusion abnormalities which could not be detected by CT scan or MRI (Table 3). When IMP was used as the radioisotope ligand, early images obtained immediately after its administration indicated perfusion abnormalities similar to those suggested by HMPAO : decreased blood flow was demonstrated in 13 patients. In 11 of them, delayed images obtained 5 hours after IMP administration showed reduced areas of ligand accumulation defect. The conditions of these 11 patients took more favorable courses than the conditions of those who showed no reductions in the area of ligand accumulation defect. None of the 40 patients included in the present study showed increased cerebral blood flow. When measured by using HSA-D, blood volume in the injured area showed increases in 2 patients examined within 10 days of the initial trauma, and decreases in 4 patients examined after the first 10 days (from 26 to 280 days).

DISCUSSION

Previously, cerebral circulation in patients with head trauma had been measured by using nitrogen oxide or radioisotopes including 133Xenon (1) or by CT scan using non-labelled Xenon (2). These methods did not come to be widely used because only a limited number of patients met the requirements to undergo such measurement. In recent years, intravenously injectabe preparations of radioisotope-labelled compounds such as HMPAO and IMP were developed. As SPECT systems became widespread, SPECT using such preparations came to be widely used for measuring cerebral blood flow. Both HMPAO and IMP can readily used for measurements in the acute phase of trauma, as well as for repetitive measurements in the subsequent course (3,4). In particular, HMPAO can be used in an emergency situation, and its high radioactivity produce a clear image within a short period of time. One of its advantages is that it is not affected by other drugs once injected intravenously. Thus, it was considered to be suitable fot the measurement of cerebral blood flow in patients with head trauma in the acute phase. However, it is difficult to predict the patient's condition based on the information from SPECT using HMPAO. Special attention should be paid for analyzing the data obtained in the subacute phase. Like HMPAO, IMP produced good early images. Patients showing decreases in the area of IMP accumulation defect in the delayed images showed a more favorable subsequent course than those showing no decreases. Thus, a patient's condition could be predicted by comparing his early and delayed images. Measurement using HSA-D in the acute phase revealed a decreased blood volume in the same area. These results were roughly consistent with those obtained by using positron emission CT (PET) (5).

REFERENCES

1. Muizelaar JP, Marmarou A, DeSalles AAF, Ward JD, Zimmerman RS, Li Z, Choi SC, Young HF (1989) J Neurosurg 71:63-71
2. Marion DW, Darby J, Yonas H (1991) J Neurosurg 74:407-414
3. Roper SN, Mena I, King WA, Schweitzer J, Garrett K, Mehringer CM, McBride D (1991) J Nucl Med 32:1684-1687
4. Sunada I, Akano Y, Yamamoto S, Kosaka H, Chibana H, Yamamoto H, Matsumura Y, Iguchi K, Kawama A, Obiya M, Muramoto T, Kawasaki M (1991) Kakuigaku 13:62-63
5. Tenjin H, Ueda S, Mizukawa N, Imahori Y, Hino A, Yamaki T, Kuboyama T, Ebisu T, Hirakawa K, Yamashita M, Nakanishi H (1990) Neurosurgery 26:971-979

Table 1
Patient list in acute phase

name	age sex	GCS	HMPAO early	delayed	IMP	GOS
S.K.	64M	10	◉	O	P	MD
H.M.	15M	14	O	O	P	GR
Y.K.	19M	14	O	O	P	GR
H.S.	20M	13	O	O	P	GR
H.Y.	39M	14	O	O	P	GR
I.K.	41M	14	O	O	P	GR
S.G.	57M	13	O	O	P	GR
T.K.	64M	14	O	O	P	GR
Y.T.	65M	13	O	O	P	GR
Y.Y.	55M	14	O	O	N	MD
H.N.	16M	14	◉			GR
M.S.	57F	4	◉			D
F.M.	63M	4	◉			D
K.O.	81M	12	◉			SD
S.I.	23M	14	O			GR
A.I.	36M	14	O			GR
S.Y.	40M	14	O			GR
S.S.	42M	12	O			GR
A.K.	64M	14	O			GR
K.T.	65M	13	O			MD
S.T.	66F	10	O			D
M.T.	16F	14	×			GR
H.K.	18M	13	×			GR
T.H.	42F	14	×			GR
T.I.	52M	14	×			GR

Table 2
Patient list in subacute phase

name	age sex	GCS	HMPAO early	delayed	IMP	GOS
K.Y.	41F	13	◉	◉	P	MD
H.W.	88F	5	◉	◉	N	VS
Y.C.	59F	14	O	O	P	GR
Y.Y.	59M	13	◉			MD
S.O.	61F	12	◉			GR
J.S.	23M	13	O			GR
M.N.	39M	5	O			VS
I.I.	41M	14	O			GR
T.O.	32M	12	×			GR
F.U.	71F	14	×			GR

Table 3
Patient list in chronic phase

name	age sex	HMPAO early	delayed	IMP	GOS
T.M.	54M	O	O	N	MD
K.K.	58M	O	O	N	MD
F.Y.	46M	O			SD
H.W.	54M	O			MD
K.C.	68M	O			MD

HMPAO:99m-Tc-HMPAO, IMP:123I-IMP
abnormal: ◉:generally, O:partially, ×:normal
P:redistribution(+),N:redistribution(-)
GCS:Glasgow Coma Scale, GOS:Glasgow Outcome Scale
GR:good recovery, MD:moderate disability
SD:severe disability
VS:persitent vegatative state, D:death

Validation Study of Skull Three-Dimensional Computed Tomographic Scans (3D-CT) in the Management of Head Injury

KENRO SUNAMI[1], SEIICHIRO HOSHI[1], SOICHI SUNADA[1], MOTOO KUBOTA[1], NAOKATU SAEKI[2], and AKIRA YAMAURA[2]

[1]Department of Neurosurgery, Kawatetsu Chiba Hospital, Chuo-ku, Chiba, 260 Japan, and [2]Department of Neurological Surgery, School of Medicine, Chiba University, Chuo-ku, Chiba, 260 Japan

SUMMARY

Recent advances of methods and software in computed tomographic scans enable us to produce three dimensional images of skull fractures from all directions. We studied the usefulness and limitations of 3D-CT in the head injured patients.

MATERIALS AND METHODS: 1) SOMATOME-PLUS(SIEMENS) is used with a radiographic technique of 210mAs and 120 kV. A 1-second scan time is employed. A scan slice thickness of 1 mm or 2 mm is used in all patients. 2) After scanning is completed, the 3D-CT images are created to obtain any view desired with a technique of lighting, removal of overlying anatomic structures and rotation. 3) Eleven cases, ages ranging from 14 to 71 years, were studied.

RESULTS: 1) 3D-CT scans can provide a great deal of detailed and valuable information about deformities present in the skull base, facial bones and the orbits. 2) Linear skull fractures without dislocation are not well visualized. 3) In the thin areas of bone, so called "pseudoforamen" artifacts are seen.

3D-CT scans are useful in the management of head injured patients by visualizing detailed skull fractures, many of which may not be apparent by conventional radiographic technique.

KEY WORDS: three dimensional surface reconstruction, computed tomography, head injury, skull fracture, optic canal fracture,

INTRODUCTION

Recent advances of methods and software in computed tomographic scans enable us to visualize three dimensional images of skull fractures from all directions. We studied the usefulness and limitations of 3D-CT in the head injured patients.

MATERIALS AND METHODS

SOMATOME-PLUS(SIEMENS) is used with a radiographic technique of 210mAs and 120 kV. A 1-second scan time is employed. A scan slice thickness of 1 mm or 2 mm is used in all patients. After scanning is completed, the 3D-CT images are created to obtain any view desired with a technique of lighting, removal of overlying anatomic structures and rotation. Eleven cases, ages ranging from 14 to 71 years, were studied.

RESULTS

A case of depressed skull fracture in the supraorbital area is shown in Fig. 1. In comparison with two dimensional CT, the exact location and the degree of the deformity, as well as bone fragments, are more accurately represented from desired angles by 3D-CT.

Figure 2 shows a case of facial injury. Multiple fractures of the facial bone, including bilateral condyle fractures and a mental fracture of the mandible were not clearly visible by the skull x-ray.

However, 3D-CT delineated these fractures more precisely from desired angles by rotation and shading.

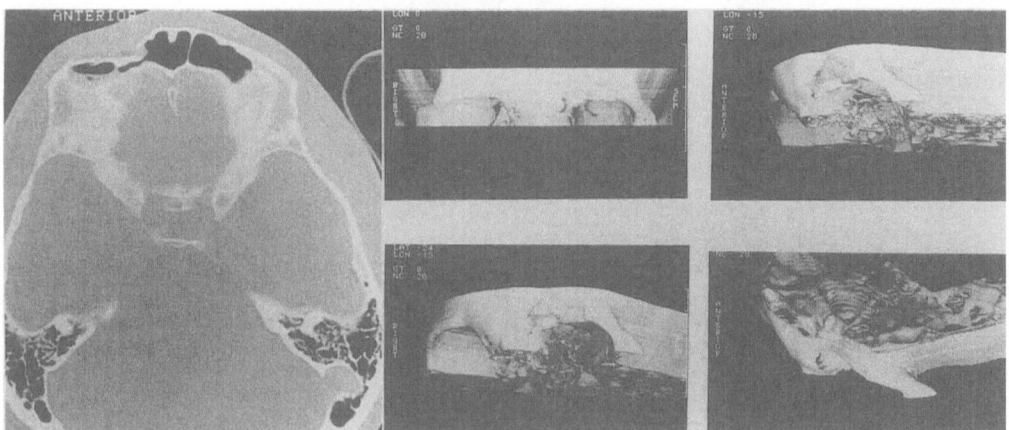

Fig. 1 An example of a depressed skull fracture in the left supraorbital area. 3D-CT reveals the degree of the deformity along with bone fragments more accurately than 2D-CT.

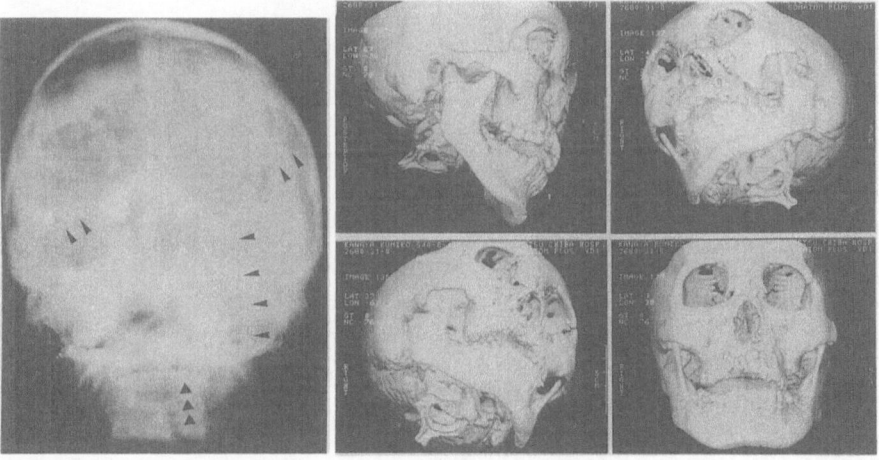

Fig. 2 A case of facial injury. Skull x-ray shows facial bone fractures including bilateral condyle fractures and a mental fracture of the mandible (arrow head). 3D-CT demonstrates clearly the fractures by rotation more clearly than skull x-ray.

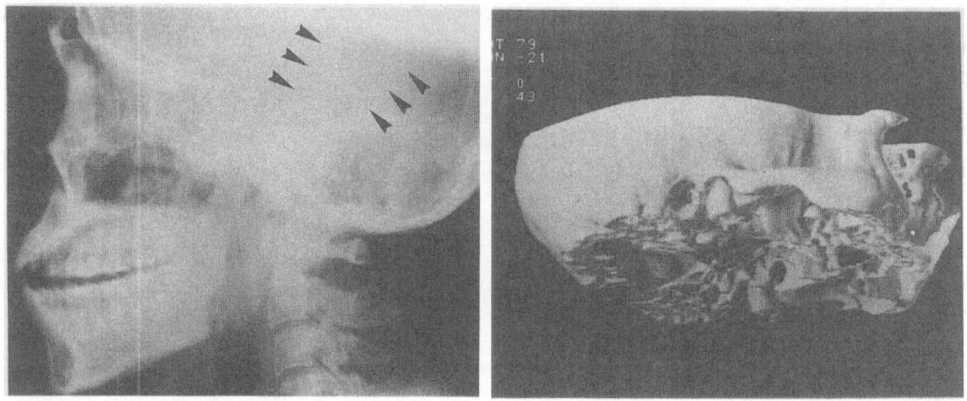

Fig. 3 Skull x-ray shows linear skull fractures in the right posterior temporal area (arrow head). 3D-CT,however, failed to reveal the fractures.

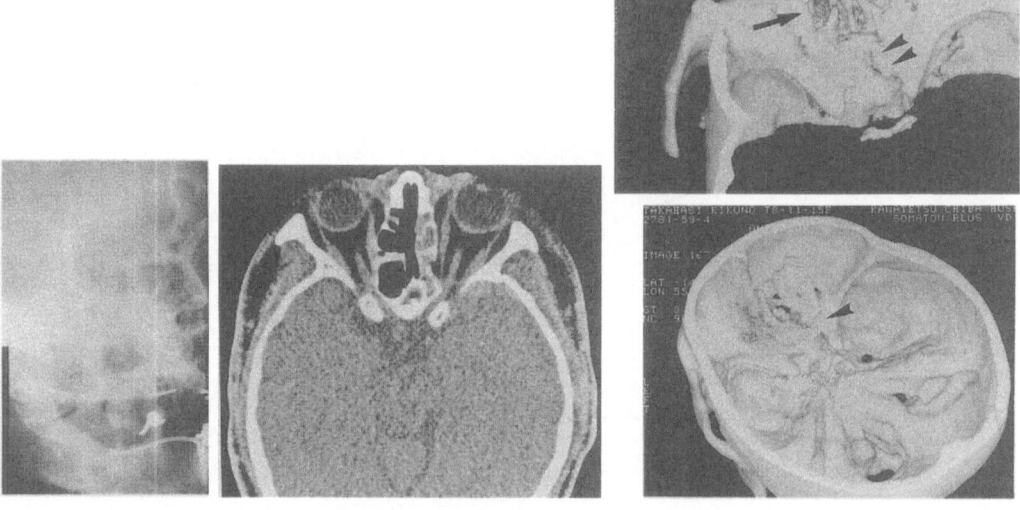

Fig. 4 A case of optic canal fracture. Skull x-ray and 2D-CT failed to show the fracture line. 3D-CT visualized the deformity and fracture at the roof of the optic canal. The "pseudoforamen" was seen at the very thin area of the bone (arrow).

An example of linear skull fractures in the right posterior temporal area is shown in Fig. 3. 3D-CT failed to visualize the fracture. At present, the fractures without dislocation or deformity are not well visualized by 3D-CT.

A case of optic canal fracture is shown in Fig. 4. Skull x-ray and 2D-CT failed to show fracture lines. 3D-CT visualized the deformity and fracture at the roof of the optic canal. The "pseudoforamen" was seen at the very thin area of the bone.

DISCUSSION

Clinical application of 3D-CT has been reported as early as 1983 by Marsh and Vanner[1,2].

Recent advances in high resolution CT scanner together with the improvement of software has been refining 3D images year by year. This resulted in greatly improved diagnostic accuracy and surgical planning by visualizing detailed skull fractures, many of which were not apparent by standard radiographic technique.

In optic nerve injury, radiographic delineation of direct optic nerve injury has been difficult by conventional techniques. Mahapatra AK and Bhatra R[3] reported 45 patients with posttraumatic unilateral blindness and the computed tomographic scan was normal in all and an optic canal fracture was recorded in only one patient. However, Stuzin JM et al.[4] showed a direct injury to the intracanalicular portion of the optic nerve by 3D-CT. If the refined 3D-CT scanner is used, the direct injury of the optic nerve could be demonstrated more frequently than expected although management of optic nerve injury is controversial.

Pseudoforamen designates bone defects seen in areas of papyraceous bone, such as the orbital roof and cribriform plate[5]. A recent developed scanner has made possible the differentiation between this artifact and an actual fracture[6].

3D images, however, cannot replace or substitute the standard radiographic technique due to their weak points, such as "pseudoforamen" artifacts and non-visualization of fractures without dislocation.

CONCLUSIONS

1) 3D-CT scans can provide a great deal of detailed and valuable information about deformities present in the skull base, facial bones and the orbits.
2) Linear skull fractures without dislocation are not well visualized.
3) In the thin areas of bone, so called "pseudoforamen" artifacts are seen.

REFERENCES

1. Marsh JL, Vannier MW (1983) The "third dimension in craniofacial surgery. Plast Reconstr Surg 71:759-767
2. Vannier MW, Marsh JL, Gado MH, Totty WG, Gilula LA, Evens RG (1983) Clinical applications of three-dimensional surface reconstruction from CT scans: Experience with 250 patient studies. Electromedica 51:122-131
3. Mahapatra AK, Bhatia R (1989) Predictive value of vusual evoked potentials in unilateral optic nerve injury. Surg Neurol 31:339-342
4. Stuzin JM, Cutting CB, McCarthy JG, Dufresne CR (1988) Radiographical documentation of direct injury of the intracanlicular segment of the optic nerve in the orbital apex syndrome. Ann Plast Surg 20:368-373
5. Hemmy DC, Tessier PL (1985) CT of dry skulls with craniofacial deformities: Accuracy of three-demenisional reconstruction. Radiology 157:113-116
6. Nishimoto H, Tsukiyama T, Nishimura J, Fujioka M, Tsubokawa T (1987) An evaluation of three-dimensional surface-reconstruction CT (3D-CT) in children with craniosynostosis. CT Kenkyu 9:543-552

6—Cell Damage and Repair in Central Nervous System Injury

Alteration of the Neurotransmitter Contens in the Rabbit Brain Functional Structures at Remote Period Following Experimental Mild Craniocerebral Trauma

I.G. Vasilyeva, N.G. Chopic, and A.P. Cherchenco
Department of Biochemistry, Research Institute of Neurosurgery, Kiev 252 052, Ukraine

SUMMARY

The paper shows results of the research into content of catecholamines in hemispheres, nucleus caudatus,hipothalamus,hippocampus of the rabbits brain 14 days, six and twelve months after easy brain injury.The investigations have shown that 14 days after the trauma there may be found only slight alterations in contents of catecholamines in the above structures.After six and twelve months the alterations are more significant: in the right and left hemispheres the content of noradrenaline fall more than 1.5 times; content of dophamine in these structures also falls:1.5 times hipothalamus and more than 4 times in nucleus caudatus.

KEY WORDS: brain injury, catecholamines

INTRODUCTION

An easy brain injury leads to various changes in functioning of the nervous tissue and the whole organism [1,2,3]. In case of an easy brain injury the pathological process in its fan-like development embraces the whole organism . The degree of involvement of some functional systems depends on individual peculiarities of the organism. The main task in studying pathogenesis of the easy brain unjury is determination of key breaks in integral interactions of the organism.The material substrate of various disturbances to which may lead an easy brain injury may be expressed in violstions of metabolism in neurotransmitter systems of brain structures irrespective of the form of neurotransmitter systems characteristic of them. The purpose of this work was to study contents of neurotransmitters in cortex of the left and right hemispheres, in hipothalamus, hippocampus and in nucleus caudatus of the brain of rabbits when checking after 6 months and one year after an easy brain injury. The selection of structures was predominated by the idea that an easy brain injury in the integral system of the brain responsible for adequacy of efferent reactions resulted in metabolic changes causing development of syndrome of higher spasmodic readiness which in some cases revealed in the form of epileptic attacks.

MATERIALS AND METHODS

Experimental Animals

Male rabbits of grey giant breed with the mass of 2.5-3 kg kept on standard ration of the vivarium have been used in the experiment.

Easy Brain Injury Simulation

To simulate an easy brain injury in rabbits a spring striker [4] was used. The impact was done in parietal region along the median line. The rabbit was not fixed. Before the impact the hair on the head was carefully cut. The spring tension was adjusted so that the impulse of the impact force, causing an experimental easy brain injury ,was equal to 2.35 + 0.04 kg.m/s. After an impact in 75% of cases animals fell on the floor with heads thrown back and with straightened extremities spread to the maximum and they remained in this position from 30 to 90 seconds.Then,after several uncoordinated sharp movements with extremities and head the rabbits rose.For 1-5 minutes their movements were listless,poorly coordinated,shaky,after which the state of animals became normal. No neurological symptomatics was observed.

Tissue Preparing

The tissue of hemispheres, nucleus caudatus,hipothalamus and hippocampus was extracted very quickly, homogenized in 0.1 of $HCLO_4$ (1:10) with addition of $K_2S_2O_5$,processed on the ultrasonic disintegrator, 50 Hz , 15 s, centrifuged at 8000 rev/min for 5 min.

Determination of Catecholamines

Determination of catecholamines was carried out by HPLC method with microcolon chromatograph "Millichrom",as it was described in [5]. Extraction of catecholamines was done in 1.0 M tris-buffer pH 4.86. The extract was added with 3,4- digidrobenzilamine HBr (DGBA) as an internal standard and alumina for adsorption of catecholamines.Test tubes were shaken for 15 minutes,after which the mixture was centrifufed fopr 3 minutes at 1000g; supernatant fluid was suctioned-off with the help of a water-jet pump.AI_2O_3 was flushed three times with redistillated water.To elute catecholamines from aluminium oxide,we used 0.2M $HCLO_4$, mixed,centrifuged for 4 minutes at 1000g; 10 ul of supernatant fluid was applied on the column.

Chromatography

100 ml of nonststionary phase contained 0.03 î of potassium-phosphate buffer, 0.03 M of citric acid, 50 mg of sodium octylsulfonate,10 mg of Na-EDTA, pH 4.86 as well as 8ml of methanol.Colon-Silasorb (Czecho-Slovakia) C-8 (2x60 mm),flow velocity-100 ul/min, working electrode potential-0.75 V.

RESULTS AND DISCUSSION

The results of the investigation on contents of catecholamines in rabbit brain structures in dynamics of an easy brain injury are shown in Table 1.
As we can se from the above data, changes concerning the contents of catecholamines in the rabbit brain in the injury dynamics are ambiguous both in relation to some neurotransmitters (noradrenaline and dophamine) and in relation to different brain structures.Thus,the contents of noradrenaline and dophamine 14 days after the injury were close to control values. 6 months and one year after the injury the contents of noradrenaline in hipothalamus,hippocampus and nucleus caudatùs were not different from those in check animals either. As to the cortex of the left and rigth hemispheres , the contents of noradrenaline in these structures were subjected to omnidirectional

changes in the period after the injury which were studied : 6 months after injury there was observed a trend towards the increase of contents , and 1 year after the injury we could see statistically significant reduction of noradrenaline contents in the cortex of the left and right hemispheres . The contents of dophamine in hippocampus 6 months and 1 year after an easy brain injury did not statistically differ from check values. In hipothalamus the dophamine contents were 1.5-fold lower as compared with check values 6 months and 1 year after the easy brain injury . Considerable (4 and 5-fold) reduction of dophamine contents after 6 months and 1 year, respectively, was found in nucleus caudatus. As to the contents of

Table 1. Contents of Catecholamines in Rabbit Brain Structures in Dynamics of an Easy Brain Injury (ng/g of tissue).

	Control	14 days	6 months	1 year
NRADRENALINE				
Hipothalamus	1047 ±209	954 ±150	890 ±136	1102 ±177
Hippocampus	382 ± 66	367 ± 57	496 ± 73	385 ± 43
Nucleus caudatus	151 ± 20	111 ± 25	157 ± 13	140 ± 31
Hemisphere(L)	195 ± 24	162 ± 20	259 ± 27	115 ± 10*
Hemisphere(R)	180 ± 14	200 ± 14	221 ± 23	110 ± 17*
DOPHAMINE				
Hipotalamus	65 ± 6	60 ± 7	43 ± 3*	45 ± 6*
Hippocampus	13 ± 2	10 ± 1	8 ± 1	17 ± 1
Nucleus caudatus	337 ± 43	280 ± 33	88 ± 29*	61 ± 32*
Hemisphere(L)	57 ± 15	55 ± 13	33 ± 8	36 ± 10
Hemisphere(R)	39 ± 5	46 ± 6	113 ± 61	26 ± 9

* - values for which P<0.05

dophamine in the cortex of the left and right hemispheres of the brain in remote period following the easy brain injury we did not find any statistically significant deviations. Thus, the findings obtained allow to the following generalizations on higher sensitivity of the brain dophaminergic system to traumatic injuries as well as on unequal sensitivity of separate brain structures to such actions. Proceeding from the well-known role of studied structures in the brain functioning we may assume that the discovered manifestation of such changes can take place at the level of the organism.
For the last time was accumulated large considerable material testifying to the supposition on important role of neostriatum and its main structure- nucleus caudatus - in high integrative functiones of the brain, in processes of higher nervous activity [6]. The neostriatum participates in integrative processes of the brain, realizing its influence mainly through cortex and subcortex motor and sensomotor system ; inhibition mechanisms both inside the nucleus itself and directed at the main target - cells (substantia nigra, globus pallidus are main mechanisms participating in realization of this striatal function [7]. Since the ways provading strio-pallido-thalamo-cortical-reactions play an important part in providing central mechanisms of spatial organization of motor functions [8,9], the discovery by us considerable reduction of dophamine contents in one of the structures of this way - nucleus caudatus - in remote period following the easy brain injury may lead to local muscular stiffnes, hyperactivity, causeles aggressiveness of animal. Besides, many researchers treat mental depression from positions of functional weacness of dophaminergic brain system [10].

Thus , on the basis of the above researches we can say that an easy brain injury leads to prolonged disturbances in main neurotransmitter system (dophaminergic and noradrenalinergic) in the cortex, nucleus caudatus and hipothalamus of animals in the experiment; the most significant they are in nucleus caudatus which may be externally manifested in behavior and muscular tension of animals and which is diagnoctic and prognostic criterion of development of an easy brain injury pathogenesis.

REFERENCES

1. Annegers J.F. Crabow J.D., Grover R.V. (1980) Neurology 30: 683-689.
2. Hauser W.A., Tapaddor K., Factor P.R., Finer C. (1984) Neurology 34: 746-751
3. Meyer C.A., Crossman B.Q.,Sarwar N.(1981) Arch.Naurol.(Clinic) 38: 623-629.
4. Lukianov T.T (1979) Racionalizatorskie predlogenia i izobretenia v medicine,Kiev ,pp 89-91
5. Boneski A.A., Fedorov V.I. (1988) Laboratornoe delo 4: 21-25. 6. Suvorov N.F.,Schapovalova K.B.(1989) Fiziologycheskiy Jurnal SSSR LXXII:1337-1356
7. Dzugaeva S.B. (1981) In: Sb. nauchnuh trudov: Talamo-strio-kortikalnie vzaimootnoshenia, Moscow, pp 36-39.
8. Budancev A. (1976) Monoaminoergicheskie sistemy v mozge. Moscow,pp 1 -206.
9. Vein A.M.,Golubev V.L., Berezin E. (1981) Parkinsonizm: clinica, etiologia, patogenez, lechenie.Riga,pp 1-304.
10. Aruschanian E.B. (1987) Jurnal nevropatologia i psihiatria LXXVII: 925-931

Traumatic Brain Damage Mediated by Excitatory Amino Acid Neurotransmitters: Glutamate Release from Contused Brain Tissue

Yoichi Katayama, Tatsuro Kawamata, Hiroaki Tanaka, Kosaku Kinoshita, Atsuo Yoshino, and Takashi Tsubokawa

Department of Neurological Surgery, Nihon University School of Medicine, Tokyo, 173 Japan

SUMMARY

Changes in extracellular glutamate was measured by microdialysis ($[Glu]_d$) within isolated and contused brain tissue, and in brain areas surrounding the cavity filled by contused brain tissue in rats. $[Glu]_d$ within contused brain tissue remained to be elevated longer than $[Glu]_d$ within isolated but non-contused brain tissue. Isolation of brain tissue can be regarded as ischemia induction. The prolonged elevation of $[Glu]_d$ within contused brain tissue may represent more efficient diffusion of glutamate which may be inhibited by shrunken extracellular space in non-contused ischemic brain. $[Glu]_d$ was also found to be elevated in brain areas surrounding the cavity filled by contused brain tissue but not non-contused brain tissue. This increase in $[Glu]_d$ was inhibited by an excitatory amino acid antagonist, suggesting that diffusion of glutamate from contused brain tissue may cause further glutamate release from surrounding brain areas. In the light of increasing evidence for neurotoxicity of glutamate, therapies for traumatic brain injury should include those for preventing glutamate release from contused brain tissue and surrounding brain areas.

KEY WORDS: cerebral contusion - excitatory amino acids - microdialysis - traumatic brain injury

INTRODUCTION

Changes in ion permeability in response to neurotransmitter release are characteristics of the neurons as an excitable cell. Neuronal firing and synaptic transmission are operated by two major classes of ion channels, voltage-dependent and ligand-dependent ion channels. There may be many events which maladaptively activate these channels in traumatic brain injury. Injury process unique to neuronal cells, if exist, may be related to ion fluxes through these channels.

Our previous studies have indicated that excitatory amino acids (EAAs) transmitters are involved in the mechanism of early ionic fluxes, cellular swelling, hypermetabolism and subsequent metabolic derangements following concussive brain injury [e.g., 5,10]. It has been suggested that indiscriminate release of EAAs from nerve terminals plays a vital role in producing these events. Little is currently known, however, regarding the role of EAAs in contusional brain injury [1]. EAAs of the brain exist not only in the transmitter pool in the nerve terminal but also in the metabolic pool within the cell. In contusional brain injury, EAAs may also be released from metabolic pool of mechanically disrupted cells in addition to transmitter pool of the depolarized nerve terminals.

Contusions demonstrate morphological evolution and progressive deterioration in clinical condition during initial 12-24 hours post-injury. EAAs may comprise important component of such changes if they are released continuously from contused brain tissue. The present study investigated the effects of EAAs released from contused brain tissue on the surrounding brain areas. Contusions are composed several pathological components including necrosis, hemorrhage, infarct and edema. In order to investigate metabolic influences of contused brain tissue on surrounding brain areas in isolation, we employed an experimental model of isolated brain contusion.

MATERIALS AND METHODS

Animal preparations

Young Sprague-Dawley rats weighing 180-250 g were employed. They were anesthetized with a mixture of oxygen (33%), nitrous oxide (66%) and enflurane (1.5-2.0 ml/min), and placed in a stereotaxic frame with the nosebar setting at 2.5 mm below the interaural level. The rectal temperature was maintained at 37.0-38.0°C with a heating pad. A precisely determined volume of brain tissue was removed from the frontal cortex of the rat using specially designed cannula (Fig. 1). The removed brain tissue was contused immediately after removal. The brain tissue was returned at 5 min after removal to the cavity from which the brain tissue had been obtained. In control experiments, gelatin of equivalent volume was placed in the cavity.

Microdialysis procedures

Microdialysis probes (O.D., 300 u; effective length, 3 mm; cut off, 20000 MW) were positioned vertically in the frontal cortex 1-4 mm from the edge of the cavity. The probes were inserted immediately after placing the brain tissue or gelatin into the cavity. In some of the animals, probes were placed in the center of the cavity which was filled by contused brain tissue or gelatin (gelfoam). The probes were perfused with Ringer solution (adjusted to pH 7.4) at a rate of 5.0 µl/min. The temperature of the perfusate was adjusted to be 37°C, and the temperature was maintained with a chamber filled with water at 37°C in which whole length of the inlet tubings was placed. Sodium kynurenate (KYN, at 0, 1, 5 or 10 mM [5,8]), a broad spectrum antagonist of EAA receptors, was administered through the probe throughout the experiment, replacing equimolar sodium chloride in the perfusate. Details of the microdialysis procedures have been described elsewhere [5,8]. Upon completion of each experiment, the position of the probe was confirmed anatomically.

Measurements of EAAs

The dialysate concentration of glutamate ($[Glu]_d$) was measured by high-performance liquid chromatography [6]. Precolumn derivatization of the amino acids with o-phthaldialdehyde was employed to form highly fluorescent reaction products which were separated using a Rainin Model HP fitted with a Rainin Microsorb Short-One C18 (4.6 mm ID x 10 cm) column and a fluorescence detector (LDC Fluoromonitor III Detector, excitation 340 nm, emission 440 nm). The concentrations of amino acids were normalized with a known concentration of isoleucine (10 µM) added to the dialysate as an internal standard.

RESULTS

EAA release from contused brain tissue

The insertion of the probe induced a transient increase in $[Glu]_d$. While re-insertion of probes through tracks previously made produces less marked increase in $[Glu]_d$, measurements of $[Glu]_d$ was always initiated after penetration of intact brain areas in the present experiment. The $[Glu]_d$ level then rapidly stabilized. No glutamate was naturally detected in dialysate obtained within gelatin.

A high $[Glu]_d$ was observed within the isolated but non-contused brain tissue immediately after the probe insertion. The $[Glu]_d$ level reached 10 times of the $[Glu]_d$ level simultaneously measured within the normal brain tissue. The $[Glu]_d$ then gradually decreased. The $[Glu]_d$ remained to be 2-3 times higher than the $[Glu]_d$ level within the normal brain tissue at 1 hours after producing lesions.

Similarly, a high $[Glu]_d$ was demonstrated within the contused brain tissue immediately after probe insertion. The $[Glu]_d$ level was approximately 10 times of the $[Glu]_d$ level simultaneously measured within the normal brain tissue. As compared to isolated but non-contused brain tissue, however, contused brain tissue remained to demonstrate high $[Glu]_d$ level for longer time. The $[Glu]_d$ at 1 hour after producing lesions was 4-5 times higher than the $[Glu]_d$ level within the normal brain tissue.

EAA increase in surrounding brain areas

The $[Glu]_d$ level was also found to be elevated within brain areas surrounding the cavity filled by contused brain tissue. Thus, dialysate collected within brain areas 1.0 mm distant from the edge of the cavity during 1 hour period after producing lesions revealed $[Glu]_d$ of 2-3 times higher than $[Glu]_d$ observed in brain areas surrounding the cavity filled by gelatin (Table 1). No such an increase in $[Glu]_d$ was demonstrated when the cavity was filled by isolated but non-contused brain tissue (Table 1). The in situ administration of KYN significantly inhibited this increase in $[Glu]_d$ within brain areas surrounding the cavity filled by contused brain tissue (Table 1).

Table 1. Dialysate concentration of glutamate ($[Glu]_d$, μM).

Content of the cavity	Center of the cavity	1 mm distant from the cavity	1 mm distant from the cavity (KYN)
Gelfoam	0.0	3.4±1.3	
Isolated, non-contused brain tissue	22.5±3.9	4.7±1.1	
Contused brain tissue	34.5±4.5	9.4±2.5	3.8±1.4

Dialysate for 1 hour. KYN, 10mM kynurenic acid in perfusate.

DISCUSSION

The isolation without inducing contusion can be regarded as induction of focal cerebral ischemia. The changes observed within brain tissue subjected to such an insult were basically similar to those observed in complete cerebral ischemia [6,7,9]. Shrinkage of the extracellular space (ECS) occurring concomitantly with massive ionic fluxes during cerebral ischemia may reduce the available volume fraction and effective surface area for dialysis [6,7,9]. The recovery rate in vivo of any substances within the ECS may therefore decrease during this period of ischemia. Furthermore, with shrinkage of the ECS, dialysis may cause a rapid depletion of glutamate from the ECS. Thus, the decrease in $[Glu]_d$ after the increase in non-contused ischemic brain appears to represent rapid depletion of glutamate from the available volume fraction for dialysis. The prolonged elevation of $[Glu]_d$ within contused brain tissue suggests that the volume fraction available for dialysis is larger and diffusion of glutamate is more efficient. $[Glu]_d$ was also found to be elevated in brain areas surrounding the cavity filled by contused brain tissue but not non-contused brain tissue, again suggesting a more efficient diffusion of glutamate within contused brain tissue.

Since the increase was inhibited by an EAA antagonist, however, the increase in $[Glu]_d$ in surrounding brain areas cannot be attributable merely to diffusion from contused brain tissue. EAAs produce massive ionic fluxes through the cell membrane [11]. If the ionic fluxes are sufficiently large, the nerve terminals may be depolarized and further release of EAA neurotransmitters may result [5,13]. Such a diffusion-reaction process appears to be involved in the increase in $[Glu]_d$ in surrounding brain areas. In the light of increasing evidence for neurotoxicity of EAAs, contused brain tissue appears to produce considerable metabolic influences to surrounding brain areas, which may render neuronal cells more vulnerable to secondary insults [2,3,4]. Therapies of traumatic brain injury should include those for therapies for preventing EAA release from contused brain tissue and surrounding brain areas, such as resection of contused brain tissue and administration of EAA antagonists.

REFERENCES

1. Faden AI, Demediuk P, Panter SS et al (1989) The role of excitatory amino acids and NMDA receptors in traumatic brain injury. Science 244: 798-800.
2. Ishige N, Pitts LH, Pogliani L et al (1987) Effects of hypoxia on traumatic brain injury in ratsa: Part 2 changes in high energy phosphate metabolism. Neurosurgery 20: 854.
3. Jenkins LW, Moszynski K, Lyeth BG et al (1989) Increased vulnerability of the mildly traumatized rat brain to cerebral ischemia. Brain Research 477: 211-224.
4. Katayama Y, Becker DP: Pathophysiology and treatment of head trauma (1990) In Aochi O, Amaha K, Takeshita H (eds): Intensive and Critical Care Medicine, Amsterdam, Excerpta Medica, pp.259-262
5. Katayama Y, Becker DP, Tamura T et al (1990) Massive increase in extracellular potassium and indiscriminate glutamte release after concussive brain injury. J Neurosurg, 73: 889-900.
6. Katayama Y, Kawamata T, Tamura T et al (1991) Calcium-dependent glutamate release concomitant with massive potassium flux during cerebral ischemia in vivo. Brain Res, 558: 136-140.
7. Katayama Y, Tamura T, Becker DP et al (1991) Calcium-dependent component of massive increase in extracellular potassium during cerebral ischemia as demonstrated by microdialysis in vivo. Brain Res, 567: 57-63
8. Katayama Y, Tamura T, Becker DP et al (1991) Inhibition of rapid potassium flux during cerebral ischemia in vivo with an excitatory amino acid antagonist. Brain Res, 568: 294-298.
9. Katayama Y, Tamura T, Becker DP et al (1992) Early cellular swelling during cerebral ischemia in vivo is mediated by excitatory amino acids released from nerve terminals. Brain Res, 577: 121-126.
10. Kawamata T, Katayama Y, Hovda DA et al (1992) Administration of excitatory amino acid antagonists via microdialysis prevents the increase in glucose utilization seen immediately following concussive brain injury. J Cereb Blood Flow Metab, 12: 12-24.
11. Mayer ML, Westbrook GL (1987) Cellular mechanisms underlying excitotoxicity. TINS 10: 59-61.
12. Sunami K, Nakamura T, Ozawa Y et al (1989) Hypermetabolic state following experimental head injury. Neurosurg Rev 12:400-411.
13. Takahashi H, Manaka S, Sano K (1981) Changes in extracellular potassium concentration in cortex and brain stem during the acute phase of experimental closed head injury. J Neurosurg 55:708-717.

Neurofunctional Changes in Thalamic Neurons After Cortical Ablation in Adult Rats: Effect of Basic Fibroblast Growth Factor upon Thalamic Neurons

KAZUO KATAOKA[1], KAZUO YAMADA[2], TATSUYA TOKUNO[1], SUMIO KONDO[1], TOSHIHARU ASAI[1], SIKO CHICHIBU[3], MAMORU TANEDA[2], TORU HAYAKAWA[2], RYOTARO KURODA[1], and MASAHIKO IOKU[1]

[1]Department of Neurosurgery and [3]First Department of Physiology, Kinki University School of Medicine, Osaka-Sayama, Osaka, 589, and [2]Department of Neurosurgery, Osaka University Medical School, Fukushima, Osaka, 553 Japan

SUMMARY

Traumatic damage to cortex results in progressive degeneration in the ipsilateral thalamus. It has recently been suggested that this degeneration is attributable to neurotrophic mechanisms. We studied the functional and morphological changes in thalamic relay neurons that occurred following traumatic cortical ablation, and also studied the effects of basic fibroblast growth factor (b-FGF), one of neurotrophic factors, on these changes.

We ablated the foreleg projection area of left sensori-motor cortex of adult Wistar rats anesthetized with chloral hydrate using a dental drill. In the b-FGF group, 1μg of b-FGF (50-100 μl) was injected into the cavity formed by cortical ablation, and the rats again received 1μg of b-FGF (50 μl) by percutaneous injection to the cisterna magna 4 days later. Fourteen days after ablation, using glass microelectrodes neuron activity of the nucleus ventralis posterolateralis (VPL) was recorded during chloral hydrate anesthesia following repetitive electrical stimulation of the contralateral forepaw at frequencies ranging from 1 to 50 Hz. The average number of firings of VPL neurons in response to 25 stimulations at 30 Hz was significantly reduced to 0.41 and 0.11 spikes per stimulus, in rats without b-FGF treatment and rats with b-FGF treatments, respectively. In normal rats, the same stimulation produced 0.72 spikes per stimulus. Histological examination demonstrated degenerating neurons and decreases in the number of neurons present in the ipsilateral thalamus in rats without b-FGF treatment following ablation. In rats treated with b-FGF, these morphological thalamic changes were somewhat less pronounced.

This study demonstrates that traumatic cortical ablation results in functional and morphologic changes. A previous study of ours showed that b-FGF treatment prevented morphological degeneration of the ipsilateral thalamus following cortical infarct [Yamada et al., *J Cereb Blood Flow Metab* 11:472-479, 1991]. In the present study, treatment with b-FGF ameliorated somewhat the morphological degeneration in VPL after ablation of sensori-motor cortex, but did not improve the unit responses of VPL neurons.

Key Words: Basic fibroblast growth factor, Cortical ablation, Thalamus, Single unit response.

INTRODUCTION

Even if injury to the brain is limited focally to a single region, neuronal structures remote from the primary lesion but related to it by neuronal pathways develop functional and/or histological changes. The thalamocortical and corticothalamic pathways very strongly connect the cerebral cortex and the ipsilateral thalamus. Cortical traumatic injury and cortical infarct therefore result in progressive degeneration in the ipsilateral thalamus [1,2,3,4]. We recently studied by recording of thalamic unit activity the sequential changes in direct function of thalamic neurons during degeneration following cortical infarct [5]. A previous study of ours demonstrated that basic fibroblast growth factor (b-FGF), one of the neurotrophic factors, prevented morphological degeneration of the ipsilateral thalamus after cortical infarct in rats [6]. It would be of some interest to study the neurological function of thalamic neurons treated with b-FGF following cortical injury. We studied the functional and morphological changes of thalamic relay neurons that occurred following traumatic cortical ablation. The effect of administration of b-FGF following cortical ablation on thalamic neurons was also studied.

MATERIALS AND METHODS

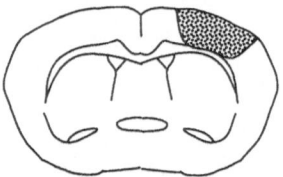

Fig.1. Schematic drawing of cotical ablation of the left sensori-motor cortex (foreleg area).

Twenty adult female Wistar rats (15 weeks of age) were studied. They were anesthetized with 400 mg/kg chloral hydrate i.p., and then were mounted on a stereotaxic apparatus. The skull was exposed, and a burr hole was made over the left sensori-motor cortex. The foreleg projection area [7] of left sensori-motor cortex was ablated using a dental drill (Fig. 1). In the 10 rats receiving b-FGF treatment, 1μg of b-FGF (diluted in 50-100 μl of 0.1 % bovine serum albumin (BSA), 0.01M phosphate buffer saline (PBS)) was injected into the cavity immediately following cortical ablation. For the untreated group (10 rats), 50-100 μl of 0.1% BSA in 0.01M PBS without b-FGF was injected into the cavity. A small piece of gelfoam was placed in the cavity prior to skin closure. The rats of the b-FGF treatment group received again 1μg of b-FGF (diluted in 50 μl of 0.1 % BSA, 0.01M PBS) by percutaneous injection of the cisterna magna 4 days after cortical ablation. Basic FGF was kindly provided by Takeda Chemical Industrial Ltd. (Osaka, Japan).

Since the level of spontaneous activity of thalamic relay neurons is relatively low in anesthetized rats, we evaluated the responses of thalamic neurons to repetitive electrical stimulation applied to the contralateral forepaw. The rats were anesthetized with chloral hydrate (400 mg/kg i.p.) 14 days after cortical ablation. As controls, 9 age matched rats were anesthetized with chloral hydrate. The method used for recording of thalamic unit activity has previously been described [5]. Briefly, the head of the rat was fixed in a stereotaxic instrument, and a small burr hole was made over the left thalamus. A glass microelectrode (4-8 mega Ω) was stereotaxically inserted into the nucleus ventralis posterolateralis (VPL) using coordinates assigned in the atlas of Paxinos and Watson [8] (A 4.7-5.7, L 3.0-3.5, H 4.5-6.0). We determined that unit activity which occurred specifically in response to electrical stimulation of the contralateral forepaw. The forepaw was stimulated repeatedly with gradually increasing frequencies from 1 to 50 Hz; at each frequency, 25 pulses were delivered. The evoked unit responses were evaluated as the firing probability at each stimulation frequency. The firing probability was calculated from the average number of spikes in response to each group of 25 stimuli. Left thalamic unit responses evoked by right forepaw stimulation were recorded from 9 normal control rats as well.

Following unit recording, the animals were perfused transcardially with 4% paraformaldehyde in 0.1 M phosphate buffer solution under deep pentobarbital anesthesia and brains were removed. We made 6 μm paraffin embedded brain sections for Hematoxylin and Eosin staining. The degree of thalamic degeneration were microscopically determined.

We used the non-parametric Mann-Whitney U test for statistical evaluation of results.

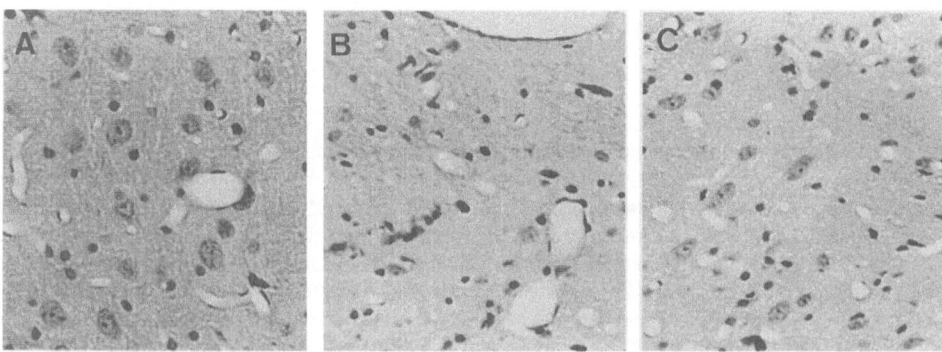

Fig. 2. Microphotography of VPL. A: Normal control, B: Cortical ablation and no b-FGF treatment, C: Cortical ablation and b-FGF treatment.

RESULTS

Paraffin-embedded brain sections stained by Hematoxylin and Eosin from the brains of untreated rats obtained 14 days after cortical ablation revealed degenerative changes in ipsilateral VPL neurons and decreases in the number of ipsilateral VPL neurons compared to contralateral VPL. Brain sections obtained from treated rats demonstrated relative preservation of the number of ipsilateral VPL neurons (Fig.2). B-FGF treatment resulted in morphological modification of the thalamic degenerative changes induced by cortical ablation.

Table *Number of rats and unit recordings*

	Total No. of rats	No. of rats with unit recording	Total No. of units
Normal control	9	9	13
Cortical ablation b-FGF (-)	10	8	13
Cortical ablation b-FGF (+)	10	6	9

Thalamic unit responses were barely measurable in 60% (6/10) of the b-FGF treated rats that had undergone ablation and in 80% (8/10) of the untreated rats that had undergone ablation. It was easy to detect thalamic unit responses in all 9 of the normal control rats. We were able to calculate firing probabilities for 35 units from 23 rats (Table). Figure 3 shows original charts of thalamic unit responses evoked by forepaw stimulation for the 3 groups. Figure 4 shows the relationship between firing probability and stimulus frequency for each of the 3 groups. In these 3 groups, VPL unit probability of firing decreased with increased stimulus frequency. The probability of firing in ablated rats with or without b-FGF treatment was lower than that in normal controls at every stimulus frequency tested. In the group of rats which had undergone ablation, the firing probability in rats treated with b-FGF was lower than that in rats without b-FGF treatment (Fig.4).

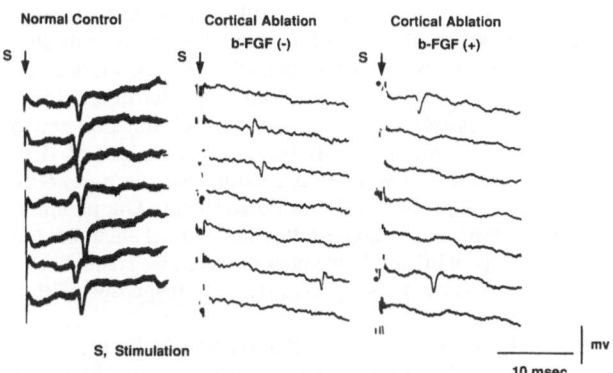

Fig.3. Unit responses to successive stiumli at 30 Hz.

DISCUSSION

Recently, several reports of efforts to ameliorate cortical lesion-induced thalamic degeneration have been made. Immediate transplantation of fetal cortex reduces the degree of thalamic atrophy occurring after cortical ablation in newborn rats [9, 10]. Autologous peripheral nerve grafts between the ipsilateral

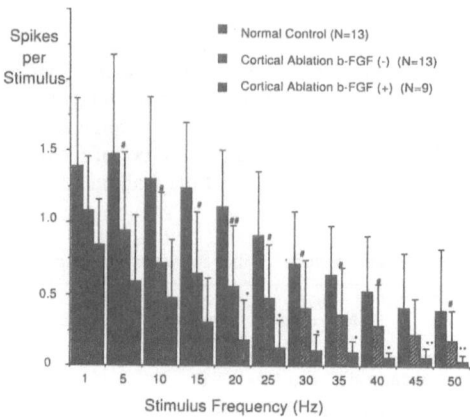

Fig. 4. Average (±SD) frequency response of somatically excited VPL neurons of 3 groups.
# p<0.05, ## p<0.01, vs Normal control.   * p<0.05, ** p<0.01, vs Cortical ablation b-FGF(-).

thalamus and the contralateral cortex possibly ameliorate the cortical lesion-induced degenerative cell changes in ipsilateral thalamus occurring after unilateral cortical ablation [11]. Immediate trials of restitution of the neuronal network by transplantation contribute to prevention of thalamic degeneration. It is well known that neurons require specific neurotrophic factors derived from the different brain areas for survival. The effects of humoral factors derived from transplant of embryonal brain tissue, which possibly contains a variety of types of trophic factors, must therefore be considered. Yamada et al. [6] clearly showed that exogenous b-FGF, itself a neurotrophic factor, prevented thalamic degeneration following cortical infarct in adult rats in the absence of establishment of new neural connections. In the present study, b-FGF treatment resulted in some amelioration of thalamic morphological changes notable 14 days after cortical ablation.

In rats, VPL neurons receive facilitative synaptic inputs from the cortex. Focal depression of somatosensory cortex induced by direct lidocaine application results in profound depression of synaptic transmission in rat VPL neurons [12]. Our previous unit recording study demonstrated that characteristic changes occurred in VPL neuron firing properties following cortical infarct. Following a profound disturbance of somatosensory transmission in VPL neurons during the acute stage (1 day after occlusion) of cortical infarct, a transient recovery of somatosensory transmission occurred 4-7 days after infarct; depression was subsequently observed again on the 14th day after infarct [5]. The initial depression of somatosensory transmission is possibly a consequence of the elimination due to ischemia of facilitative corticofugal influences on VPL neurons. Recovery from the acute phase of depression may be due to an unknown compensatory mechanism. The late depression may be a consequence of morphological degenerative changes themselves associated with functional silence. Our preliminary study showed that the time-course of changes in thalamic unit response following cortical ablation seems to be similar to that of changes observed following cortical infarct. In the present study, we studied neuronal unit changes present 14 days after cortical ablation because we suspected that unit responses on the 14th day might possibly reflect morphological changes.

Even without b-FGF treatment, some ipsilateral VPL neurons could respond to contralateral forepaw stimulation 14 days after ablation, though those neurons might be during degeneration. Although b-FGF treatment resulted in some amelioration of the morphological degeneration of thalamic neurons occurring after cortical ablation, these neurons nevertheless seemed to differ from normal. The methods used in the present study permit only qualitative evaluation of neurons. Results obtained from study of neurons capable of responding to peripheral stimulation demonstrated that the treatment of b-FGF rather disturbed the firing probability of VPL neurons. The present study has shown that functional recovery does not follow morphological improvement achieved by treatment with a neurotrophic agent in the absence of restitution of damaged neuronal networks. Related work has shown that the γ-aminobutyric acid agonist muscimol prevents the degeneration of SNR neurons that occurs following placement of ipsilateral striatal lesions in rats [13]. However, amelioration of the morphological condition of SNR neurons induced by the muscimol injection was not associated with functional recovery, but rather with deterioration of striato-nigral function [14].

Acknowledgements:Authors thank Takeda Chemical Industrial Ltd. for the supply of b-FGF. We thank Ms. Ryuko Esaki for excellent technical assistance. This work was supported in part by a grant-in-aid for scientific research from the Ministry of Education (02670641), Japan.

REFERENCES

1. Cooper RM, Thurlow GA, Rooney BJ (1984) 2-Deoxyglucose uptake and histologic changes in rat thalamus after neocortical ablations. *Exp Neurol* 83:134-143
2. Kataoka K, Hayakawa T, Yamada K, Mushiroi T, Kuroda R, Mogami H (1989) Neuronal network disturbance after focal ischemia in rats. *Stroke* 20:1226-1235
3. Fujie W, Kirino T, Tomukai N, Iwasa T, Tamura A (1990) Progressive shrinkage of the thalamus following middle cerebral artery occlusion in rats. *Stroke* 21:1485-1488
4. Tamura A, Tahira Y, Nagashima H, Kirino T, Gotoh O, Hojo S, Sano K (1991) Thalamic atrophy following cerebral infarction in the territory of the middle cerebral artery. *Stroke* 22:615-618
5. Tokuno T, Kataoka K, Asai T, Chichibu S, Kuroda R, Ioku M, Yamada K, Hayakawa T (1992) Functional changes in thalamic relay neurons after focal cerebral infarct. A study of unit recordings from VPL neurons after MCA occlusion in rats. *J Cereb Blood Flow Metab* in press
6. Yamada K, Kinoshita A, Kohmura E, Sakaguchi T, Taguchi J, Kataoka K, Hayakawa T (1991) Basic fibroblast growth factor prevents thalamic degeneration after cortical infarction. *J Cereb Blood Flow Metab* 11:472-478
7. Hall RD, Lindholm EP (1974) Organization of motor and somatosensory neocortex in the albino rat. *Brain Research* 66:23-38
8. Paxinos G, Watson C (1986) The Rat Brain in Stereotaxic Coordinates. Sydney, Academic Press, Inc.
9. Sharp FR, Gonzalez MF (1986) Fetal cortical transplants ameliorate thalamic atrophy ipsilateral to neonatal frontal cortex lesions. *Neurosci Lett* 71:247-251
10. Sørensen J Chr, Zimmer J, Castro AJ (1989) Fetal cortical transplants reduce the thalamic atrophy induced by frontal cortical lesions in newborn rats. *Neurosci Lett* 98:33-38
11. Cossu M, Martelli A, Pau A, Viale S, Siccardi D, Viale GL (1987) Axonal elongation into peripheral nerve grafts between thalamus and somatosensory cortex of the rat. An experimental study. *Brain Research* 415:399-403
12. Yuan B, Morrow TJ, Casey KL (1985) Responsiveness of ventrobasal thalamic neurons after suppression of S1 cortex in the anesthetized rat. *J Neurosci* 5:2971-2978
13. Saji M, Reis DJ (1987) Delayed transneuronal death of substantia nigra neurons prevented by γ-aminobutyric acid agonist. *Science* 235:66-69
14. Schallert T, Jones TA, Lindner MD (1990) Multilevel transneuronal degeneration after brain damage. Behavioral events and effects of anticonvulsant g-aminobutyric acid-related drugs. *Stroke* 21(suppl III):III-143-III-146

An Experimental Study of the Evolution of Focal Axonal Injury

GIUSTINO TOMEI[1], DIEGO SPAGNOLI[1], ROBERTO VILLANI[1], GUIDO FUMAGALLI[2], CARLO SALA[2], T.A. GENNARELLI[3]

[1]Institute of Neurosurgery, [2]CNR Department of Cytofarmacology, University of Milan, Milan, Italy, and [3]Department of Neurosurgery, University of Pennsylvania, Philadelphia, USA

SUMMARY

Uniaxial stretch of the optic nerve of the albino guinea pig can reproduce the axonal damage as demonstrated in prolonged traumatic coma in humans and primates. By morphological and neurophysiological approaches we have demonstrated that in the acute phase (24 hrs after injury) axonal lesions are characterized by terminal clubs and focal axonal enlargements along with an elongation of visual evoked potentials (VEPs). In this model, in which the lesion is distributed along the entire nerve, the velocity of the fast phase of axoplasmic transport in injured nerves was increased (218 mm/day vs. 176 mm/day in controls) and so was the amount of transported proteins. There was no accumulation and a block of protein uptake at the site of the lesion as demonstrated in other biological models. One week after injury, axonal lesions observed in the acute phase and alterations of VEPs disappeared, whereas the rate of axonal transport and the amount of protein uptake were persistently increased. Therefore in this model, an increase of anterograde fast transport was demonstrated both in acute and chronic phases. Since regeneration of optic axons was never evident on morphological study, the restoration of axonal function and the persistence of active axonal transport one week after injury support that spontaneous reparative processes occurred in lesioned axons.

KEY WORDS: optic nerve, axonal injury, axonal transport, guinea pig

INTRODUCTION

A model of axonal injury has been developed in our laboratories [1,2]. Uniaxial stretch of the optic nerve of the albino guinea pig reproduced the axonal damage demonstrated in prolonged traumatic coma in humans and primates [1,2]. Whereas other trauma models use a direct mechanism of lesion (crush, ligation, transection) that is followed by complete axotomy and vessel disruption, this model produces an indirect and non invasive lesion. As a result, a pure axonal damage involving the entire optic nerve is induced.

Here we study the axonal transport and its modifications in relation to the presence of axonal lesion during the acute and chronic phases.

MATERIALS AND METHODS

Animal preparation, biomechanics , injury apparatus, morphological and neurophysiological study methods were described in detail elsewhere [1,2] . For axoplasmic transport study, animals were deeply anaesthetized and the right eye globe and optic nerve were mobilized. Twenty µl of (3,4-3H)L-Proline (48

Ci/mM-1mCi/ml-I.C.N. Radiochemicals, Irvin,Ca) were injected using a 50 µl Hamilton syringe into the vitreous of the eye. Injury was performed few minutes before injection. At 3,6,12,24, hrs after injection, animals were deeply re-anaesthetized and killed. Right optic nerve was cut into 4 tracts of 2 mm of lenght, called 2mm (first tract), 4mm (2nd tract), 6 mm(3rd tract) and 4mm (4th tract). Left lateral geniculate body (LGB) and superior colliculus (SC) were isolated from the brain. Specimens of optic nerve, LGB and SC were homogenized at 4°C in 50 mM Tris-HCl (pH 7.2) containing 2% Triton X-100 in glass to glass potters. The homogenate was centrifugated at 75000 g for 20 minutes at 4°C. Pellets were resolubilized in 1N NaOH. Tritium activity was measured by a Beckman model LS 7500 after addition of 10 ml of scintillation fluid. Specific activity was expressed in DPM (mean +SD). Twenty control and 22 injured animals were used. To evaluate axonal transport velocity, the lenght of optic nerve, chiasm, optic tract and LGB-SC distance were measured and resulted in 10 mm, 2 mm, 10 mm and 3 mm respectively. The entire lenght of the optic system was 25 mm. Data obtained within 24 hours from injection permitted considerations on the fast phase of axonal transport. The study of fast axonal transport was also carried out in animals 1 week after injection: animals were killed 3 and 6 hrs after injection of proline.

RESULTS

(a) Control animals

Three hours after injection, the largest amount of tritium activity was present in the first tract of the optic nerve. Activity was then spreading down and decreasing from the 2nd to the 4th tract. (Fig.1). In the following post-injection intervals (6,12,24 hrs), radioactivity was progressively increasing along the nerve: at 6 hrs, mean DPM value of the entire nerve was almost twice than at 3 hours. At 12 and 24 hours after injection, radioactivity was 3.6 and 4.6 times larger respectively.

Three hours after injection,. the front of the leading wave was evident at the level of LGB (Fig.1). In the subsequent intervals there was a progressive increase of activity in LGB and SC; at 24 hrs it was 4.3 and 11.3 fold larger respectively than that measured at the level of the last segment of the nerve. Activity measured at the level of SC was always significantly greater than that measured at the level of LGB (p<0.001) (Fig.1).

The front of the leading wave was evident at the level of LGB 3 hours after the injection. The lenght from the globe to the LGB is 22 mm: the calculated rate of the fast phase of axonal transport in control animals was therefore 176 mm/day.

(b) Injured animals

In injured animals, the profile of tritium activity along the optic nerve paralleled that seen in controls at all the post-injection intervals studied; yet the amount of aminoacid incorporation and the velocity of fast axonal transport were different. In fact, the amount of radioactivity in various segments at different time points (3,6,12,24 hours) was always larger in lesioned than in control animals. Activity counted in the last 3 segments of the nerve, in LGB and SC was 70%, 80% and 140% of the control values at 6,12 and 24 hrs intervals.

At 3 hrs interval, the more striking evidence was the early appearance of activity at the level of SC.: the difference of values calculated at the level of terminal fields was no more evident (ratio LGB/SC=0.90). In injured animals, the front of the leading wave 3 hours after injection was therefore at the level of SC. Since the LGB-SC tract is covered by non retinal ganglionic cells, some assumptions must be take into account to measure the fast axonal transport rate in the injured optic nerves. At the first time point (3 hours), the presence of high amounts of radioactivity in SC suggests that the front wave had reached the LGB earlier than in controls. By subtracting from the 3 hours time point the time theoretically required for transport from LGB to SC, we could calculate indirectly the fast axonal transport rate in injured axons. This value was 218 mm /day, i.e. much higher than controls (p<0.01).

Similar results were obtained in animals injected one week after the lesion, suggesting that, in this model, the changes in fast axonal transport persisted for at least one week after injury.

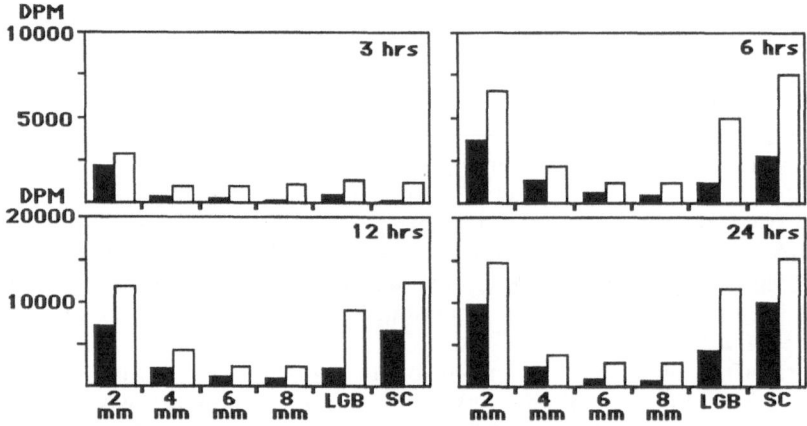

Fig. Fast axoplasmic transport in guinea pig optic nerve. Profile and distribution of L-Proline along the nerve and terminal fields at 3,6,12,24 hrs after injection in control (filled bars) and injured (open bars) nerves.

DISCUSSION

Our experiments have demonstrated that the intensity and the rate of the fast axonal transport are markedly increased in injured guinea pig optic nerve both in the acute (3-24 hours after injury) or chronic (1 week) phases. This confirms morphological studies which showed, in the acute phase, an increased accumulation of HRP and membrane bound bodies at the level of axonal enlargements [2]. Membraneous and soluble materials are known to move along the axons at velocity within the range of rapid phase of transport. [3].

Our results differ from other biological models of CNS nerve lesion, in which a considerable decrease of proteins transport occurred [4]. In these experiments and in other peripheral nerve models of lesioning, the rapid decline in transport was referred to anoxia due to interruption of blood supply [4,5]. In our model, injury is provided by an indirect and non invasive mechanism with no vascular involvement. Besides, the injury is distributed along the entire optic nerve and, in the acute phase, axotomized and lesioned in continuity axons are intermingled with normal axons [2]. Marked accumulation of organelles and disruption of the cytoskeletal network observed at the level of swollen and disrupted axons in the acute phase disappeared one week after injury. At this time point, an important reduction of axonal lesions became apparent and was paralleled by the improvement of neurophysiological data. In fact, VEPs recordings, abnormally reduced in the acute phase, improved and normalized one week after injury. The most striking result of this study is that the changes in fast axoplasmic transport do not parallel the morphological and neurophysiological changes occuring after one week from injury.

In our model, morphological evidence of regeneration both in acute and chronic phases was not achieved [2]. Although there is no firm evidence for or against the hypothesis that modifications in fast transport regulate nerve regeneration [4], an increase of rapid axoplasmic transport delivering materials from the cell body to the surface of sprouting neurons has been hypotetized [6]. The concept that CNS neurons do not regenerate has been recently denied and the presence of persistent regeneration of rat optic nerve after cold injury has been demonstrated [7]. On the other hand, the changes in the fast transport proteins occurring during post-axotomy regeneration of peripheral nerve or during maturation of visual system in mammalians ("growth associated proteins"), have not been seen in injured rabbit optic nerve axons [4].

Results of our prevoius and present research can lead to the following considerations. The active and persistently increase of transport one week after injury suggest that the changes in fast axoplasmic transport support the reparative processes in those axons which were lesioned in continuity and not axomized.

REFERENCES

1. Gennarelli T.A., Thibault L.E.,Tipperman R., Tomei G., Sergot R.,Brown M., Maxwell W.L., Graham D.I.,Adams J.H., Irvine A.,Gennarelli L.M.,Duhaime A.C., Boock R., Greenberg J. (1989) - J.Neurosurg , 71:244-253

2.Tomei G.,Spagnoli D.,Ducati A.,Landi A., Villani R.,Fumagalli G.,Sala C.,Gennarelli T.A. (1990) - Acta Neurophatol 80:506-513

3.Baitinger C.,Levine J.,Lorenz T.,Simon C.,Skene P.,Willard M. (1982) - In:Axolpasmic transport. Weiss D.G. (Ed),Springer-Verlag, pp 110-120

4. Bisby M.A. (1982) - In: Axoplasmic transport in physiology and pathology.- Weiss D.G. and Gorio A.(Eds)-Springer Verlag, pp 70-76

5. Sjostrand J.,Graham McLean W.,Rydevik B. (1982)- In: Axoplasmic transport in physiology and pathology.- Weiss D.G. and Gorio A.(Eds)-Springer Verlag, pp 140-145

6.Pfenninger K.H. (1982)- In: Axoplasmic transport in physiology and pathology.- Weiss D.G. and Gorio A.(Eds)-Springer Verlag, pp 52-61

7. Marakami M.,Ide C.,Kanaya H. (1989) - J Neurosurg, 71:254-265

Physiological Roles of Neurotrophic Factors in Brain Injury

MUTSUO FUJISAWA[1], TOSHIFUMI ITANO[2], OSAMU MIYAMOTO[2], YOSHITAKA YAMAMOTO[3], OSAMU HATASE[2], and SEIGO NAGAO[1]

[1]Department of Neurological Surgery, [2]Department of Physiology, and [3]Department of Neuropsychiatry, Kagawa Medical School, Kagawa, 761-07 Japan

SUMMARY

Basic fibroblast growth factor (bFGF) and nerve growth factor (NGF) were administered into the cerebral cortex of rat brain following unilateral fimbria fornix transection. Both bFGF and NGF stimulated the sprouting of acetylcholinesterase (AChE) positive fibers in the lesioned side hippocampus. Furthermore, a small number of AChE-positive fibers were regenerated in rats with making only cavity. In the b-FGF treated rats, the diameters of AChE-positive fibers were significantly thicker as compared with the NGF treated rats. The regeneration pattern of cholinergic fibers was similar to that in rats by the formation of cavity with only vehicle. These results suggest that b-FGF may affect cholinergic neurons by different mechanisms as compared with NGF.

KEY WORDS: bFGF, NGF, Regeneration, Acetylcholinesterase positive fibers, Hippocampus

INTRODUCTION

Neurotrophic factors (NTFs) may play important roles in the nervous system [1,2]. Nerve growth factor (NGF), which was originally found as a neurite-promoting factor for peripheral sensory and sympathetic neuron [3,4], has recently been revealed to be produced and be functioning as a NTF in the CNS [5]. In the normal brain, NGF synthesized in the target neurons are retrogradely transported to the NGF sensitive neurons and act as a maturation and maintenance factor [6,7]. Basic fibroblast growth factor (bFGF), which was originally purified from pituitary gland as potent mitogen for fibroblast [8], also has trophic effect on neurons in vivo and in vitro [9,10]. For example, bFGF promotes survival of dissociated hippocampal neurons [11] and prevents death of fimbria-fornix lesioned cholinergic neurons in vivo [12]. However there is no direct evidence that bFGF act on neurons directly after brain injury. In the present study, we have examined the effect of NGF and b-FGF on the regeneration of cholinergic fibers in hippocampus after fimbria-fornix transection.

MATERIALS AND METHODS

Young adult female Sprague-Dawley rats weighing between 220-250g at the beginning of the experiment were used. The animals were anesthetized with ether and pentobarbital, and placed in a stereotaxic apparatus. They received unilateral transection of the right fimbria-fornix (FF-lesion) by aspiration through the medial parietal cortex and corpus callosum, 1-2mm posterior to bregma. This procedure transects cholinergic afferent reaching the hippocampus via the two dorsal routes though the cingulate bundle and the fimbria fornix. Sterile pieces of gel form (4x4x6mm) were soaked in $25\mu l$ of Dulbecco's modified Eagle's medium(DMEM) with or without the addition of the following additives:1) $20\mu g$ of NGF from mouse submaxillary gland and 2) $12.5\mu g$ of bFGF from bovine brain. A piece of gel form was placed into a cavity made by aspiration in the right parietal cortex. Four weeks after fimbria fornix transection, these animals received transcardial perfusion of 0.9% saline followed by ice cold buffered 4% paraformaldehyde(PH7.4) under barbiturate anesthesia. The brains were removed and post fixed at 4°c in the fixative for 4h, and then immersed in 30% sucrose at 4°c until they sank. Hippocampal areas were serially sectioned in the coronal planes at 50μm thickness. These sections were collected for acetylcholinesterase(AChE) staining based on the thiocholine methods, using ethoproprazine as the inhibitor of non specific esterases and with 0.25% silver nitrate to enhance the sulfide reaction product. Counter-staining was lightly done with Cresyl Violet. The diameter of AChE-positive fibers in hippocampus was measured by image analysis system-IBAS at magnification x1000. The measurement of fiber diameter in the hippocampus was done on two sections per animal at location of 3.3mm and 5.3mm caudal to Bregma (n=5, per group).

RESULTS

In FF-lesion rat, complete loss of AChE-positive fibers in the hippocampus of lesion side was seen (Fig. 1A and B) 4 weeks after unilateral fimbria fornix transection. However, exogenous NGF or bFGF treatment stimulated the sprouting of AChE-positive fibers in hippocampus (Fig. 2C, D, E and F). A small number of AChE-positive fibers were regenerated even in the DMEM treated rats. (Fig. 2A and B). Furthermore, in the bFGF treated rat (Fig. 2E and F), some AChE-positive fibers showed a thicker and knottier appearance as compared with the other groups . AChE-positive fibers were not regenerated in the hippocampus in the case of administrating a gel foam with anti NGF antibody into the cavity following FF lesion (data not shown). Fig. 3 shows the diameter of AChE-positive fibers in the hippocampus 4 weeks after FF lesion. As indicated in the figure, the diameter of AChE-positive fibers in bFGF treated rats was significantly thicker as compared with the other groups. There were no significant differences between DMEM and NGF treated group.

DISCUSSION

Fimbria-fornix transection showed complete loss of AChE-positive fibers in lesioned side hippocampus. Exogenous administration of NTFs stimulated the sprouting of AChE-positive fibers in denervated hippocampus. However, it is not clear where cholinergic fibers regenerate from. There are three separate routes via which cholinergic afferents reach to the hippocampus: a supracallosal pathway, a subcallosal pathway, and a ventral pathway [13,14]. In the present study, the two dorsal pathways were transected, but the ventral pathway was intact. There is a possibility that AChE-positive fibers in dorsal hippocampus

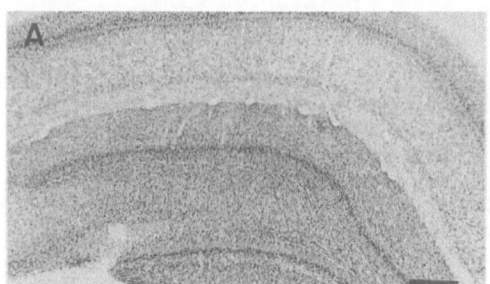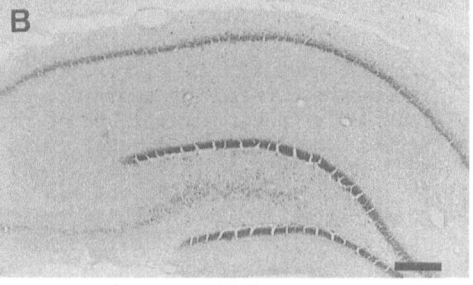

Fig.1 AChE-positive fibers in the hippocampus 4 weeks after unilateral fimbria-fornix transection (FF lesion). A: normal side, and B: lesion side. complete loss of AChE-positive fibers was seen. Scale bar=250μm

regenerate through ventral pathway. We can not neglect the possibility that sprouting of cholinergic fibers generate from contralateral hippocampus through the commisures. Some amount of fibers were regenerated in the hippocampus of DMEM treated rats. There were no significant differences of the diameters of regenerating fibers between DMEM treated group and NGF treated group. These results suggest that NGF may function as one of intrinsic neurotrophic factors after brain injury. Yoshida et al. reported that FGFs (both acidic and basic)

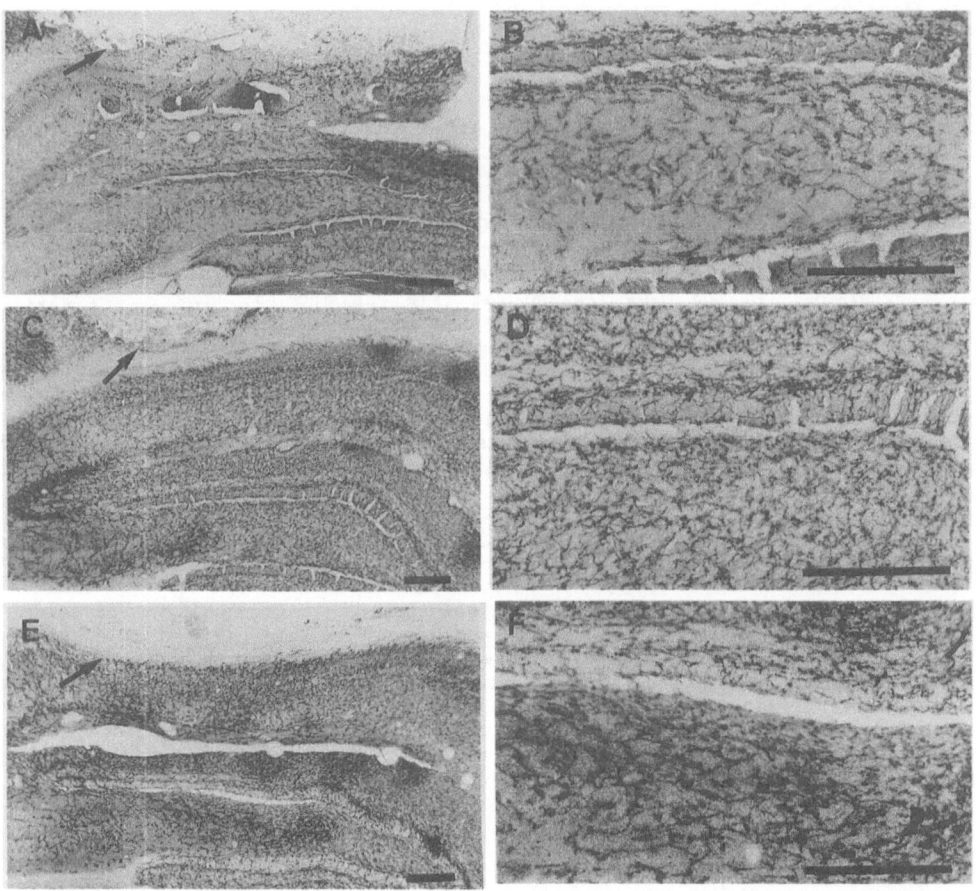

Fig. 2 AChE-positive fibers in the hippocampus after FF lesion and implantation of gel foam with following additives, A,B: DMEM only (control). C,D: NGF. E,F: b-FGF. A,C,D: low power micrographs of the hippocampus. B,D,F: higher magnification of CA4 and dentate gyrus. A small number of AChE-positive fibers regenerated even in the case of DMEM only treatment, and the regeneration pattern of AChE-positive fibers in the b-FGF treated rat was different from the other groups. The arrow indicates the cavity in which the gel foam was implanted. Scale bar = 0.25μ m

might stimulate proliferation of and NGF secretion by astrocytes and act as an autocrine growth factor in the case of brain damage [15]. In our data, however , not only thin fibers but also thick fibers were regenerated in b-FGF treated group, while NGF and DMEM regenerated only thin fibers. The diameters of AChE-positive fibers in b-FGF group were significantly thicker as compared with the other groups. These results suggest that b-FGF may act on cholinergic neurons directly and stimulate NGF secretion by astrocytes. These observations open the possibility that exogenous administration of NTFs must be used for therapy of the brain injury.

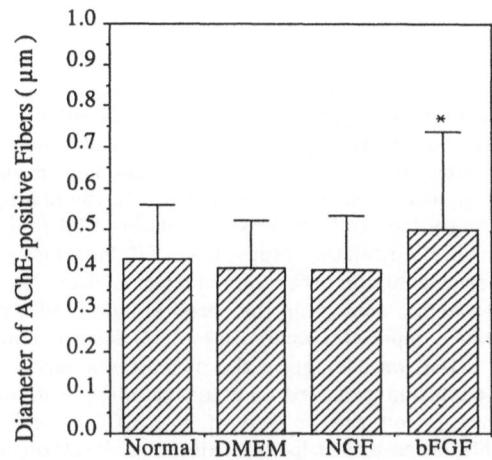

Fig. 3 The diameters of AChE-positive fibers in the hippocampus 4 weeks after FF lesion are shown in this figure. X-axis represents the diameters in micrometers (μm) and Y-axis represents the total fibers (%). * $P < 0.001$.

REFERENCES

1. Cattaneo E, Mckay R (1990) Nature 347: 762-765
2. Walicke P, Cowan WM, Ueno N, Baird A, Guillemin R (1986) Proc Natl Acad Sci USA 83: 3012-3016
3. Bueker ED, (1948) Anat Rec 102: 369-390
4. Levi-Montalcini R, Meyer H, Hamberger V (1954) Cancer Res 14: 49-57
5. Korsching S, Auburger G, Heumann R, Scott J, Thoenen H (1985) EMBO J 4: 1389-1393
6. Hatanaka H, Tsukui H, Nihonmatsu I (1988) Brain Res 467: 85-95
7. Johnson EM, Taniuchi M, Clark B, Springer JE, Koh S, Tayrien MW, Loy R (1987) J Neurosci 7: 923-929
8. Gospodarowicz D, Jones KL, Sato G (1974) Proc Natl Acad Sci USA 71: 2295-2299
9. Morrison RS, Sharma A, de Vellis J, Bradshaw RA (1986) Proc Natl Acad Sci USA 83: 7537-7541
10. Otto D, Frotcher M, Unsicker K (1989) J Neurosci Res 22: 83-91
11. Walicke P, Cowan WM, Ueno N, Baird A, Guillemin (1986) Proc Natl Acad Sci USA 83: 3012-3016
12. Anderson KJ, Dam D, Lee S, Cotman CW (1988) Nature 332: 361-361
13. Gage FH, Bjöklund A, Stenevi U (1983) Brain Res 268: 27-37
14. Gage FH, Bjöklund A, Stenevi U, Dunnett SB (1983) Brain Res 268: 39-47
15. Yoshida K, Gage FH (1991) Brain Res 538: 118-126

Effect of the Kappa Agonist CI-977 on Ischaemic Brain Damage and Cerebral Blood Flow After Middle Cerebral Artery Occlusion in the Rat

Kazuhiro Kusumoto[1], Kenneth B. Mackay[2], James McCulloch[2], David I. Graham[2], and Tetsuhiko Asakura[1]

[1]Department of Neurosurgery, University of Kagoshima, Kagoshima, Japan, and [2]Wellcome Surgical Institute, University of Glasgow, Glasgow G61 1QH, Scotland, UK

SUMMARY

The effects of the kappa opioid receptor agonist CI-977 upon the volume of ischaemic brain damage (defined with quantitative neuropathology) and local cerebral blood flow (CBF) (defined with [^{14}C]iodoantipyrine autoradiography) after permanent middle cerebral artery (MCA) occlusion have been examined in halothane-anaesthetised rats. In the neuropathological study, CI-977 (0.3mg/kg s.c.) or vehicle (saline, 1ml/kg) was administered 30 min before and 30 min after MCA occlusion. In the cerebral circulatory study, CI-977 (0.3mg/kg s.c.) was given 30 min pre-occlusion only, and CBF measured 30 min after the induction of ischaemia. Treatment with CI-977 reduced the volume of ischaemic damage in the cerebral hemisphere and cerebral cortex (by 27% and 32% respectively when compared to controls; P<0.05) despite a marked and sustained hypotension, with only minimal effect on damage in the caudate nucleus. The administration of CI-977 30 min prior to MCA occlusion produced no effect on either the level of local CBF in any of the 24 regions examined or on the volume of low CBF determined by frequency distribution analysis in the hemispheres either ipsilaterally or contralaterally to the occluded MCA. These results suggest the observed anti-ischaemic effects of CI-977 in this model cannot be attributed to improvement of blood flow to the hypoperfused cerebral tissue.

KEY WORDS: Focal cerebral ischaemia; Kappa agonist; Neuroprotection; Infarction.

INTRODUCTION

Agonists at the kappa opioid receptor subtype have been shown to ameliorate ischaemic neuronal degeneration in animal models of global and focal cerebral ischaemia [1,2,3]. A precise mechanistic basis for the neuroprotective effects displayed by kappa agonists is presently unknown. However, although kappa agonists may presynaptically attenuate excitotoxic mechanisms [4], it has been the ability of such drugs to reduce cerebral oedema and secondary neuronal damage via a drug-induced water diuresis which has attracted greatest speculation with respect to mechanism of action [3]. Thus, in the present study we have investigated the ability of a highly selective kappa agonist CI-977 [5] to reduce the volume of ischaemic brain damage in a rat model of focal ischaemia, in which key physiological variables (blood pressure, rectal temperature etc.) which are though to influence lesion size, were assessed throughout, and to establish whether cerebral circulatory effects contribute to, or confound, the neuroprotective effects of kappa agonists.

MATERIALS AND METHODS

Surgical Preparation

The investigations were carried out in 29 adult male Sprague Dawley rats weighing between 352 and 443g. The animals were anaesthetised initially with 2%, and thereafter ventilated mechanically with a nitrous oxide-oxygen mixture (70%:30%) containing 0.5 to 1% halothane. A tracheostomy was performed and polyethylene catheters inserted into both femoral arteries and one femoral vein to allow the continuous monitoring of mean arterial blood pressure (MABP), repeated sampling of arterial blood and administration of radioactive tracer. Body temperature was monitored by a rectal thermometer, and the animals maintained normothermic via a heating blanket controlled by the thermometer. The stroke volume of the ventilator was adjusted to maintain arterial carbon dioxide at approximately 37mmHg. Adequate oxygenation (P_aO_2 >100mmHg) was maintained throughout. The left MCA in each animal was then permanently occluded as described previously [1].

CI-977 and Infarction Volume

CI-977 (0.3mg/kg) or vehicle (saline, 1ml/kg) were given as subcutaneous injections 30 min before and 30 min after occlusion of the MCA. Four hours after the induction of ischaemia, the animals (n=14) were sacrificed by transcardiac perfusion fixation with 40% formaldehyde, glacial acetic acid and absolute methanol (FAM 1:1:8 v/v/v), and the brains processed histologically for evaluation of ischaemic lesion volume as previously described [6].

CI-977 and Local CBF

CI-977 (0.3mg/kg) or vehicle (saline, 1ml/kg) were given as a single subcutaneous injection 30 min before MCA occlusion. Local CBF was assessed 30 min after the induction of ischaemia using the [^{14}C]iodoantipyrine quantitative autoradiographic technique described by Sakurada and colleagues [7]. The resultant autoradiograms were then analysed quantitatively using two densitometric strategies described previously (for full methodological details see [8]).

RESULTS

CI-977 and Infarction Volume

The administration of CI-977 (0.3mg/kg) induced a marked and sustained hypotension. Five min after the pre-occlusion injection, MABP was reduced to approximately 70% of control levels (control: 93 ± 5mmHg; CI-977: 64 ± 3mmHg, P<0.001). Post-occlusion, marked hypotension persisted throughout the experimental period, with the second injection of CI-977 producing no further reduction. The administration of the vehicle did not alter MABP. There were no differences between the two groups with respect to respiratory blood gas status or rectal temperature, but CI-977 induced a 10% reduction in arterial plasma glucose in the post-occlusion period. Pre- and post-occlusion administration with CI-977 reduced the volume of ischaemic brain damage in the cerebral hemisphere and cerebral cortex (reduced by 27% and 32% respectively which compared to controls; P<0.05; Fig. 1). The volume of ischaemic damage in the caudate nucleus was minimally influenced by treatment with CI-977 (Fig. 1).

In the hemispheres ipsilateral and contralateral to the occluded MCA, the administration of CI-977 30 min prior to the occlusion produced no marked effects in the level of CBF in any of the 24 neuroanatomically defined regions analysed (e.g. caudate nucleus and sensory motor cortex; Fig. 2). Similarly, cumulative frequency distribution analysis reveals that CI-977 has no major effect on the volume of cerebral blood flow in either the ischaemic or the non-ischaemic hemisphere e.g. control: $118 \pm 20mm^3$; CI-977: $92 \pm 14mm^3$ of the ipsilateral hemisphere had a cumulative volume of CBF <25ml/100g/min.

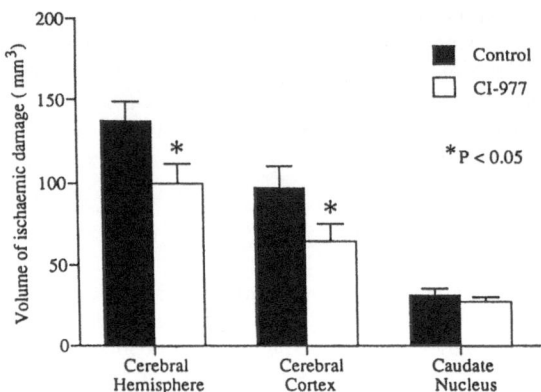

Fig. 1   Effect of CI-977 upon the volume of ischaemic brain damage after permanent MCA occlusion. Data are mean ± SEM.

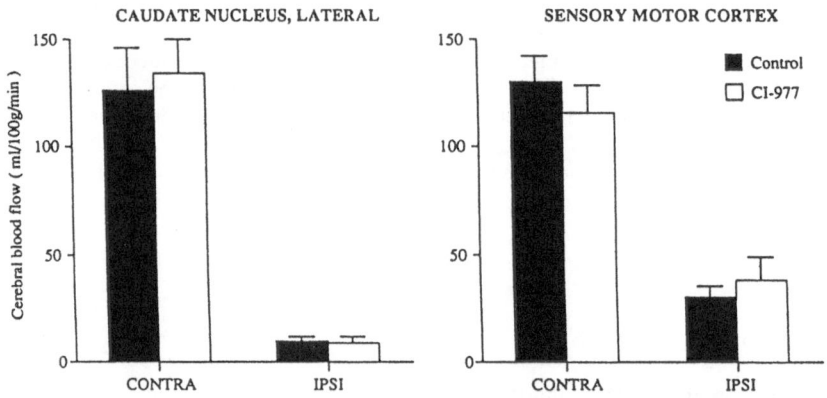

Fig. 2   Effect of CI-977 on local CBF 30 min after permanent MCA occlusion. CI-977 has no effect on CBF either with the contralateral areas or on the low flows in the ipsilateral regions. Data are mean ± SEM.

DISCUSSION

These experiments add to the growing evidence that systemic administration of a kappa opioid agonist can ameliorate the consequences of cerebral ischaemia [1,2,3]. The present study provides two important features into a possible mechanistic basis underlying such an effect. First, the reductions in the amount of ischaemic brain damage which CI-977 effected cannot be attributed to alterations in critical systemic variables (e.g. core temperature, MABP, blood gas status) which were regulated or monitored throughout the post-ischaemic period. Second, CI-977 has minimal effects on CBF, indicating that effects of the drug on cerebral tissue perfusion are unlikely to contribute to its neuroprotective effects in this model.

The neuroprotective effect of kappa agonists is commonly attributed to a reduction in cerebral oedema [3]. However, comparison of the potency of CI-977 as a diuretic [5] and a neuroprotective agent in the rat [1], indicate that at the dose producing maximum diuresis, CI-977 has no significant effect on the volume of infarction following MCA occlusion. Indeed, in the gerbil model of global ischaemia, CI-977 is neuroprotective despite the absence of diuresis [2]. Furthermore, CI-977 has been shown to reduce the volume of brain swelling precisely in parallel with the volume of infarction [1], suggesting no primary reduction of swelling relative to infarction.

CI-977 may modulate the neurotoxic effects of glutamate by presynaptically attenuating its release. *In vitro* studies suggest that kappa agonists inhibit the evoked release of glutamate from rat cortical slices [4] and guinea-pig hippocampal mossy fibre synaptosomes [9], putatively by closing N-type Ca^{2+} channels [10] or enhancing Ca^{2+} extrusion [11]. Thus, kappa agonists may be neuroprotective by reducing the Ca^{2+}-dependent component of glutamate released following an ischaemic episode.

In conclusion, these results indicate that CI-977 reduces ischaemic brain damage in a model of focal ischaemia, in the absence of any alterations in cerebral circulatory effects.

REFERENCES

1. Kusumoto K, Mackay KB, McCulloch J (1992) The effect of the kappa-opioid receptor agonist CI-977 in a rat model of focal cerebral ischaemia. Brain Research, 576:147-151.
2. Hayward NJ, McKnight AT, Woodruff GN (1992) The neuroprotective action of k-opioid agonists in the gerbil. Mol Neuropharmacol (in press).
3. Silvia RC, Slizgi GR, Ludens JH, Tang AH (1987) Protection from ischemia-induced cerebral edema in the rat by U-50488H, a kappa opioid receptor agonist. Brain Research 403:52-57.
4. Lambert PD, Woodruff GN, Hughes J, Hunter JC (1991) Inhibition of L-glutamate release: A possible mechanism of action for the neuroprotective effects of the k-selective agonist CI-977. Mol Neuropharmacol 1:77-82.
5. Hunter JC, Leighton GE, Meecham KG, Boyle SJ, Horwell DC, Rees DC, Hughes J (1990) CI-977, a novel and selective agonist for the k-opioid receptor. Br J Pharmacol 101:183-189.
6. Osborne KA, Shigeno T, Balarsky A-M, Ford I, McCulloch J, Teasdale GM, Graham DI (1987) Quantitative assessment of early brain damage in a rat model of focal cerebral ischaemia. J Neurol Neurosurg Psychiat 50:402-410.
7. Sakurada O, Kennedy C, Jehle J, Brown JD, Carbin GL, Sokoloff L (1978) Measurement of local cerebral blood flow with iodo[^{14}C]antipyrine. Am J Physiol 234:H59-H66.
8. Gotoh O, Mohamed AA, McCulloch J, Graham DI, Harper AM, Teasdale GM (1986) Nimodipine and the haemodynamic and histopathological consequences of middle cerebral artery occlusion in the rat. J Cereb Blood Flow Metab 6:321-331.
9. Gannon RL, Terrian DM (1991) U-50,488H inhibits dynorphin and glutamate release from guinea pig hippocampal mossy fiber terminals. Brain Research 548:242-247.
10. Xiang J-Z, Adamson P, Brammer MJ, Campbell IC (1990) The k-opiate agonist U50488H decreases the entry of ^{45}Ca into rat cortical synaptosomes by inhibiting N- but not L-type calcium channels. Neuropharmacol 29:439-444.
11. Olson KG, Welch SP (1991) The effects of dynorphin (1-13) and U50,488H on free intracellular calcium in guinea pig cerebellar synaptosomes. Life Sci 481:575-581.

Roles of Free Radicals in the Self-Propagating Injury Within Injured Spinal Cord Tissue

Nariyuki Hayashi[1], Joseph More[2], Richard Bunge[2], and Barth A. Green[2]

[1]Nihon University Critical & Emergency Center, Itabashi-ku, Tokyo, 173 Japan, and [2]Department of Neurological Surgery, University of Miami, Miami FL. 33136, USA

SUMMARY

Two patterns of sequential changes in the quantitative distribution of superoxide anion free radicals in spinal cord injury were demonstrated in relation to further expansion of the lesions, changes in the tissue ATP, NADH, pH, and free radical scavengers. Following spinal cord injury, the free radical scavenger, α-tocopherol was consumed until at 2 hours after injury. At this early stage, the loss of tissue ATP and development of tissue acidosis were limited to the small directly injured area. The initial role of free radicals in the self-propagating tissue damage occurring around the lesions was first evident at 2 hours and continued with 8-16 hours after injury. The progressive loss of tissue ATP and development of tissue acidosis were closely correlated increasing levels of superoxide anion radicals. However, the late activated free radical reactions as seen at 24-72 hours, which were maximal at 48 hours after injury, appeared to be involved in the development of spinal cord edema. These late free radical reactions were correlated with increasing amounts of neutrophils in the injured cord.

KEY WORDS: spinal cord injury, free radical, superoxide anion, free radical scavenger, edema

INTRODUCTION

The major issue for successful treatment of spinal cord injury is the prevention of secondary tissue damage in the injured tissue. Recent studies have been focused on free radical reactions in the injured tissue as a possible major cause of secondary tissue damage [1,4]. In fact high-dosage free radical scavenger therapy at the acute stage has produced good results. However, the precise location, characteristics and magnitude of the free radical-induced changes in the injured tissue, and the reason why membrane-acting free radical scavengers are of limited useful at the acute stage are not yet known with certainly. We recently developed a new technique for the simultaneous mapping of the distribution of superoxide anion radicals, energy metabolism, tissue pH, and vascular permeability in frozen tissue sections [2,3]. In this paper, we present data concerning sequential changes in the localized increases of free radicals in injured spinal cord tissue, and discuss their role in the self-propagation mechanism for the development of secondary tissue damage.

MATERIALS AND METHODS

Animal preparation

Thirty-nine male Sprague Dawley rats weighing 250-300 g were fasted overnight but given free access to water. Anesthesia was begun with 12 mg/kg pentobarbital sodium (I.P.) and 60 mg/kg ketamine (I.M.). Subsequently, 2 mg/kg pentobarbital sodium was injected regularly and intravenously in order to maintain the anesthesia. The animals were placed in stereotaxic frames and were mounted on an Aquamatic K module heating pad (German Rupp Industries, Ont.). The body temperature was measured rectally and maintained at $37.0 \pm 0.5°C$.

Spinal cord injury was investigated as follows. To evaluated the metabolic changes, laminectomy was performed between Th 5 and Th9. Irreversible spinal cord injury was determined at its center, i.e., at Th 7, by the weight drop method with 100 gcf, employing a modification of Allen's procedure.

The experimental animals were divided into a non-injured group and an injured group.

Group I (n=9). After recording a stable baseline for the systemic arterial blood pressure and blood gases, a sham operation was performed. The localized distribution of free radicals was studied in the non-injured spinal cord tissue.

Group II (n=30). Following spinal cord injury, the sequential changes in the quantitative distribution of superoxide anions, changes in tissue ATP, NAD/NADH redox state, tissue pH were studied until 72 hours after injury. At the acute stage, the changes in the free radical scavenge, α-tocopherol in the lesions were measured by high-performance liquid chromatography method in order to assess the protective mechanism against to tissue damage by free radical anions.

Sampling techniques

At the end of each experiment, the spinal cord was frozen in situ by pouring liquid nitrogen via a funnel onto the spinal vertebral column. The spinal cord tissue was chiseled out during irrigation with liquid nitrogen, and the tissue was kept at -80°C until being subjected to in vitro experiments. The tissues were sliced at a thickness of 15 μm thickness with cryostats for mapping of the superoxide anions, tissue ATP with analysis of the NADH and tissue pH. For measurement of the α-tocopherol in the lesions, spinal cord tissue was removed as a cylinder which included the lesion and some parts of the non- injured tissue as a heterogeneous sample.

Technique for mapping superoxide free radicals

The distribution of superoxide anions in the CNS was determined, the basis of on the 380-nm chemiluminescence of 2-methyl-6-phenyl-3,7-dihydroimidazo[1,2a]pyrazin-3-one (CLA-phenyl, A5307, Tokyo Kasei Kogyo Co., Ltd., Tokyo, Japan), which reacts with superoxide anions.

Each 15-μm sliced frozen tissue section was mounted on a millipore filter paper (CA 250/0, Schleicher & Schuell Co., Germany) saturated with CLA-phenyl solution in the millipore holes.

The frozen tissue section was first melted, and was then trapped in the filter pores at room temperature. Superoxide-CLA-phenyl photochemical reactions occurred immediately within the 1-μm diameter pores of the millipore filter paper. The paper was pasted on the thin cover glass and then placed directly onto ASA-20000 Polaroid film in a dark room. The light emitted by the superoxide-CLA-phenyl photochemical reactions in the pores of the filter paper was recorded on the Polaroid film as picture produced by exactly 2 minutes of exposure.The densities of superoxide anion radicals on the Polaroid films were determined by scanning with a densitometer. The localized changes in superoxide free radical density in the ischemic lesions are presented as percent (%) changes from the normal brain tissue density for the same sites [2,3].

RESULTS

1. Non-injured spinal cord tissue : group I

Normal brain tissue exhibited very low intensity CLA-chemiluminescence by superoxide free radicals. Topical applications of superoxide dismutase (10 units) on sampling inhibited the CLA-chemiluminescence.The α-tocopherol in the spinal cord tissue could be not separated for the gray and white matter without altering the metabolism which still remained, so we were only able to obtain mean values for the combination of gray and white matter. These were 11.7 ± 42 μg/g and 12.6 ± 58 μg /g, respectively.

2. Spinal cord injury; group II

Macroscopic examinations revealed the immediate occurrence of small hemorrhages in the gray matter as well as in the interface zone between the gray and white matter. Such vascular damage began to become magnified at 4-8 hours after the spinal cord injury. Hematomyelia with spinal cord edema was observed most severely at 48 hours after injury.

a. Localized changes of tissue ATP and pH: Energy crisis developed immediately at the lesion sites in the gray matter and dorsal white matter. These metabolic changes began to become magnified and developed more widely distributed from 2 hours after injury. At the end of 4 hours after injury, areas with loss of tissue ATP extended to 2-3 vertebral cord segments from the directly injured site towards the caudal and cranial directions.

The changes in tissue pH revealed a similar pattern to the loss of tissue ATP in the injured cord Severe tissue acidosis developed and extended into the perifocal area from 2 hours after injury. The necrotic tissue pH showed a maximum at 6.6.

b. Changes of free radical scavengers at the acute stage: The α-tocopherol level was not markedly changed until 1hour after injury, being 12.2±0.36 μg/g at 5-30 minutes and 11.4± 1.60 μg/g at 1 hour,or 96% and 90% of the control value, respectively. However, at 2 hours after injury, the α-tocopherol in the injured cord rapidly declined by 47%, to a level of 6.6 ± 1.42 μg/g. Thereafter, the α-tocopherol values continued to decline to 6.3± 0.82 μg/g at 3 hours and 6.4 ±1.01 μg/g at 4 hours without recovery .

c. Localized changes of free radicals in the injured spinal cord tissue: The sequential changes of superoxide anion free radicals in the injured cord demonstrated two different patterns. Superoxide free radicals were evidently not produced immediately in the injured tissue except in the white matter. The initial free radical reaction in the gray matter appeared at 2-3 hours after injury. Disturbance of energy metabolism (loss of tissue ATP) was closely correlated with increasing amounts of superoxide anions at 2 hours after injury. This relationship is illustrated in Fig.1. The critical level of free radicals which led to ATP crisis was 2.5 times higher than the normal values. A second rebounding increase of superoxide anions in the injured tissue was observed after 24 hours. Such free radical reactions were prolonged for more than 72 hours and were most severe at 48 hours after injury. The distribution patters of free radicals were correlated with the areas of loss of tissue ATP. Quantitative two-dimensional analysis of the concentration of superoxide free radicals in the lesions at 48 hours after injury, revealed a specific magnified pattern of free radicals and propagation around the lesions as shown in longitudinal spinal cord sections (Fig.2). The highest density of superoxide anions was located at the center of each lesion in most cases. These specific distribution pattern of superoxide anions in injured cord were closely correlated with amount of infiltration of neutrophils and macrophagus which were observed in pathological studies. Tissue necrosis and multiple hemorrhages were involving in the lesions.

DISCUSSION

Recent studies have demonstrated that oxygen free radicals involving superoxide anions, and hydroxy radicals, can facilitate damage of endotherial and parenchymal cell membranes by disrupting their structure and functions [4]. This process leads to puncture and damage to the enzymatic regulation of ion transport system. Subsequently, vasogenic edema, cytotoxic edema and neutrophils aggregation may cause ischemic lesions to expand further [1,4]. Despite this conceptual framework, previous studies have failed to elucidate the precise location, characteristics, and magnitude of free radical-induced alterations of injured tissue in vivo. The present experiments revealed specific quantitative distribution patterns of superoxide free radicals in relation to changes of the tissue ATP, NADH, pH, and the free radical scavengers, α-tocopherol, and further expansion of spinal cord injury [3].

The initial magnification of the spinal cord tissue damage by free radical reactions was protected by the consumption of free radical scavengers in the cord until 2 hours after injury. At this early stage, loss of tissue ATP and development of tissue acidosis were in fact limited to the directly injured small tissue area.

The initial role of free radicals in the self-propagating tissue damage occurring around the lesions could thus first be evident at 2 hours after injury. The distribution of superoxide free radicals in the injured tissue was severe in the gray matter and watershed zone of the centrifugal and centripetal spinal cord feeding arteries, as compared to that in the white matter. This localized increase of superoxide anions was closely correlated with a progressive loss of tissue ATP and the development of tissue acidosis. Previous studies have demonstrated that superoxide anion itself represents a low toxic radical. However, when it becomes changed into the form of hydroxy radicals by proton activation in tissue acidosis, the hydroxy radicals induce severe tissue damage, cell membrane perturbation and endotherial damage with the production of arachdonic acid conversion to prostaglandin synthesis, and the production of lipoxygenase stimulating neutrophils.Such tissue damage mechanisms were demonstrated in the present experiments to start from 2 hours after injury.

A late rebounding increase of superoxide free radicals was observed at 24-72 hours, with a maximum at 48 hours after injury. Such late activated free radical reactions appeared to be involved in the development of spinal cord edema.

Various sources of superoxide anions have been reported in biological systems. These include the oxidization of ubisemiquinone radicals in the respiratory chain, prostaglandin synthesis, conversion from available nucleotides (NADPH), purine degradation with oxidization of xanthine oxidase, conversion of xanthine to urea, and activation of neutrophils. As a possible mechanism for the secondary tissue damage occurring in the area around the lesion focus, progressive production of free radicals from the reperfusion oxygen supply has been suggested.

In the present study, the initial free radical reaction was correlated with consumption of scavengers and production of prostaglandin. These specific cell membrane perturbation mechanisms could be accounted for at short times within 8 hours. However, the fact that the highest density of free radicals was observed at the center of the necrotic tissue at 48 hours after reperfusion and infiltration of neutrophils in the injured tissue, indicated that the sources of free radicals might involve the activation of neutrophils (intravascular generating factors) instead of processes of oxygen metabolic origin such as ubisemiquinone oxidization, conversion from available nucleotides, and degradation of ATP to xanthine. From the clinical standpoint for the treatment of these free radical reactions, cell membrane-acting, free radical scavengers could be available for use when they applied within 8 hours and be most effective within 2 hours. However, neutrophil-induced delayed free radicals, associated with intracellular NADPH-radicals, could not be protected against with cell membrane-acting scavengers. Further studies are need on the regulation of neutrophils.

REFERENCES

1. Chan PH, Schmidley W, Fishman RA, Longer SM (1984) Brain injury, edema, and vascular permeability induced by oxygen-derived free radicals. Neurology 34: 315-320
2. Hayashi N, Tsubokawa T, Watson B, More J, and Green BA (1990) A new mapping study of superoxide free radicals, vascular permeability, and energy metabolism in the central nervous system. Brain Edema VIII 51: 31-33
3. Hayashi N, Prado R, More J, Bunge R, and Green BA. (1991) Regional changes of free radicals in photochemically induced ischemic injury in the central nervous system. Laser in the Life Science 4: 1-7
4. Kontos, H.A., Wei, E.P (1986) Superoxide production in experimental brain injury. J. Neurosurg. 64: 803-807

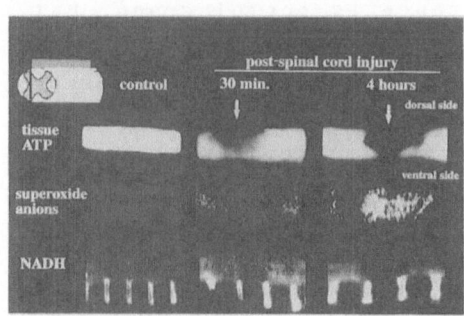

Fig. 1 Changes of tissue ATP, NADH and super-oxide anion radicals in the gray matter after spinal cord injury at the acute stage.

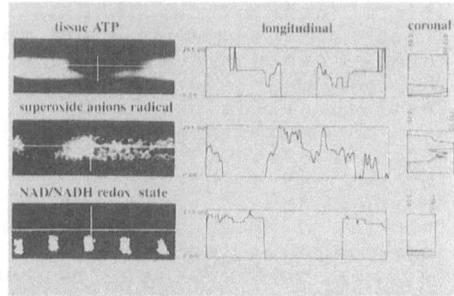

Fig. 2 Delayed increase of superoxide anions radicals at 48 hours after injury. Two-dimenstional analysis of the tissue ATP, superoxide anions, and NADH showed a clear relationship.

Transient Hypotension Induces Remote Neuronal Damage from the Primary Concussion in the Rat

KAZUYA SHIRAISHI, SHIRO KOBAYASHI, MITSUYOSHI SASAKI, SHOZO NAKAZAWA[1], and HIRONOBU ITO[2]

[1]Department of Neurosurgery, and [2]Anatomy, Nippon Medical School, Bunkyo-ku, Tokyo, 113 Japan

Key Words; Concussion, delayed neuronal damage, hypotension, rat, 2-DG

Abstract
    In order to evaluate effects of hypotension in the experimantal concussion model, a conventional fluid percussion method was combined with transient hypotension in the rat. Over the right dorsal cortex, fluid percussion apparatus was located. After the insults(average 4.3 atm.), venous blood was evacuated until the mean blood pressure fell down to sixty mmHg for six minutes. Sixty minutes after the insults, glucose utilization was studied by 14-C-2-Deoxyglucose (2-DG) method. Other rats were sacrificed under general anesthesia by transcardiac perfusion of 4% paraformaldehyde to make Nissl preparations after twenty four, seventy two hours, or seven days of postinsult survival. Although 2-DG of control group(percussion only) showed normal glucose utilization values, that of hypotension loaded group had hypermatabolic lesions at the ipsilateral cortex and hippocampus and hypometabolic lesions at the ipsilateral basal ggl.. The Nissl sections of control group had minor cortical contusion throughout seven days after. Those of hypotension group sacrificed twenty four hours after had the almost same appearance as contol group. But, seventy two hours after, specimens revealed picnotic changes of the ipsilateral cortex and the hippocampus and the depletion of ipsilateral thalamic neurons. Seven days later, these lesions were deteriorated and accompanied by the contralateral cortical neuronal damage. Hypermatabolic lesions in 2-DG might be due to the excessive release of excitatory amino acids(EAA), but the neuronal damage was retarded and revealed three days after the insults, which should be one day after in the middle cerebral artery occlusion ischemic model. And the hypometabolic lesions also revealed delayed type neuronal damage. According to these results, hypotension could induce delayed neuronal injury in the rat, but 2-DG values of early phase did not fully correspond with the lesion in Nissl preparations. The etiology is unknown but this model would contribute to investigation of the delayed damage after traumatic brain injury.

Introduction
    Although the clinical brain injury is usually followed by several kinds of insults; transient hypotension, dyspnea, epilepsy, or shock, we can seldom depict them as ischemic brain damage at the time patients arrive at hospitals. Brain damage

resulting from ischemia seems to add to that inflicted by the primary injury (Graham and Adams) and actually remote neuronal damage, which is distant from the primary injury, usually develops later in multisystem trauma. We designed to study the effects of transient hypotension in mild brain concussion model in the rat.

Material and Methods

Sprague-Dawly male rats, weighing 330-380 gm, were anesthetized with chloral hydrate (350 mg/kg). The left femoral artery and vein were catheterized with PE-50 (Clay & Adams) and body temperature was kept at 37.5C with a heating pad(ATB-1100, Nihon Koden). Over the right dorsal cortex, fluid percussion apparatus was located. The average of the fluid pulse was 4.3 atm. Control group(N=12) had that percussion only. In hypotension loaded group(N=12), after the percussion venous blood was immediately evacuated through the femoral vein until the mean blood pressure fell down to sixty mmHg for six minutes. Then, evacuate blood was heparinized(2U/ml) and transfused gradually to the same rat and the mean blood pressure was maintained around 95-110 mmHg. Thiry minutes later, the arterial blood gas analyses were performed. Sixty minutes after the percussion, three rats of each group were studied about glucose utilization with 2-DG method. Details were described before (Shiraishi et al.). Rats for pathological specimens were given free access to food and water after insults. Twenty four, seventy two hours, and seven days after the percussion, each three rats of both groups were sacrificed under general anesthesia by transcardiac perfusion of 4% paraformaldehyde (0.1M PBS, pH7.2), making Nissl preparations.

Results

All rats survived and did not have any epileptic signs. Values of the arterial blood gas were within normal limits. As to glucose utilization described below.

umolglucose /100g min.	Rt cortex	Lt.cortex	Rt basal ggl.	Rt. Hipc.
control	79.6+10.8	75.2+4.6	65.2+8.8	51.0+6.7
tr. hypo.	102.2+11.0	69.3+5.6	41.4+5.8	88.9+10.5

	Rt.thalmus	Lt.thalamus
control	73.3+6.2	74.4+2.4
tr. hypo.	69.8+3.5	72.5+5.5

In control group, 2-DG values were normal as reported before and the site of percussion was not clear. Transient hypotension loaded group had hypermatabolic changes at the ipsilateral cortex and the hippocampus and hypometabolic one at the ipsilateral basal ggl. Nissl preparations showed minor contusion in the right dorsal cortex in the control group even seven days after. Hypotension group had the same appearance like those of control group in twenty four hours after, though seventy two hours later picnotic changes of neurons developed at the ipsilateral cortex

and the hippocampus. And the thalamic neurons were partially
depleted and extinguished. Seven days after, those changes were
deteriorated and the contralateral cortical neurons revealed picnotic changes.

Discussion
    As to the glucose metabolism it has been reported that glucose
uptake is high in cortex and low in subcortical tissue (Shah and
West) And recently Kawamata et al. have published that diffuse
hypermatabolism develops immediately after the percussion. In
this experiment, control group showed minor contusion in
specimens but could not increase glucose uptake one hour after
the percussion as previously reported(Sunami et al.) Hypotension
group developed diffuse and remote neuronal damage though 2-DG
could not fully reveal early metabolic changes in glucose
utilization. The additional effects of posttraumatic secondary
insult such as ischemia have published(Jenkins, Ishige) and mentioned excitotoxic hypothesis. And NMDA antagonists were also
reported to be able to protect injured cell from cell
death(Tecoma). But the relationship between the early glucose
utilization and pathological changes has not been discussed in
the experimental traumatic model. Shiraishi et al. reported that
excitotoxic cell death following focal ischemia (middle cerebral
occlusion) should be performed in glucose utilization within one
hour after insults. We have not yet finished sequential study for
glucose utilization in this model. Our own preliminary study has
failed to detect definite metabolic changes of glucose in the ipsilateral thalamus and the contralateral cortex. Transsynaptic
degeneration may cause such lesions, but we do not have any data
about it. In conclusion present study suggests that mild concussion followed by transient hypotension could induce delayed type
brain injury, which is not always corresponding with early metabolic changes in glucose. Although etiology is still unknown, we
hope that this model will offer an experimental material for
delayed or secondary brain injury.

References
Graham DI et al. J. Neurological Sciences 39, 213-34, 1978
Shiraishi K et al. J. Cereb. Blood Flow Metab. 9, 765-773, 1989
Shah KR et al. Neurosci. Lett. 40, 287-291, 1983
Kawamata T et al. J Cereb. Blood Flow & Met 12, 12-24, 1992
Sunami K et al. Neurosurg. Rev. 12, 400-411, 1989
Tecoma ES et al. Neuron 2, 1541-1545, 1989
Jenkins LW et al. Brain Res. 477, 211-224, 1989
Ishige N et al. J Neurosurg. 68, 129-36, 1988

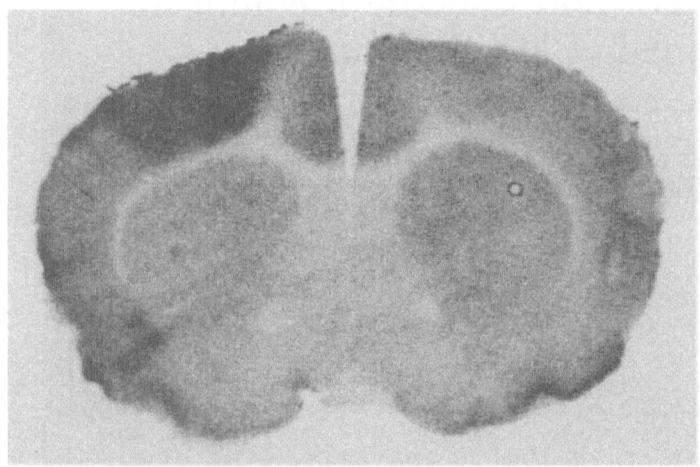

Fig.1 2-DG study
coronal section
at basal ggl.

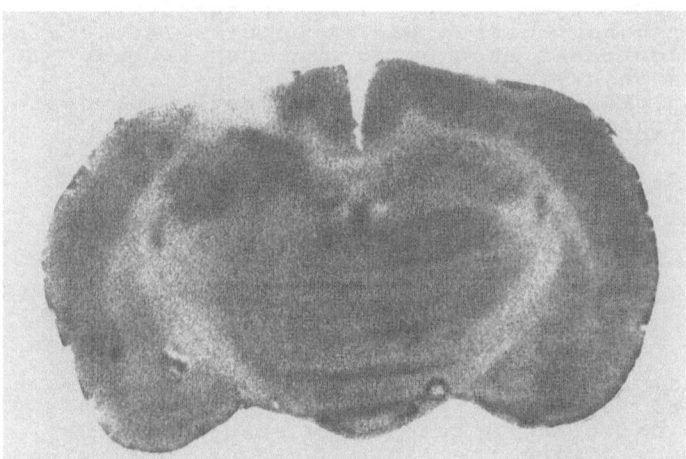

Fig.2 2-DG study
coronal section
at the hippocam-
us and thalamus

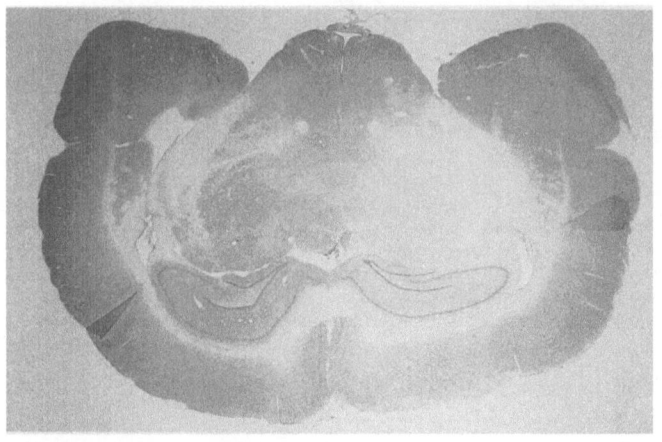

Fig.3 Nissl section
seventy-two hrs.
after insults.
Rt. dorsal cortex
and thalamus,
stained palely

Cerebral Blood Flow and Glucose Metabolism Following Experimental Head Injury

KATSUJI SHIMA[1], YUJI SAITOH[1], HIROSHI NAWASHIRO[1], HIROO CHIGASAKI[1], and ANTHONY MARMAROU[2]

[1]Department of Neurosurgery, National Defense Medical College, Tokorozawa, Saitama, 359 Japan, and
[2]Division of Neurosurgery, Medical College of Virginia, Richmond, Virginia 23298, USA

SUMMARY

Local cerebral blood flow(lCBF) and glucose metabolism were measured with the autoradiographic techniques in rats subjected to concussive closed head injury. Following moderate injury, a varied increase in lCBF occurred in 5 of 23 structures measured at 15 min postinjury. These structures located in the brain stem and diencephalon. These variedly changed lCBF showed a tendency to return to control values by 4 h postinjury. In the severe injury group, lCBF in survivors was decreased(20-40 %) throughout widespread structures. At 40 min postinjury, lCGU was decreased much more than lCBF in many structures. At 4 h postinjury, there was an insignificant recovery of 5-35 % in lCGU in many areas. The results demonstrate that concussive brain injury provokes heterogeneous changes of lCBF and lCGU among many neural structures during the acute stage of the injury with a global trend toward hypometabolism.

KEY WORDS: concussion, cerebral blood flow, glucose utilization, calcium, blood-brain barrier

INTRODUCTION

Only a few experimental studies of local CBF and metabolism in the acute phase of head injury are reported. The objective of the present study was designed to detect the changes in lCBF, lCGU and neuronal damage during the acute phase of concussive brain injury.

MATERIALS AND METHODS

Sixty male Sprague-Dawley rats, each weighing 300 to 450 g, were anesthetized with 1.5-2 % halothane by mask. Femoral artery and vein catheters were inserted, and the animals were partially restrained by a plaster cast around hindquarters. A stainless steel disc(10 mm in diameter) was secured at the vertex for protecting the skull. Soon after discontinuing anesthesia, the animal was placed horizontally on the foam bed. The blunt head injury was delivered by dropping a weight(450 g) from the tubing positioned above the steel helmet. Two levels of the injury were selected by varying the height of the weight drop; moderate injury from 1 m and severe injury from 2 m.

Local cerebral blood flow (lCBF)

Following head injury, the animal was restrained and autoradiographic studies were done as follows. Fifteen min and 4 h after the injury, 100 microcuries/kg of ^{14}C-iodoantipyrine was infused over 30 sec and timed arterial samples were obtained. At 30 sec the rat was decapitated, the brain rapidly removed, frozen and cut into 20 micron-thick sections. LCBF was calculated according to Sakurada et al[1].

Local cerebral glucose utilization (lCGU)

LCGU was measured using the technique designed by Sokoloff et al[2]. The measurement of lCGU was initiated by the intravenous injection of 100 microcuries/kg ^{14}C-2-deoxyglucose(^{14}C-DG). Timed blood samples were obtained for analysis of ^{14}C activity and glucose concentration. The animals were decapitated 40 min and 4 h after trauma, respectively 30 min and 45 min after the injection of ^{14}C-DG. Autoradiographs were prepared in the same manner as for lCBF, and lCGU was calculated using the lumped constant for the normal rat determined by Sokoloff et al[2].

Posttraumatic neuronal damage was determined by [45]Ca autoradiography[3]. Rats subjected to trauma were injected with [45]Ca (100 microcuries/100 g) either 10 min, 1 day, 3 day, 7 day and 10 days after trauma. The [45]Ca was allowed to circulate for 4 h, and the brains were removed and autoradiographed in the same manner as for lCBF.

Traumatic changes of blood-brain barrier(BBB) permeability were assessed by intravenous injection of Evans blue(2 % in saline) at 5 min pre- or post-injury.

RESULTS

The mean arterial blood pressure(MABP) transiently increased by 29 % in moderate injury, 60 % in survivors of severe injury and 77 % in nonsurvivors of severe injury over each baseline value, and returned to baseline value within 30 sec in both levels of injury. MABP in the severe injury group was significantly greater($p < 0.01$) than in the moderate injury group at 2-8 sec postinjury. However, there were no significant differences in MABP, body temperature, hematocrit, blood gases, or blood glucose between both injury groups during the autoradiographic studies.

Subarachnoid hemorrhage around the ventral brain-stem was seen in 38(6/16) % of moderate injury group and in 79(23/29) % of severe injury group. Macroscopic intraparenchymal hemorrhage was not found in any animals of both injury groups. There was no visible extravasation of Evans blue in the brains of all animals measured at 15 min or 4 h post-injury. The abnormal accumulation of [45]Ca was not seen by 72 h after moderate injury and 4 h after severe injury. After 7 days the light accumulation of calcium was seen in the hippocampus.

Compared with mean values of sham-operated control rats (n=3), moderate injury resulted in mean lCBF increases of 44 % in substantia nigra ($p < 0.05$), and 10-15 % in hypothalamus, septal nucleus and pontine gray, while there were decreases of lCBF in many others (Table 1). In moderate injury group, there was a tendency for variedly changed lCBF to return to control values by 4 h after the injury. In severe injury, lCBF was markedly decreased throughout widespread areas, and none of the areas measured showed any increases in lCBF.

At 40 min post-injury, lCGU showed a significant decrease in all structures examined and the percent changes from control values was more than those of lCBF (Table 2). At 4 h post-injury, there was an insignificant recovery of 5-35 % in lCGU in all regions studied excluding hippocampus and mamillary body.

Table 1 Percent changes in lCBF after head injury compared with control values.

Representative Structures	Moderate Injury		Severe Injury	
	15 min posttrauma (n=4)	4 h posttrauma (n=5)	15 min posttrauma (n=6)	4 h posttrauma (n=2)
Frontal Cortex	-27.4 %	- 6.0 %	-29.9 %	-35.6 %
Med. Geniculate Body	-13.5	-23.5	-46.2#	-45.5
Thalamus(Ventral N.)	- 6.3	-31.8*	-31.7	-46.4
Hypothalamus	15.2	-19.1	-35.2#	-29.0
Amygdala	-16.6	-36.5*	-34.2	-35.7
Septal N.	9.7	0.0	- 8.3	-16.9
Hippocampus(Ammon)	-19.1*	-23.3	-29.3	-39.2
Substantia Nigra	44.4*	16.9	-15.7#	-16.2
Pontine Gray	10.0	- 4.9	-23.1#	-34.7

*=p<0.05 vs sham control(n=3); #=p<0.05 vs moderate injury

Table 2 Percent changes in lCGU after head injury compared with control values.

Representative Structures	Moderate Injury	
	40 min posttrauma (n=4)	4 h posttrauma (n=4)
Frontal Cortex	-44.9**	-10.9 %
Med. Geniculate Body	-37.1*	- 8.3
Thalamus(Ventral N.)	-33.8	-25.0*
Hypothalamus	-31.9	5.9
Amygdala	-39.8*	-12.9
Septal N.	- 3.6	18.2
Hippocampus(Ammon)	-37.5	-26.6*
Substantia Nigra	-25.6	2.8
Pontine Gray	-44.3*	-2.5

*=p<0.05, **=p<0.01 vs sham control(n=5)

DISCUSSION

There are many reports as to the relationship between CBF and metabolism following head injury, but the results are inconsistent. In the early posttraumatic period cerebral metabolic rate of oxygen is reported to be reduced associated with an increase in CBF[4] or relatively unchanged[5]. In the present study, it was found that a varied increase in lCBF in the brain stem and diencephalon at 15 min postinjury and an extensive decrease in lCGU at 40 min postinjury. This flow-metabolic uncoupling at the acute phase of brain injury has been also obtained clinically by Obrist et al[6]. They argued that the uncoupling was due to a decrease in cerebral vasomotor tone, which was suggested by impaired CBF autoregulation to blood pressure changes.

Previous studies have demonstrated variable lCGU after experimental head injury. Nakamura et al[7] reported using fluid-contusion model that the lCGU in the lesioned cortex commonly decreased to 70-80 % of the control at 1 h postinjury, then returned to preinjury level by 2 h. However, some animals showed a 150 % increase in lCGU as a result of spreading depression. Kawamata et al[8] utilized a fluid-percussion model and found a remarkable increase(up to 181 %) in glucose uptake at 45 min postinjury. Such an increase in lCGU can be attributed to the changes in blood pressure and BBB immediately postinjury resulted from the administration of 14C-DG at 30 sec preinjury. A basic assumption of the 14C-DG method is that the plasma concentration of glucose and that the rate of glucose consumption are constant throughout the experimental period[2]. On the basis of our studies we conclude that the metabolic changes are heterogeneous, however, there is a global tendency toward hypometabolism with 4 h postinjury. This observation is consistent with the clinical experience.

REFERENCES

1. Sakurada O, Kennedy C, Jehle J, Brown JP, Carbin GL, Sokoloff L (1978) Measurement of local cerebral blood flow with [^{14}C]-iodoantipyrine. Am J Physiol 234:H59-H66
2. Sokoloff L, Reivich M, Kennedy C, DesRosiers MH, Patlak CS, Pettigrew KD, Sakurada O, Shinohara M (1977) The [^{14}C]-deoxyglucose method for the measurement of local cerebral glucose utilization: Theory, procedure, and normal values in the conscious and anesthetized albino rat. J Neurochem 28:897-916
3. Dienel GA (1984) Regional accumulation of calcium in post-ischemic rat brain. J Neurochem 43:913-925
4. Nilsson B, Nordstrom, C-H (1977) Experimetal head injury in the rat. Part 3: Cerebral blood flow and oxygen consumption after concussive impact acceleration. J Neurosurg 47:262-273
5. Unterberg AW, Andersen BJ, Clarke GD, Marmarou A (1988) Cerebral energy metabolism following fluid-percussion brain injury in cats. J Neurosurg 68:594-600
6. Obrist WD, Langfitt TW, Jaggi JL, (1984) Cerebral blood flow and metabolism in comatose patients with acute head injury. Relationship to intracranial hypertension. J neurosurg 61:241-253
7. Nakamura T, Namba H, Sunami K, Kubota M, Ozawa Y, Yamaura A, Makino H (1987) Study of local cerebral glucose utilization in experimental head injury. Neurol Med Chir(Tokyo) 27:396-403
8. Kawamata T, Katayama Y, Hovda DA, Yoshino A, Becker DP (1992) Administration of excitatory amino acid antagonist via microdyalysis attenuates the increase in glucose utilization seen following concussive brain injury. J Cereb Blood Flow Metab 12:12-24

Secondary Damage of the Cerebral Cortex: Blood Flow and Metabolic Studies

Hiroshi K. Inoue, Satoshi Kobayashi, Masaru Nakamura, Satoru Horikoshi, and Chihiro Ohye

Department of Neurosurgery, Gunma University School of Medicine, Maebashi, 371 Japan

SUMMARY

Secondary degeneration is obvious in special sensory systems after destruction of that system's major input. We have reported secondary damage of the cerebrum (hemiatrophy) due to lesions in the basal ganglia. In this study the changes of cerebral blood flow and metabolism were examined quantitatively in order to analyze the relationship between such changes and neuronal damage followed by cerebral hemiatrophy. Five cases with lesions in the basal ganglia (pallidum) were studied by PET scan using O-15 labelled CO2 and O2 and/or F-18 labelled FDG. Five cases with thalamic lesions were also examined as a comparative study. Only one case with the thalamic lesion showed local decrease of oxygen metabolism in the ipsilateral cerebral cortex. All cases with pallidal lesions showed extensive decrease of blood flow and metabolism in the cortex. Compared with the contralateral cortex there was a 20-27% decrease of blood flow , a 10-20% decrease of oxygen metabolic rate, and a 15-32% decrease of glucose metabolic rate. It is concluded that pallidal lesions cause an extensive decrease in blood flow and metabolism of the ipsilateral cerebral cortex and this contributes to neuronal damage as shown by cerebral hemiatrophy. Metabolic depression shown by the ratio of asymmetry (affected side/normal side) may reflect the decreased number of cortical neurons.

KEY WORDS: neuronal damage, cerebral cortex, blood flow, metabolism, hemiatrophy

INTRODUCTION

Secondary damage of neurons after brain insult is well known. Laboratory and clinical studies have revealed the causes to be brain edema, hypoxia, acidosis and excessive release of excitatory neuro-transmitters in the acute phase of injury. However, little information is available concerning prolonged secondary damage in the chronic phase. We have found prolonged changes of cerebral blood flow and metabolism in cases with pallidal lesions. These cases showed cerebral hemiatrophy after several months [1]. In this study the secondary blood flow - metabolic changes in the cerebrum were examined quantitatively using PET·scan in order to analyze how these changes relate to prolonged neuronal damage followed by hemiatrophy.

CLINICAL CASES AND METHODS

Five patients with basal ganglia lesions consisted of 4 men and one woman ranging in age from 15 to 78 years (mean 52.0 years). Clinical diagnoses were primary brain tumors (one germinoma and 4 lymphomas). Four tumors were on the left side and one on the right side. Five patients with thalamic lesions (4 gliomas and one lymphoma) were all male ranging in age from 12 to 78 years (mean 48.4 years). Two tumors were on the left side and three on the right side. The location of the lesions was evaluated by MR imaging and/or CT scans.

Changes of cerebral blood flow and oxygen metabolism associated with the lesions were studied by PET scan using O-15 labelled CO_2 and O_2 according to the method of Frackowiak, et al[2]. During the continuous inhalation of CO_2 (10 mCi/min) or O_2 (10 mCi/min), arterial blood samples were collected from the radial artery 3 times for each scan. Changes of cerebral glucose metabolism were studied using F-18 labelled fluoro-2-deoxy-D-glucose according to the method of Sokoloff, et al[3]. After the venous injection of the deoxyglucose (5 mCi), arterial blood was collected 30 times in 60 minutes and the kinetic rate constant of Phelps, et al[4] was used for calculation. In all patients, the PET study was done before treatment and two of them had second studies after treatment.

The quantitative studies of regional cerebral blood flow (rCBF), regional cerebral metabolic rate for oxygen (rCMRO2) and regional cerebral metabolic rate for glucose (rCMRGL) were performed on the plane including the thalamus and the basal ganglia. This plane was compatible with the slice 48 mm from the orbito-meatal line on the CT scan. Four regions of interest (ROI) in the cerebral hemisphere were measured on both sides and the ratio of asymmetry (affected side/normal side) was calculated. ROIs were in the frontal, anterior temporal, middle temporal and occipital lobes.

RESULTS

Changes of rCBF

CBF studies were performed in three cases. The mean cortical rCBF values of the normal side were 26.8 (range from 23.7 to 29.7), 32.2 (range from 28.1 to 40.7) and 42.8 (range from 36.5 to 55.2) ml/100g/min, respectively. The values for the affected side were 21.4 (range from 19.0 to 24.3), 23.8 (range from 19.2 to 33.1) and 30.8 (range from 22.6 to 37.3) ml/100g/min, respectively. The mean ratios of asymmetry were 0.80, 0.73 and 0.74, respectively. CBF studies showed a 20% to 27% decrease on the affected side compared with the normal side. CBF of patients with thalamic lesions were measured in four cases. No apparent changes were observed in these patients.

Changes of rCMRO2

CMRO2 studies were performed in three cases. The mean cortical rCMRO2 values on the normal side were 250.2 (range from 233.8 to 260.8), 285.4 (range from 235.4 to 340.0) and 323.5 (range from 300 to 337.5) ml/10l/min, respectively. The values on the affected side were 226.2 (range from 191.5 to 268.5), 228.6 (range from 194.5 to 299.1) and 287.5 (range from 212.5 to 362.5) ml/10l/min, respectively. The mean ratios of asymmetry were 0.90, 0.80 and 0.89, respectively. There was a 10% to 20% decrease on the affected side. CMRO2 was measured in five patients with thalamic lesions. Only one patient showed a local decrease in oxygen metabolism.

Changes of rCMRGL

CMRGL studies were performed in four cases. The mean cortical rCMRGL values on the normal side were 12.9 (range from 11.8 to 14.6), 21.9 (range from 19.6 to 23.3), 24.1 (range from 22.1 to 27.5) and 44.5 (range from 40.1 to 46.2) µmol/100g/min, respectively. The values on the affected side were 10.1 (range from 5.1 to 12.9), 17.6 (range from 15.4 to 21.4), 16.5 (range from 13.3 to 20.2) and 38.0 (range from 32.1 to 43.5) µmol/100g/min, respectively. The mean ratios of asymmetry were 0.77, 0.85, 0.68 and 0.80, respectively. There was a 15% to 32% decrease in the affected side (Fig. 1A,B). In patients with thalamic lesions CMRGL was measured in one cases and no apparent change was observed.

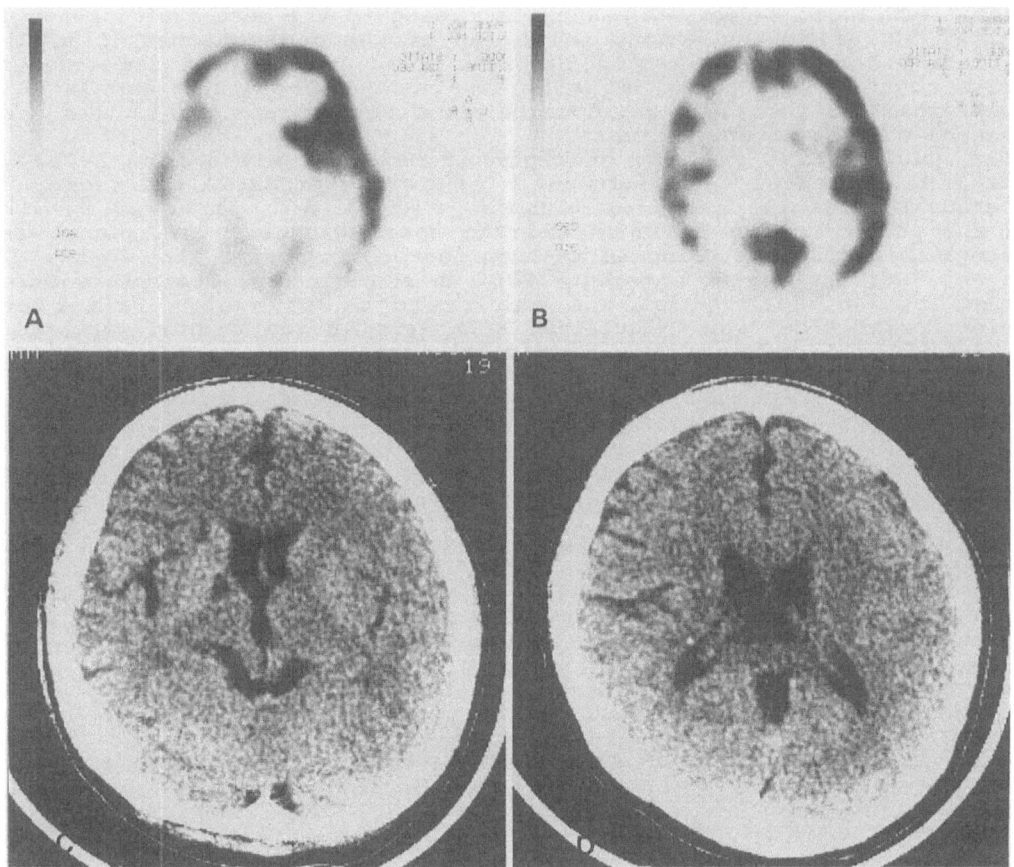

Fig. 1. A,B: PET study of CMRGL showing decreased metabolism on the right side of the cerebral hemisphere. C,D: CT scan demonstrated cerebral hemiatrophy after 8 months.

Second Studies after Treatment

Follow-up studies of CBF and CMRO2 were performed in two cases and CMRGL was also measured in one of them after several months. Progressive changes were observed in both cases. CBF decreased from 27% to 30% in one case and from 26% to 29% in the other case. CMRO2 decreased from 20% to 28% in one case and from 12% to 24% in the other case. A decrease on CMRGL from 20% to 27% was observed.

DISCUSSION

Secondary degeneration is obvious in special sensory systems after destruction of the major input [5,6]. Secondary damage after only partial input ablation has also been reported in the midbrain central gray [7]. Moreover we have found secondary degeneration in the cerebral cortex of a rat model of Alzheimer's disease, reported as transneuronal degeneration [8]. In the rat model, a 14% to 27% decrease of neuronal density was reported in the cerebral cortex [9]. In this study we found a 20% to 27% decrease in blood flow on the affected side of the cortex, a 10% to 20% decrease of oxygen metabolic rate and a 15% to 32% decrease of glucose metabolic rate. The variability of the absolute values of rCBF, rCMRO2 and rCMRGL in each individual case made it difficult to determine the critical values for the development of secondary damage. Moreover, the changes had progressed at the time of the second studies performed in 2 cases. Thus secondary degeneration may require as long a time as the transneuronal degeneration of the rat model, in which hemiatrophy of the cerebral cortex may appear on radiological examinations after as much as several months (Fig. 1C,D).

Kiyosawa, et al. reported the changes of CMRGL in baboons with unilateral lesions of the basal nucleus. They found recovery of the metabolic depression within 6 to 13 weeks despite sustained cholinergic denervation [10]. Pallidal lesions in this study are large enough for destruction of the basal nucleus and other neighboring structures. Prolonged changes of the cerebrum may require not only cholinergic denervation but also other factors. The above-mentioned baboon study showed that the metabolic depression was most prominent in the frontal and frontotemporal regions and least marked in the parietal and occipital regions. However, we could not find significant differences related to the anatomical region. Exact evaluation of the lesions in the basal ganglia and meticulous calculations of ROIs in the cerebrum are required for better understandings of the secondary damage of the cortex.

We thank Dr. Jeremy C. Ganz for reviewing the manuscript. This study was supporting by the Grant-in-Aid for Scientific Research from the Ministry of Education, Science and Culture in Japan.

REFERENCES

1. Inoue HK, Kobayashi S, Nakamura M, Horikoshi S, Ohye C (1991) Adv Neurotrauma Res 3: 26-31
2. Frackowiak RSJ, Lenzi GL, Jones T, Heather JD (1980) J Comput Assist Tomogr 5: 727-736
3. Sokoloff L, Reivich M, Kennedy C, DesRosiers MH, Patlak CS, Pettigrew KD, Sakurada O, Shinohara M (1977) J Neurochem 28: 897-916
4. Phelps ME, Huang SC, Hoffman EJ, Selin CS, Sokoloff L, Kuhl DE (1979) Ann Neurol 6: 371-388
5. Wong-Riley MTT (1972) J Comp Neurol 144: 61-92
6. Jean-Baptiste M, Morest DK (1975) J Comp Neurol 162: 111-134
7. Chung SK, Cohen RS, Pfaff DW (1990) Neuroscience 38: 409-426
8. Inoue HK, Nakamura M, Mouton PR, Olson L (1992) J Clin Electron Microscopy 25: in press
9. Arendash GW, Millard MJ, Dunn AJ, Meyer EM (1987) Science 238: 952-956
10. Kiyosawa M, Baron JC, Hamel E, Pappata S, Duverger D, Riche D, Mazoyer B, Naquet R, MacKenzie ET (1989) Brain 112: 435-455

Basic Fibroblast Growth Factor Prevents Retrograde Degeneration of the Thalamic Neurons After Ablation of the Somatosensory Cortex

EIJI KOHMURA, TAKAMICHI YUGUCHI, KAZUO YAMADA, TAKEO SAKAGUCHI, and TORU HAYAKAWA

Department of Neurosurgery, Osaka University Medical School, Fukushima-ku, Osaka, 553 Japan

SUMMARY

We studied whether a recombinant human basic fibroblast growth factor (bFGF), could prevent retrograde degeneration after neuronal injury. Four weeks after ablation of the somatosensory cortex of young female rats, extensive neuronal degeneration of the lateral ventroposterior nucleus (VPL) of the ipsilateral thalamus could be observed. When bFGF (1µg/0.1ml) soaked in gelfoam was applied topically at the time of surgery, this neuronal degeneration in the VPL was markedly reduced. However, the same dose of bFGF failed to save the thalamic neurons from retrograde degeneration, when it was given 3 days later. Cellular response to bFGF was analyzed with BrdU incorporation.

KEY WORDS: Degeneration, Fibroblast growth factor, Injury, Neuron, Thalamus

INTRODUCTION

Neuronal loss following axotomy eliminates the possibility of regeneration and might be a hindrance to functional recovery from severe head injury. We studied thalamic degeneration after cortical ablation as an experimental model for retrograde neuronal degeneration, that has been known since the late 1800s [1]. Recent reports showed that neurotrophic factor, such as nerve growth factor (NGF), can modulate neuronal degeneration [2]. However, NGF is known to act only on a restrictive neuronal system in the central nervous system (CNS), while bFGF has its range [3,4,5]. We investigated whether CS23, a stabilized form of the recombinant human bFGF, could save the thalamic neurons from retrograde degeneration.

METHODS

Animal Model

We used female Wistar rats (100–150g) for the subsequent experiments. Under general anesthesia with ketamine hydrochloride, the left primary somatosensory cortex [6] was exposed and removed by sliding a slightly-curved razor blade along the craniectomy edge. After hemostasis was achieved, we placed a gel foam, soaked either with bFGF(CS23) (1µg/0.1ml) or with vehicle only (0.1ml of normal saline with 0.2% of albumin), into the cavity to cover the entire lesion. In bFGF(CS23), two cysteine residues (Cys^{69} and Cys^{87}) are replaced by serine residues to stabilize the molecule while preserving its activity [7]. The skin was closed and animals were returned to their cage [8].

In the second experiment, we applied bFGF(CS23) 3 days after ablation. In this time we closed the wound initially placing a gel foam without bFGF into the cavity. We reopened the wound 3 days from then on under the same anesthesia. We replaced the gel foam with another one, soaked either with bFGF(CS23) (1µg/0.1ml) or with vehicle only.

Evaluation of Thalamic Atrophy

Four weeks after the surgery, those animals were deeply anesthetized with intraperitoneal injection of sodium pentobarbital and perfused with 4% paraformaldehyde in 0.1M phosphate buffer (pH 7.4). The brains were removed and immersed in the same fixative for 24 hours. The fixated brains were dehydrated and embedded in paraffin, and serial coronal sections (6 μm thick) obtained from an area 3 mm posterior to the bregma. These sections were used for staining with luxol fast blue and cresyl violet. To evaluate macroscopic atrophy, sections were projected on white paper at a fixed magnification rate and relevant regions (VPL+VPM) were traced. The sectional area of these regions was measured with a planimeter. This procedure was done by technical assistants who were not informed experimental protocol. The atrophic ratio (percentage) was calculated as follows:

$$\frac{\text{(Sectional area on contralateral side)}-\text{(sectional area on lesion side)}}{\text{(Sectional area on contralateral side)}} \times 100$$

Data were analyzed with Student's t-test.

BrdU Labeling

We gave 5-bromo-2'-deoxyuridine (BrdU) on day 3 to investigate cell-proliferating activity induced by bFGF application. These animals were fixated 90 minutes after intravenous BrdU administration (20mg BrdU/ 100g BW). This time 70% ethanol was used as fixative. Paraffin sections were made and incorporated BrdU was visualized by immunohistochemistry with mouse monoclonal anti-BrdU IgG (Becton Dickinson) as a primary antibody. Labeling index was displayed as a percentage of BrdU positive cells to total cells in the region of interest.

RESULTS

Prevention of Retrograde Degeneration

Four weeks after ablation of the somatosensory cortex of young female rats, we observed extensive neuronal degeneration or loss of neurons in the VPL of the ipsilateral thalamus. Other region that does not project directly to the removed cortex, such as the mediodorsal nucleus, showed no degenerative change. When bFGF(CS23) (1μg/ 0.1ml) soaked in gel foam was applied topically at the time of surgery, this neuronal degeneration in the VPL was markedly reduced and many neurons showed normal morphological appearance. The atrophic ratio for (VPL+VPM) could be significantly reduced by bFGF(CS23) {atrophic ratio: bFGF(-); 45.6±10.4%(n=7), bFGF(+); 26.9±8.0% (n=10), p<0.01} (Fig. 1). However, the same dose of bFGF(CS23) failed to save the thalamic neurons from retrograde degeneration, when it was given 3 days later. The atrophic ratio for (VPL+VPM) showed this time no statistical difference despite bFGF(CS23) treatment {atrophic ratio: bFGF(-); 53.0±8.3%(n=8), bFGF(+); 57.7±14.5%(n=9), NS} (Fig. 1). These results showed clearly that bFGF (CS23) can prevent the thalamic degeneration after ablation of the somatosensory cortex and that administration of bFGF is only effective in the early period after injury.

BrdU Labeling

In the group without bFGF(CS23), BrdU positive cells were confined to the peri-ablation area (labeling index; 6%). In contrast, wide distribution of BrdU positive cells were observed in the group with bFGF(CS23). Labeling index was 18.3% in the peri-ablation area. High labeling index was observed also in the bilateral corpus callosum (ipsilateral: 16.6%, contralateral: 10.8%). Double staining with glial fibrillary acidic protein (GFAP) showed most of the BrdU positive cells were negative for GFAP (data not shown).

DISCUSSION

We showed that bFGF(CS23) can prevent retrograde degeneration of thalamic neurons after ablation of the somatosensory cortex [8]. Moreover, the treatment is not effective unless it is given in the very early phase after ablation.

If retrograde degeneration is caused by failure of trophic factors to be transported from the axonal terminals, how can a single application of bFGF prevent neuronal loss? Does bFGF really constitute a trophic factor for the thalamic neurons or for the septal cholinergic neurons [9]? Basic FGF may act directly on neurons as a trophic factor or indirectly through modification of the surrounding environment. Wanaka and Johnson reported recently that the FGF receptor mRNA was not detectable in the basal forebrain cholinergic neurons or in most of the thalamus in adult rats [10]. This strongly suggests indirect action of bFGF on the septal cholinergic neurons and the thalamic neurons.

We observed more increased GFAP expression around the ablation site in bFGF-treated animals in 3 days and one week than that of without bFGF [8]. This increase in GFAP reaction was assumed to have been induced by the topically-applied bFGF. Experiments with BrdU showed that the distribution of BrdU positive cells were more extensive in the group treated with bFGF. Most cells incorporating BrdU were negative for GFAP. These results showed that single application of bFGF can modulate the microenvironment around injury. Following topical application of bFGF, neuronal sprouting might be accelerated, either directly or indirectly, by bFGF, to create a new pathway to obtain a continuous supply of trophic factors. Ineffectiveness of delayed bFGF administration showed that bFGF cannot alter degenerative change once it has started.

Since the first requirement for nerve regeneration is preserved neuronal cell bodies, we hope that prevention of retrograde degeneration may lead to reduction of neurological sequelae after trauma to the CNS. Therapy with growth factors should become a new approach to be investigated also in neurotraumatology.

ACKNOWLEDGMENT

The authors are very grateful to Takeda Chemical Industries for their kind donation of bFGF(CS23).

REFERENCES

1. White EL (1979) Brain Res Rev 1: 275–311
2. Hefti F (1986) J Neurosci 6: 2155–2162
3. Kromer LF, Bjørklund A, Stenevi U (1981) Brain Res 210: 153–171
4. Unsicker K, Reichert-Preibsch H, Schmidt R, Pettmann B, Laboudette G, Sensenbrenner M (1987) Proc Natl Acad Sci USA 84: 5459–5463
5. Walicke PA (1988) J Neurosci Res 8: 2618–2627
6. Hall RD, Lindholm EP (1974) Brain Res 66: 23–28
7. Seno M, Sasada R, Iwane M, Sudo K, Kurokawa T, Ito K, Igarashi K (1988) Biochem Biophys Res Comm 151: 701–708
8. Kohmura E, Yuguchi T, Yamada K, Hayakawa T (1990) Advances in Exp Neurotrauma Res 2:58–63
9. Otto D, Froetscher M, Unsicker K (1989) J Neurosci Res 22, 83–91
10. Wanaka A, Johnson EMJr (1990) Neuron 5: 267–281

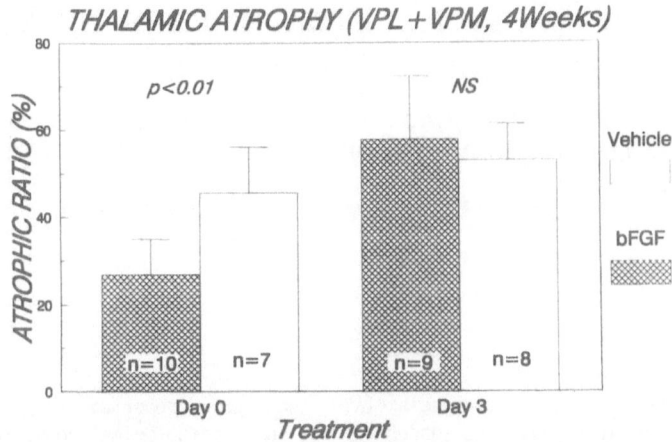

Fig. 1 Atrophic rate of the ipsilateral (VPL+VPM) 4 weeks after ablasion. The atrophic ratio for (VPL+VPM) could be significantly reduced by bFGF(CS23) when it was given at the time of ablation. However, the same dose of bFGF(CS23) failed to save the thalamic neurons from retrograde degeneration, when it was given 3 days later.

Treatment of Vasogenic Brain Edema by V_1 Receptor Antagonist of Arginine Vasopressin

MASAHIRO KAGAWA[1], SEIGO NAGAO[1], TSUYOSHI KUNIYOSHI[1], TOMOYA OGAWA[1], TERUKAZU ITO[1], YUTAKA HONMA[1], HIDEYUKI KUYAMA[1], TOSHIFUMI ITANO[2], and OSAMU HATASE[2]

[1]Department of Neurological Surgery, and [2]Physiology, Kagawa Medical School, Kagawa, 761-07 Japan

SUMMARY

Centrally released arginine vasopressin (AVP) has been reported to increase the water permeability of brain capillaries under normal and pathological conditions. In present experiment, we divided cold-injured brain into cortical and deep structure, and studied the effect of central administration of V_1 receptor antagonist (5 ng, 50 ng, and 500 ng per rat) on vasogenic brain edema. Cold injury induced significant increases in brain water and tissue sodium content of bilateral cortical structures, but no changes in bilateral deep structures. Intraventricular administration of V_1 receptor antagonist (50 ng) significantly reduced this accumulation of water and sodium in cortical structures without any change in plasma osmolality. A large quantity of this antagonist (500 ng) showed no changes in brain water content of bilateral cortical structures. It is suggested that this antagonist has an optimal concentration of this antagonist for inhibiting vasogenic brain edema.

KEY WORDS : brain edema, arginine vasopressin, receptor antagonist, cold injury

INTRODUCTION

Central administration of arginine vasopressin (AVP) was reported to increase brain capillary permeability to water[8] and brain water content[1,2].
In cold-injured cat brains, we previously showed that electric stimulation of the medullary reticular formation (MORF) for 40 minutes induced a high concentration of AVP in the cerebrospinal fluid (CSF)[7] and significant increases in brain water content in the white matter of the injured hemisphere[6]. We suggested that central AVP released by the stimulation of MORF was the promotion of vasogenic brain edema.
It is not known, however, whether AVP regulates the permeability of brain capillaries via a V_1 receptor or V_2 receptor. We had conducted an experiment to clarify the effects of centrally administering V_1 and V_2 receptor antagonists of AVP in cold-induced vasogenic brain edemas, and to determine whether these AVP blockades have a significant therapeutic effect on vasogenic brain edemas. Our results suggested that a centrally administered AVP receptor antagonist, especially a V_1 receptor antagonist, prevented the increment of brain water content induced by cold injury in rats[5].
We undertook this study to clarify an optimal concentration of a V_1 receptor antagonist for reducing vasogenic brain edema induced by cold injury.

MATERIALS AND METHODS

The experiments were performed on male Sprague-Dawley rats that ranged in weight from 250 to 350 g. During operations and before decapitation, the animals were anesthetized with an intraperitoneal injection of pentobarbital sodium (30mg/100g body weight). A linear incision was made over the sagittal suture. A burr hole was drilled over the left cerebral convexity. An AVP V_1 receptor antagonist ([deamino-Pen^1,O-Me-Tyr^2,Arg^8]-Vasopressin) in 1 μl of a Ringer solution was administered into the left lateral ventricle with the following stereotactic coordinates: A=-1.0 mm from bregma, L=1.5 mm from midline, V=4 mm below the skull. Ten minutes after intraventricular administration (i.v.a.), a cold injury was induced in the left hemisphere of the brain by applying a copper rod (5 mm in diameter) cooled by liquid nitrogen to the exposed bony skull for 20 seconds. The skin incision was sutured and the animals were placed in cages and fed freely. Twenty-four hours after the injury, animals were killed by decapitation. The brain was removed immediately and both injured and contralateral hemispheres were divided into the cortical and deep structure. The brain water content of each part was measured using the dry-weight method (at 110 ℃ for 24 hours). The brain tissue sodium and potassium were extracted with 2 N nitric acid for 48 hours and analyzed using atomic absorption spectrophotometry. Before decapitation, a blood sample was taken from the femoral artery, and plasma osmolality was measured using freezing point depression.
Statistical analysis was performed using the Student's t-test.
The experimental protocols for each groups were as follows :
Group A : normal rats. (n=25)
Group B : 1 μl of a Ringer solution (i.v.a.) + cold lesion (n=20)
Group C : 5 ng of a V_1 receptor antagonist (i.v.a.) + cold lesion (n=16)
Group D : 50 ng of a V_1 receptor antagonist (i.v.a.) + cold lesion (n=17)
Group E : 500 ng of a V_1 receptor antagonist (i.v.a.) + cold lesion (n=13)

RESULTS

Changes in the brain water content of all groups are presented in Fig. 1. The administration of 50 ng of V_1 receptor antagonist caused a significant reduction in the brain water content of both the injured and non-injured cortical structures without any change in plasma osmolality (Table 1). In group C, the brain water content of the bilateral cortical structures showed a slight decrease, but this change was not statisticaly significant.
In the injured cortical structure, the level of sodium was significantly increased with decreases of potassium 24 hours after the cold-induced lesion. These changes were inhibited by the administration of 50 ng of a V_1 receptor antagonist (Fig. 2). There were no significant changes in the tissue sodim and potassium content in the deep structures.

Table 1 The plasma osmolality in centrally administered V_1 receptor antagonist was studied 24 hours after cold injury. No significant differeces were found between all groups. Values are means ± standard error.

	A	**B**	**C**	**D**	**E**
Osmolality (mOsmol/kg)	304.5±0.8	305.9±1.2	307.3±1.0	307.8±0.9	303.5±2.0

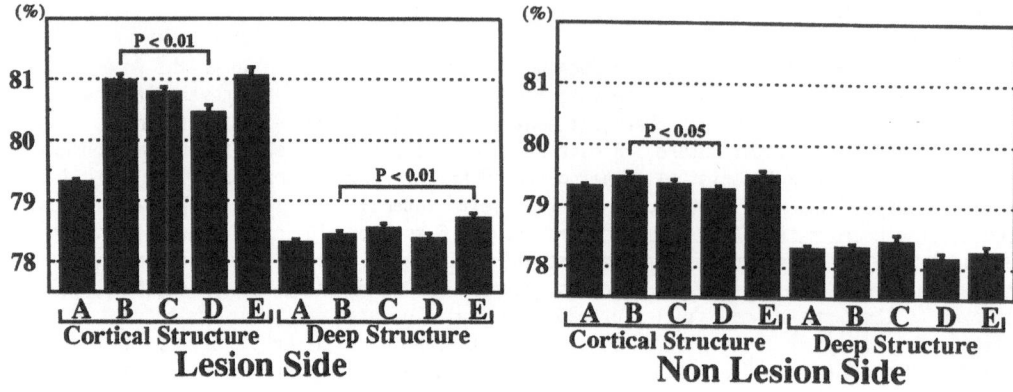

Fig. 1 Changes in the brain water content of both cold injured and non-injured hemispheres.
Cold injury induced significant increases in brain water content of bilateral
cortical structures without any change in deep structures. Fifty ng of V_1 antagonist
significantly reduced the increases of brain water content, but not 5 ng and 500 ng.
Values are means ± standard error.

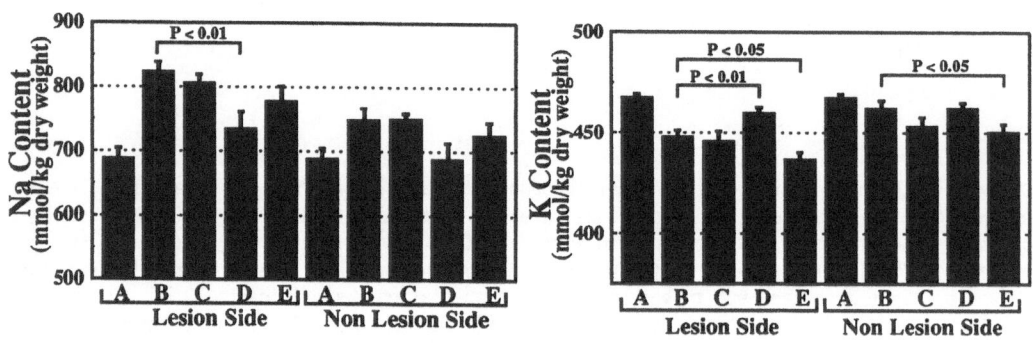

Fig. 2 Changes in the brain tissue sodium and potassium of bilateral cortical structures.
Cold injury induced significant increases in sodium with decrease of potassium. These
changes were significantly reduced by 50 ng of V_1 receptor antagonist in the injured
cortical structure, but it was not significant in the contralateral side. Values are
means ± standard error.

DISCUSSION

Elevated AVP levels in the CSF were reported in association with raised intracerebral pressure
(ICP), including stroke, subarachnoid hemorrhage, benign intracranial hypertension, and
bacterial meningitis.
Centrally administered AVP has been reported to increase brain water permeability in the
capillaries of normal monkeys[8] and brain water content with and without water accumulation
in rats[1]. Furthermore, central infusion of AVP in conscious goats led to a rise in ICP[12].

Reeder et al. reported that intraventricular administration of pharmacological doses of AVP facilitated cold-induced vasogenic edemas and concluded that this facilitation resulted from an AVP-induced increase in capillary permeability[9]. Our previous experiments showed that stimulation of the MORF resulted in a significant increase in CSF-AVP levels and water content in the cold-injured hemisphere (1.5%to 3%) within a short period of time (40 and 80 minutes, respectively)[6,7]. We suggested that increases in brain water content were associated with centrally released AVP.

In the rat model of both common carotid arteries occlusion, the subcutaneous injection of an AVP V_2 receptor antagonist reduced the ischemic-induced cerebral edema[14]. However, the reduction of the edema was associated with an increase in plasma osmotic pressure. On the other hand, the increase in brain water content induced by the infusion of AVP into bilateral caudates of normal cats was blocked by the simultaneous infusion of an AVP V_1 receptor antagonist[10,11]. This suggests that the increase in capillary permeability was mediated by the V_1 receptor.

We speculated that the content of AVP in the CSF may increase by three pathways. First, AVP is released from vasopressinergic neuronal terminals. A widespread innervation of AVP-containing fibers in the brain has been reported in anatomical studies[13]. AVP-containing neural processes in contact with blood vessels corresponded mainly to dendritic structures upon immunoelectronhistochemical study[4], and the pial artery revealed scattered vasopresin-immunoreactive nerve fibers[3]. Second, the paraventricular nucleus, the suprachiasmatic nucleus, and the nucleus of the stria terminalis appear to be the source of AVP. These nuclei directly release AVP into the ventricular system. A high concentration of AVP in plasma was reported in patients with intracranial hypertension. A third explanation is that a disruption of the blood-brain barrier induces an influx of this circulating AVP.

Five ng and 500 ng of this antagonist were not effective dosages for preventing increases in brain water content. This antagonist was reported to behave as a partial agonist as well as antagonist[15]. A large quantity, that is 500 ng, of this antagonist may possibly play a role as an agonist. This antagonist has an optimal concentration for exerting maximum effect on vasogenic brain edema.

Our results suggest that an optimal concentration of V_1 receptor antagonist may reduced vasogenic brain edema in clinical cases. Further experiment will reveal that the central administration of the V_1 receptor antagonist of AVP is an effective therapeutic agent for vasogenic brain edema.

REFERENCES

1. Doczi T, Szerdahelyi P et al. (1982) Neurosurgery 11:402-407
2. Doczi T, Laszlo FA, Szerdahelyi P et al. (1984) Neurosurgery 14:436-441
3. Itakura T et al. (1988) J Cereb Blood Flow Metab 606-608.
4. Jojart I, Joo F et al. (1984) Neurosie Lett 51, 259-264
5. Kagawa M, Nagao S et al. (1991) Advances in Neurotrauma Research 3:75-79.
6. Nagao S, Ogawa T, Kuniyoshi T et al. (1989) Advances in Experimental Neurotrauma Research 1:35-40
7. Nagao S, Kuniyoshi T, Ogawa T, et al. (1990) Advances in Experimental Neurotrauma Research 2:82-86
8. Raichle ME, Grubb RL (1978) Brain Res 143:191-194
9. Reeder RF, Nattie EE, North WG (1986) J Neurosurg 64:941-950
10. Rosenberg GA, Estrada E, Kyner WT (1988) Neuroscie Lett 95:241-245
11. Rosenberg GA, Estrada E, Kyner WT (1990) In : Long D et al. (eds) Advances in Neurology. pp 149-154
12. Seckle JR, Lightman SL (1987) Brain Res 423:279-285
13. Swanson LW, Kuypers HGJM et al. (1980) J Comp Neurol 194:555-570
14. Tang AH, Ho PM (1988) Life Sciences 43:399-403
15. Vallejo M, Lightman SL (1987) Brain Res 422:295-302.

7—Experimental Studies

The Acceleration-Deceleration Fractures of the Skull Base – An Experimental Study

MIODRAG A. POPOVIC[1], BORIS KLUN[2], NIKO HERAKOVIC[3], and DRAGICA NOE[3]

[1]Institute of Pathology, Medical Faculty, University of Ljubljana, 61000 Ljubljana, Slovenia, [2]University Clinic of Neurosurgery, University Clinic Centre of Ljubljana, 61000 Ljubljana, Slovenia, and [3]Faculty of Mechanical Engineering, University of Ljubljana, 61000 Ljubljana, Slovenia

SUMMARY

In the research work on acceleration-deceleration fractures, 25 cadavers of patients of the average age of 68 were used. The death of patients was not caused by injury. All ethical and moral principles were fully observed.

The selection of areas in which the experiments were carried out depended on those predominantly exposed to injuries: forehead, occiput and temples, which were divided due to the position of the fossa cranii media, according to the action of force upon the temporal-frontal, temporal-parietal and temporal-occipital areas.

During experimental work, the deformation of the skull were measured with computer aided testing (CAT). Computer aided testing and the graphic output presentation were performed by means of our own software.

KEY WORDS: Skull of base, blow, deformation, fracture, computer

INTRODUCTION

The fractures of the skull base and the skull or both can generally be caused by an adequately strong force acting on the head [1]. In view of this we researched the action of force on the head and its consequences on the skull base [2].

MATERIAL AND METHOD

Twenty-five cadavers were needed. For the selection of a cadaver it was important that the patient had not died due to an injury and the experiment was carried before the autopsy. The selection of 11 female and 14 male bodies, with an average age of 68, was accidental.

The experiments were conducted by means of a special pneumatic cylinder in an experimental set-up, constructed for this purpose at the Faculty of Mechanical Engineering (Fig. 1).

The pressure in the air reservoir of the cylinder was from 6.5 to 7 bars. The piston weighted 9 kg with average speed 2 m/s.

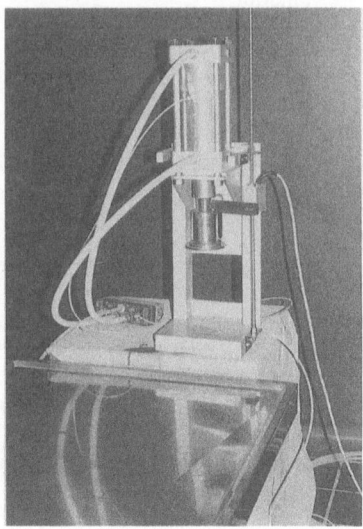

Fig. 1 Pneumatic cylinder

During the action of dynamic force on the head, skull deformation was measured using computer aided testing (CAT). Computer data processing and the graphic output presentation were performed with our own software.

RESULTS

Fractures of the base in the fossa anterior et posterior resulted from the blows on the forehead or occiput (Fig. 2, 3).

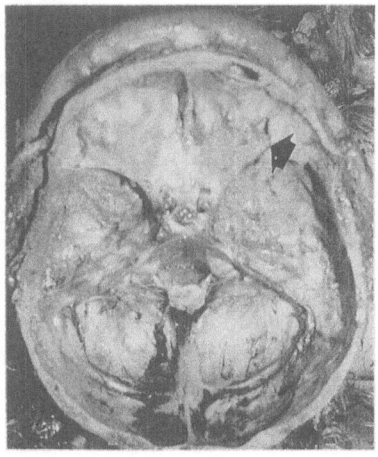

Fig. 2 Fracture of the base in fossa anterior

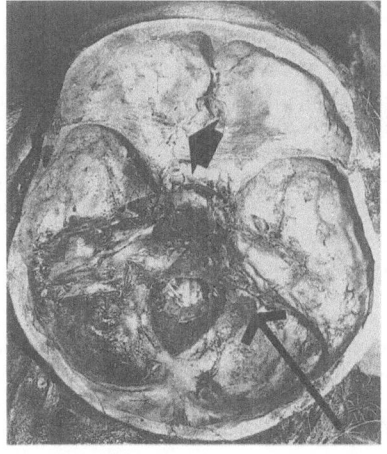

Fig. 3 Fracture of the base in fossa anterior et posterior

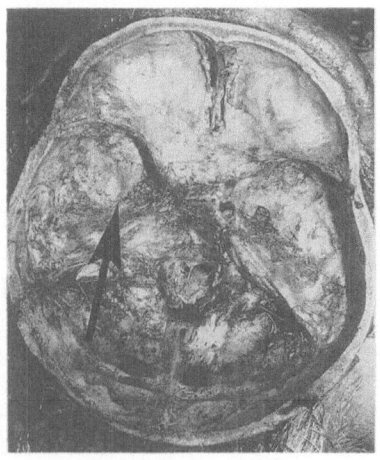

Fig. 4 Fracture of the base in fossa media and anterior

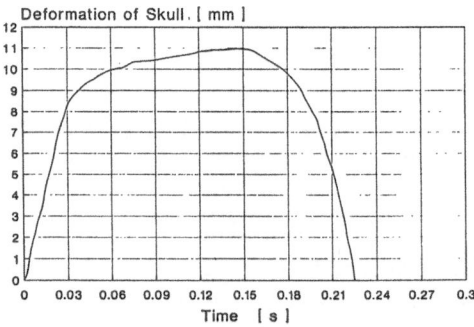

Fig. 5 Skull deformation by blow on the forehead

Blows on the occiput led to two more fractures of the skull.

Base fractures in the fossa media and anterior as well as three fractures of the skull were caused by blows on the temporal sides (Fig. 4). By each blow on the head, skull deformation was measured and the graphic output was produced with computer aided testing (CAT) equipment, (Fig. 5, 6, 7).

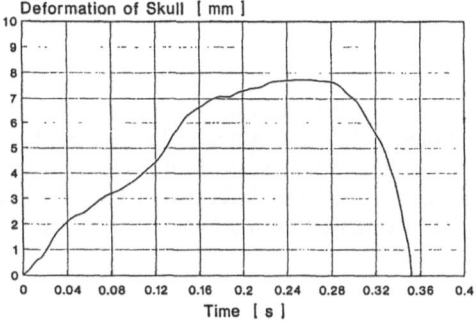

Fig. 6 Skull deformation by blow on the occiput

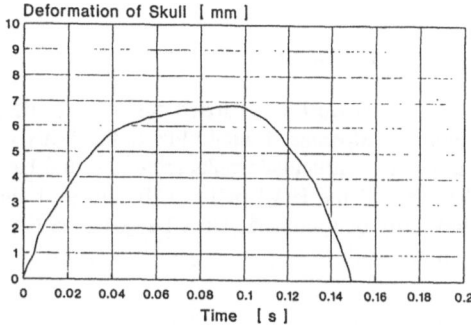

Fig. 7 Skull deformation by blow on the temple

DISCUSSION

The blow on the forehead did not cause any fracture of the skull whereas fractures occurred on the base at every single experiment. Linear fissure in the fossa anterior frequently run through the orbital part of the frontal bone, less frequently through the lamina cribrosa or the region of the sphenoidal bone [1, 2, 3]. According to our findings such fractures more often damage some of sinuses than the first or second cranial nerve [4, 5]. The diagram of the skull deformation by the blow on the forehead has showed the longest way, what is the results of very good amortization on the base in fossa anterior [1, 5, 6, 7].

The fissures on the base in fossa posterior partly run as a ring like fracture around the big foramen and partly in the direction of the sigmoidal sinus [1, 8]. If the blow on the occipital side causes a fracture in the fossa anterior, injuries of afore-mentioned occur in the same fossa. The diagram shows that the skull deformation usually lasts longer.

A blow on the temporal side can also cause a fracture of the skull if it comes from the frontal or parietal direction. A blow from the frontal direction regularly causes a fracture of the Turkish saddle as well as a fracture of the pyramid in its upper third [9, 10, 15]. However, a blow from the parietal direction does not cause any fracture of the Turkish saddle, but only a fracture of the pyramid in its lower third. A completely different picture is obtained on the base in case of a blow on the temporal side from the occipital direction. In this case fractures occur in the projection of the crista alaris. The diagram with the shortest time and way of skull deformation can arise if a blow on the temple comes from the parietal direction. If a blow on the temple comes from the occipital side, then the diagram can be similar to the diagram of skull deformation in the occipital region.

CONCLUSION

Our findings have showed that the fractures in the fossa anterior and fossa posterior are the most dangerous for lesions of the sinuses. The fractures of the Turkish saddle can injure the hypophysis and hypothalamus as well as the carotid veins and the cavernous sinus. In the case of the pyramid fractures, injuries of the substances around the pyramid and in it can occur. In the region of crista alaris the fractures can cause the injuries of the venous sinus of the little wings as well as the cranial nerves in the upper orbital fissure.

ACKNOWLEDGEMENTS

The research work was carried out at the Institute of Pathology at the Medical Faculty, University of Ljubljana, Slovenia. I would like to thank my mentor, Professor Dr. Boris Klun for his precious help and advice. Particular thanks are due to the Head of the Institute of Pathology, Professor Dr. Dusan Ferluga and the Head of the Laboratory of Pneumatics at the Mechanical Faculty of Engineering, University of Ljubljana, Doc. Dr. Dragica Noe, to my family as well as to all who have helped me with my work.

REFERENCES

1. Prokop O.: Forensiche Medizin. Zweite Auflage. Berlin: Veb Verlag Volk und Gesungheit, 1986: 192-204.
2. Wolf Heidegger G.: Atlas der systematische Anatomie des Menshen.   Dritte Auflage. Basel Munchen Paris London New York Sydney Karger S., 1972
3. Ferre J.C., Chevalier C., Robert B., Degrez J., Le Cloarec A.Y., Legoux R., Orio E., Barbin J.Y.: Reflections on the mechanical structure of the base of the skull and on the face. Surg. Radiol. Anat., 1989; 11: 41-48.
4. Raveh J., Vuillemin F., Sutter F.: Subcranial management of 395 combined frontobasal midface fractures. Arch Otolaryngol Head Neck Surg., 1988; 134: 1114-1122.
5. Gwyn F.: Facial fractures, associeted injuries and complications. Plastic and Reconstructive Surgery, 1971; 47: 225.
6. Sturla F., Absi D., Buquet J.: Anatomical and mechanical fractures. An experimental study. Plastic and Reconstructive Surgery, 1980; 66: 815-820.
7. Richard R.: Ocular motility disturbance following trauma. Adv Ophthalmic Plast Reconstr Surg., 1987; 7: 133-147.
8. Gerhard V., Goran S.: Ring fracture of the base of the skull. The Journal of Trauma, 1974; 14: 494-505.
9. Griffin J.E., Altenau M.M., Scaefer S.D.: Bilateral longitudinal temporal bone fractures. Laryngoscope, 1980; 89: 1432-1435.
10. Bartynski W.S., Wang A.M.: Cavernous sinus air in a patient with basilar skull fracture et CT identification. J Comput Assist Tomogr., 1988; 12: 141-142.

Experimental Study in Cerebral Venous Circulatory Disturbance: With Special Reference to Venous Hemorrhage

Masaki Gotoh[1], Toru Fukuhara[1], Takeshi Shirakawa[1], Shigeki Nishino[1], Toshikazu Saijyo[1], Masamitsu Kawauchi[1], Takashi Ohmoto[1], and Hideyuki Kuyama[2]

[1]Department of Neurological Surgery, Okayama University Medical School, Okayama, 700 Japan and
[2]Department of Neurological Surgery, Kagawa Medical School, Kagawa, 761-07 Japan

SUMMARY

Using a new devised model of dural sinus occlusion, we investigated the pathophysiology including venous hemorrhage. Sixteen cats received the occlusion of superior sagittal sinus(SSS) and diploic veins(DV). Intracranial pressure(ICP), cerebral blood volume(CBV) and regional cerebral blood flow(rCBF) were measured for 12 hours. At sacrifice, cerebral water content was determined. Other 8 cats received the additional occlusion of cortical veins(CV). In both groups, the blood-brain barrier(BBB) permeability was evaluated with Evans blue. The SSS and DV occlusion produced a significant increase in ICP and CBV and a significant decrease in rCBF. Cerebral water content also increased significantly. However, neither extravasated Evans blue nor venous hemorrhage could be observed, when thrombus was defined within SSS. Contrarily, the additional CV occlusion produced hemorrhagic infarctions in 6 cats, where Evans blue dye extravasated. These data suggest that dural sinus occlusion led to an increase in CBV and cerebral water content resulting in intracranial hypertension, and decreased rCBF. The brain edema in this model seemed to be hydrostatic edema. The obstruction of CV might be essential in the development of hemorrhage in this model, and the BBB was disrupted in these areas.

KEY WORDS: dural sinus occlusion, cortical vein occlusion, venous hemorrhage, hydrostatic edema

INTRODUCTION

Impairment of cerebral venous drainage plays a significant role in the pathogenesis of severe head injuries. Several authors have reported dural sinus thromboses after closed head injuries[1-4]. However, the pathophysiology of venous circulatory disturbance is poorly understood.
We devised a new experimental model of dural sinus occlusion. Using this model, we investigated the pathophysiology of dural sinus occlusion and the pathogenesis of venous hemorrhage.

MATERIALS AND METHODS

Experiment 1: Dural Sinus Occlusion

Under general anesthesia, 16 cats received the exposure of bilateral parietotemporal bone. Two burr holes were made over the anterior end of superior sagittal sinus(SSS) and the posterior end near the confluens. Outer table of the skull was also scraped all along the circumference of calvaria to exposure diploic veins(DV). SSS and DV were occluded by coagulating through the burr holes and packing bone wax, respectively. Intracranial pressure(ICP), cerebral blood volume(CBV), regional cerebral blood flow(rCBF) were measured for 12 hours after the occlusion. Cerebral water content also measured 12 hours after the occlusion.

Experiment 2: Occlusion of the Dural Sinuses and Cortical Veins

In the same manner as Experiment 1, 8 cats received the exposure of SSS and DV. After DV occlusion by packing bone wax, 0.3-0.5ml cyanoacrylate was injected into SSS to occlude SSS and cortical veins.

In both experiments, Evans blue was injected intravenously 11 hours after the occlusion to evaluate blood-brain barrier(BBB) permeability. Histological examinations were performed after the experiments.

RESULTS

Experiment 1

The changes in ICP, CBV, rCBF, and cerebral water content after the occlusion are shown in Table 1. ICP increased gradually for 12 hours. CBV also increased, but the degree of increase after 6 hours was small. rCBF decreased gradually, but the degree of reduction was more prominent within 6 hours. Cerebral water content increased significantly in both the gray and the white matter 12 hours after the occlusion.

Table 1 Changes in ICP, CBV, rCBF, cerebral water content after the dural sinus occlusion.

hours after occlusion	ICP (n=9, mmHg)	CBV (n=8, %)	rCBF (n=9, ml/100g/min)	Water Content (n=8, %) gray matter	white matter
control	6.1±4.4	(-)	50.4±5.6	79.2±0.4	67.6±0.6
1hr	8.5±6.5	11.9±6.5	39.4±8.3[b]		
2hrs	10.7±7.2[a]	14.3±6.5	38.1±9.5[b]		
3hrs	13.5±7.8[b]	15.8±5.5	33.0±8.1[c]		
4hrs	15.6±8.9[b]	16.7±6.3	30.4±7.1[c]		
5hrs	17.5±8.8[b]	21.3±11.9	25.7±4.0[c]		
6hrs	18.8±7.0[c]	25.6±12.8	23.0±4.8[c]	81.7±0.5[b]	73.3±1.5[b]
7hrs	24.7±9.1[c]	27.4±12.3	23.0±4.6[c]		
8hrs	27.8±9.7[c]	28.5±11.5	22.4±4.0[c]		
9hrs	32.0±12.6[c]	30.7±10.1	21.2±4.3[c]		
10hrs	35.1±10.2[c]	30.3±10.2	21.2±3.5[c]		
11hrs	34.8±11.4[c]	30.2±10.2	20.6±3.3[c]		
12hrs	36.3±12.3[c]	29.8±9.9	19.8±4.6[c]	83.4±1.2[c]	76.8±1.6[c]

Values are means±SD
[a] Significantly different from control (p<0.05).
[b] Significantly different from control (p<0.01).
[c] Significantly different from control (p<0.001).

Macroscopically, Evans blue extravasation was visualized only in the injured area due to surgical procedure(Fig. 1). Light microscopic findings showed edematous changes in both the gray and the white matter. However, no hemorrhage could be seen.

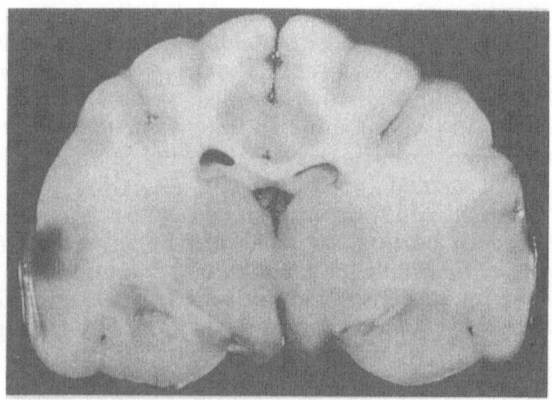

Fig. 1 Coronal section of the brain in Experiment 1. Evans blue extravasation was limited in the injured area due to surgical procedure.

Experiment 2

Macroscopic examinations showed hemorrhagic infarctions in the parasagittal cortex in 6 cats(Fig. 2). The hemorrhage was restricted to the territory of occluded cortical veins. Evans blue extravasated mainly around the gray matter accompanied by hemorrhages. Light microscopic study revealed multiple foci of petechial hemorrhages.

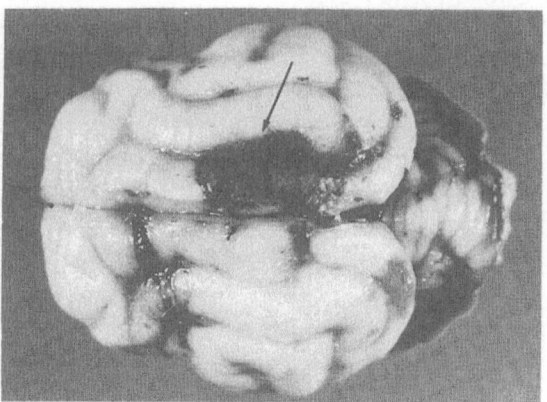

Fig. 2 Postmortem photograph of the brain in Experiment 2 showing hemorrhagic infarction(arrow) in the parasagittal cortex.

DISCUSSION

The present study suggested that the cerebral venous system occlusion led to an increase in CBV and cerebral water content resulting in intracranial hypertension. The occlusion also decreased rCBF. Wagner and Traystman examined rCBF responses to elevated jugular venous pressure and found that rCBF decreased significantly when cerebral perfusion pressure(CPP) decreased to value below 60 mmHg[5]. We supposed that decreased rCBF resulted from both lowered CPP and cerebral edema. These parameter changes were more prominent within 6 hours after the occlusion. The deep venous system, which was preserved in this model, might drain venous blood as a collateral circulation.

The histological findings in Experiment 1 did not demonstrate Evans blue extravasation, suggesting that a dural sinus occlusion for 12 hours did not cause the BBB disruption. The brain edema in this model seemed to be hydrostatic edema[6].

Concerning hemorrhagic factors following sinus occlusion, several authors reported that the extended occlusion to cortical veins might be essential in the development of hemorrhage[7, 8]. We confirmed the conception and supposed that the BBB was disrupted in these areas. From the microscopic findings, hemorrhages might occur at capillaries and venules when the occlusion involved confluent portions of collecting venules and veins.

REFERENCES

1. Carrie AW, Jaffe FA (1954) Thrombosis of superior sagittal sinus caused by trauma without penetrating injury. J Neurosurg 11: 173-182
2. Martin JP (1955) Signs of obstruction of the superior longitudinal sinus following closed head injuries(traumatic hydrocephalus). Br Med J 2: 467-470
3. Stringer WL, Peerless SJ (1982) Superior sagittal sinus thrombosis after closed head injury. Neurosurgery 12: 95-96
4. Hesselbrock R, Sawaya R, Tomsick T, Wadhwa S (1985) Superior sagittal sinus thrombosis after closed head injury. Neurosurgery 16: 825-828
5. Wagner EM, Traystman RJ (1983) Effects of cerebral venous and cerebrospinal fluid pressure on cerebral blood flow. In: Auer LM, Loew F (eds) The Cerebral Veins. Springer-Verlag, Wien New York, pp 223-230
6. Miller JD (1979) The management of cerebral oedema. Br J Hosp Med 21: 152-165
7. Bousser MG, Chiras J, Bories J, Castaigne P (1985) Cerebral venous thrombosis-A review of 38 cases. Stroke 16: 199-213
8. Fujita K, Kojima N, Tamaki N, Matsumoto S (1985) Brain edema in intracranial venous hypertension. In: Inaba Y, Klatzo I, Spatz M (eds) Brain edema. Springer-Verlag, Berlin Heiderberg New York Tokyo, pp 228-234

Amelioration of Septal Cholinergic Neuronal Degeneration After Nerve Growth Factor Deprivation by Cytokine-Activated Astrocytes

Kazunari Yoshida[1], Masachika Sagoh[1], Hirooki Wakamoto[1],
Takahito Yazaki[1], Mitsuhiro Otani[1], Shigeo Toya[1], and Fred H. Gage[2]

[1]Department of Neurosurgery, School of Medicine, Keio University, Shinjuku-ku, Tokyo, 160 Japan, and
[2]Department of Neurosciences, University of California, San Diego, La'Jolla, California 92093, USA

SUMMARY

Nerve growth factor (NGF) synthesis and secretion from astrocytes is cooperatively regulated by various cytokines including fibroblast growth factors, interleukin-1β (IL-1β), tumor necrosis factor-α (TNF-α), and transforming growth factor-β1 (TGF-β1). The present study was performed to determine the effect of NGF produced by cytokine-activated astrocytes on NGF-deprived septal neurons *in vitro*. Enzymatically dissociated septal neurons from E-16 rat fetuses were grown on monolayered astrocytes obtained from neonatal rat hippocampi in a serum-free defined medium. Effects of the various combinations of IL-1β, TNF-α and TGF-β1 on septal cholinergic neurons cocultured with astrocytes were examined. A combination of IL-1β and TNF-α increased choline-acetyltransferase (CAT) activity via NGF produced by astrocytes. NGF-treated septal cholinergic neurons were found to degenerate following NGF deprivation. However, a combination of IL-1β and TNF-α significantly reduced the degeneration of NGF-deprived septal cholinergic neurons by activating astrocytes. The cytokines, which regulate NGF synthesis and secretion in astrocytes, are considered to play an important role in neuronal regeneration following brain injury.

KEY WORDS : nerve growth factor, astrocytes, cholinergic neurons, cytokines,
cell culture

INTRODUCTION

Astrocytes are known to possess exclusive neurotrophic effects which are thought to be mediated by neurotrophic factors (NTFs), cell surface molecules and extracellular matrix. Although astrocytes are likely to produce many kinds of NTFs, NGF is the only NTF which has been demonstrated to be secreted by astrocytes [1]. The cholinergic neurons of the basal forebrain are NGF-sensitive in the central nervous system. NGF increases CAT activity and promotes survival and axonal growth *in vitro* [2]. Exogenous NGF prevents cholinergic cell death following the intrinsic NGF deprivation by the transection of the septo-hippocampal pathway in vivo [3,4]. NGF produced by hippocampal neurons is considered to act as a target-derived growth factor for septal cholinergic neurons[5,6]. Although the functions of NGF produced by astrocytes are not clear, NGF production by astrocytes following injury has been suggested by *in vivo* experiments [7,8]. Furthermore, we have shown that NGF production by astrocytes is cooperatively regulated by various cytokines, *i.e.*, FGFs, IL-1ß, TNF-α and TGFß1, which are likely to be present in the brain following injury, while platelet-derived growth factor, IL-3, IL-6, TGF-α and epidermal growth factor have no or a very small effect [9,10]. In the present study, we examine the function of NGF produced by cytokine-activated astrocytes.

MATERIALS AND METHODS

Cell Cultures

Astrocytes: Astrocyte-enriched cultures were prepared as previously described [9]. Hippocampi were dissected out from newborn rats, and the meninges, blood vessels, and choroid plexus were carefully removed under a dissection microscope. The brain fragments made by passing through a stainless steel mesh (pore size 200 μm) were suspended in Dulbecco modified Eagle's medium (DME) supplemented with 10% fetal calf serum (FCS), 2.5 mg/l Fungizone, and 40 mg/l gentamicin, and were seeded in poly-L-lysine coated culture flasks (25 cm^2, Corning). Astrocyte-enriched culture obtained after two passages with the enzymatic treatment was used for the present study.

Neurons: Septal area was dissected from rat fetuses (E-16), and meninges and blood vessels were carefully removed under a dissecting microscope. The brain fragments obtained by passing through a stainless steel mesh (pore size 200 μm) were incubated in 0.25% trypsin in Hank's balanced salt solution for 10 min at 37 °C. Undissociated tissues were removed by passing through stainless steel mesh (pore size 100 μm) after neutralization of trypsin by adding the same amount of 10% FCS-DME. The dissociated cells were spun down, washed with Dulbecco's phosphate buffered saline (PBS), and suspended in N2 medium supplemented with 40 mg/ml Gentamicin, 2.5 mg/ml Fungizone and 750 mg/ml bovine serum albumin (N2-BSA). These cells were grown on subcultured astrocytes grown in poly-L-lysine (Sigma) treated 24-well culture plates.

CAT assay

CAT activity was measured by the Fonnum's method [11] modified by Hatanaka et al. [12]. Cells were homogenized by sonication in 100 ml of 50 mM Tris-HCl buffer, pH 7.4, with 0.1% Triton X-100. Protein levels were measured by Coomassie protein assay reagent (Pierce). Aliquots (20 ml) of the supernatants of homogenates (10,000 rpm for 2 min) were mixed with the same amount of substrate solution (200 mM [^{14}C]acetyl coA (4.00 mCi/mmol, New England Nuclear), 10mM choline chloride, 200mM eserine salicylate, 300mM NaCl in 50mM PB), and incubated for 45 min at 37 °C. The enzyme reaction was stopped by adding 0.5 ml of 5:2 mixture of 20 mM PB containing 0.1 mM p-chloro-mercuribenzoic acid and acetonitrile containing 5 mg/ml of sodium tetraphenylborate. Subsequently, 1 ml of toluene-based scintillation cocktail was added for the measurement of radioactivity.

RESULTS and DISCUSSION

Because astrocytes are ideal substrates for neurons, the neurons can be kept healthy for a long time, even at a low cell density when cocultured with monolayered astrocytes. In this coculture system, effects of IL-1ß and TNF-α on septal cholinergic neurons were

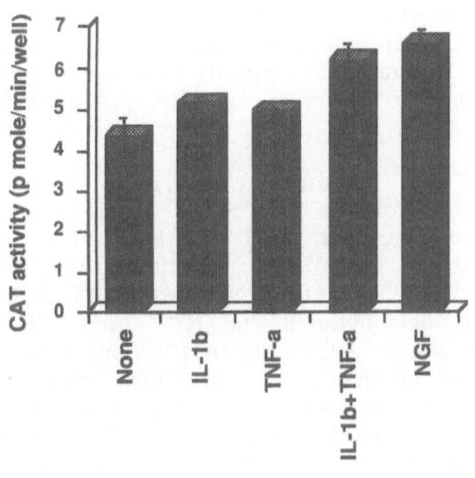

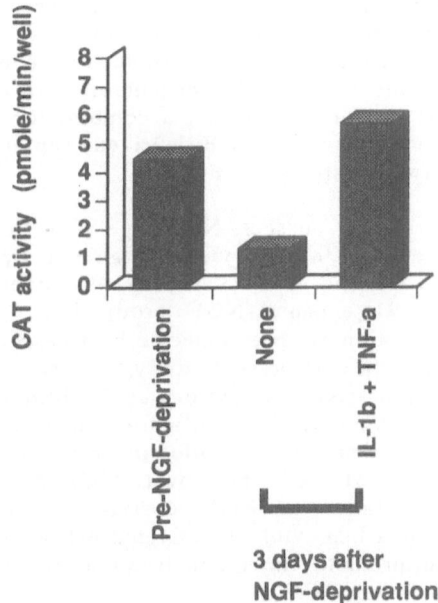

Fig. 1. Effects of IL-1ß (30 unit/ml) and TNF-α (100 ng/ml) was examined by using a coculture system of hippocampal astrocytes and septal neurons. Effect of NGF (100 ng/ml) was examined as control. Values represent means ± S.D. of three determinations.

Fig. 2. Effect of a combination of IL-1ß (30 unit/ml) and TNF-α (100 ng/ml) of NGF-deprived septal cholinergic neurons cocultured with hippocampal astrocytes was examined. Values represent mean of duplicated determinations.

examined (Fig. 1). The cultures were treated with cytokines for four days from the second day of culture. Each of these cytokines had a very slight effect on CAT activity. However, the CAT activity of septal neurons stimulated by a combination of IL-1ß and TNF-α approached the level of that stimulated by an optimal dose of NGF. Although CAT immunoreactivity in non-stimulated cultures was very weak, some cholinergic neurons stimulated by NGF or a combination of IL-1ß and TNF-α were clearly detected by immunocytochemistry (not shown). The cholinergic neurotrophic effect of a combination of IL-1ß and TNF-α was significantly reduced by anti-NGF neutralizing antibody, and this combination failed to increase CAT activity in the presence of a full dose of NGF (not shown). This combination had no direct effect on CAT activity of glia-deprived septal neuronal cultures in the presence of Ara-C (not shown). Therefore, IL-1ß and TNF-α enhance the CAT activity in septal cholinergic neurons by stimulating NGF production by astrocytes.

Subsequently, the effect of IL-1ß and TNF-α on NGF-deprived septal cholinergic neurons was examined. The septal neurons cocultured with astrocytes were treated with

NGF for 4 days from 1 day after seeding. On the fifth day of culture, the cells were rinsed three times with PBS to remove NGF. These cultures were grown three more days in the presence or absence of a combination of IL-1ß and TNF-α. The cholinergic neurons were found to degenerate following NGF deprivation as indicated by decease of CAT activity. However, a combination of IL-1ß and TNF-α significantly reduced the degeneration of NGF-deprived septal cholinergic neurons via NGF produced by activated astrocytes (Fig. 2).

Astrocytes possess NGF-type and non-NGF-type neurotrophic activity [13]. NGF production in astrocytes is regulated by various cytokines, i.e., FGFs, IL-1ß, TNF-α, TGF-ß1 and EGF [9,10,14-18]. Among those cytokines, aFGF, IL-1ß, TNF-α and TGF-ß1 enhance NGF production cooperatively [9,10]. The regulation of NGF production has been detected by measuring mRNA^{NGF} [14,16] or NGF protein [9,10,14-18]. In the present study, we have clearly demonstrated that NGF produced by cytokine-activated astrocytes is functionally active. NGF may not be involved in neurotrophic activity in astrocytes in the normal brain; however, cytokines, which are likely to be released following brain injury stimulate astrocytes to produce a significant amount of NGF. Moreover, NGF released from activated astrocytes ameliorates the degeneration of NGF-deprived septal cholinergic neurons. These results strongly suggest that cytokine-activated astrocytes may support the survival of damaged neurons and promote the reconstruction of damaged neural-network for a short period by producing NGF.

REFERENCES

1. Furukawa S., Furukawa Y., Satoyoshi E., and Hayashi K. (1986) *Biochem. Biophys. Res. Com.* **136**, 57-63.
2. Honegger P. (1983) *Monogr. Neurol. Sci.* **9**, 36-42.
3. Hefti F. (1986) *J. Neurosci.* **6**, 2155-2162.
4. Williams L.A., Varon S., Peterson G.M., Wictorin K., Fischer W., Bjorklund A., and Gage F.H. (1986) *Proc. Natl. Acad. Sci. USA* **83**, 9231-9235.
5. Ayer-Lelievre C., Olson L., Ebendal T., Seiger A, and Persson H. (1988) *Science* **240**, 1339-1341.
6. Whittemore S.R., Friedmann P.L., Larkammer D., and Persson H. (1988) *J. Neurosci. Res.* **20**, 403-410.
7. Gage F.H., Olejniczak P., and Armstrong D.M. (1988) *Exp. Neurol.* **102**, 2-13.
8. Lu B., Yokoyama M., Dreyfus C.F., and Black I.B. (1991) *J. Neurosci.* **11**, 318-326.
9. Yoshida K., and Gage F.H. (1991) *Brain Res.* **538**, 118-126.
10. Yoshida K., and Gage F.H. (1991) *Brain Res.* **569**, 14-24.
11. Fonnum F. (1975) *J. Neurochem.* **24**, 407-409.
12. Hatanaka H., and Tsukui H. (1986) *Dev. Brain Res.* **30**, 47-56.
13. Lindsay R.M. (1979) *Nature* **282**, 80-82.
14. Spranger M., Lindholm D., Bandtlow C., Heumann R., Guahn H., Näher-Noé M., and Thoenen H. (1990) *Europ. J. Neurosci.* **2**, 69-76.
15. Gadient R.A., Cron K.C., and Otten U. (1990) *Neurosci. Lett.* **117**, 335-340.
16. Lindholm D., Hengerer B., Zafra F., and Thoenen H. (1990) *NeuroReport* **1**, 9-12.
17. Fukumoto H., Kakihana M., and Suno M. (1991) *Neurosci. Lett.* **122**, 221-224.
18. Carman-Krzan M., Vige X., and Wise B.C. (1991) *J. Neurochem.* **56**, 636-643.

HSP72-Like Immunoreactivity After Fluid Percussive Brain Injury in the Rat: Relationship to Cell Type

HIROKAZU TANNO, RUSS P. NOCKELS, LAWRENCE H. PITTS, and L.J. NOBLE

Department of Neurosurgery, University of California and San Francisco General Hospital, San Francisco, California 94110, USA

SUMMARY

We have previously developed a model of fluid percussive head injury in the rat and focussed on alterations in permeability of the blood-brain barrier (BBB) to plasma proteins [1]. In the present study we examined the immunolocalization of the stress protein HSP72 after brain injury and relate these findings to the pattern of breakdown of the BBB. Rats were subjected to a lateral fluid percussive brain injury (4.5-5.2 atm., 20 msec.) and HSP72-like immunoreactivity was evaluated in brain sections at the light microscopic level. At the impact site, which typically exhibits prolonged barrier breakdown, the superficial cortex exhibited necrotic changes. Within this necrotic area immunoreactivity was restricted to blood vessels. In the adjacent cortex, numerous neurons and glia as well as pia arachnoid and blood vessels were immunostained. In other brain regions such as parasagittal cortex, deep cortical layer, and CA3 in the posterior hippocampus, which express transient abnormal permeability and no obvious pathological changes, only a limited number of neurons and glia were immunostained. Vessels exhibited no immunoreactivity. These results suggest that sites of breakdown of the BBB correspond to cell populations that are stressed and /or injured, as defined by expression of HSP72. Differential expression of HSP72 is correlated in part with the duration of breakdown of the BBB, and probably with the magnitude of local tissue injury.

Key Words : Experimental brain injury, Blood-brain barrier breakdown, HSP72, Cellular injury

INTRODUCTION

Our previous study demonstrated that barrier breakdown after this injury was prominent and widespread within the injured hemisphere. In this model, the impact site typically exhibits *prolonged* barrier breakdown, whereas other brain regions such as parasagittal cortex, deep cortical layer, and CA3 of the posterior hippocampus express *transient* abnormal permeability [1]. The relationship between post-traumatic BBB disruption and cellular injury is unclear. We hypothesize that areas of the brain that exhibit marked extravasation of plasma proteins may be injured or stressed and thus express HSP72-like immunoreactivity. It is believed that denatured proteins activate heat shock factors that stimulate heat shock transcription [2,3]. To begin to test this hypothesis we examined the expression of HSP72-like immunoreactivity, a marker of cellular stress/injury [4,5,6,7,8], after mild fluid percussive brain injury and relate these findings to the known pattern of barrier breakdown after a similar brain injury.

MATERIALS AND METHODS

7 adult male Sprague-Dawley rats (350-400g) were prepared for lateral fluid percussive brain injury as previously described [9]. Briefly each animal was anesthetized with 4% chloral hydrate (8ml/kg, b.w., I.P.). A lateral 4mm diameter craniotomy was made in the right temporal region just above the zygoma. A polyethylene tube (PE 350) filled with isotonic saline was

placed over the dura, fixed to the skull, and then connected to a fluid percussive device. Animals were subjected to an impact pressure of 4.8-5.2 atm. for 20 msec. and sacrificed at 24 hours by intracardiac perfusion with 4% paraformaldehyde. Each brain was removed and 100 um sections were cut on a vibratome. Sections from each brain were prepared for immunolocalization of HSP72. Adjacent sections were stained with cresyl violet in order to examine general morphology.

Immunocytochemical techniques were used to localize HSP72. Vibratomed sections were incubated in; 1) mouse anti-human HSP72 (Amersham), 2) biotinylated horse anti-mouse IgG, rat adsorbed (Vector Labs), 3) avidin-biotin-HRP complex (Vector Labs). The final reaction product was visualized using 0.05% 3,3-diaminobenzidine tetrachloride (DAB) as the chromogen in the presence of 0.02% H_2O_2. Immunolocalization of HSP in brain sections was evaluated at the light microscopic level.

RESULTS

In general, hemorrhage was restricted to the ipsilateral external capsule. Cellular necrosis, as assessed by cresyl violet, was restricted to the superficial cortex at the impact site. Other brain regions showed no abnormal findings.

HSP72 immunoreactivity in the injured brain was noted at the impact site as well as in other brain regions including the parasagittal cortex, deep cortical layer and hippocampus (Fig. 1). *Impact site (Fig.2)* In the necrotic area (Zone 1) only blood vessels were immunostained. The adjacent cortex bordering this necrotic area (Zone 2) was characterized by prominent HSP72-like immunoreactivity. HSP72-like immunoreactivity was observed in both cell bodies and processes of numerous neurons and glia (Fig. 3). Immunostaining was also present in pia-arachnoid and in certain blood vessels (Fig. 4).
Other brain regions (Fig.5) HSP72 like immunoreactivity was restricted to a few neurons in the ipsilateral parasagittal cortex and to neurons and glia in the deep cortical layer and CA3 in hippocampus. In several animals, immunoreactivity was also present in the contralateral parasagittal cortex.

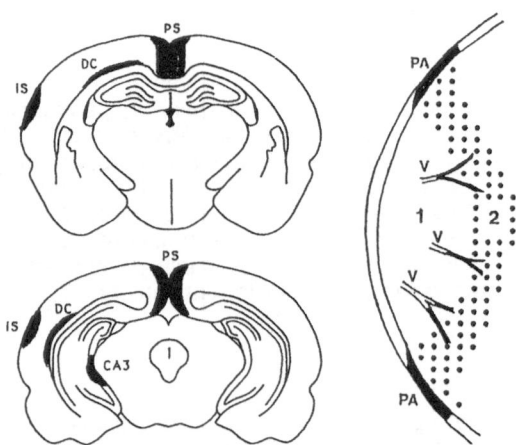

Fig. 1 (left) The distribution of HSP72-like immunoreactivity. IS: impact site, PP: parasagittal cortex, DC: deep cortical layer, CA3: hippocampus

Fig. 2 (right) Schematic illustration of the distribution of HSP72-like immunoreactivity at the impact site. Zone 1 (area of necrosis), Zone 2 (adjacent cortex). Blackened areas of pia arachnoid (PA) and blood vessels (V) define typical immunoreactivity Immunoreactive neurons and glia (designated by dots) are restricted to Zone 2.

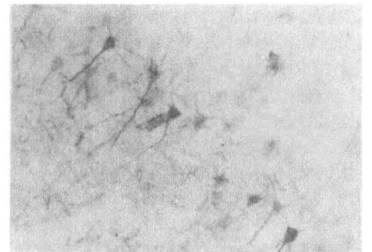
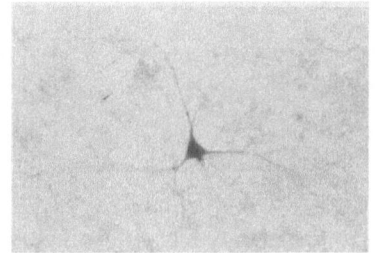
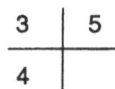
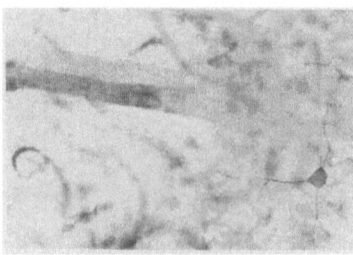

Fig. 3 and 4. Immunoreactivity is noted in numerous neurons and glia in Zone 2 as well as blood vessels in Zone 1 and 2 at the impact site. The immunoreactivity is localized in both the cell bodies and their processes.

Fig. 5. Immunoreactive neuron in the parasagittal cortex.

DISCUSSION

This study demonstrates that the impact site, characterized by a prolonged barrier breakdown, exhibits prominent HSP72 expression in neurons and glia. In contrast, transient breakdown, noted in other regions, is associated with less HSP72 expression in cells. The expression of HSP72 immunoreactivity in blood vessels parallels the pattern of prolonged breakdown of BBB but is not associated with transient barrier breakdown. These findings suggested that the duration of the breakdown may be correlated with HSP72 expression in neurons and glia and that prolonged abnormal permeability may reflect a state of stress or injury in blood vessels.

The apparent selective expression of HSP72 in blood vessels in the necrotic region and the regional distribution of HSP72 beyond the area of necrosis most likely reflects severity of injury and relative vulnerability of each cell type to injury. The most pronounced expression occurred in neurons, glia and blood vessels that bordered the necrotic area. In the deep cortical layer and CA3 in the hippocampus, immunolabelled neurons and glia were evident, whereas in the parasagittal cortex label was restricted to a limited number of neurons. Based upon several studies [5.6,10], it is thought that neurons are the most vulnerable to injury followed by glia and then endothelial cells. Such a criteria, applied to the present study, would suggest that severity of injury would be as follows;
impact site >> deep cortical layer and CA3 in the hippocampus > parasagittal cortex.

Breakdown of BBB results in the unrestricted entry of humoral agents that can be injurious to brain tissue. Sites of barrier breakdown may thus define populations of cells that are stressed and/or injured. There is, for example, evidence that certain neurons accumulate extravasated plasma proteins at sites of vascular disruption [1,11,12,13,14] These proteins are localized in a diffuse pattern throughout the cytoplasmic compartment. This particular localization suggests that the plasma membrane of the cells may be injured or irreversibly damaged.

The factors leading to the induction of HSP72 remain unclear. We can, however, speculate on several interrelated events. First, mild fluid percussive brain injury may deliver a direct physical insult that is of sufficient magnitude to elicit the heat shock response. Second, breakdown of the blood-brain barrier may result in the entry of plasma components that either directly or indirectly injure cells. An example of the latter would be cell excitation leading to glutamate release and subsequent cell injury [7]. Third, extravasated plasma proteins may become denatured. These denatured products if taken up into cells could then activate heat shock factors that stimulate heat shock transcription.

In summary, this study presents the following findings. 1) brain regions associated with breakdown of the BBB express differing degrees of cell injury. 2) differential expression in cell types of HSP72 is correlated in part with the duration of breakdown of the BBB, and probably with the magnitude of local tissue injury. 3) transient breakdown of the BBB is not accompanied by expression of HSP72 in blood vessels. Taken together, these results suggest that sites of breakdown of the BBB correspond to cell populations that are stressed and /or injured, as defined by expression of HSP72.

REFFERENCES

1. Tanno H, Nockels RP, Pitts LH, Noble LJ (1992) Breakdown of the blood-brain barrier after fluid percussive brain injury in the rat. Part 1. Distribution and time course of protein extravasation. J Neurotrauma 9: 21-32
2. Ananthan J, Goldberg AL, Voellmy R (1986) Abnormal proteins serve as eukaryotic stress signals and trigger the activation of heat shock genes. Science 232:522-524
3. Pelham HRP (1986) Speculations on the functions of the major heat shock and glucose-regulated proteins. Cell 49:959-961
4. Gonzalez MF, Shiraishi K, Hisanaga K, Sagar SM, Mandabach M, Sharp FR (1989) Heat shock proteins as markers of neural injury. Mol Brain Res 6:93-100
5. Gonzalez MF, Lowenstein D, Fernyak S, Hisanaga K, Simon R, Sharp FR (1991) Induction of heat shock protein 72-like immunoreactivity in hippocampal formation following transient global ischemia. Brain Res Bull 26:241-250
6. Sharp FR, Lowenstein D, Simon R, Hisanaga K (1991) Heat shock protein hsp72 induction in cortical and striatal astrocytes and neurons following infarction. J Cereb Blood Flow Metab 11:621-627
7. Vass K, Welch WJ, Nowak TSJr (1988) Localization of 70-kDa stress protein induction in gerbil brain after ischemia. Acta Neuropathol 77:128-135
8. Welch WJ, Suhan JP (1986) Cellular and biochemical events in mammalian cells during and after recovery from physiological stress. J Cell Biol 103:2035-2052
9. Ishige N, Pitts LH, Berry I, Carlson SG, Nishimura MC, Moseley ME, Weinstein PR (1987) The effect of hypoxia on traumatic head injury in rats: Alterations in neurologic function, brain edema, and cerebral blood flow. J Cerebral Blood Flow Metab 7:759-767
10. Ferriero DM, Soberano HQ, Simon PR, Sharp FP (1990) Hypoxia-ischemia induces heat shock protein like (HSP72) immunoreactivity in neonatal rat brain. Dev Brain Res 50:145-150
11. Brightman MW, Klatzo I, Olsson Y, Reese TS (1970) The blood-brain barrier to proteins under normal and pathological conditions. J Neurol Sci 10:215-239
12. Povlishock JT, Becker DP, Miller JD, Jenkins LW, Dietrich WD (1979) The morphopathologic substrates of concussion. Acta Neuropathol 47;1-11
13. Loberg EM, Torvik A (1991) Uptake of plasma proteins into damaged neurons. An experimental study on cryogenic lesions in rats. Acta Neuropathol 81:479-485
14. Sokrab TEO, Johansson BB, Kalimo H, Olsson Y (1988) A transient hypertensive opening of the blood-brain barrier can lead to brain damage. Extravasation of serum proteins and cellular changes in rats subjected to aortic compression. Acta Neuropathol 75:557-565

8—Monitoring

Contribution of Increased Cerebral Blood Volume to Post-Traumatic Intracranial Hypertension

ROBERT J. HARIRI, ANDREW D. FIRLIK, VICTOR A. CHANG, PHILIP S. BARIE, and JAMSHID B.G. GHAJAR

The Aitken Neurosurgery Laboratory, Division of Neurosurgery, Department of Surgery, Cornell University Medical College, New York, NY 10021, USA

SUMMARY

Cerebrovascular dysfunction following traumatic brain injury (TBI) may be the critical mediator of excess morbidity and mortality after TBI. Despite aggressive therapy, death is often due to refractory intracranial hypertension (IH). Cerebral cortical reflectance photoplethysmoghraphy and radioactively labeled red blood cells were employed to study cerebral blood volume (CBV) changes associated with increased intracranial pressure (ICP) after TBI in miniature swine. An early elevation in ICP immediately after TBI (t=0) was accompanied by a large increase in CBV compared to pre-TBI levels (19.2 ± 4.9 vs 8.9 ± 2.7 mL/100g tissue, $p<0.05$). Decreased CBV corresponded to lower ICP within 1 hour, followed by a slow rise that paralleled the increase in ICP. CBV (16.1 ± 3.3 vs 8.9 ± 2.7, $p<0.05$) and ICP (23 ± 2.2 vs 9 ± 0.6, $p<0.05$) were higher at 6 hours than at baseline. Based on compartmental analysis, the data indicate that ICP changes immediately after TBI and within 6 hours are predominantly due to increased CBV.

INTRODUCTION

It is well accepted that uncontrollable intracranial hypertension is the single most frequent cause of death in aggressively managed head-injured patients. [1] However, the sequence of events and contributing factors leading to elevated ICP are not well understood. We hypothesized that the acute cerebrovascular response to TBI is characterized by increases in cerebral blood volume (CBV) that may account, at least in part, for the ICP changes observed clinically. To specifically analyze the contribution of CBV to post-traumatic intracranial hypertension, we employed continuous cerebral cortical reflectance photoplethysmography, combined with determinations of brain compliance and cerebral oxygen extraction, in a porcine fluid percussion model.

MATERIAL AND METHODS

The model of frontal brain injury by fluid percussion is described in detail elsewhere [2]. Miniature swine were allowed to equilibrate following surgical preparation for a 30 minute period prior to experimental injury. The following physiologic variables were continuously monitored using an analog-to-digital conversion data acquisition system: mean arterial blood pressure (mABP), CVP, SSP, ICP, heart rate (HR), inspired (FiO_2) and expired (FeO_2) oxygen concentrations, expired isoflurane concentration, end tidal CO_2 ($PetCO_2$), and core temperature.

Since cerebral blood flow and volume increase linearly with $PaCO_2$ the rate of ventilation was manipulated to produce varying $PaCO_2$ ($etCO_2$) levels determine the changes in CBV as measured by cerebral cortical reflectance photoplethysmography and Technetium-99m labeled red blood cells. These correlation experiments were conducted in four control ani-

A 14 mm burr hole was made in the frontal region, contralateral to the injury screw, in all animals for epidural placement of a flexible reflectance photoplethysmography probe. The probe consisted of miniature red and infrared light-emitting diodes (LED's) and a silicon photodetecting diode mounted on a flexible circuit board. Output from the photodetector was selectively tuned to provide data on photostimulation by specific wavelengths. The probe was connected to a photodemodulation circuit and an analog-to-digital converter connected to a microcomputer. Reflected red and infrared photoplethysmograms were employed to evaluate cerebral cortical blood volume and oxygen saturation of hemoglobin (SaO_2). Amplitudes of the reflected signals were used in the calculation of SaO_2 (oximetry) [3] and as an index of cerebral blood volume. Cerebral blood volume (CBV) changes were simultaneously measured using radioactively (Technetium-99m) labeled red blood cells (RBCs) and detected by a gamma collimator placed over site of the reflectance probe in some animals to calibrate the reflectance photoplethysmographic technique. Brain compliance was determined using the single injection method described by Marmarou, et al.[4]

RESULTS AND DISCUSSION

To evaluate the accuracy of the photoplethysmographic technique for determining CBV changes in real time, simultaneous determinations were made by counting radioactively labeled RBCs in the same tissue region. Both 99m Tc decay from labeled RBCs and the red a.c. amplitude derived from reflectance photoplethysmography were well correlated to changes in CBV that occurred in response to variations in end-tidal CO_2. This relationship was significant (p = 0.00001) throughout the range of photodetector sensitivity of the system, and when counts were corrected for decay. Total counts were then converted to a blood volume measurement based on the results of direct counting of whole blood specimens drawn during the experiment. From this relationship, calculation of CBV was made from the red a.c. amplitude alone.

Physiologic data, obtained 30 minutes following surgical preparation, demonstrated no statistically significant differences in baseline ICP, mABP, CVP, or SSP between groups. Arterial blood gases and temperature were unchanged from baseline values throughout the duration of the experiment in both groups. Animals in Group I developed a significant, transient systemic hypertension following TBI that lasted approximately 30 minutes and then returned to baseline values.

Intracranial hypertension occurred immediately following TBI in injured animals (Figure 5), rising to significantly higher levels from baseline (24±2 vs 9±1, p<0.001) within minutes of injury, and returning to near baseline within 30 minutes. A more gradual increase in ICP developed over the next several hours, achieving significance (p<0.05) from 90 minutes after TBI to the end of the experimental period. Notably, the immediate post-injury rise in ICP that occurred during the period of systemic arterial hypertension was accompanied by an increase in CBV to more than double the baseline values (19.2 ±1.4 vs 8.9±1.1 mL/100 g tissue, p<0.05) at the time of the greatest rise in ICP (Figure 1). Although CBV decreased from this peak at the time of injury, it remained significantly elevated above baseline levels throughout the experimental period.

Arteriovenous oxygen content difference across the brain significantly decreased (1.9±0.1 vs 3.8±0.3 mL/dL, p<0.05) during the immediate post-traumatic rise in ICP and CBV (Figure 2), and was inversely related to the photoplethysmographically calculated cerebral cortical SaO_2. Oxygen extraction then gradually increased during the post-traumatic period and was significantly higher than baseline values from 3 to 6 hours following injury. Calculated cerebral cortical SaO_2 initially rose after injury and then gradually declined to significantly lower than baseline values after 4 hours.

Brain compliance measurements made prior to and at 6 hours after experimental TBI were used to predict volumetric changes that corresponded to the rise in ICP immediately after TBI and at the end of the experiment. The increase in CBV immediately after TBI accounted for 95% of the expected volumetric increase necessary to cause the observed elevation in ICP. At six hours, the change in CBV accounted for 75% of the volumetric increase responsible for the elevation in ICP observed.

Compartmental analysis of the intracranial space allows one to predict pressure changes from volumetric changes, and to attribute these fluxes to the individual intracranial compartments. From the pressure-volume index determined by bolus injection and the CBV as estimated by photoplethysmography, we calculated the increases in ICP that were expected to occur as a result of the CBV increases we measured. Our results indicate that in the period immediately following TBI, elevations in ICP can be accounted for, almost entirely, by concomitant increases in CBV. At the conclusion of the experimental period, however, CBV was responsible for only 75 percent of the elevation in ICP. Higher measured ICP than that predicted from our CBV measurements could be explained by mechanisms such as volumetric increases in the cerebrospinal fluid or interstitial compartments (cerebral edema).

The relationships between ICP, CBF, and CBV are complex; many previous data are conflicting. Intracranial hypertension in post-traumatic coma has been associated with a variety of CBF measurements, ranging from marked hyperemia to extremely low flow states[5-6]. Knowledge of the CBV may be important in the management of severely-head injured patients because it can be used together with measurements of brain compliance to determine the proportion of the ICP elevation that can be directly attributed to arterial and venous blood volumes and, by extension, to non-vascular components of ICP such as parenchymal edema or volumetric increases in cerebrospinal fluid. This method may alter treatment patients with intracranial hypertension who could be treated based upon whether their ICP change was due mainly to brain edema or to an increase in CBV.

REFERENCES

1. Miller JD, Becker DP, Ward JD, Sullivan HG, Adams WE, Rosner MJ (1977) Significance of intracranial hypertension in severe head injury. J Neurosurg 47:503-516.

2. Sullivan HG, Martinez J, Becker DP, Miller JD, Griffith R, Wist AO (1976) Fluid percussion model of mechanical brain injury in the cat. J Neurosurg 45:520-523.

3. Hampson NB, Piantadosi Ca, (1990) Near infrared optical responses in feline brain and skeletal muscle tissues during respiratory acid-based imbalance. Brain Res 519:249-254.

4. Callahan RJ, Froelich JW, McKusick KA, Leppo J, Strauss W, (1982) A modified method for the in vivo labeling of red blood cells with TC-99m: Concise Communication. J Nucl Med 23:315-318.

5. Kontos HA, Wei EP, Navari RM, Levasseur JE, Rosenblum WI, Patterson JL (1978) Responses of cerebral arteries and arterioles to acute hypotension and hypertension. Am J Physiol 234:H371-H383.

6. Obrist WD, Gennarelli TA, Segawa H, Dolinskas CA, Langfitt TW (1979) Relation of cerebral blood flow to neurological status and outcome in head injured patients. J Neurosurg 51:292-300.

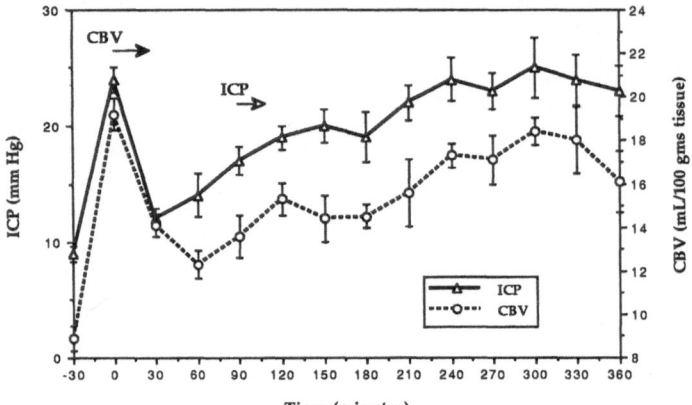

FIGURE 1

Changes in intracranial pressure (ICP) (solid lines) closely paralleled the increases in cerebral blood volume (CBV) (dashed lines) following fluid percussion-induced closed head injury. The marked increases in ICP and CBV attendant to the injury (given at time T=0) are reflective of the marked systemic hypertension and cerebral vasodilatation that occurs immediately following injury. Increased CBV was noted ($p<0.05$, two-w ANOVA) beginning immediately after injury and for the duration of the experiment (depicted by the solid arrow). Increased ICP was noted ($p<0.05$, two-way ANOVA, open arrow) immediately and again beginning 90 minutes after injury and for the duration of the experiment.

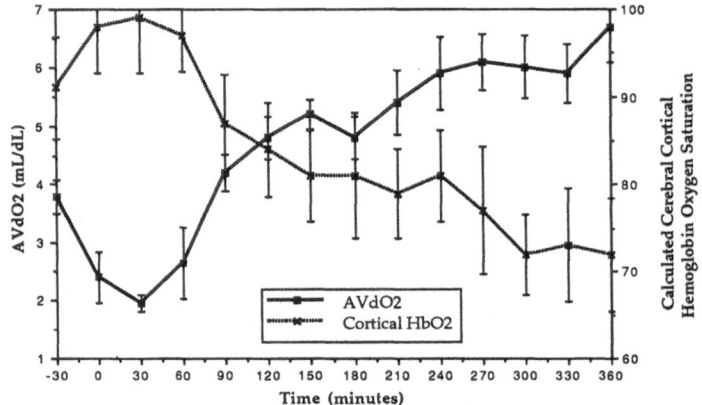

FIGURE 2

Cerebral arteriovenous oxygen difference ($AVdO_2$, solid line) and cortical blood oxyhemoglobin saturation (HbO_2, dotted line) are shown with respect to time following induction of a closed head injury using the fluid percussion technique. The injury stimulus was applied at time = 0

292

Cerebral Perfusion Pressure Management of Head Injury

MICHAEL J. ROSNER and SHEILA D. ROSNER

The University of Alabama at Birmingham, Birmingham, Alabama, USA

SUMMARY

Management of intracranial pressure per se as the primary therapeutic end point in the traumatically brain injured patient has produced little change in mortality or morbidity over the last two decades. As a result, we have evaluated the management and active manipulation of cerebral perfusion pressure (CPP = SABP - ICP) to a level of 70-80 mmHg or greater.

117 patients (GCS = 5.1±1) have been managed titrating CPP to 70-80 mmHg or higher. Methods of CPP management included volume expansion, nursing patients in the flat position, and catecholamine infusions to maintain the SABP side of the CPP equation. CSF drainage and mannitol were used for their effects on the ICP side of the equation. CPP was maintained at an average of 83 ± 14 mmHg, ICP = 24 ± 11 mmHg and SABP = 106 ± 14 mmHg. CVP averaged 8.6 ± 4.1 mmHg and PCWP averaged 16 ± 2 mmHg. Average fluid intake was 5.1 ± 3.5 L/d; output was 4.6 ± 3.4 L/d. Albumin 25% (53 ± 55 gm/d) and packed red cells enhanced vascular expansion. Hemoglobin averaged 11.7 ± 1.5 gms. Patients were maintained normocapneic and hyperventilation was only used for acute, transient periods of intracranial hypertension. These values are mean value for fourteen days.

Results: Overall mortality was 31% with PVS = 4%. 80% of survivors (53% of total series) made a good recovery (GOS = 4.7 ± .1 at 10.7 months). The results in those patients with surgical mass lesions (27%) were identical to those not requiring craniotomy.

We conclude that CPP management produces both superior mortality and morbidity when compared to previous methods of management and that the patient with a surgical mass lesion benefits to a proportionately greater degree than even those with simpler closed head injuries.

KEY WORDS: Traumatic Brain Injury, Cerebral Perfusion Pressure, Intracranial Pressure, Therapy, Closed Head Injury

INTRODUCTION

We have developed a therapeutic model for treatment of severe traumatic brain injury based upon management of cerebral perfusion pressure (CPP) rather than ICP alone.[7] The CPP model grew out of observations relating low or unstable CPP to the genesis of ICP waves.[4,5,6]

HYPOTHESES

CPP Management will be associated with

    1.   Improved survival
    2.   Improved morbidity

MATERIALS AND METHODS

I.   Frontal Ventriculostomy
    - ICP Monitoring
        Therapeutic CSF drainage-drained prn to maintain
        CPP $\geq$ 70 torr.
II.   Ventilation
    - Muscle paralysis
    - $PaO_2 \geq 70$ ($SaO_2 \geq 90\%$)
    - $PaCO_2$ 35-40 torr
    - Reserve "hyperventilation" for acute situations
III. Phenylephrine or norepinephrine used to maintain CPP $\geq$ 70 torr--
        try to limit < 4 μg/kg/min or 0.4 μg/kg/min respectively
    - Dopamine 2 μg/kg/min to protect renal function
IV. Mannitol
    - 0.5-1.0 gm/kg/prn CPP < 70 torr
    - try to limit to q4h
    - replace diuresis cc/cc if patient euvolemic
V.   Hydration
    - Euvolemia
    - Maintain CVP 8-10 torr, PCWP 12-15 torr
    - Avoid
        - Over hydration
        - Positive Na^+ balance
    - Packed red cells, concentrated (25%) albumin used frequently
    - Many IV orders: "I=O + losses" to avoid wide swings in
        hydration
    - Daily weights
VI. Patients nursed flat
VII. CPP level:
        Start $\geq$ 70 torr
        Increase as needed to eliminate pressure waves and minimize
          ICP
        May require CPP 90-100 torr in acute situation
VIII. Nutritional support withheld until ICP controlled by CSF
        drainage alone

RESULTS

Overall mortality in this series was 32% (Table I) and average GCS was
5.1 (Table II). Equally important was the very low rate of persistent
vegetative state (3%) accompanied by a 55% rate of "favorable"
outcome. Outcome of the 27% undergoing craniotomy was identical to
those with "closed head injury".

Approximately 20% of the deaths represent deaths due to progressive
intracranial hypertension; many of these included management errors.
Another 20% represented gross management error. Sixty percent were
"non-cerebral" deaths or "elective withdrawal of support".

Table I: Comparison of Outcome of Cerebral Perfusion Pressure Management with ICP Therapy[*]

OUTCOME[**]	GCS = 3		GCS = 4		GCS = 5		GCS = 6		GCS = 7		Total	
	CPP	ICP	CPP	ICP	CPP	ICP	CPP	ICP	CPP	ICP	CPP	ICP
Good	10.5	4.1	16.7	6.3	20.0	12.1	60.6	29.2	68.8	46.6	35.9	22.3
Moderate	15.8	3.1	25.0	8.1	20.0	17.1	18.2	21.2	12.5	22.3	18.8	15.1
Severe	10.5	10.3	16.7	18.9	16.0	23.2	3.0	31.2	6.2	11.5	10.2	16.9
PVS	5.2	4.1	4.2	10.8	4.0	7.3	3.0	5.3	0.	2.0	3.4	5.6
Dead	58.	78.4	37.5	55.9	40.0	40.2	15.2	21.2	12.5	17.6	31.6	40.1

[*] "ICP Therapy" data from Marshall et al, 1991
[**] All values as %

Table II: Patients with traumatic brain injury of GCS ≤ 7

N =	117
Age	27.4 ± 12.0 years
GCS	5.10 ± 1.35
CSF lactate	4.35 ± 3.15 mmol/L
Multiple injury	50%
Operative Mass Lesion	27%

No patient entered if GCS > 7 by 24 hours post-injury

DISCUSSION

CPP management has shown itself to improve mortality and probably morbidity when compared to traditional ICP management. ICP deaths have typically accounted for ≥ 50% deaths after head injury in previous series and this "malignant intracranial hypertension" has yielded very slowly if at all to traditional ICP management. The regimen presented here deviates significantly from the "traditional" management schemes and is, in fact, incompatible with most components (Table III) of "standard" ICP management. However, our results have been consistently better than most prior reports [1,2,3] and the techniques are now used throughout our intensive care unit for all ICP

Table III: Comparison of "Traditional" vs "CPP Management"

MODALITY	TRADITIONAL ICP THERAPY	CPP MANAGEMENT
Position flat (4)	Elevate HOB ≥ 30°	HOB=0° : Patient
Fluids	2/3 Maintenance BUN 35mg%	Hydrate normally I=0 + losses
Hypertension	Prevent -use sedatives -use antihypertensives -use blockers -avoid stimulation	Facilitate -vascular expansion -vasopressors -active stimulation
Mannitol (5)	Osmolality 310-320 Replace 2/3 diuresis	Normal osmolality Replace cc/cc if patient euvolemic I=0 + losses
Barbiturates	Burst suppression	Avoid-cardiac depressants
Hyperventilation	pCO_2 25-28 torr	pCO_2 35-40 torr -"Bag" acutely only

"problems".[4-7] We feel that nearly 50% of our "current" death rate is potentially avoidable and mortality can be reduced further. More importantly, morbidity is far superior to that achieved using ICP management alone and can probably be further reduced.

CONCLUSION

1. CPP management has resulted in greatly improved ICP control and markedly reduces the occurrence of "malignant" intracranial hypertension.
2. Mortality has been reduced to 75% compared to "traditional" ICP treatment regimes used for management of traumatic brain injury.
3. Morbidity as measured by "favorable outcome" was 55% vs 37% for CPP vs. ICP therapy: More than a 50% improvement in "favorable outcome" over previous therapy.
4. The "surgical mass lesion" patient benefits to a proportionately greater extent than the "closed head injured" patient.

REFERENCES

1. Gennarelli, TA, Spielman, GM, Langfitt, TW, et al (1982) Influence of the type of intracranial lesion on outcome from severe head injury. J Neurosurg 56:26-31
2. Colohan, WMA, Gross, CR, Torner, JC, et al (1989) Head injury mortality in two centers with different emergency medical services and intensive care. J Neurosurg 71:202-207
3. Marshall, LF, Gantille, T, Klauber, MR, et al (1991) The outcome of severe closed head injury. J Neurosurg (Suppl) 75:S28-S36
4. Rosner, MJ, Becker, DP (1984) The origin and evolution of plateau waves: Experimental observations and a theoretical model. J Neurosurg 60:312-324
5. Rosner, MJ, Coley, I (1986) Cerebral perfusion pressure, intracranial pressure, and head elevation. J Neurosurg 65:636-641
6. Rosner, MJ, Coley, I (1987) Cerebral perfusion pressure: A hemodynamic mechanism of mannitol and the post mannitol hemogram. Neurosurgery, 21:147-156
7. Rosner, MJ, Daughton, S (1990) Cerebral perfusion pressure management in head injury. J Trauma 30:933-941

Continuous Monitoring of Transcranial Doppler, Jugular Venous Oxygen Saturation, and Quantitative EEG in Severe Head Injury

TOSHIYUKI SHIOGAI, EISHI SATO, YOSHIKI FUJII, KAZUO TAKEUCHI, and ISAMU SAITO

Department of Neurosurgery, Kyorin University School of Medicine, Mitaka, Tokyo, 181 Japan

SUMMARY

To prevent neuronal brain damage caused by circulatory and metabolic disturbances following severe head injury, we have introduced a continuous monitoring system of transcranial Doppler (TCD), jugular bulb venous oxygen saturation (SjO2), and quantitative EEG (qEEG). The clinical significance was evaluated in terms of autoregulation (decreased cerebral perfusion pressure, CPP), CO2 reactivity (hyperventilation), vasospasm and delayed focal ischemic lesions (CT), hyperemia and diffuse brain swelling (CT), and patients' outcome at one month after injury. The TCD, qEEG, and SjO2 (8 cases) of 46 comatose patients (ages 7-75, mean 46; 38 with focal and 8 with diffuse injuries) were monitored in acute phase for 2-14 days (mean, 6).

1) Decreased mean and end-diastolic velocity (VM, VD), and increased pulsatility index (PI) of TCD were significantly correlated with decreased CPP and EEG total power in patients with defective autoregulation. Zero VD was observed even below an abrupt CPP breakpoint of 40 mmHg, and indicated grave prognosis (all cases but one fatal). 2) Elevated VM and SjO2 (hyperemia) was associated with increased CPP but not always diffuse brain swelling (CT). Elevated VM and PI (vasospasm) and decreased CPP rarely resulted in delayed focal ischemic lesions (CT). 3) During hyperventilation, close coupling was identified in the order of flow (VM) and metabolism (SjO2), metabolism and function (qEEG), and flow and function. Barbiturates might alter the correlation between metabolism and function. In conclusion, continuous monitoring of TCD, SjO2, and qEEG has a complementary role in evaluating ischemia, hyperemia, and ensuing neuronal brain dysfunction in patients with severe head injury.

KEY WORDS: transcranial Doppler, jugular bulb venous oxygen saturation, quantitative EEG, computerized monitoring system, severe head injury

INTRODUCTION

Disturbances of cerebral circulation and metabolism play an important role of ensuing neuronal damage to the brain in patients with severe head injury (SHI). In order to accomplish early detection of neuronal dysfunction caused by derangements of cerebral blood flow (CBF) and oxygen metabolism, we have introduced a continuous monitoring system of TCD, SjO2, and qEEG. The clinical significance was evaluated in terms of autoregulation (decreased CPP), CO2 vaso-reactivity (hyperventilation, HV), vasospasm and delayed focal ischemic lesions, hyperemia and diffuse brain swelling (DBS), and patients' outcome.

PATIENTS AND METHODS

Forty-six comatose patients (Ages 7-75, mean 46; Glasgow coma scores 3-8, mean 4;38 with focal and 8 with diffuse injuries) were analysed. Decompressive craniotomy was performed for 30 patients. Pentobarbital was administered in 10 cases to control intracranial pressure (ICP). TCD and qEEG were monitored in all 46 cases, CPP in 36, and SjO2 in 8. Monitoring periods were every 10 minutes (2 minutes for CO2 reactivity test). The duration of monitoring was 2-14 days (mean 6) in the acute phase of SHI. TCD was measured in the middle cerebral artery (MCA) and three parameters were analyzed;1) VM, 2) VD, 3) PI = peak systolic velocity (VS)-VD/VM. EEG was recorded in parietal scalp (P3-A1 or P4-A2 montage) ipsilateral to TCD monitoring. The qEEG was calculated bypower spectral analysis:1) total power (TP) and mean frequency (MF), 0-30 Hz; 2) absolute and relative power densities, δ(0-4 Hz), θ(4-8 Hz), α(8-12 Hz), β(12-30 Hz).

Two major conditions were assessed on the basis of TCD findings and related to the patient's outcome at one month after injury (25 survivors, 21 dead). The first, comprising cerebrovascular autoregulation and CO2 reactivity, was analyzed during decreased flow velocity (FV) caused by decreased CPP and HV, respectively. Critical threshold of autoregulation to fatal brain damage and coupling of flow, metabolism, and function during HV also were assessed. The second, increased FV was evaluated in terms of the relationship between hyperemia and DBS revealed by CT and also between vasospasm and delayed focal ischemic lesions visualized by CT.

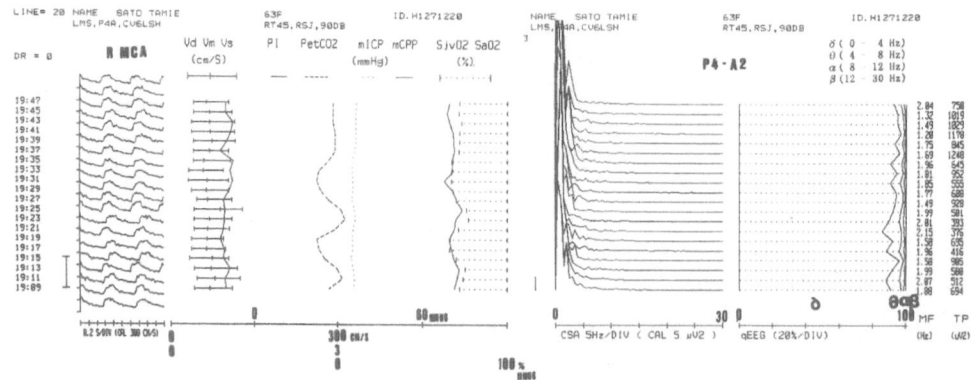

Fig. 1 Postoperative continuous monitoring during HV of a 63-year-old patient with acute subdural hematoma. The abbreviations used in the text were omitted.
Sequential changes recorded every two minutes are listed from bottom to top. From left to right: TCD waveforms in the right (R) MCA; parameters of TCD (Vd, Vm, Vs, PI); end-tidal CO2 partial pressure (PETCO2); mean ICP and CPP; SjO2; arterial oxygen saturation, SaO2; compressed spectral arrays (CSA) at right parietal scalp (P4-A2 montage), relative power spectral bands and parameters (MF, TP) of qEEG.

RESULTS

Critical Autoregulation Threshold to Fatal Brain Damage

Decreased VM and VD tended to correlate with decreased CPP in acute phase after SHI. In survivors, these correlations were not temporally stable because of individual or daily variance of physiological parameters. In fatal cases, however, significant close correlations were identified between, and in the order of, VM and CPP (maximal correlation coefficient, R = 0.93), PI and CPP (R = -0.73), and VD and CPP (R = 0.71). Furthermore, EEG TP significantly correlated with CPP (R = 0.81), with VM (R = 0.92), and with VD (R = 0.87). In the relationship between CPP and VD, especially, zero VD indicated an abrupt CPP breakpoint even below 40mmHg. This breakpoint differed in accordance with changes in individual physiological parameters. Of 20 cases in which zero VD was demonstrated during monitoring, all but one were fatal (95% mortality rate).

Increased Flow Velocity, Hyperemia, and Diffuse Brain Swelling

The relationship in 30 cases between increased maximal VM during all monitoring periods and mean CPP had a significant correlation (R = 0.48, p <0.01, n = 30). Almost all cases of increased VM (>100cm/s) demonstrated CPP of over 40 mmHg. Moreover, in a case of increased VM (>100 cm/s), there was a close correlation between VM and SjO2 (R = 0.54, p < 0.001, n = 69). DBS as demonstrated by CT, however, was identified only in three of 17 cases of increased VM (>100 cm/s). All three cases were eventually fatal.

Increased Flow Velocity, Vasospasm, and Delayed Focal Ischemic Lesions

Delayed focal ischemic lesions in the MCA territory without relation to cerebral contusion demonstrated by follow-up CT scans in 3 of 17 cases of increased VM (> 100cm/s). In one of the cases, three dimensional TCD mapping showed focal increases of VM (>100 cm/s) in M1 portion of the MCA three days after evacuation of acute subdural hematoma. Increased PI and decreased CPP were associated. Two of the three cases were survived.

Coupling Between VM, SjO2, and qEEG during Hyperventilation

CO2 vasoreactivity during HV ($\triangle$VM/$\triangle$CO2) was preserved in all six cases unrelated to age and therapy. There was a closer coupling of VM and SjO2 than of SjO2 and qEEG in all but one fatal case (TS, Table 1). However, coupling of qEEG and VM was not always obvious. In two patients who received barbiturates, a negative correlation between SjO2 and qEEG was detected.

Table 1 Correlations between VM, SjO2, qEEG during hyperventilation.

Case	Age	Type of injury	Days*	BT**	CO2 reactivity ($\triangle$VM/$\triangle$CO2)	Correlation coefficients (r)***		
						VM/SjO2	SjO2/qEEG	qEEG/VM
TS	15	diffuse	1	−	2.03	NS	0.73 (rα)	NS
TS	63	focal	5	−	3.70	0.74	NS	NS
SS	72	focal	4	−	3.04	0.58	0.36 (rα)	0.67 (rα)
TT	53	diffuse	5	+	1.27	0.71	0.52 (aα)	NS
MY	50	focal	3	+	2.87	0.62	−0.52 (rα)	NS
SI	40	focal	6	+	2.53	0.86	−0.74 (rβ)	−0.86 (rβ)

* days after injury; ** barbiturate therapy; *** NS = not significant,
rα = relative α activity, rβ = relative β activity, aα = absolute α power.

DISCUSSION

Decreased Flow Velocity, Critical Autoregulation Threshold, and Fatal Brain Damage

Cerebral pressure autoregulation in the acute phase of SHI is not only always impaired but is unrelated to outcome [1]. However, in terms of a lower limit of autoregulation, a relatively stable value of 40-60 mmHg CPP has been known [2]. In the fatal cases of our series, there were close correlations between TCD parameters and CPP below 40 mmHg, especially in between VM and CPP. This critical value was supported by other TCD studies [3]. Recently, a critical CPP value of 70 mmHg was pointed out in the relationship between CPP and PI or SjO2 [4]. In related to outcome, zero VD indicated by an abrupt breakpoint of even below 40 mmHg CPP [5] had a close relationship with fatal outcome [6]

Increased Flow Velocity, Hyperemia, and Diffuse Brain Swelling

Hyperemia after SHI is believed to be a highly association with intracranial hypertension [7]. Hyperemia with increased CBF, also is an important factor in developing increased FV of TCD. In our series, there was a significant relatinship of VM with CPP and SjO2. Moreover, increased FV rarely was associated with DBS determined by CT. These results suggested that increased FV caused by hyperemia is not always associated with severe intracranial hypertension. A lack of correlation between CBF and cerebral blood volume in hyperemic children has been pointed out [1].

Increased Flow Velocity, Vasospasm, and Delayed Focal Ischemic Lesions

Vasospasm is another important cause of increased FV in head injuries, especially traumatic subarachnoid hemorrhage [8]. Increased FV should be differentiated vasospasm (narrowing of vessel diameter) from hyperemia (increased CBF). To overcome this problem, measurement of the cervical internal carotid artery velocity [8] or of SjO2 [9] has been introduced. In this series, three dimensional TCD also was useful in detecting a focal increase of FV caused by vasospasm. Follow-up CT scan rarely delineated cerebral infarction in MCA territory. A relationship between development of delayed focal ischemic lesions and decreased CPP also has been suggested [9].

CO2 Reactivity and Coupling of Cerebral Circulation, Metabolism, and Function

It is generally believed that there is a strong coupling among the electrical activity of the brain, CBF and metabolism. In our SHI series during HV, close coupling was observed in the order of flow (VM) and metabolism (SjO2), metabolism and function (qEEG), and flow and function. In normal subjects, it has been pointed out that the coupling of metabolism and function was closer than flow and function during HV [10]. The coupling of flow and metabolism was especially strong irrespective of age, type of injury, and barbiturate therapy in this series. HV, therefore, is effective for such hyperemic patients.

REFERENCES

1. Muizelaar JP, Ward JD, Marmarou A, Newlon PG, Wachi A (1989) Cerebral blood flow and metabolism in severely head-injured children. part 2: autoregulation. J Neurosurg 71: 72-76
2. Miller JD, Bell BA (1987) Cerebral blood flow variations with perfusion pressure and metabolism. In:Wood JH (ed) Cerebral Blood Flow. McGraw-Hill Book Co. New York pp 119-130
3. Lunder T, Lindegaad K-F, Nornes H (1990) Continuous recording of the middle cerebral artery blood velocity in clinical neurosurgery. Acta Neurochir (Wien) 102: 85-90
4. Chan KH, Miller JD, Dearden NM, Andrews PJD, Midgley S (1992) The effect of changes in cerebral perfusion pressure upon middle cerebral artery blood flow velocity and jugular bulb venous oxygen saturation after severe brain injury. J Neurosurg 77: 55-61
5. Shiogai T, Tomita Y, Hara M, Takeuchi K, Saito I (1992) Estimation of cerebral perfusion pressure and intracranial pressure from transcranial Doppler sonography in comatose patients. In: Oka M, von Reutern G-M, Furuhata H, Kodaira K (eds) Recent Advances in Neurosonology. Elsevier Science Publishers BV. Amsterdam. pp 225-231
6. Shiogai T, Sato E, Tokitsu M, Hara M, Takeuchi K (1990) Transcranial Doppler monitoring in severe brain damage: Relationships between intracranial hemodynamics, brain dysfunction, and outcome. Neurol Res 12: 205-213
7. Obrist WD, Lagfitt TW, Jaggi JL, Cruz J, Gennarelli TA (1984) Cerebral blood flow and metabolism in comatose patients with acute head injury. J Neurosurg 61: 241-253
8. Weber M, Grolimund P, Seiler RW (1990) Evaluation of posttraumatic cerebral blood flow velocities by transcranial Doppler ultrasonography. Neurosurgery 27: 106-112
9. Chan KH, Dearden NM, Miller JD (1992) The significance of posttraumatic increase in cerebral blood flow velocity: a transcranial Doppler ultrasound study. Neurosurgery 30: 697-700
10. Kraaier V, Van Huffelen AC, Wieneke GH, Van der Worp, Baer PR (1992) Quantitative EEG changes due to cerebral vasoconstriction. Indomethacin versus hyperventilation-induced reduction in cerebral blood flow in normal subjects. Electroenceph clin Neurophysiol 82: 208-212

Cerebral Hyperemia Prior to Acute Cerebral Swelling in Patients with Severe Brain Injuries:
The Role of Transcranial Doppler Monitoring

Zainal Muttaqin[1], Tohru Uozumi[1], Satoshi Kuwabara[1], Kazunori Arita[1], Kaoru Kurisu[1], Sinji Ohba[1], Hiroaki Kohno[1], Hidenori Ogasawara[1], Minako Ohtani[2], and Takashi Mikami[2]

[1]Department of Neurosurgery and [2]Division of Emergency Medicine and Intensive Care Medicine, Hiroshima University School of Medicine, Hiroshima, 734 Japan

SUMMARY

Acute cerebrovascular congestion after a closed head injury is significantly related to intracranial hypertension. As an indirect method of cerebral blood flow measurement, transcranial doppler sonography (TCD) provides a rapid and noninvasive assessment of cerebral hemodynamic, including hyperemic condition.

TCD examination was serially performed in 35 patients with severe head injury with intact cerebral circulation; i.e. the mean flow velocity (MFV) patterns of the middle cerebral artery (MCA) didn't show signs of cerebral circulatory arrest such as systolic spike, to and fro, or no flow. The results showed that the MFV of the MCAs and ipsilateral extracranial internal carotid arteries (ICAs) in 9 of these patients increased sharply and pulsatility index decreased during 48-96 hours after the injury. This was soon followed by pattern of high intracranial resistance, consistent with elevated ICP in monitored patients and acute brain swelling on repeated computed tomographic (CT) scans. Correlation between increased MFVs, decreased PIs, and cerebral hemodynamic changes leading to acute brain swelling is discussed.

The number of patients who ended with severe disability, vegetative state, or death was 66% in these group of 9 patients, compared to only 34% for the overall 35 patients with severe head injury. Though the morbidity and mortality rates largely depend on the primary injury, the presence of acute cerebral swelling aggravate the grave course in these patients. And the ability of TCD to monitor the hyperemic state prior to edema should lead us to adjust the therapy in order to minimize the secondary insult related to intracranial hypertension.

KEY WORDS

Cerebral hyperemia, transcranial doppler, severe head injury, cerebral edema.

INTRODUCTION

Diffuse cerebral swelling after a closed head injury is mainly due to cerebral hyperemia and subsequent increase in cerebral blood volume, and not due to brain edema (1,2,3,4.5). This acute cerebrovascular congestion or hyperemia is significantly related to intracranial hypertension and unfavorable outcome (2,6). Several methods had been introduced to measure this hyperemic state, such as by measuring Hunsfield Unit on computed tomography (CT) (2,6), or by studying the cerebral blood flow (3,5,7).

The recent development of transcranial doppler (TCD) sonography had provided a rapid and noninvasive assessment of cerebral hemodynamic, especially blood velocity and pulsatility in the basal cerebral arteries (8,9,10). Aaslid et al (9) and Hennerici et al (11) reccommended the use of mean flow velocity (MFV) values to discriminate normal from abnormal, since it is less dependent on systemic cardiac factors. This measured velocities are proportional to flow in most circumstances (8,9,12,13,14). It therefore serves as a continuous index of cerebral blood flow in the measured vessels. Recently, Shigemori et al (5) using TCD sonography found that increase of MFV in TCD recording is strongly related to the development of diffuse cerebral swelling.

In order to examine the value of TCD monitoring in predicting hemodynamic phenomenas early after head injury, we presented 9 cases of severe head injury in whom acute increase of MFV and decrease of PI values preceded the acute cerebral swelling as clinically assessed and proved by CT examination and/or intracranial pressure (ICP) monitoring.

MATERIALS AND METHODS

Patients

54 patients with severe head injury (Glasgow coma scale 8 or less) were admitted to our emergency unit during four -year- period (April 1988 to March 1992) All patients were evaluated using TCD sonography starting from admission, and then every 12 hours during critical period and then daily until it is not needed anymore. Among these, 19 patient were admitted with an already compromised cerebral perfusion pressure, in whom TCD showed patterns of intracranial circulatory arrest (15). This group were excluded from further evaluation. The other 35 patients had their first TCD evaluation between 2 to 6 hours after the trauma, and they were considered as the base of our study. Among them, 9 patients (25.7%) were found to have abnormally elevated flow velocity of the middle cerebral arteries, more than 100 cm/second, during their course of treatment, and are presented here. There were 5 men and 4 women and their ages ranging from 4 to 49 years (mean 23.6 years). Glasgow Coma Scale (GCS) scores after non surgical resuscitation were 5 in 7 patients, 7 and 3 in the other 2 patients.

Examination technique

TCD studies were performed using a TC2-64 transcranial doppler (EME, Uberlingen, Germany). Transtemporal windows were used for insonation of the middle cerebral arteries (MCAs) in all patients. Simultaneous measurement of distal portion of the extracranial internal carotid artery, high in the neck, were also done in all cases. The measured MFV were displayed in centimeters per second (cm/sec.). Gosling's pulsatility index (13) (peak systolic velocity - end diastolic velocity / mean velocity) for each measurement was also calculated. CT scan was performed at admission and then repeated serially at regular intervals and when clinically indicated. ICP were monitored in 5 of these patients, using an epidural fluid filled-device (Nihon Kohden Corporation, Japan), or a fiberoptic device (Camino Laboratories, California). In two patients, carotid angiography was performed at the time when their TCD showed acute increase of MFV.

RESULTS

TCD evaluation on this group of 9 patients showed that MFVs on admission was 57.8+6.4cm/sec (mean+SE). It was then quickly increased and peaked during 48 to 96 hours after the injury, which was 132.4+5.9 cm/sec (mean+SE). The course of this change for each case is shown in Fig.1a. The MFVs of the distal extracranial portion of the internal carotid artery ,high in the neck, were simultaneously increased to about 72-82 cm/second. The normal range of which is 36.3+8.6cm/second (16). The pulsatility index (PI) value was 1.0+0.09 (mean+SE)on admission and soon went down into 0.65+0.06 (mean+SE) when the MFVs reached their peak values. The course of this change for each case is shown in Fig.1b. These high MFVs were soon followed by patterns of high intracranial resistance,i.e. diastolic flow velocity decreased and systolic peaks became more spiky, in 6 cases, and patterns of cerebral circulatory arrest leading to brain death- in one case, consistence with elevated ICPs on monitored patients. Repeat CT scans were taken within 24 H after the presence of this high resistance patterns, and acute swelling was noted from the absence or compression of cerebral cisterns in these 7 cases (Fig.2). This pattern of high intracranial resistance, observed in 6 patients, quickly worsened into patterns of cerebral circulatory arrest which led to brain death in 3, and normalized in the other 3 cases (case1, case8, and case9). Case1, with severe bilateral frontal contusion, ended up vegetative, while cases 8 and 9 were discharged two months later with mild disability.
The other two patients, case2 and case6, whom the high flow velocities on TCD were soon normalized and never had any pattern of high intracranial resistance, showed a better pictures regarding to edema on their repeat CTs. Case 2 was discharged with mild disability, and case 6, probably related to primary contusion of the brainstem, was bed-ridden with severe neurological deficit.

DISCUSSION

High flow velocity during TCD measurement has two possible interpretations, an absolute increase of cerebral blood flow (CBF) or a decrease of the vessel diameter without changes of the absolute CBF (compensatory increase of MFV during arterial spasm). Weber et al (17) and Lindegaard et al (16) excluded the possibility of intracranial arterial spasm by using ratio of MCA flow velocity to that of distal extracranial portion of ipsilateral internal carotid artery (ICA) high in the neck. Our data on these 9 patients showed that the MFV of both, the MCAs and ipsilateral ICAs, simultaneously increased sharply during the first 3 days after trauma and they reached more than twice above their initial values. Weber et al (17) assumed a spasm of MCA if the ratio of blood flow velocity in the MCA (VMCA) to the blood flow velocity in the ICA (VICA) exeeded 3 (normal value 1.7+0.4). In our cases, the highest value of this ratio was 2, observed in case 8, while the mean value for all cases was 1.91. Therefore, acute cerebrovascular hyperemia , rather than spasm, was assumed to occur in these patients. Angiography was performed in case 1 and case 2, during their peak of MFVs, and revealed no arterial spasm. Rozsa et al (4) studied traumatic brain swelling seen on CT using measurement of Hunsfield Unit, and found that in the first hours and days after head injury, diffuse swelling was caused more frequently by cerebrovascular congestion. Mchedlishvili (18,19), using experimental brain injury in dogs found that circulatory changes play a crucial role in the course of brain edema development, particularly the major cerebral arteries and pial arterial networks. Resistance to blood flow decreases as the pial networks dilates during pre-edematous period following brain trauma. This will soon changes to constriction as soon as edema has already developed. In our cases, the mean PI value decreased to about 63% of its initial value, suggesting changes of vascular resistance. Concerning cerebral vascular resistance, a very important fact explained by the Poiseulle formula (8) said that " flow resistance is inversely proportional to diameter in the fourth power ". This means that a modest increase of 10% in vessel diameter will result in about 32% decrease in resistance. As much of the resistance within the cerebral circulation is found within the arterioles, the decrease of PIs in our cases is believed to be related to the dilatation of cerebral arterioles, including pial arterial network, during pre-edematous period.

Any incremental increase in cerebral arterial blood volume gives an additional volume to the total intracranial volume i.e. increases the intracranial pressure. This and the vascular constriction observed by Mchedlishvili (19) caused the increase of PI values after edema has already developed. The results of ICP monitoring in 4 patients revealed that it fluctuated in a similar trend as the changes of PI values on TCD (Fig.3). ICP increased following the hyperemic phase, while at the same time the majority of TCD showed patterns of high intracranial resistance. We assumed this TCD pattern to be related to a critical value of the cerebral perfusion pressure (CPP) as also observed by Hassler at al (15). A further drop in CPP will change this pattern into a cerebral circulatory arrest, i.e. systolic spike, to and fro, or no flow, as exhibited by 4 out of our 9 cases.

The number of patients who ended with severe disability, vegetative, or dead were rather high, 6 out of 9 cases or 66%, in this group with abnormally high MFVs, compared with its reference group, which is only 12 out of 35 cases or 34%. Although the outcome of these severely head injured patients largely depend on the primary injury of the neural structures, this indirect measurement of CBF using TCD should lead us to accurately adjust the therapy in order to prevent and not to exacerbate the deleterious effect of acute cerebral swelling. Some modes of therapy such as dehydration cannot exert a beneficial effect in hyperemic condition, but it is good in edematous phase, while hyperventilation, suitable for hyperemic condition, is dangerous in edematous swelling for decreasing the already compromised CBF.

REFERENCES

1. Bruce DA, Langfitt TW, Miller JD, Shutz A, Valpalahti MP, Stanek A, Goldberg H (1973) Regional cerebral blood flow. intracranial pressure, and brain metabolism in comatose patients. J Neurosurg 38: 131-144.
2. Bruce DA, Alavi A, Bilaniuk L, Dolinskas C, Obrist W, Uzzell B (1981) Diffuse cerebral swelling following head injuries in children: the syndrome of "malignant brain edema". J Neurosurg 54: 170-178.
3. Muizelaar JP, Ward JD, Marmarou A, Newton PG, Wachi A (1989) Cerebral blood flow and metabolism in severely head-injured children. Part 2: Autoregulation. J Neurosurg 71: 72-76.
4. Rozsa L, Grote EH, Egan P (1989) Traumatic brain swelling studied by computerized tomography and densitometry. Neurosurg Rev 12: 133-140.
5. Shigemori M, Moriyama T, Harada K, Kikuchi N, Tokutomi T, Kuramoto S (1990) Intracranial hemodynamics in Diffuse and Focal Brain Injuries. Evaluation with Transcranial Doppler (TCD) Ultrasound. Acta Neurochir (Wien) 107: 5-10.
6. Yoshino E, Yamaki T, Higuchi T, Horikawa W, Hirakawa K (1985) Acute brain edema in fatal head injury : Analysis by dynamic CT scanning. J Neurosurg 63: 830-839.
7. Obrist WD, Langfitt TW, Jaggi JL, Cruz J, Genarelli TA (1984) Cerebral blood flow and metabolism in comatose patients with acute head injury. J Neurosurg 61: 241-253.
8. Aaslid R (ed) (1976) Transcranial Doppler Sonography. Springer-Verlag, Wien New York.
9. Aaslid R, Markwalder T-M, Nornes H (1982) Noninvasive transcranial doppler recording of flow velocity in basal cerebral arteries. J Neurosurg 57: 769-774.
10. Harders A (1986) Neurosurgical applications of Transcranial Doppler Sonography. Springer-Verlag, Wien New York.
11. Hennerici M, Rautenberg W, Sitzer G, Schwartz A (1987) Transcranial Doppler Ultrasound for the Assessment of Intracranial Arterial Flow Velocity- Part 1. Examination technique and normal values. Surg Neurol 27: 439-448.
12. Bishop CCR, Powell S, Rutt D, Browse NL (1986) Transcranial Doppler measurement of middle cerebral artery blood flow velocity: A validation study. Stroke 17: 913-915.
13. Gosling RG, King DH (1974) Arterial assessment by Doppler-shift ultrasound. Proc R Soc Lond (Biol) 67:447-449.
14. Kontos HA (1989) Validity of cerebral arterial blood flow calculations from velocity measurements. Stroke 20:1-3.
15. Hassler W, Steinmetz H, Gawlowski J (1988) Transcranial Doppler Ultrasonography in raised intracranial pressure and in intracranial circulatory arrest. J Neurosurg 68: 745-751.
16. Lindegaard KF, Nornes H, Bakke SJ, Sorteberg W, Nakstad P (1989) Cerebral vasospasm diagnosis by means of angiography and blood velocity measurements. Acta Neurochir (Wien) 100: 12-24.
17. Weber M, Grolimund P, Seiler RW (1990) Evaluation of Posttraumatic Cerebral Blood Flow Velocities by Transcranial Doppler Ultrasonography. Neurosurgery 27: 106-112.
18. Mchedlishvili G (1986) Arterial Behavior and Blood Circulation in the Brain. Plenum Publishing Corporation, New York-London.

19. Mchedlishvili G (1988) Pathogenetic role of circulatory factors in brain edema development. Neurosurg. Rev. 11: 7-13.

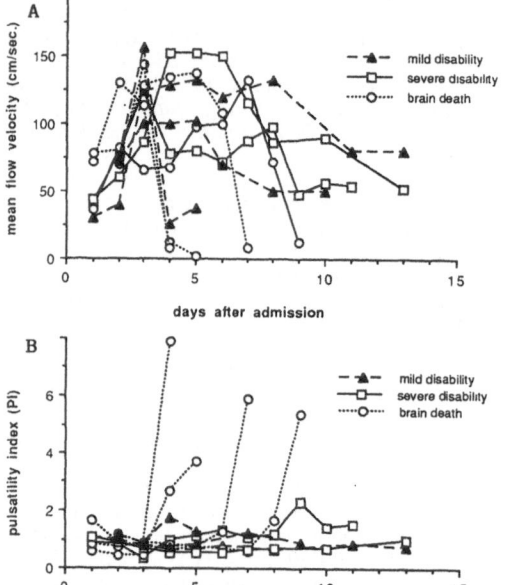

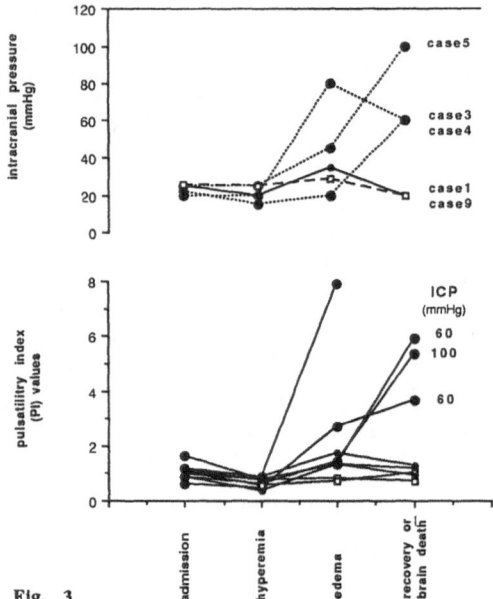

Fig. 1
A. Changes of mean flow velocities. of MCAs. Abnormally high flow velocities,showing hyperemic condition, were noted from the second admission day. They then decreased as edema has developed. In four cases (open circle) they ended up with cerebral circulatory arrest /brain death.

B. Changes of pulsatility indexes. They decreased until the third admission day, then began to increase as edema has developed, creating a TCD patterns of high intracranial resistance in 7 cases before ended up with brain death in 5.

Fig. 3
Pattern of changes of TCD pulsatility (lower graph) for all 9 cases, and changes of ICP in 4 monitored cases (upper graph). Note the similar trends in the fluctuation of ICP and TCD pulsatility during different phase of intracranial hemodynamics. They tend to stay low during hyperemia, and increased after edema has developed. Their normalization leads to recovery (open box and small solid circle), regardless of neurological status, and their progressivity leads to intracranial circulatory arrest and brain death (solid large circle).

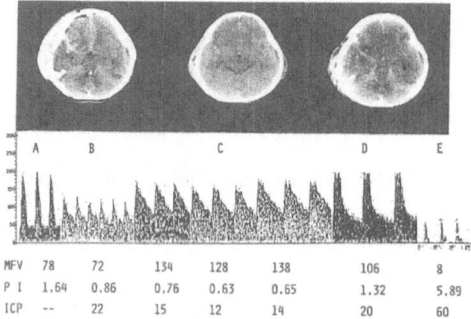

MFV	78	72	134	128	138	106	8
P I	1.64	0.86	0.76	0.63	0.65	1.32	5.89
ICP	--	22	15	12	14	20	60

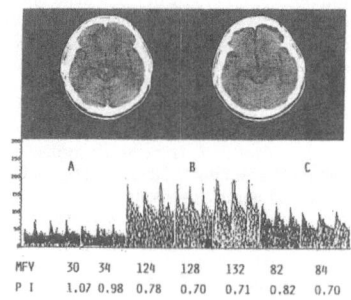

MFV	30	34	124	128	132	82	84
P I	1.07	0.98	0.78	0.70	0.71	0.82	0.70

Fig. 2a
Upper: CT scans of case 4; on admission (left), during the presence of high flow velocity on TCD (middle), and after high resistance pattern appeared on TCD (right). Note that the ambien cistern was initially tight, then loose, and finally obstructed during acute brain swelling. Lower: Results of TCD monitoring in case 4. The high resistance pattern seen on admission (A) was improved after non-surgical resuscitation i.e. controlled ventilation and mannitol administration (B), then changed into high flow velocity (C) on the third admission day, followed by high resistance (D) on the fifth day, before quickly progressed into cerebral circulatory arrest (E) on the same day. ICP increased progressively from 20 to 60 mmHg when this D pattern was observed.

Fig. 2b
Upper: CT scans of case 2; on admission (left) and when the high flow velocity was observed on TCD monitoring (right). High intracranial resistance pattern had never been observed in this case, which was discharged with only mild disability. Lower: Results of TCD monitoring in case 2. High flow velocity pattern appeared from the third until the seventh admission day (B), and then gradually normalized (C). High resistance pattern had never been observed during its course.

Investigation of Intracranial Haemodynamics by Means of Transcranial Doppler Ultrasonography After Severe Head Injury – A Clinical Study

László Novák, László Rózsa, Sándor Szabó, and Róza Gombi

Department of Neurosurgery, University School of Medicine, Debrecen, Hungary

SUMMARY

54 head injured patients were monitored by means of transcranial Doppler (TCD) ultrasonography. The diffuse brain swelling was evaluated by CT (15 mild, 9 moderate, 28 severe), 2 patients had only focal laesions. We assessed the Glasgow Coma Scale (GCS) by admission and the Glasgow Outcome Scale (GOS). The flow velocity (FV) in the middle cerebral artery (MCA) was monitored by admission and repeatedly depending on clinical state.

At the time of admission 20 patients (37%) showed decreased (lower than 50 cm/sec) FV in MCA[1]. However in group of severe brain swelling 18 patients (64.2%) had marked FV reduction. The TCD follow up revealed FV increase in 13 cases (more than 120 cm/sec) referring to definite vasospasm. There was no correlation between the occurence of vasospasm and the degree of brain swelling. At the time of admission in 6 patients TCD proved oscillating flow. All of them died.

Authors discuss the correlation between the vasospasm, main clinical characteristics and CT findings. They emphasize the prognostic value of TCD monitoring in severe head injury.

KEY WORDS: head injury, intracranial haemodynamics, transcranial Doppler ultrasonography, vasospasm, brain swelling

INTRODUCTION

Head injury requires continuous intensive monitoring. Transcranial Doppler sonography may have unique role to follow up the blood flow velocity changes and semiquantitatively the intracranial hypertension [1]. We examined the blood flow velocity changes following severe head injury and its correlation with CT, clinical condition and outcome.

MATERIALS AND METHODS

We monitored 54 severe head injured patients whose mean GCS score was 6.2 at the time of admission.

---

1 Abbreviation. TCD, transcranial Doppler; FV, mean flow velocity; MCA, middle cerebral artery; GCS, Glasgow Coma Scale; GOS, Glasgow Outcome Scale.

The Table 1. shows the summary of ages, sex and focal injury of patients.

Table 1. Age, sex distribution and focal injury of patients.

Total	n=45	
Age	4-82 years	
Average age	41 years	
Sex	male n=45	
	female n=9	
Focal injury	epidural haematoma	11
	acute subdural haematoma	13
	chronic subdural haematoma	2
	contusion	22
	intracerebral haemorrhage	11
	depressed skull fracture	6

The degree of diffuse brain swelling was evaluated in a modification of Ito et al. [2] according to Rózsa et al. [3] and classified into three categories.

1. **Mild**, when the cortical sulci, Sylvian fissure, third ventricle and perimesencephalic cistern were compressed, but visible, in CT scans.
2. **Moderate**, when one or two of the above structures were not visible.
3. **Severe**, when three or four of these structures were not visible.

We used a transcranial Doppler TC 2-64B device with a 8 MHz probe. The FV were recorded from MCA on both sides. The measurement were performed at the time of admission and repeatedly daily or more frequently depending on clinical state. The technique of TCD ultrasonography as well as normal results have been documented well before [4]. According to Aaslid [4] and to our earlier results [5] the normal FV ranged from 50 to 70 cm/sec. More than 120 cm/sec FV was regarded as vasospasm limit [6]. The outcome of patients was evaluated by Glasgow Outcome Scale. The patients were divided into groups according to degree of brain swelling. The mean velocities were calculated and significancy was determined by student's test.

RESULTS

15 patients had mild, 9 moderate and 28 severe diffuse brain swelling at the time of admission. 2 patients had only focal laesions. At the time of hospitalisation 20 patients (37%) showed decreased (lower than 50 cm/sec) FV in MCA , 20 patients (37%) had normal (50-70 cm/sec) and 8 patients (14.9%) had accelerated FV. In 6 patients (11.1%) TCD ultrasonography proved oscillating flow. All of them died. Figure 1. shows the mean FV in groups of patients with various degrees of brain swelling.

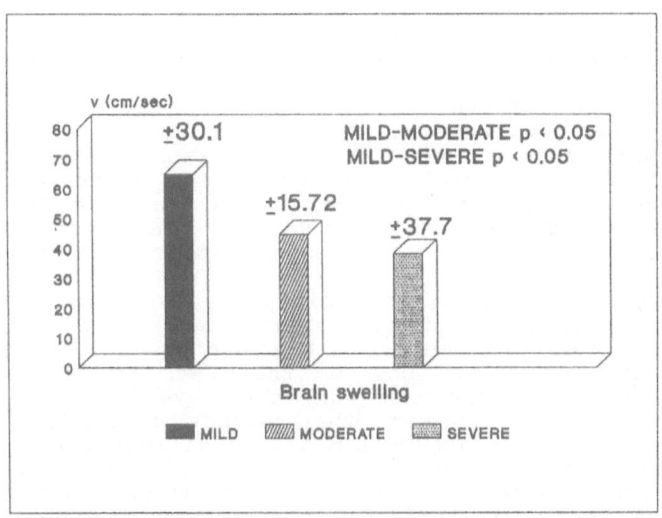

Fig. 1. Correlation of mean FV in MCA of patients with various degrees of brain swelling.

The mean FV in the group of patients with moderate diffuse brain swelling is significantly lower than in the group of mild diffuse brain swelling. The same correlation was observed between groups of mild and severe diffuse brain swelling. There was no significant correlation between moderate and severe diffuse brain swelling group. The mean FV value in group of mild diffuse brain swelling stayed within normal limits. The mean FV value is lower than 50 cm/sec in groups of moderate and severe diffuse brain swelling. 21 patients died. 6.6 % from mild (1 patient), 33.3 % from moderate (3 patients) and 60.71% from group of severe diffuse brain swelling (17 patients).

The TCD follow up revealed FV increase (more than 120 cm/sec) in 13 cases (3 /20%/ from mild, 4 /44.4%/ from moderate and 6 /21.4%/ from group of severe diffuse brain swelling) referring to definite vasospasm. 9 of these patients had contusion or intracerebral bleeding, 1 epidural , 2 chronic subdural, 1 acute subdural haematomas. The major clinical characteristics of patients with and without vasospasm are shown in Table 2.

Table 2. Major clinical characteristics of patients with and without vasospasm.

Vasospasm	Case Number	Mean Age /years/	GCS /mean/	GOS 1	2	3	4	5
present	13	35/10-56/	5.77	1	6	2	0	4
no	41	42.85/4-82/	7.02	13	8	5	0	17

GOS: 1, good; 2, moderate disability; 3, severe disability; 4, persistent vegetative state; 5, dead.

DISCUSSION

The FV in patients with severe diffuse brain swelling markedly decreased at the time of admission comparing with the group of patients with mild diffuse brain swelling. Certainly the elevated intracranial pressure can be the major cause of it. Thus TCD monitoring may closely refer to the intracranial pressure. The significantly higher mortality rate in the severe diffuse brain swelling group let us draw the conclusion that the decreased FV in MCA measured with TCD ultrasonography and the severe diffuse brain swelling seen on CT scans together suggest poor outcome.

The time course of vasospasm in severe head trauma is similar to that of following aneurysmal subarachnoidal haemorrhage [7]. Remarkable that 9 (70%) of patients with vasospasm had intracerebral haemorrhages or contusions. However there was no strict correlation between incidence of vasospasm and the severity of diffuse brain swelling. There is a tendency that higher incidence of vasospasm could be expected in the group of moderate diffuse brain swelling.
No significant difference was found in the clinical state and outcome between patients with and without vasospasm. The severity of vasospasm was not as serious as in aneurysmatic subarachnoid haemorrhage probably because the amount of blood entering into subarachnoid space is not as significant. Vasospasm could worsen the already existing ischaemia, therefore TCD monitoring is very important in planning of adequate therapy.

REFERENCES

1. Hassler W, Steinmetz H, Gawlowski J (1988) J Neurosurg 68:745-751
2. Ito U, Tomita H, Yamazaki S (1986) Acta Neurochir 79:120-124
3. Rózsa L, Grote EH, Egan P (1989) Neurosurg Rev 12:133-140
4. Aaslid R, Markwalder I, Nornes H (1982) J Neurosurg 57:769-744
5. Rózsa L, Gawlowski J (1987) Hung Radiol 61:154-162
6. Aaslid R, Huber P, Nornes H (1984) J Neurosurg 60:37-41
7. Seiler RW, Grolimund P, Aaslid R, Huber P, Nornes H (1986) J Neurosurg 64:594-600

Outcome of Patients with Severe Head Injury – Evaluation by Cerebral Perfusion Pressure

Akira Yoshida[1], Takeshi Shima[2], Yoshikazu Okada[2], Masahiro Nishida[2], Kanji Yamane[2], Shinji Okita[2], and Hidehiro Matsumoto[1]

[1]Department of Critical Care Medicine and [2]Neurosurgery, Chugoku Rousai Hospital, Kure, 737-01 Japan

Key words: head injury, intracranial pressure, cerebral perfusion pressure, barbiturate

INTRODUCTION

The outcome of patients sustaining head injury is affected by many factors: type of injury (diffuse or focal), coma level, age, intracranial pressure (ICP), cerebral perfusion pressure (CPP) and so on [1]. Of these factors, CPP is considered to be the most important because much of secondary brain insults are caused by ischemia through the reduction in CPP. One purpose of this study was to clarify the influence of CPP on the outcome of severely head injured patients. Another was to examine the effect of barbiturate therapy upon the outcome.

CLINICAL MATERIAL AND METHODS

This study population consisted of 32 patients admitted to our ICU within six hours after severe closed head injury. The mean age was 45.7 ± 20.0 years and the mean Glasgow Coma Scale (GCS) score was 7.4 ± 3.5 at the time of admission. Twenty-three patients had an initial GCS$\leq$7, while the remainder with an initial GCS>8 deteriorated to GCS$\leq$7 after entrance to the ICU because brain swelling or hematomas increased. Twenty-seven patients underwent emergency surgery, primarily for reduction of hematomas.

The monitoring of ICP was started using an epidural transducer (Ladd/Steritek) within 24 hours of the injury, and the epidural pressure (EDP) was continuously recorded. Systemic arterial pressure (SABP) was monitored from an indwelling radial artery catheter and CPP was calculated from the difference of SABP and EDP. The average EDP value (CPP value) of a 4-hour "block" was obtained by averaging the mean EDP (mean CPP) over four hours. All patients were treated with osmotic agent (10% glycerol 400–1600 mℓ/day), and the excessive urine volume was corrected by infusing electrolyte solutions. All patients were intubated, and $PaCO_2$ was controlled to about 30 mmHg. Barbiturate therapy (thiamylal 3–6 mg/kg/min) was initiated when EDP could not be controlled below 25 mmHg. The outcomes of the patients were determined by Glasgow Outcome Scale (GOS) six month after the injury.

RESULTS

The EDP monitoring period was 9.1 ± 5.3 days. Barbiturate therapy was performed in 22 patients for 7.7 ± 4.9 days, and dopamine (3-15 μg/kg/min) was added in 17 of them to maintain the CPP level. Three patients developed neurological deterioration following the reduction in the dosage of barbiturates.

Six patients died within 10 days after the injury (total mortality rate 19%), and seven were classified as persistent vegetative state or severe disability. The remainder (59% of the total) had good outcomes (good recovery or moderate disability). The time course changes of the 4-hour "block" mean EDPs and mean CPPs were as follows:

Dead group: Six patients died of uncontrolled intracranial hypertension within 10 days after the injury. All patients underwent surgery and five of them were treated with barbiturates. The initial EDP and the initial CPP in this group was 42.3 ± 13.0 and 49.2 ± 10.2 mmHg respectively. The EDPs increased above 50 mmHg and the CPPs decreased below 40 mmHg in all of this group (Fig. A, B). The five patients developed fully dilated and non-reactive pupils when the EDPs exceeded 50 mmHg (Fig. A).

Persistent vegetative state (PV) - Severe disability (SD) group: Seven patients were classified into this group. Six patients underwent emergency surgery and five were treated with barbiturates. One patient presented hypoxemia and shock at the time of admission. Three patients temporarily recovered well but later deteriorated because of systemic complications. The initial EDP was 19.6 ± 14.0 mmHg in this outcome group and the EDPs increased above 50 mmHg in two patients (Fig. C). The initial CPP was 73.6 ± 17.8 mmHg, and the CPPs never decreased below 40 mmHg during the monitoring periods (Fig. D).

Good recovery (GR) - Moderate disability (MD) group: Nineteen patients belonged to this outcome group. Emergency surgery was performed in 15 patients. Barbiturates were administered in the twelve (defined as the barbiturate group). The initial EDP was 15.2 ± 8.7 mmHg in the barbiturate group and 15.6 ± 8.8 mmHg in the non-barbiturate group. The EDPs tended to be higher in the barbiturate group, but never exceeded 50 mmHg (Fig. E, F). The initial CPP was 62.7 ± 10.5 mmHg in the barbiturate group, which was significantly lower than the value of the non-barbiturate group (81.1 ± 10.4 mmHg) [p<0.01]. The CPPs could be maintained above 70 mmHg in the non-barbiturate group (Fig. G), while they were in the 40-100 mmHg (mostly 40-70 mmHg) range in the barbiturate group (Fig. H).

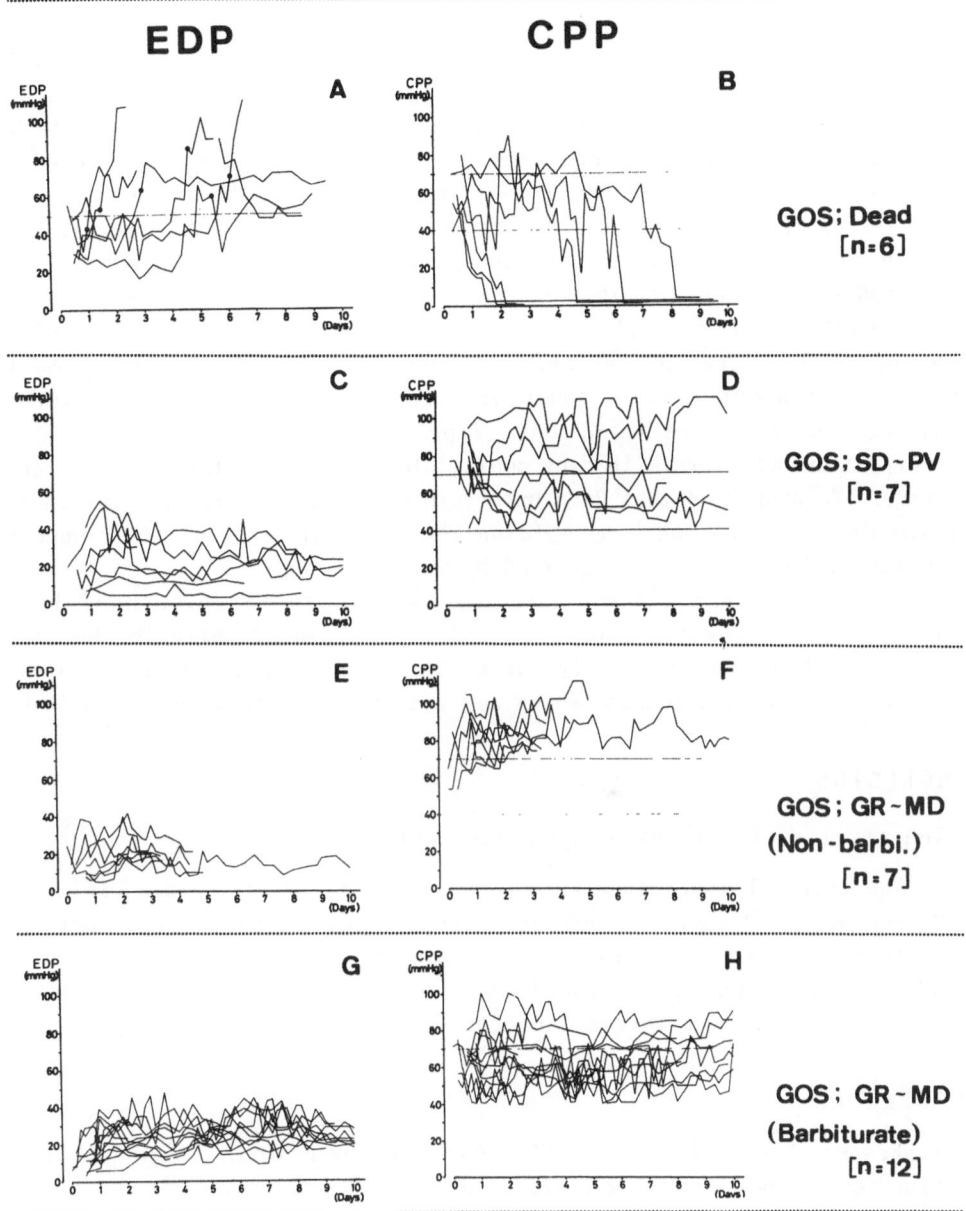

EDP

CPP

GOS; Dead
[n=6]

GOS; SD~PV
[n=7]

GOS; GR~MD
(Non-barbi.)
[n=7]

GOS; GR~MD
(Barbiturate)
[n=12]

Fig. A–H.   Time course changes of 4-hour "block" mean EDPs and CPPs in each outcome group.   Fig. A, B: GOS = Dead (n=6);   Fig: C, D. GOS = PV or SD (n=7); Fig. E, F: GOS = MD or GR without barbiturate therapy (n=7)   and   Fig. G, H: GOS = MR or GR with barbiturate therapy (Fig. G, H).   Closed circles in Fig. A represent the onsets of fully dilated and non-reactive pupils.

DISCUSSION

This study indicated that the mean CPP level of 40 mmHg was critical, which was quite consistent with the value reported by Tsutsumi et al.[2]. Although the optimal level of CPP in severely head injured patients is controversial, our results suggested that the mean CPP constantly greater than 70 mmHg was necessary for a good outcome when barbiturates were not administered. Rosner et al. advocate that the reduction in CPP promotes an increase in cerebral blood volume through the vasodilatory response of the brain, and thus causes a further increment in ICP and decrement in CPP [3]. The threshold of this vasodilatory "cascade" is considered to be about 70 mmHg for head injury (90-100 mmHg in more severe injury) [4], which is consistent with our results concerning the patients without barbiturate therapy. On the other hand, our 12 patients who accomplished a good recovery under barbiturate therapy could tolerate a lower level of CPP (40-60 mmHg). We suspected that deep barbiturate therapy lowered the threshold for vasodilatory "cascade" by holding the cerebral vascular resistance at a constant and high level as reported by Gray et al.[5].

Our results demonstrated that barbiturate therapy was useful for improving the outcomes of some severely head injured patients, but that barbiturate should be cautiously administered, because it often produces a potent circulatory suppression which may lead to a critical reduction in CPP.

CONCLUSION

The results of this study suggests that;

1. The mean CPP lower than 40 mmHg is critical in severe head injury.
2. The mean CPP above 70 mmHg is necessary for a good outcome, but this threshold can be lowered by barbiturate therapy.
3. Arterial hypotension should be avoided by vigorous treatment in practice of barbiturate therapy.

REFERENCES

1. Vinken PJ, Bruyn GW, Klawans HL (1990) Handbook of Clinical Neurology. Elsevier Science Publishers. Amsterdam, pp 367-395
2. Tsutsumi H (1986) Intracranial Pressure VI. Springer-Verlag. Berlin, Heidelberg. pp 661-666
3. Rosner MJ (1986) Intracranial Pressure VI. Springer-Verlag. Berlin, Heidelberg. pp 137-141
4. Gray WJ (1987) J Neurosurg 67: 377-380
5. Rosner MJ (1990) J Trauma 30: 933-941

Toxicity of Nutritional Support in the Traumatic Brain Injured

MICHAEL J. ROSNER and SHEILA D. ROSNER

The University of Alabama at Birmingham, Birmingham, Alabama, USA

SUMMARY

We have observed patients with severe traumatic brain injuries
deteriorate after institution of parenteral nutrition. We established
a protocol designed to test the hypothesis that "institution of
nutritional support would be associated with increased difficulty in
the maintenance of ICP/CPP and/or neurologic function."

Patients were managed using cerebral perfusion pressure as the primary
end point of therapy. After CPP was maintained by CSF drainage alone,
TPN at 1,000 KCal/d was begun. These calories were 60% glucose, 25%
protein and 15% lipid. Total fluid intake was maintained constant.
CSF drainage and pressor requirements, mannitol and other
interventions for management of changing neurologic or ICP/CPP status
were monitored and compared with "prenutrition" trends.

RESULTS: Complete data from 55 patients (GCS = 5.1 ± 0.1) were
available. Average CSF drainage requirements increased 45% (105 to
152 cc/day) over 72-96 hours after institution of alimentation. CPP
management index (mannitol + phenylephrine + CSF output) was
calculated for each patient and increased by 55%. Serum glucose
increased from 134 ± 69 to 149 ± 51 mg%. If nutritional support were
discontinued, the index reverted to baseline. Nine patients
deteriorated sufficiently to require cessation of nutritional support
and subsequently improved. Seven patients deteriorated slightly but
nutritional support was continued. The remainder of the patients
demonstrated alteration in physiologic trends but did not clinically
deteriorate and nutritional support was continued throughout.

Total mortality was 32% which represents superior results over prior
series. We conclude that early nutritional support in these patients
was not necessary for reduced mortality or morbidity and indeed this
"therapy" may potentiate intracranial hypertension and clinical
deterioration in 20% or more of the severely brain injured. Putative
mechanisms for this deterioration include glucose loading and
potentiation of "excitotoxin" mechanisms of brain injury. The
prejudice for early "feeding" in traumatically brain injured patients
must be re-examined.

KEY WORDS: Traumatic Brain Injury, Closed Head Injury, Excitotoxin,
Hyperalimentation, Glucose

INTRODUCTION

While the interest in alimentation of brain injured patients has increased, little attention has been given to the potentially adverse effects of caloric and amino-acid loading. Both toxicity of glucose loading [4,8,11] and amino acids which potentiate "excitotoxin" release [1,7] have been described. At the same time, enthusiasm for alimenting brain injured patients is based upon a demonstrated "hypermetabolic" state [2,3,9] and relatively minor systemic changes with alimentation rather than demonstrating improved neurologic recovery [5,6,12].

We have observed clinical deterioration in brain injured patients concommitant with the institution of alimentation. As a result of these observations, we have withheld additional caloric support in severely brain injured paitents until ICP had been controlled by CSF drainage alone. This has allowed us to prospectively test the following hypotheses.

1. Additional caloric support would be associated with an increase in intracranial pressure or effort required to maintain cerebral perfusion pressure at 70 mmHg or above.
2. A subset of patients would be identified who
   a. Clinically worsened and/or
   b. Required termination of alimentation in order to control ICP.

MATERIALS AND METHODS

Patients
   Traumatic brain injury GCS $\leq$ 7
   All patients CPP protocol (CPP $\geq$ 70 mmHg)
      Normovolemia
      Pressors used freely
      P_aCO_2 35 torr
      Fluids Intake = Output + constant
      Head of bed = 0°
Daily or qod measures of
   CSF output
   CSF lactate
   Mannitol
   Phenylephrine
   Albumin
   Electrolytes
   Glucose
   Others (Table I)
CPP "Index 1" calculated as
   Index 1 = CSF output (cc) + mannitol (gms) + phenylephrine (mg)

Table I: General Characteristics

	N	GCS INITIAL	CSF LACTATE INITIAL	AGE (YEARS)	NUTRITION BEGUN (HOSP DAY)
Overall Sample*	116	5.0±0.1	4.1±0.4	27.8±1.2	- - -
Study Sample**	71	5.3±0.1	4.4±0.1	27.5±1.6	11.5±0.8
Deteriorating Sample**	16	5.5±0.2	4.3±0.2	27.9±3.5	11.3±1.5
-TPN Stopped**	9	5.8±0.3	4.2±0.3	26.0±4.2	8.8±1.1
-TPN Continued**	7	5.1±0.4	4.4±0.3	30.4±6.0	9.3±2.2

*   Consecutively admitted to CPP protocol
**   Patients still with ventriculostomy at time alimentation begun

RESULTS

Table II provides representative values for selected parameters at the outset of alimentation (Nday=0), the four days prior (Nday=4) and immediately following (Nday=4) alimentation. Glucose rose from 121 mg% (Nday=0) to 150 mg% over the next four days. The gradual decline from Nday - 4 to -1 was reversed (131 mg% to 121 mg%). The effort required for ICP-CPP management increased 100% (94 to 182 "Index 1").

The group that deteriorated (Table III, N=16) demonstrated similar patterns of increasing hyperglycemia altering the previous trend toward normality, and an increase in ICP-CPP control index of 30-40%.

The group deteriorating to the point of withholding TPN (N=9) showed their highest ICP concomitant with feeding (Nday = 0), ceased their clinical improvement (GCS static $\leq$ 8.4) and some worsened. Index 1 increased 40-50%.

All groups demonstrated a slight (some individuals $\geq$ 50%) increase in CSF lactate.

DISCUSSION

Alimentation leads to an increase in the effort necessary to maintain intracranial pressure and cerebral perfusion pressure. This increase is frequent in the brain injured population though variable. It is severe enough to warrant withholding of nutritional support in the majority of patients until ICP is controlled by CSF drainage alone. Even at that point, the response to alimentation may lead to an increase in intracranial pressure and the effort required for its control in about 20% of patients. In 2/3 of these, the response may be severe enough to warrant discontinuation of alimentation until the patient is further stabilized.

The putative mechanism for this response is caloric loading via glucose [4,9,11] and potentiation of excitotoxin activity [1,7]. While increasing caloric intake may lead to hyperglycemia, the use of insulin or a natural tolerance to increased calories may limit the level of hyperglycemia yet not necessarily the adverse response.

The morbidity and mortality of this group of patients is superior to similar series [10] and brings into question the conclusions of those who feel alimentation is necessary.[2,3,5,6,12]

CONCLUSIONS

1. ICP/CPP "index" increases 50% or more after instituting an additional 1000 Kcal/day as parenteral nutrition. The putative mechanism is caloric loading via glucose or "excitotoxin" increase.
2. There is a subset of patients more susceptible to these effects which may relate to a lower "glucose tolerance".
3. Delaying alimentation until CSF drainage alone controls ICP does not deleteriously affect outcome, and brings into question the "dogma" or bias that early alimentation is necessary for a "good" outcome.

315

REFERENCES

1. Baethmann, A, Maier-Hauff, K, Schürer, et al (1989) Release of glutamate and of free fatty acids in vasogenic brain edema. J Neurosurg 70:578-591
2. Clifton, GL, Robertson, CS, Choi, SC (1986) Assessment of nutritional requirements head-injured patients. J Neurosurg 64:895-901.
3. Clifton GL, Robertson, CS, Contant, CF (1985) Enteral alimentation in head injury. J Neurosurg 62: 186-193
4. Ginsberg, MD, Welsh, FA, Budd, WW (1980) Deleterious effects of glucose pretreatment on recovery from diffuse cerebral ischemia in the cat. I local cerebral blood flow and glucose utilization. Stroke II:347-354
5. Grahm, TW, Fadrozm, DB, Harrington, T (1989) The benefits of early jejunal hyperalimentation in head-injured patients. Neurosurg 25:729-735
6. Hadley, MN, Grahm, TW, Harrington, T, et al (1986) Nutritional support and neurotrauma: A critical review of early nutrition in forty-five acute head injury patients. Neurosurg 19:367-373
7. Kempshi, O, von Andrian, V, Schurer, L, Baethmann, A (1990) Intravenous glutamate enhances edema formation after a freezing lesion. In Dong, et al (eds), Advances in Neurology 52:219-223
8. Rosner, MJ, Becker, DP (1984) Experimental brain injury successful therapy with the weak base, tromethamine with an overview of CNS acidosis. J Neurosurg 60:961-971
9. Rosner, MJ, Newsome, HH, Becker, DP (1984) Mechanical brain injury: The sympatho-adrenal response. J Neurosurg 61:75-85
10. Rosner, MJ, Rosner, SD (1990) Cerebral perfusion pressure management in head injury. J Trauma 30:933-941
11. Waters, DC, Hoff, JT, Black, KL (1986) Effect of parenteral nutritional on cold-induced vasogenic edema in cats. J Neurosurg 64:460-465
12. Young, B, Oh, L, Twyman, D, et al (1987) The effect of nutritional support on outcome from severe head injury. J Neurosurg 67:668-676

Table II: Patients tolerating nutritional support (N = 55)

(Nday *) Nutrition Day	-4	-3	-2	-1	0	1	2	3	4
GCS	8.09± 0.4	8.5 ± 0.4	9.2 ± 0.5	9.1 ± 0.5	9.6 ± 0.5	9.9 ± 0.5	9.7 ± 0.5	9.7 ± 0.5	9.9 ± 0.5
Highest ICP	28.1 ± 1.4	26.7 ± 1.1	27.4 ± 1.2	26.0 ± 1.1	27.1 ± 1.3	25.1 ± 1.0	27.7 ± 1.7	27.4 ± 2.3	29.8 ± 3.6
SABP	104.2 ± 2.2	105.6 ± 1.8	104.3 ± 1.4	103.3 ± 1.4	103.2 ± 1.7	103.2 ± 2.0	105.4 ± 2.1	104.9 ± 2.1	105.6 ± 2.1
ICP	20.8 ± 0.9	19.8 ± 0.7	19.6 ± 0.6	19.9 ± 0.6	19.9 ± 0.7	19.6 ± 0.8	19.8 ± 0.9	18.8 ± 1.1	19.8 ± 1.3
CPP	84.2 ± 1.9	86.8 ± 1.9	85.4 ± 1.7	85.1 ± 1.5	83.9 ± 1.9	85.8 ± 2.4	87.6 ± 2.6	86.9 ± 3.1	87.4 ± 4.1
Serum Glucose	131.2 ± 5.6	126.7 ± 4.8	122.0 ± 4.3	121.2 ± 4.3	121.1 ± 4.9	133.4 ± 4.5	139.6 ± 6.6	152.5 ±10.6	150.1 ±12.3
CSF Lactate	2.5 ± 0.2	2.5 ± 0.2	2.6 ± 0.2	2.4 ±0.2	2.4 ± 0.2	2.6 ± 0.3	2.3 ± 0.3	2.2 ± 0.3	2.7 ± 0.6
Net I&O	284.0 ±239.8	364.6±160.5	237.3±113.0	767.6±492.4	395.0 ±140.8	423.0±135.7	594.6±154.5	132.8±390.3	540.3±165.4
CSF Out	127.8 ± 16.8	123.1 ±13.8	101.7 ±14.8	2.4 0.2	84.4 ± 16.7	81.1 ±17.0	92.1 ±19.1	137.6 ±24.1	180.1 ±23.2
ICP Therapy Index	167.5 ± 19.4	150.8 ±17.2	119.0 ±17.3	122.9 ±18.2	94.0 ± 18.8	87.6 ±17.8	104.2 ±21.1	140.1 ±25.3	181.9 ±23.5

* Nday 0 = day alimentation was begun

317

Table III: Patients who deteriorated after alimentation (N = 16)

(Nday*) Nutrition Day	-4	-3	-2	-1	0	1	2	3	4
GCS	7.4 ± 0.8	8.5 ± 0.6	8.5 ± 0.5	8.8 ± 0.5	8.8 ± 0.7	9.2 ± 0.7	9.6 ± 0.7	9.6 ± 0.6	9.5 ± 0.5
Highest ICP	27.6 ± 2.3	26.1 ± 2.1	27.0 ± 1.6	29.0 ± 1.6	29.7 ± 1.8	33.2 ± 3.5	28.9 ± 2.5	24.6 ± 2.3	26.2 ± 1.9
SABP	107.3 ± 4.3	105.8 ± 4.2	104.5 ± 3.7	103.3 ± 2.0	102.6 ± 2.8	104.4 ± 3.1	103.5 ± 3.2	105.3 ± 3.1	104.0 ± 2.
ICP	19.9 ± 1.8	20.6 ± 1.4	19.8 ± 1.1	20.5 ± 0.8	20.9 ± 1.0	21.9 ± 1.2	19.8 ± 1.5	18.7 ± 1.3	19.8 ± 1.4
CPP	86.9 ± 3.6	86.2 ± 3.6	85.2 ± 3.8	83.5 ± 2.3	82.1 ± 2.9	84.1 ± 2.8	84.4 ± 2.8	87.5 ± 3.8	85.7 ± 3.
Serum Glucose	151.9 ± 12.4	135.7 ± 6.9	129.4 ±10.6	119.5 ± 8.6	118.5 ± 7.1	136.1 ± 7.8	135.3 ±11.2	138.3 ± 6.8	150.9 ±13.
CSF Lactate	2.9 ± 0.6	2.8 ± 0.3	2.6 ± 0.3	2.3 ± 0.2	2.3 ± 0.2	2.4 ± 0.3	2.5 ± 0.2	2.2 ± 0.2	2.1 ± 0.2
Net I&O	649.4 ±245.6	538.3±326.4	873.6±276.9	592.2±374.1	582.4 ±314.3	744.6±302.3	855.6±214.1	717.3±205.9	1094.7±36.
CSF Out	117.7 ± 22.3	117.8 ±20.8	136.4 ±27.6	133.5 ±24.0	109.8 ± 27.3	97.1 ±23.8	90.6 ±24.4	146.1 ±33.5	137.4 ±36.
ICP Therapy Index	157.0 ± 32.3	174.1 ±31.5	167.4 ±34.4	145.9 ±24.6	121.3 ± 30.0	110.5 ±27.7	114.5 ±24.9	164.1 ±40.0	154.3 ±40.

* Nday 0 = day alimentation was begun

A New Potential Therapy for Treatment of Posttraumatic Brain Oedema Based on Haemodynamic Principles for Brain Volume Regulation

PER-OLOF GRÄNDE[1,2], BOGI ASGEIRSSON[1,2], and CARL-HENRIK NORDSTRÖM[3]

[1]Departments of Anaesthesia and Intensive Care, [2]Physiology and Biophysics, and [3]Neurosurgery University Hospital and University of Lund, Sweden

SUMMARY

The therapy of brain oedema described is based on the haemodynamic effects of an increase in capillary permeability of the semipermeable blood-brain barrier (BBB). The transcapillary fluid fluxes are normally controlled by the crystalloid osmotic pressure differences. After a trauma when the BBB is more open for solutes these fluxes will instead be controlled by the colloid osmotic and hydrostatic capillary pressures and will tend towards a Starling fluid equilibrium causing an interstitial or vasogenic oedema. Therefore, an aim of a potential therapy of posttraumatic brain oedema should be to decrease hydrostatic capillary pressure and to preserve a normal colloid osmotic pressure. We present a clinical application of this hypothesis by reducing hydrostatic capillary pressure via precapillary vasoconstriction as obtained by infusion of dihydroergotamine and, if necessary, also by decreasing blood pressure by means of β_1-blockade and α_2-stimulation (clonidine). Colloid osmotic pressure is maintained with albumin infusions. Preliminary results indicate that this treatment of brain oedema after a head trauma is effective in decreasing ICP, increasing survival rate and improving outcome.

KEY WORDS: brain oedema, head trauma, blood-brain barrier, capillary pressure, colloid osmotic pressure

INTRODUCTION

For proper function, the volume regulation must be more precise in the brain than in other tissues to prevent compromized increase in intracranial pressure (ICP), the brain being enclosed in a rigid cranium. Brain volume variations are normally buffered by variations in cerebral blood and cerebrospinal fluid (CSF) volumes, but this buffer capacity is quite small and, when it is consumed, compliance of the brain is significantly reduced [1]. Even a moderate increase in brain volume will now cause a large increase in ICP. A raised ICP may have deleterious circulatory effects in terms of decrease in cerebral blood flow related to the decrease in cerebral perfusion pressure (CPP) with jeopardized tissue nutrition. Herniation at high ICP is a dreaded and often lethal complication. A high ICP and a low CPP are two prognostic factors discussed contributing to poor outcome after a head trauma [1-5].

Though therapy of brain oedema varies between different centres it always aims at reducing ICP and always at preserving a high CPP. A high CPP is considered to be important for assuring adequate nutrition as ischaemia is considered to be a main triggering factor for the development of oedema [3-6]. It is even suggested that a decrease in ICP at the expense of CPP should be avoided [4,6] and a CPP above 70-80 mmHg is a common recommendation [4-7]. ICP can be reduced by reduction of intracranial blood volume, by mobilizing fluid from brain tissue to blood and by decreasing the CSF volume. In clinical practice, blood volume is reduced by inducing arterial vasoconstriction as obtained by hyperventilation (hypocapnic vasoconstriction) [1] or by high doses of barbiturate infusions (hypometabolic vasoconstriction), most often down to a so called "burst supresssion pattern" [1,8] or, as lately suggested, by infusion of indomethacin [9]. Infusion of hyperosmotic agents like mannitol, urea [1,9,10] and, lately, hyperosmolar sodium chloride [11] is used to mobilize fluid from the brain tissue to blood via osmotic absorbtion. CSF volume can be decreased by diuretics like furosemide and carbon anhydrase inhibitors

[1] and more directly by CSF drainage via an intraventricular catheter.

No doubt all these therapies are initially effective in reducing a raised ICP, but objections can be made both from a theoretical point of view and from clinical experience regarding their long-term effects. Thus, mortality is high in severely head injuried patients (correlated to Glascow Coma Scale sum score below 5) in spite of optimal use of available therapies, with a mortality in most materials above 50% [5,12]. The arterial blood volume buffer capacity is small as most of the blood in a tissue (70%) is located on the venous side. As soon as the arterial vasoconstriction has occured, the capacity of this tool to decrease ICP is consumed. An uncontrolled arterial vasoconstriction may also lead to an undesired decrease in blood supply with risk of hypoxia.

The vascular effect of hyperventilation is transient and tonus will return towards the initial vasodilator state within 4-6 hours in spite of continuing hypocapnia [1]. The capability to further increase ventilation from this hypocapnic state must be restricted. Also the vasoconstrictor effect of high dose treatment with barbiturates may turn towards vasodilation due to paralyzed and relaxed vascular smooth muscle, and a paradoxical increase in cerebral blood volume may occur [13]. The beneficial effect of osmotic agents on ICP is also transient as supported both from a theoretical point of view and from clinical experience [9,10,14]. The small urea molecule in particular quite easily penetrates the damaged blood-brain barrier (BBB) and the osmotic driving force for absorbtion will disappear. It may even be followed by a rebound increase in ICP due to osmotic filtration by accumulation of the osmotic drug [9,14]. The clinical experience of CSF drainage at a fixed pressure level is beneficial if used with caution. Still, there might be a risk of ventricular collapse after consumption of the whole natural CSF volume buffer capacity and this may lead to herniation.

Thus, objections can be made against the traditional treatment of brain oedema after a head trauma, not only from clinical experience, but also on a theoretical basis. A new treatment of these patients based on haemodynamic principles for normal tissue volume regulation is presented below.

THEORETICAL CONSIDERATIONS

Brain Volume Control with Intact BBB

A main difference between the brain and other tissues regarding normal volume control is the existence of a BBB which is impermeable not only for large molecules like albumin and other proteins, but also for solutes [14]. Therefore, fluid transfer across the capillary membrane is mainly controlled by the transcapillary crystalloid osmotic pressure differences; the much smaller colloid osmotic and hydrostatic capillary pressures (via Starling fluid equilibrium) may be more or less neglected [14]. The impermeability of the BBB implies that a filtrate passing through the capillaries is dilute with a low osmolarity and will successively lower total osmotic capacity on the interstitial side making such fluid transport self-limiting. This sophisticated interplay between solutes, water flows and crystalloid osmotic gradients effectively controls brain volume within accepted limits. It can also be argued, quite hypothetically, that the brain volume to some extent is "autocontrolled" in the sense that increased tissue pressure will counteract further transcapillary filtration by reducing transcapillary hydrostatic driving force.

Brain Volume Control with Disrupted BBB

The transcapillary fluid fluxes in areas with disrupted BBB are no longer controlled by the crystalloid osmotic pressure differences as solutes more or less freely pass across the capillary membrane. Instead, the fluids must strive towards a pressure force equilibrium between the colloid osmotic and hydrostatic capillary pressures (Starling fluid equilibrium), as in organs with high capillary permeability for solutes. The existence of fluid filtration indicates a driving force from the hydrostatic transcapillary pressure difference that is larger than that from the colloid osmotic pressure difference.

320

Pathophysiological Aspects of a Posttraumatic Brain Oedema

Haemodynamic studies in patients with severe traumatic brain lesions show that blood flow varies from low to very high values [15,16]. When relating blood flow to metabolic demand of the tissue, blood flow is rarely so low that global ischaemia will occur [15,16]. No doubt, there are contusion areas after a trauma with a significant decrease in blood perfusion [5,16]; still both hyper and hypoaemia are described in the margin zones [17]. Impairment of cerebral autoregulation may also be indicative of hyperaemia (and increase in capillary pressure) as this alone must imply vasodilation.

The "tight" BBB increases its permeability after a trauma [18]. Most likely, there is a great variation in this respect within the damaged brain, ranging from less injured areas with preserved and impermeable BBB and normal volume regulation up to the most injured areas where even large molecules like albumin may penetrate [18]. In any case, there is a dysfunction of the normal volume control of the brain in areas where solutes can freely pass the capillary membrane and this implies that hydrostatic capillary pressure as a driving force for filtration can be significant and contribute to the oedema development. A low colloid osmotic driving force may contribute to the filtration as depressed S-albumin is common in patients with severe head injury [19].

The New Concept for Treatment of Posttraumatic Brain Oedema

Based on these considerations, the perfect therapy would be restitution of the damaged BBB. There is no drug available, however, with such features, even though various types of cytokine inactivators may have such potentially beneficial effects. Instead, we introduce a concept for treatment of brain oedema based on a Starling fluid equilibrium at a brain volume which is acceptable regarding the ICP level. The concept aims at decreasing hydrostatic capillary pressure and preserving a normal colloid osmotic pressure.

CLINICAL APPLICATION AND RESULTS

This concept is applied in our ICU (approved by ethical committee) on the most severely head injured patients with lack of so called cerebral blood flow response to hyperventilation where mortality is shown to be close to 100 %.[20]. Dihydroergotamine (1.5µg/kg/h i.v.) is used as a potential drug to decrease hydrostatic capillary pressure via precapillary vasoconstriction as discussed in a previous paper [21]. If necessary, capillary pressure can be further decreased by active reduction of arterial blood pressure as obtained by ß1-blockade (max 20 µg/kg/h i.v) and clonidine (max 1µg/kgx8 i.v.); 50 mmHg (40 mmHg in small children) was stated as the lowest accepted perfusion presssure value with a zero baseline for both ICP and arterial pressure defined at the forehead. The colloid osmotic pressure, as evaluated by S-albumin, was maintained with albumin (20%) infusions. Moreover, the brain metabolism was decreased by thiopental but at a low dose (max 1-2mg/kg/h i.v) to avoid the well-known side-effects of this treatment [13,22]. The patients were slightly hyperventilated ($PaCO_2$ 4.0-4.5kPa). Temporary ICP peaks after suction etc were damped prophylactically by i.v. bolus doses of thiopental or xylocain.

Preliminary results show that ICP is effectively reduced in most patients and to values below 20 mm Hg within a few hours. 9 of the 11 patients survived and to good recovery or moderately disabled rated according to the Glasgow Outcome Scale (12) six month after the accident. Patients with preserved response to hyperventilation with an ICP above 20 mmHg are nowadays also given this therapy and preliminary results show an overall mortality rate below 20 % also in this group (n=18).

DISCUSSION

The results indicate that this new therapy of posttraumatic brain oedema may be a valuable complement to traditional treatments and that the interstitial oedema (vasogenic oedema) is significant. It may be that the intracellular component of the oedema has been overemphasized as well as ischaemia as a triggering factor. A high perfusion pressure may in fact induce further capillary filtration, aggravating the oedema (cf 15). No doubt, there is a lower limit for blood pressure below which ischaemia will appear and must be avoided, but apparently this level is not reached at perfusion pressures above 50 mmHg (40 mmHg in small children). The optimal therapy may be to strike the balance between a low perfusion pressure level below which ischemia will appear and a high level above which the oedema will increase due to filtration.

DHE is known to be a constrictor of venous capacitance vessels [21]. We have shown that DHE is also a precapillary vasoconstrictor causing decrease in capillary hydrostatic pressure and fluid absorbtion [21]. DHE thus has the dual effect of reducing blood volume both via arterial and capacitance constriction and via fluid absorbtion. The significant increase in urine production during the first hours after start of the DHE infusion seems to verify these features. A slow-down of this voluminous urine output by ADH analogue is contraindicated as water balance in these patients must be negative. The decrease in blood pressure was instituted by administration of ß1-blockade and α2-stimulation (clonidine) as only these hypotensive mechanisms lower blood pressure without a simultaneous cerebral vasodilation. Cerebral vasodilation may counteract the purpose of decreasing capillary pressure.

Even though this concept for treatment of a posttraumatic brain oedema seems to be promising on a theoretical basis and from the preliminary clinical results, it is for the future to show show if it is a valuable complement to or superior to the traditional treatment.

REFERENCES

1) Borel C, Hanley D, Diringer MN and Rogers MC (1990) Chest 98:180-189
2) Marshall LF, Smith RW, Shapiro HM (1979) J Neurosurg 50:20-25.
3) Becker DP, Miller JD, Ward JD, Greenberg RP, Young HF and Sakalas R (1977) J Neurosurg 47:491-502
4) Rosner MJ and Daughton S (1990) The J of Trauma 30,8:933-941
5) Marmarou A, Anderson RL, Ward JD, Choi SC, Young HF, Eisenberg HW, Foulkes MA, Marshall LF and Jane JA (1991) J Neurosurg 75:S59-S66
6) Miller JD (1985) Br J Anesth 57:120-130
7) Chan KH, Miller JD, Dearden M, Andrews P and Midgley S (1992) J Neurosurg 77:55-61
8) Marshall LF, Smith RW and Shapiro HM (1979) J Neurosurg 50:26-30
9) Astrup J (1991) Curr opinion in Anaesth 4:653-656
10) Abou-Madi H, Trop D, Abou-Madi N, Ravussin P (1987) Br J Anaest 59:630-639
11) Todd MM, Tommasino C and Moore S (1985) J Neurosurg 63:944-948
12) Marshall LF and Bower Sa (1985) Outcome prediction in severe head injury: In Wilkin RH, Rengachary SS (eds). Neurosurgery New-York. Mc Graw-Hill 1605-1608
13) Grände PO, Gustafsson D and Lindberg L (1990) Intensive Care Med 16:399-404
14) Fenstermacher JD (1984) Volume regulation of the central nervous system IN:Staub NC,Taylor AE (eds). Oedema. Raven Press, New York pp 383-404
15) Obrist WD, Langfitt TW, Jaggi JL, Cruz J and Gennarelli TA (1984) J Neurosurg 61:241-253
16) Marion DW, Darby J, Yonas H (1991) J Neurosurg 74: 407-414
17) Overgaard J, Tweed WA (1983) J Neurosurg 59:439-446
18) Todd NV and Graham DI (1990) Acta Neurochirurgica Suppl 51:296-299
19) Craig J, McClain MD, Henning B, Ott LG Goldblum S and Young AB (1988) J Neurosurg 69:386-392
20) Schalén W, Messeter K and Nordström CH (1991) Acta Anaesthesiol Scand 35:113-122
21) Grände PO. Intensive Care Med 15:523-527
22) Schalén W, Messeter K and Nordström CH (1992) Acta Anaesthesiol Scand 36

ACKNOWLEDGEMENTS

The study was supported by grants from the Swedish Medical Research Council (2210), Faculty of Medicine University of Lund, Sweden and the Swedish Society of Medicine.

How Low ICP Should Be Controlled in Acute Stage of Severe Head Injury Cases

KINJIRO IWATA, TOMOMI KOJIMA, KIYOSHI TAMAI

Department of Neurological Surgery, Aichi Medical University, Aichi, 480-11 Japan

SUMMARY

To care for acute stage of severe cerebral contusion cases, we have been using our ICP controller, which administers osmotic ICP reducer such as mannitol, whenever ICP rises above the "threshold level" and discontinues when ICP is reduced below the level by servo-mechanism.

We report 26 cases in which we monitored the ICP and evaluated the outcome of these patients. All 14 cases (54%), whose ICP could be controlled below 25 mmHg made good recovery, while all 8 cases (31%), whose ICP could not be controlled below 25 mmHg died or became vegetated. Therefore, 25 mmHg is the critical ICP level, and when it can be controlled below it continuously, the patients will have good prognosis.

KEY WORDS: ICP, ICP controller, head injury, mannitol

INTRODUCTION

The treatment of closed head injury, severe cerebral contusion type, sill remains a serious problem (1,2,3,5). The senior author and his group, previously monitored intracranial pressure (ICP) in a series of closed head injury and observed that some cases died without any increase of ICP. They were the victims of primary brain stem injury. In many cases, ICP elevation play an important role in pathology. Clinical endeavour should be aimed at the proper control of ICP during acute stage for better prognosis.

In addition, we investigated the efficacy of mannitol vs CBF autoregulation in these series. We observed that mannitol showed significantly less reduction of ICP, as well as, the rebound phenomenon of ICP rise afterwards (2).

ICP should be kept in physiological range to maintain sufficient cerebral perfusion pressure (CPP) continuously, day and night. At the same time, risk of cerebral herniation should be prevented from the abrupt rise of ICP (1).

For the better method of administration of mannitol to avoid physical complication, we have been advocating "intermittent and minimal dose fashion" under ICP monitoring. Therefore, we have developed the "automatic ICP controller" system for this purpose. From the experiences using our system, as well as, survey of the outcome of the cases, we report the issue of ICP level control for better prognosis with minimal complication.

MATERIALS AND METHODS

26 cases, 13 males and 13 females with average age of 33.5 y.o. (1 year old to 66 years old) were subjected to the ICP controlling system.

Table 1   26 cases with ICP controller

Head injury	16 cases
9 acute subdural hematoma	
6 contusion (DAI type)	
1 cranial compression	
Cerebral hemorrhage	6 cases
Brain tumors	4 cases
2 metastatic	
1 chondroma with hemorrhage	
1 cerebellar astrocytoma	

16 were head injury cases of which 9 were acute subdural hematoma, 6 contusion (diffuse axonal injury type), and 1 was cranial compression with parenchymal cerebral damage. All cases were comatose immediately after the accident, and all acute subdural hematoma cases had the evacuation procedure. The subdural pressure transducer was left in for subsequent cerebral swelling. All 6 contusion cases, CT showed significant intraventricular bleeding, and ventricular drainage were made together with the intraventricular CSF pressure monitoring beside the drainage tube. One severe cranial compression case with cerebral contusion was monitored by the epidural sensor, and ICP was successfully controlled. The patient made good recovery and returned to his previous occupation. Hematoma evacuation or stereotaxic drainage were performed on 6 cases of hypertensive cerebral hemorrhage, and ICP was monitored postoperatively because of predicted ICP rise. 4 cases of brain tumor were subjected to this treatment in their acute postoperative days.

In all cases, the families were well-informed of the procedure and gave their consent with strong request.

As the ICP monitoring method, the photofiber sensor of Camino 420 (Camino, U.S.A.) or semiconductor pressure transducer of Galtec (Company, Scotland) was used for brain surface ICP and parenchymatous pressure. Stathum's pressure transducer was used for CSF pressure from the ventricular tube.

Automatic ICP controller system (Iwata)(4)
As previously reported, this system is composed of 3 main devices, namely, 1) ICP monitor, 2) ICP controller, and 3) intravenous infusion pump. ICP controller contains the servo-mechanism which gives "on" signal to IV infusion pump when ICP exceeds a certain level (threshold) for 2 minutes. This works to control ICP plateau waves. This controller stops the IV infusion when the ICP becomes lower than the set threshold. Again when ICP rises above the threshold for 2 minutes, the device will signal "on". The rate of infusion is 100

ml/hr of 20% mannitol solution. ICP threshold must be set, in reality, to minimize the dosage of needed amount of mannitol according to the severity and dynamics of ICP pathology in each individual case.

Cerebral contusion in ICP controller

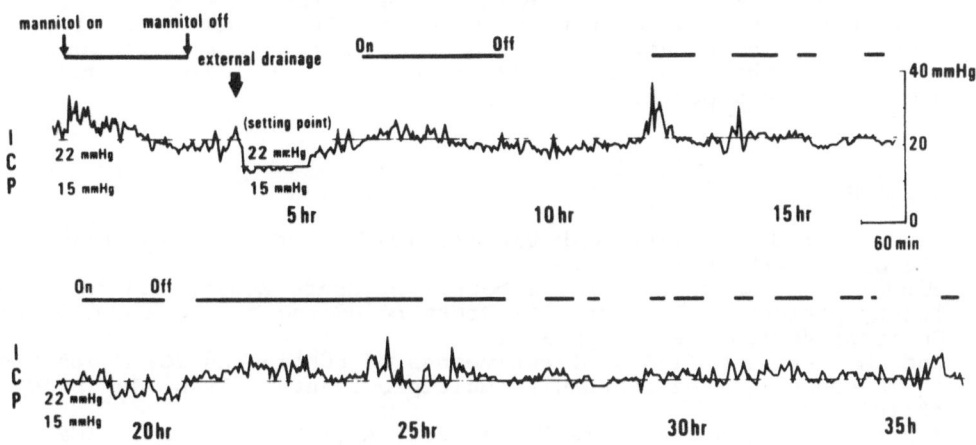

This figure shows the course of ICP controlled by the Iwata's device, administrating mannitol solution with ICP threshold of 22 mmHg high and 15 mmHg low. When ICP exceeds 22 mmHg for 2 minutes, drip of IV mannitol starts and stops immediately after ICP is reduced down to 15 mmHg. This patient recovered completely after ICP control treatment and went back to his previous occupation.

RESULTS

Table 2   Outcome of 26 cases treated with ICP controller

Outcome	Cases	Initial ICP mmHg	Threshold level mmHg				Uncontrollable
			<20	<25	<30	<35	
Good	14	20.3(10-25)	6	8			
Poor	4	30.5(28-35)	1	1	2		
Dead	8	36.7(27-70)		1		1	6

14 cases out of 26 (53.8%) had good outcome with ICP controller. Their initial ICP appeared to average 20.3 mmHg (10-25). 6 cases were controlled with less than 20 mmHg of threshold level, and in 8 cases it was possible to control with threshold of less than 25 mmHg. In 4 cases, whose initial pressure average 30.5 mmHg (28-35), their ICP could be controlled, 1 case less than 20 mmHg, 1 case less than 25 mmHg, and 2 cases had to be raised up to 30 mmHg. 8 cases died in the acute stage in which 6 cases the ICP could not be controlled by this method.

DISCUSSION AND CONCLUSION

There are few clinical literatures (3,4,5) discussing at what level ICP should be kept. This issue is still controversial. One thinks that CPP is an important parameter, but BP fluctuates so much that BP is another parameter to be controlled in those cases.

Our conclusion is that our experience using the automatic ICP controller with various setting of threshold level and the analysis of the outcome of those patients are relevant source of information. The conclusion is that ICP should be kept under 25 mmHg so that good prognosis can be expected.

REFERENCES

1. Iwata K (1974) Increased intracranial pressure. Neurosurgery (Japanese) 2(9):587-590
2. Tindall GT, Iwata K (1972) Subdural pressure monitoring in head injury patients. Intracranial Pressure edited by Brock and Dietz. Springer Verlage Berlin pp 9-14.
3. Endo M, Takano M (1989) Effectiveness of continuous ICP monitoring in management of patients with multiple injury. Iryo (Japanese) 43:1010-1013.
4. Iwata K, Yuasa H, Sugiyama T, Yamazaki A (1983) Automatic ICP controller: A new device. Intracranial Pressure V edited by Ishii S Spinger-Verlag Berlin, Heidelberg pp 157-159.
5. Marmarou A (March 1992) Increased intracranial pressure in head injury and influence of blood volume. J. Neurotrauma 9 suppl 1 pp 5327-32.

Improved Outcome from Traumatic Coma Using Ventricular CSF Drainage

Jamshid B.G. Ghajar, Robert J. Hariri, Katrina Schreiber, Kathryn Ko, Kaveh Bahramian, Laura A. Iacono, and Russell H. Patterson

The Aitken Neurosurgery Laboratory, Division of Neurosurgery, Department of Surgery, Cornell University Medical College, New York, NY 10021, USA

SUMMARY

The use of intracranial pressure (ICP) monitoring and the treatment of intracranial hypertension (IH) in severe head injury remain controversial. Hyperventilation, osmotic diuretics, barbiturates and steroids may contribute to secondary cerebral hypoperfusion in the traumatized brain. Ventricular cerebrospinal fluid (CSF) drainage, in contrast, is thought not to contribute to ischemia and may improve cerebral blood flow. This treatment, however, has never been evaluated as the sole therapeutic modality for IH.

Forty-nine patients with severe head injuries (Glasgow Coma Scale score ≤7) were entered into a prospective randomized study to assess the efficacy of ICP monitoring and CSF drainage for the treatment of IH. One group received ICP monitoring by ventriculostomy and CSF drainage for ICP greater than 15 mm Hg, while the control group received neither ICP monitoring nor specific treatment of IH. The mortality rate in the treated group was 12% compared to 53% in the control (p< 0.0001). Morever, 59% of patients returned to functional independence, based on their Glasgow Outcome Score (GOS), in the treated group compared to 2.% of the untreated patients (p< 0.0001). The percentages of vegetative and severely disabled patients did not differ significantly between groups. Outcomes for the treated group compared favorably with those of several previous studies of severe head injury.

This study demonstrates that ICP monitoring and treatment of IH in post-traumatic comatose patients significantly reduces mortality and increases the percentage of patients living independently. A graded approach to the management of IH, with CSF drainage as the principal treatment, is advocated.

Key Words: traumatic brain injury, intracranial hypertension, ventricular csf drainage, outcome, intracranial pressure monitoring

INTRODUCTION

Although it is clear that intracranial hypertension (IH) in severely head injured patients is associated with a poor prognosis,[1,2] and it is commonly assumed that treating IH can improve outcome, no prospective randomized clinical study has compared the efficacy of ICP monitoring and specific therapies aimed at reducing ICP to a control group with no monitoring and no treatment. Thus, while mortality from severe head injury has been reduced from 50 to 35% over the past 15 years,[3] the contribution of the treatment of IH has never been isolated from the contributions of advances in surgical management, diagnostic radiology, and critical care.

MATERIALS AND METHODS

The patient population for this study consisted of patients between the ages of 16 and 70 admitted to the New York Hospital-Cornell Medical Center or to the Jamaica Hospital-Cornell Trauma Center with non-penetrating severe head injuries during the three year period from January 1989 through December 1991. Severe head injury was defined as Glasgow Coma Scale (GCS) score $\leq$ 7 for at least 24 hours following initial resuscitation. Patients who met brain death criteria within 24 hours of admission were excluded.

Patients were assigned to one of two groups depending on the neurosurgeon on call for the day. Group I patients underwent placement of ventricular catheters for ICP monitoring and were treated by CSF drainage when their ICP exceeded 15 mm Hg. Group II patients had no ICP monitoring device placed and were not treated for IH. All patients were managed by a neurotrauma protocol that included intubation and ventilation to a PaO_2 of 100 mm Hg and a $PaCO_2$ of 35 mm Hg, CT scans, and prompt evacuation of significant subdural hematomas. Some patients were given 1 gm/kg mannitol on admission if they exhibited signs of impending cerebral herniation, but thereafter, mannitol was not administered for ICP management.

Patients in Group I received a frontal ventriculostomy, performed using the right angle technique,[4] within four hours of their arrival to the emergency room. CSF was drained at 15 mm Hg pressure to a desired endpoint of 10 mm Hg. Intracranial pressure was measured every hour and was averaged over an eight hour shift. Intracranial hypertension was defined as the average ICP greater than 20 mm Hg over an eight-hour shift.

RESULTS AND DISCUSSION

Forty-nine consecutive patients were entered into the study: 34 in Group I and 15 in Group II. The larger number of patients in Group I compared to Group II reflects the larger proportion of on-call days by neurosurgeons admitting patients for Group I protocol (ICP monitoring and treatment).
Demographics and specific clinical features are seen in Tables 1 & 2. The average GCS in Group I (5), was significantly ($p < 0.05$) lower than in Group II (6). There was no difference between groups in the percentage of patients who required craniotomies for evacuation of acute subdural hematomas. Ventricular ICP was monitored on an average for 4.3 days. ICP was effectively controlled by CSF drainage with the average, 13.3 mm Hg, below the clinical target of 15 mm Hg (Table 2). The incidence of IH (ICP greater than 20 mm Hg) was low (10%).

The Glasgow Outcome Score (GOS) for both groups at 6 months to 3 years following discharge is shown in Table 3. A 100% follow-up review was obtained. Mortality in Group I patients was approximately one-fourth the mortality in Group II patients ($p < 0.0001$), and the percentage of Group I patients living independently was approximately three times higher than the percentage of Group II patients living independently ($p < 0.0001$). The percentage of patients who were vegetative or dependent was not significantly different between the two groups

This study indicates that ventricular ICP monitoring and CSF drainage for IH in severely head-injured patients significantly decreases mortality without significantly increasing the percentage of vegetative or dependent patients, compared to a control group that was neither monitored nor treated for IH. We believe that the improved outcome observed in the treated group of severely head-injured patients presented in this study is attributable to a definitive, systematic approach to ICP management, with CSF drainage as the modality employed first , in contrast to multimodality treatments. CSF drainage alone was sufficient to control IH in the majority of patients and obviated the need to resort to additional methods of treatment in this study population. In addition, initiation of CSF drainage at an ICP of 15 mm Hg, in contrast to many other protocols that initiate treatment at an ICP above 20 or 25 mm Hg appears to be of valve. In summary, we recommend ICP monitoring in all comatose, head-injured patients. Our management protocol (Fig. 1) is based on early ventricular CSF drainage instituted at 15 mm Hg. Other treatment modalities are initiated in a stepwise manner only if IH is not responsive to CSF withdrawal.

Table 1   Demographics and Clinical Features

Factor	Group I	Group II
number of patients	34	15
average age(years)	33	41
motor vehicle accident(%)	76	53
evacuated acute subdural hematoma(%)	29	27
average GCS post resuscitation	5	6

GCS = Glasgow Coma Scale score

Table 2   Ventricular ICP and $PaCO_2$ Parameters

Factor	Group I	Group II
avg.duration of ICP monitoring(days)	4.3	N/A
avg.ICP during treatment(mm Hg)	13	N/A
incidence of intracranial hypertension(%)	10	N/A
ventricular CSF infection rate(%)	6	N/A
avg.$PaCO_2$ during ICP monitoring (mm Hg)	33	34

ICP = intracranial pressure, CSF = cerebrospinal fluid

Table 3   Discharge Outcome

Status	GOS	Group I(%)	Group II(%)
Dead	1	12	53
Vegetative	2	9	7
Dependent	3	20	20
Living Independently	4/5	59	20

GOS = Glasgow Outcome Scale score

REFERENCES

1. Marmarou A, Anderson RL, Ward JD, Choi SC, Young HF (1991) Impact of ICP instability and hypotension on outcome in patients with severe head trauma. J Neurosurg (suppl) 75:S59-S66

2. Miller JD, Becker DP, Ward JD, Sullivan HG, Adams WE, Rosner MJ (1977) Significance of intracranial hypertension in severe head injury. J Neurosurg 47:503-516

3. Miller JD (1991) Changing patterns in acute management of head injury. J Neurol Sci 103:S33-S37

4. Ghajar JBG (1985) A guide for ventricular catheter placement. A technical note. J Neurosurg 63:985-986

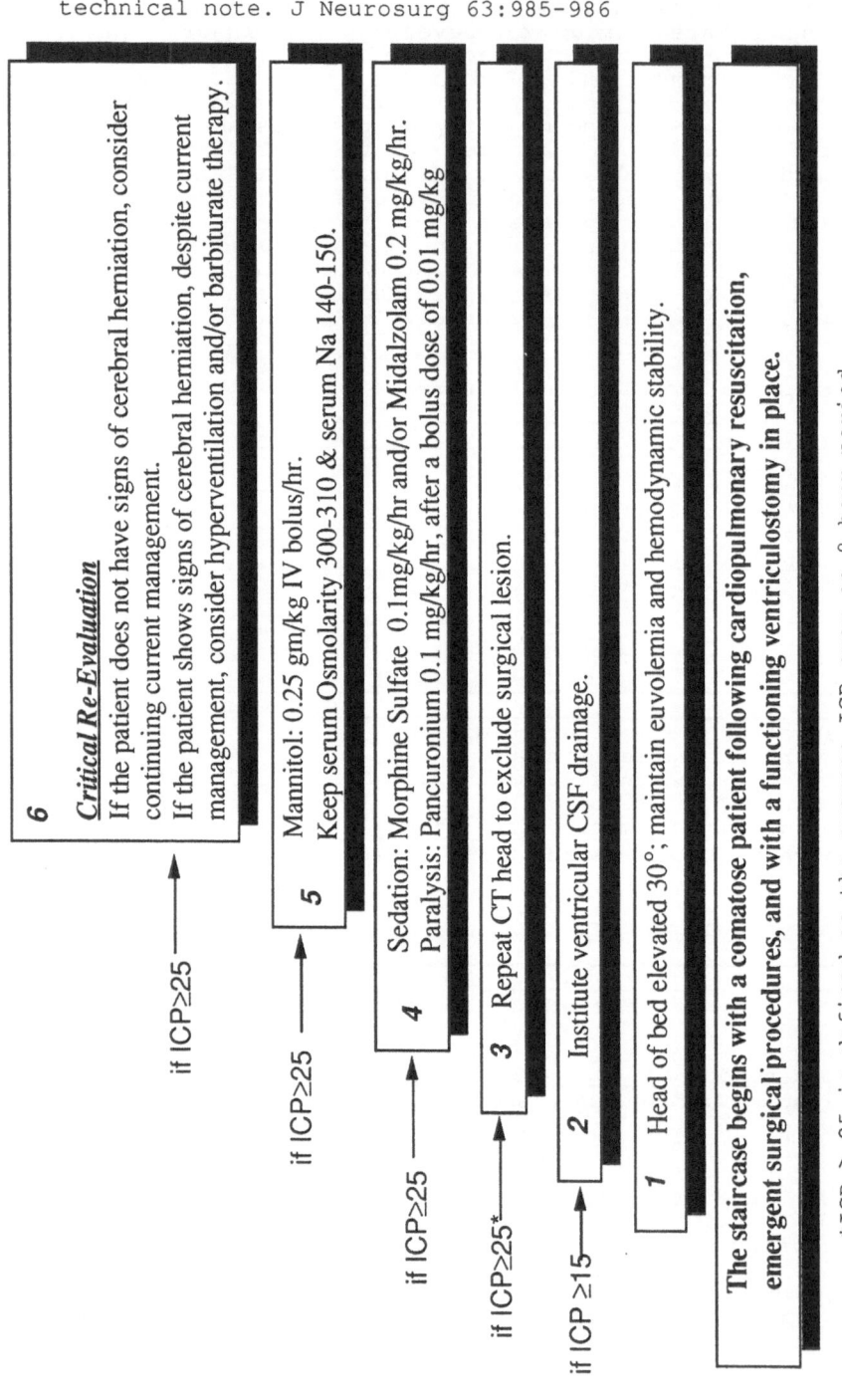

6 *Critical Re-Evaluation*
If the patient does not have signs of cerebral herniation, consider continuing current management.
If the patient shows signs of cerebral herniation, despite current management, consider hyperventilation and/or barbiturate therapy.

if ICP≥25

5 Mannitol: 0.25 gm/kg IV bolus/hr.
Keep serum Osmolarity 300-310 & serum Na 140-150.

if ICP≥25

4 Sedation: Morphine Sulfate 0.1mg/kg/hr and/or Midalzolam 0.2 mg/kg/hr.
Paralysis: Pancuronium 0.1 mg/kg/hr, after a bolus dose of 0.01 mg/kg

if ICP≥25

3 Repeat CT head to exclude surgical lesion.

if ICP≥25*

2 Institute ventricular CSF drainage.

if ICP ≥15

1 Head of bed elevated 30°; maintain euvolemia and hemodynamic stability.

The staircase begins with a comatose patient following cardiopulmonary resuscitation, emergent surgical procedures, and with a functioning ventriculostomy in place.

*ICP ≥ 25 is defined as the average ICP over an 8 hour period.

Fig.1 The ICP Management Climb

Legend: The Cornell University Medical Center protocol for intracranial pressure management utilizing a stepwise approach.

330

9—Focal Injury

Near-Infrared Spectroscopic Localization of Intracranial Hematomas

SHANKAR P. GOPINATH[1], CLAUDIA S. ROBERTSON[1], ROBERT G. GROSSMAN[1], and BRITTON CHANCE[2]

[1]Department of Neurosurgery, Baylor College of Medicine, One Baylor Plaza, Houston, Texas, 77030, USA, and
[2]Department of Biochemistry and Biophysics, University of Pennsylvania, Philadelphia, Pennsylvania, 19104, USA

SUMMARY

Near-infrared spectroscopy (NIRS) of the cerebral hemispheres, applied transcranially through the intact scalp and skull, was evaluated for its ability to detect the presence of an intracranial hematoma in 64 head injured patients. Fifty-seven of the patients had intracranial hematomas which were identified on CT scan (32-subdural, 15-epidural, 10-intracerebral). In all 57 cases, NIRS demonstrated greater absorbance of light at 760 nm on the side of the hematoma. In 51 patients, the asymmetry in light absorbance resolved after surgical evacuation of the hematoma or with spontaneous resorption of the hematoma. Six patients who developed postoperative or delayed hematomas exhibited persistence of the asymmetry in light absorbance. Seven patients, who had only diffuse injuries, exhibited only minor differences in optical density between the hemispheres, similar to 10 control patients with no head injury. Near-infrared spectroscopy appears to be useful in the initial examination of the head injured patient, as an adjunct to CT scanning, and in following patients postoperatively in the intensive care unit.

KEYWORDS: head injury, subdural hematoma, epidural hematoma, intracerebral hematoma, near-infrared spectroscopy

INTRODUCTION

Intracranial hematoma is one of the major treatable complications in patients with severe head injury. Early detection and surgical evacuation of intracranial hematomas is essential to reduce the mortality. Although the unenhanced CT scan is clearly the diagnostic procedure of choice in the acute evaluation of the head-injured patients, difficulties can exist in obtaining a timely CT scan. Also, the decision as to when and how often a CT scan should be repeated after surgery can be difficult particularly in the critically ill patient that may be difficult to transport to radiology. There is a need for an alternative simple yet rapid method of detecting the development of intracranial hematomas.

Transcranial near-infrared spectroscopy (NIRS) has been used to monitor cerebral oxygenation as well as changes in cerebral blood volume based on the physical property of light absorption by oxyhemoglobin, and deoxyhemoglobin. The potential of NIRS to localize intracranial hematomas has not been systematically studied. The present study tested the hypothesis that extravascular collections of blood should strongly absorb NIR light compared to the brain tissue because of the greater concentration of hemoglobin, and that asymmetry in the absorption of the NIR light would suggest a hematoma on the side of greatest light absorption.

MATERIAL AND METHODS

NIRS was used to identify and localize a potential intracranial hematoma in 64 patients with head injury admitted to Ben Taub General Hospital between August 1991 and August 1992. The age of the patients ranged from 4 months to 101 years. Fifty-four of the patients were studied in the emergency room prior to obtaining a CT scan, while the remaining patients were examined in the operating room prior to surgery or in the ICU if surgery was not required. In all cases, the NIRS examiner was unaware of the results of the CT Scan.

A dual wavelength NIRS unit (RunMan, manufactured by NIM, Inc.) was used to quantitate hemispheric differences in light absorbance. The probe of the NIRS unit consists of 2 tungsten filament lamps 3.5 cm on either side of a 760 and 850 nm light detector. The 3.5 cm separation of light source and detector allows measurement of NIR light absorbance in a volume of tissue approximately 2 cm wide by 2-3 cm deep. The detector measures the intensity of the unabsorbed or reflected light. Optical density is calculated from the formula:

$$OD = \log_{10}\frac{I_0}{I_A}$$

where I_0 = the intensity of the illuminating beam and I_A = the intensity of the reflected light.

The probe of the RunMan was placed successively in various regions of the scalp on both sides of the head. The intensity of reflected light at 760 nm was recorded in each of these regions. The difference in optical density (ΔOD) between the hemispheres in each of these regions was calculated by the formula:

$$\Delta OD = \log_{10}\frac{I_0}{I_N} - \log_{10}\frac{I_0}{I_H} = \log_{10}\frac{I_N}{I_H}$$

where I_0 = the intensity of the illuminating light beam, I_N is the intensity of the reflected light on the normal side, and I_H is the intensity of the reflected light on the hematoma side.

The admission CT scan diagnosis of the 64 patients included: subdural hematoma (SDH) in 32 patients, epidural hematoma (EDH) in 15, intracerebral hematoma (ICH) in 10, and diffuse brain injury (DBI) in 7. Fifty patients had surgery for evacuation of hematomas and a repeat CT scan was performed 24-48 hours postoperatively. The NIRS exam was also repeated during first few days following surgery. The remaining few patients was treated conservatively. All had follow-up CT scans and NIRS exams at regular intervals until the hematoma resolved.

RESULTS

The patients with DBI (n=7) had only minor differences in OD between the right and left sides (0.02 ± 0.01), similar to a group of 10 control patients who had no head injuries (0.02 ± 0.01). In all of the patients who had an intracranial hematoma on CT scan, a significant increase in light absorption was detected on the side of the hematoma (Table 1). The ΔOD was highest in the patients with an EDH, intermediate in the patients with a SDH, and smallest in the patients with ICH. However, there was sufficient overlap of the ΔOD between the different types of lesions that they could not be distinguished by the ΔOD alone. The preoperative ΔOD was significantly related to the thickness of the hematoma measured on the initial CT scan (n=48, r=0.59, p=0.00001).

Of the 32 patients with a SDH, 28 patients underwent surgical evacuation of the hematoma. Postoperatively the ΔOD returned to the near normal values (0.02±0.01) in the 25 who had uncomplicated courses. In the remaining 3 patients, there was a persistence of the asymmetry, suggesting the presence of a recurrent or a new hematoma which was in each case confirmed by a CT scan.

Of the 15 patients with an EDH, 13 patients underwent evacuation of the hematoma. Postoperatively the ΔOD was 0.02±0.01 in the 10 who had no postoperative complications. In 3 patients with recurrent or new hematomas, the ΔOD averaged 0.86+0.31 postoperatively.

Of the 10 patients with ICH, 8 had surgical evacuation and 2 were treated medically. The asymmetry of light absorption resolved in all of these patients.

Table 1. Hemispheric difference in optical density (ΔOD) in patients with different types of intracranial lesions.

Type of Lesion	Preoperative ΔOD (ipsi -contralateral)	Postoperative ΔOD (patients without post-op hematomas)	Postoperative ΔOD (patients with post-op hematomas)
Subdural hematoma (n=32)	0.87 ± 0.30	0.02±0.01	1.01±0.19
Epidural hematoma (n =15)	1.09 ± 0.29	0.02±0.01	0.86±0.31
Intracerebral hematoma (n =10)	0.40 ± 0.11	0.03±0.01	
Diffuse brain injury (n= 7)	0.02 ± 0.01		
p value (ANOVA)	.0001		

DISCUSSION

Transcranial NIRS has been used to detect silent cerebral hypoxia and changes in cerebral blood volume in infants [1-6]. It is sensitive in evaluating the metabolic brain injury in the infant [7]. Using NIRS, measurement of CBF has been performed in preterm infants [8].

Our study demonstrates the usefulness of NIRS in localizing intracranial hematomas in patients with severe head injury. NIRS was sensitive enough to recognize all extracerebral and intracerebral collections of blood identified on CT scan although the differences between the types of hematomas could not be distinguished with certainty. NIRS appears to be useful in the initial examination of the head injured patients, as an adjunct to CT scanning, and in following patients postoperatively in the intensive care unit.

REFERENCES

1. Brazy JE, Lewis DV, Mitnick MD, et al (1985) Noninvasive monitoring of cerebral oxygenation in preterm infants. Preliminary observations Pediatrics 75:217-225

2. Brazy JE, Lewis DV (1986) Changes in cerebral blood volume and cytochrome aa3 during hypertensive peaks in preterm infants J Pediatr 108:983-987

3. Brazy JE (1988) Effects of crying on cerebral blood volume and cytochrome aa3 J Pediatr 112:457-461

4. Brazy JE (1991) Cerebral oxygen monitoring with near infrared spectroscopy: clinical applications to neonates J Clin Monit 7:325-334

5. Deply DT, Cope MC, Cady EB, et al (1987) Cerebral monitoring in newborn infants by magnetic resonance and near infrared spectroscopy Scand J Clini Lab Invest 47(suppl 188):9-17

6. Wyatt JS, Cope M, Delpy DT, et al (1986) Quantification of cerebral oxygenation and hemodynamics in sick newborn infants by near infrared spectrophotometry. Lancet II:1063-1066

7. Chance B, Smith DS, Delivoria-Papadopoulos M, Younkin DP (1989) New techniques for evaluating metabolic brain injury in newborn infants. Crit Care Med 17:465-471

8. Edwards AD, Wyatt JS, Richardson C, et al (1988) Cotside measurement of cerebral blood flow in ill newborn infants by near infrared spectroscopy. Lancet II:770-771

CT – Guided Stereotactic Aspiration of Traumatic Intracerebral Hematomas

Lu Yun-Jian and Bao Yu-Hai

Department of Neurosurgery, Xinjiang Medical College, Urumqi, China

SUMMARY

It is not well known whether traumatic intracerebral hematoma could be treated safely and effectively through aspiration up to now. In the past six months, we performed CT—guided stereotactic aspiration of traumatic intracerebal hematomas which had produced a shift of the brain midline structures of less than 5mm and which were generally not considered to need a craniotomy. We inserted a brain needle accurately into the hematoma cavity through a burr hole or a twist drill hole made directly through the scalp and bone. With a syringe, we then aspirated the clotted or liquified hematoma as much as possible. Then we injected 10,000u Urokinase diluted with 2ml isotonic saline solution into the hematoma cavity in order to liquify the remaining hematoma. According to the condition of the patients, aspiration was performed 1 to 3 times. Their hematomas ranging in volume from 10ml to 32ml totally disappeared within 10 days. All the patients who received this treatment were discharged without any complications and returned to normal life. Compared to conservative treatment, the advantages of this treatment is that the intracranial hypertension and mass effect are reduced more rapidly, promoting the improvement of clinical symptoms and the recovery of neurological deficits; and that damage to the brain is minimal. In our opinion, this treatment is suitable for some intracerebral hematomas which produced only a little brain shift, in which ICP was not too high, or where the hematomas were in a deeper or functional area.

KEY WORDS: aspiration, intracerebral hematoma, trauma, Urokinase

INTRODUCTION

The management of the traumatic intracerebral hematoma which produced a slight shift of the brain midline structures or compression of the unilateral ventricle is a controversial problem when the patient had not deteriorated in conscious level or developed new neurological deficits since injury. In the past six months, we successfully treated six patients with the traumatic intracerebral hematoma, using CT—guided stereotactic aspiration surgery not adopting "wait and see". Now we reported our methods and results below.

MATERIALS AND METHODS

During the past six months, 6 male patients with traumatic intracerebral hematomas were admitted to the Department of Neurosurgery of the Xinjiang Medical College. The diagnoses were confirmed by CT scanning on admission. The patients ranged from 19 to 53 years of age (mean 31.7 years). Their hematomas ranged in volume from 10ml to 32ml (mean 24.3ml). The duration from trauma to admission, the chief symptoms and signs, and the location of hematomas are listed in Table 1.

Table 1. Age,sex and hematoma location,chief symptoms and signs ,hematoma volume and duration from trauma to admission of these patients with traumatic intracerebral hematomas.

Case No.	Age	Sex	Chief symptoms and signs	Duration	Hematoma location	Volume
1	53	M	Headache Vomiting Hemiplegia	60 hours	Left basal ganglia	32 ml
2	20	M	Headache Vomiting Hemiplegia	16 days	Deep region of right frontal lobe	29 ml
3	36	M	Headache Vomiting	11 days	Subcortical region of left frontal lobe	30 ml
4	34	M	Headache Vomiting	48 hours	Subcortical region of right parietal lobe	25 ml
5	28	M	Headache Hemiplegia	4 days	Deep region of right frontal lobe	10 ml
6	19	M	Headache Vomiting Hemiplegia	13 days	Deep region of right parietal lobe	20 ml

As soom as the hematoma was confirmed and its location was measured by CT scanning, a burr hole or a twist drill hole was made at the point nearest to the hematoma, avoiding damage to the functional regions and vessels. Then we inserted a brain needle accurately into the hematoma cavity according to the CT measurement. After it was confirmed that the tip of the brain needle was exactly in the hematoma cavity, we aspirated the clotted or liquified hematoma as much as possible with a ordinary syringe. Then we injected 10, ooou Urokinase diluted with 2ml isotonic saline solution into the hematoma cavity in order to liquify the hematoma. The same procedure was repeated every other day untill the hematoma had been almost totally evacuated.

RESULTS

In our series of 6 patients suffering traumatic intracerebral hematomas after closed head injury, 3 patients whose duration from the trauma to admission of the hematoma was longer than 11 days just received aspiration one time because their hematomas were liquified. The other 3 patients received aspiration 2 to 3 times and their hematomas totally disappeared within 10 days.   The No. 2 patient´s hemiplegia dramatically recovered on the third day after the first aspiration. All the patients received this treatment were discharged home without any complications and neurological deficits except the No. 1 patient whose hemiplegia did not totally recover because of the location of the hematoma [Fig. 1,2].

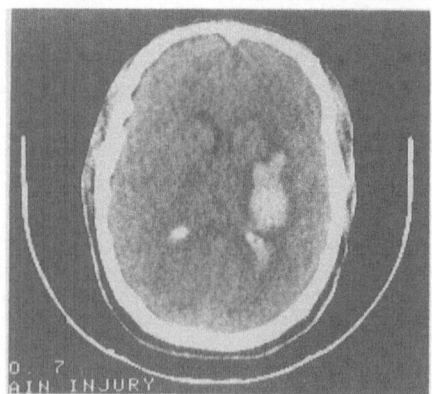

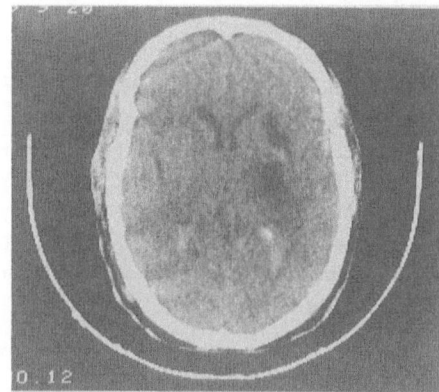

Fig. 1 The No. 1 patient´s CT scan shows a hematoma of the left basal ganglia 60 hours after the trauma.

Fig. 2 A new CT scan of the No. 1 patient shows that the hematoma has disappeared on the fifth day after the first aspiration.

DISCUSSION

A patient with a traumatic intracerebral hematoma who has not deteriorated or developed any new neurological deficit since the injury often make it difficult for the neurosurgeon to decide whether to remove the hematoma or not. Some authors believe that conservative treatment can abtain good results if the patient´s consciousness level is in the range of 13—15 GCS score and does not become worse during the treatment [1]. But Bullock,etc. reported that some patients would suddenly deteriorate or die during the course of conservative treatment because of a late sudden rise in intracranial pressure. Even the intracranial pressure monitoring could not predict the sudden change and the need for surgery[2]. Yamamoto,etc. reported that they successfully treated a 6—year—old boy with a massive traumatic hematoma of the basal ganglia with CT—guided stereotactic aspiration surgery in 1990[3]. Nguyen,etc . also reported that they treated 3 cases with post—traumatic intracerebral hematomas with Backlund´s needle under X—ray computerized tomography [4]. Encouraged by their experiences,we treated 6 patients with CT—guided stereotactic aspiration. Due to the use of Urokinase to liquify the hematoma,the aspiration surgery was made more effective and we achieved good results. Compared to conservative treatment,the main advantage of this treatment is that the intracranial hypertension and mass effect are reduced more rapidly,promoting the improvement of clinical symptoms and the recovery of neurological deficit. In our opinion,this treatment is suitable for some traumatic intracerebral hematomas which only produces a little brain shift,in which ICP was not too high,or where the hematomas were in a deeper or functional region.

Because this treatment brings almost no damage to the brain and its procedure is simple,we believe that the combination of the CT—guided aspiration surgery and conservative treatment can remarkablely improve the quality of life of the patient. For some of those hard—to—decide—on patients,we believe we can now take a positive measure and avoide the risks of "wait and see".

REFERENCES

1. Koziarski A (1991) Conservative treatment of post—traumatic intracerebral hematoma. Neurol—Neurochir—pol 25(2):230—237
2. Bullock R, Golek J, Blake G (1989) Traumatic intracerebral hematoma —which patients should undergo surgical evacuation? CT scan features and ICP monitoring as a basis for decision making. Surg—Neurol 32 (3):181 —187
3. Yamamoto F, Eguchi G, Yoshimura k, Shigemori M, Kuramoto S (1990) Massive traumatic hematoma localized in the basal ganglia:treated by CT—guided stereotactic aspiration surgery. No—Shinkei—Geka 18 (6):563—565
4. Nguyen JP, Gaston A, Brugieres P, Nallino J, Rostaing S, Decq P, Leguerinel C, Keravel Y(1991) Intracerebral hematoma surgically treated under X—ray computed tomography with Backlund´ s needle. A series of 15 cases . Neurochirurgie 37(1):50—57

Missile Brain Injuries: An Approach to the Management on the Basis of Experience with 106 Wounded Patients in Osijek General Hospital over the 15 Month Period of War

DJURO VRANKOVIĆ[1], IVAN HEĆIMOVIĆ[1], BRUNO SPLAVSKI[1], and BRANKA KRISTEK[2]

Divisions of [1]Neurosurgery, and [2]Radiology, Osijek General Hospital, Osijek, Croatia

SUMMARY

This article is based on data gathered from 106 patients with penetrating brain injuries. They were admitted and treated at the Neurosurgical division of Osijek General Hospital over the 15 month period of war (May 16, 1991 to August 16, 1992). The patients, from region of east Slavonia & Baranya (north eastern Croatia), sustained their injuries during the enforced and brutal war of Serbian aggressor troops and the Yugoslav Federal Army (army of former Yugoslavia) against Croatia.

These patients were divided into four groups dependent of their state on admission, neurosurgical management and to the early results obtained.

We paid most attention to the preservation of the brain tissue. We removed all foreign bodies (cloth, hairs, particles of soil, stone, etc.), and we took away only the accessible bone and shell fragments. We never reoperated bacause of retained bone fragments therefore, our approach was less radical regarding the removal of indriven and retained small bone fragments.

General mortality was 50%. During the early postoperative period, of the survived patients (53 cases) two had brain abscess (3.77%), two meningitis, and six epilepsy (11.3%), despite retained bone fragments in 28 patients, ie. in 62.2%. These findings strenghtened us in the opinion that a less aggressive approach to surgical managment is appropriate.

KEY WORDS: missile brain injuries, less aggressive approach, retained bone fragments.

INTRODUCTION

In the neurosurgical treatment of penetrating craniocerebral missile injuries a dilemma exists between taking an aggressive approach to the removal of indriven small bone fragments, or a more conservative one, especially when a postoperative computed tomography (CT) scan indicates the presence of retained bone fragments. [1,2] The question of whether to reoperate, or not then arises.

Many articles related to this problem have accentuated the need for early reoperation and removal of retained bone fragments. [3,4] Recently, however, more and more articles have appeared which present an opposing view. Our data lead us to conclude that less radical practice is advisable.

It is the purpose of this article to describe our neurosurgical managment and attitude toward patients with missile brain injuries, with particular attention to the indriven small bone fragments.

MATERIALS AND METHODS

During the 15 months (May 16, 1991-August 16, 1992) in Osijek Hospital 4.169 the war wounded were admitted. 2.253 were treated as out-patients and 1.916 were hospitalized. 106 patients with missile brain injuries were admitted to the Divison of Neurosurgery, the incidence of 5.53% of hospitalized patients. Out of 106 patients 53, ie. 50% survived. They were the subjects of our study.

Eight patients were treated nonoperatively (no craniotomy). Forty five wounded underwent surgery. Diagnostics consisted of a complete neurological evaluation by a neurosurgeon and a clinical examination by a general surgeon, as well as a two-plane x-ray of the head, and a chest x-ray in each case. In some cases a CT of the brain was taken (but all that has been applied after standard resuscitative measures).

Surgical debridement of the edges of the scalp wound, the dura mater and bone flap , suction of necrotic brain tissue; evacuation of hematomas, and extraction of all organic foreign bodies, but the bone and shell fragments only the accessible, ones have been our usual practice. Defect on the dura was covered by a graft (mostly autologous). [5] Closure of scalp wounds was performed with full thickness of the skin and without tension (sometimes by the rotation of a scalp flap).

In the early postoperative period a control CT scan of the brain was made. Throughout the stay in Hospital, as well as on the follow-up, we looked out for the possible development of complications: dehiscence of wounds, cerebrospinal fluid (CSF) leaks on the skin wound, meningitis, abscess formation, intracranical (i.c.) hypertension, epilepsy, osteitis.

Among the non-survived patients (53 cases) the first group of 11 wounded, admitted to Hospital with the severe head injury, had simply the missile wounds on the scalp closed. They died within 24-48 hours after admission. The second group of 9 wounded expired on the operating table during surgery.

The majority of the remaining 33 patients, had the Glasgow Coma Scala (GCS) score 3-7, and three of them had 10-14 (one was a 80 years old woman). Although most of them had minimal chances to survive all were surgically managed. Some had multisystem injuries. The majority (90.9%) were autopsied. The principal cause of death was primary destruction of brain tissue.

RESULTS

Half of all patients with penetrating brain injuries survived. We can only present data on the early results (complications and outcome) obtained from these patients. Some of our patients (23 of them) were lost to follow-up, because after hospital discharge they were evacuated to safer places in the country and abroad. Of the survived, 30 of them were continued to be followed-up at our Hospital.

We had 45 patients with indriven bone fragments. In 17 patients these fragments were completely removed and in 22 only partially. Six of these patients were conservatively treated. The other 2 patients treated nonoperatively and 6 by surgery had no indriven bone fragments. /Table 1./

Table 1 Forty five survived (of 53) with indriven bone fragments

	cases	percentage
with indriven bone fragments	45	84.9%
managed nonoperatively	6	13.3%
treated surgically	39	86.7%
completely removed bone fragments	17	43.6%
partially removed bone fragments	22	56.4%
retained bone fragments (6 n.op. + 22 op.)	28	62.2%

n. op. = nonoperatively, op. = operatively

In the early period after injury and operation, we had 2 cases with brain abscess around the bone fragments (3.77%). On the follow-up (2 and half months after injury and operation) one patient was discovered with a brain abscess (a patient with removed bone fragments).

Five patients developed epileptic seizures. One more case was diagnosed on the follow-up.

Dehiscence of the scalp wounds were found in 7 patients. All healed in a short time.

CFS leaks from the scalp wound were evident in 11 wounded. By resuturing the dehiscenced wounds and by repeated lumbar punctures CSF leaks stopped.

Meningitis developed in the 4 wounded (2 associated with brain abscess), ie. 7.66%, although some were treated with three antibiotics (penicillin-G, gentamycin, metronidazol). By the administration of appropriate antibiotics (after testing the sensitivity of the microorganisms) and operating on the 2 wounded, with brain abscess, they were cured.

One patient with an epidural and one with a subdural hematoma were discowered and operated on.

One case (the posterior fossa missile injury) developed hydrocephalus, which was treated by CSF shunting procedure. He died, in spite of treatment, because of a primary lesion of the brain.

Outcome (based on Glasgow Outcome Scale - GOS) of the patients followed-up by us is: good recovery 19, moderate disability 6, severe disability 4, and persistent vegetative state 1 case.

Thirty of 33 non-survived patients (who died between 1 and 21 days of being operated) were autopsied. The results showed: one case of subdural empyema, three of meningoencephalitis and 1 of meningitis. The others did not have any signs of infection, although they had retained bone and/or shell fragments. The incidence rate of complications being 15.1%.

DISCUSSION

Thanks to quick organization in response to the war conditions, adequate facilities and to the ability of personnel to admit a large number of the wounded, we were able to accomplish early surgery for each patient admitted to the Neurosurgical division, regardless to their number and admission time.

Injuries of the brain and tissues of the head, by bullets and shell fragments were large, both in the missile track as well as in the brain surrounding the track, due to the shock waves, temporary and permanent cavitation effects, and in some ricocheting as well as deformation of the missile. [6,7,8,9] In such cases early surgery is essential if a successful outcome is to be achived. The provision of prompt treatment depends on the time taken over the transportation of the wounded to hospital. For our patients, the average time elapsed between being wounded and being admitted to hospital was 1.35 hours (the fastest transport time was 5 minutes - a man injured in the hospital yard, and the longest was 24 hours). In spite of that we had a slightly higher percentage of mortality. This can be explained by the fact that our Hospital, being situated on the front-line, received more critical cases in a relatively short time. Therefore, there was no selection of patients as e.g., in hospitals on the second-fire line, where to reach them more time for transportation was needed.

We have divided the wounded into four groups. We shall analyze the data obtained from groups 1. and 2., the survived patients. The first group (8 patients) consisted of those who were treated by conservative measures (antibiotics, anticonvulsants, antiedematous agents). Those patients were without signs of i.c. hematomas having mass-effect, elevated intracranial pressure (ICP) and fully conscious. All had good outcome.

The remained of the survived patients belong to group 2. and together with group 1. (53 patients) they form the basis for this study.

Standardized surgical protocol for missile war penetrating brain wounds, applied during past and in some recent wars (Korea, Vietnam) was termed "aggressive", radical approach, because of the policy of this protocol, regarding postoperative discovery of retained bone fragments. This policy is: "early reoperation to remove retained bone fragments". [2] An alternative option which deals with this problem is presented in recent literature, and defends the so called "less aggressive" approach. [1,2,8,10] We adopted this policy and after examination of our findings, we are convinced of the validity of this approach.

Surgical debridement of necrotic tissues, starting form the entry wound on the scalp to the end of the missile track in the brain, as well as the removal of all foreign bodies (particles of cloth, hairs, dirt, soil, stone, etc) is the policy accepted by all neurosurgeons. We, as the followers of the less radical approach to this problem, removed only those bone and shell fragments which were easily accessible. [11] Therefore, we never were surprised when, on the postoperative CT scan of the brain, retained bone fragments were found. This is because our priority was to preserve the vital brain tissue. Today, especially, with the possibility for monitoring these patients by CT scanning, and with the availability of newer broad-spectrum antibiotics we feel confident in taking this standpoint. Our results confirm this opinion. Out of 53 survivors (group 1. and 2.) there were 28 cases with retained bone chips, ie. an incidence of 62.2%. One reason for such a high number of retained bone fragments is, that many of these cases had a tangential injury and some fragments were driven into brain tissue out of missile track, so even with finger palpation we were unable to feel them. [7] Up to now (for some patients this is a follow-up perod of 15 months) we have had 2 cases of patients with brain abscess and 2 with meningitis. The other group (25 wounded) was without indriven bone fragments (8 were admitted without fragment and 17 had fragments surgically removed). Of these 1 case developed brain abscess and 2 cases developed meningitis. There is evidently no difference between patients with retained and removed bone fragments. /Table 2./

Table 2: Retained small bone fragments, early results

	8 patients treated n.op.		45 patients surgicaly treated			
	No b.f.	With b.f.	completely removed b.f.	partially removed b.f.	shell fragment only	Total
Patients	2	6	17	22	6	53
Infection: brain abscess	0	0	1	2	0	3
meningitis	0	0	2	2	0	4
Epilepsy	0	0	3	3	0	6

b.f. = bone fragment, n.op. = nonoperatively

The 28 patients with retained bone fragments are in good condition (no increase of neurological deficits, infection, brain edema) and none of them has died. The aforementioned could have occured had we followed the aggressive approach and reoperated on them. M.E. Carey described some cases with complications which developed after reoperation for retained bone fragments. [10]

We believe that the problem of intracerebral bone fragments could be solved with the use and help of intraoperative ultrasound scanning. This would facilitate the removal of the indriven fragments without damaging the brain tissue. [1,12]

This report deals with the early results so, in making a connection between epilepsy and retained bone fragments, we can only refer to early seizures. In our series there were 6 cases with epilepsy. In 3 of them with no retained bone fragments. /Table 2./ Now, the question may arise as to whether these seizures are caused by these fragments or not. Location of damaged brain cortex (motor area) and formed glial scars and hypoxic tissue around are already sufficient to act as epileptiform discharges, regardless to retained or removed fragments. [13]

Another possible complication, described in literature, is neoplastic growth in the region of retained bone and shell fragments (glioma, meningioma). [14,15,16] We shall not be able to report on this for some years, although in our opinion the results will be the same as those observed in the relationship between epilepsy (meningitis) - bone chips - glial scars.

In conclusion, it is important, with regard to neurological deficits, to cause as little harm as possible to brain tissue. Therefore, our policy is to take the less radical approach regarding the indriven bone fragments, i.e. never to perform reoperation solely because of the presence of such fragments, except in cases of infection and abscess formation. We presume that the use of intraoperative ultrasonography could play a major role in the non-traumatic removal of indriven bone fragments.

REFERENCES
1. Kaufman HH, Schwab K, Salazar AM (1991) Surg Neurol 36: 370-377
2. Brandvold B. Levi L, Feinsod M, George ED (1990) J Neurosurg 72: 15-21
3. Hagan R (1971) J Neurosurg 34: 132-141
4. Lewin W, Gibson RM (1965) Br J Surg 43: 628-632
5. Vranković Dj, Hećimović I, Splavski B, Dmitrović B (1992) Neurochirurgia 35: 1-6 (in print)
6. Dufour D, Jensen SK, Own-Smith M, Salmela J, Stenning GF, Zetterström B (1988) Surgery for victims of war. Geneva: International Committe of the Red Cross
7. Kirkpatrick JB, Di Maio V (1978) J Neurosurg 49: 185-198
8. Byrnes DP, Crockard HA, Gordon DS, Gleadhill CA (1974) Br J Surg 61: 169-176
9. Lindenbreg R (1968) In: Minkler J (Ed) Pathology of the Nervous System. New York: McGraw-Hill, pp 1705-1765
10. Carey ME, Young HF, Rish BL, Mathis JL (1974) J Neurosurg 41: 542-549
11. Hubschmann O, Shapiro K, Baden M, Shulman K (1979) J Trauma 19: 1-12
12. Chandler WF (1990) In: Rubin JM, Chandler WF (Eds) Ultrasound in Neurosurgery. Raven Press, New York, pp 102-105
13. Raimondi AJ, Samuelson GH (1970) J Neurosurg 32: 647-653
14. Zülch KJ (Ed) (1986) In: Brain Tumors. Their Biology and Pathology. 3rd Edition. Berlin, Springer-Verlag, pp 70-77
15. Troost D, Tulleken CAF (1984) Clinical Neurophatology 4: 139-142
16. Russell DS, Rubinstein LJ (1989) In: Pathology of the Nervous System. Fifth Edition. London Melbourne Auckland, Edward Arnold, pp 19-20 and 454-455

Prognosis in Patients with Post-Traumatic Intracerebral Hemorrhage Vs Contusion

N. Muthukumar, U.S. Srinivasan, M. Sampathkumar, and R. Gajendran

Department of Neurosurgery, Madurai Medical College and Government Rajaji Hospital, Madurai, India

SUMMARY

The outcome in 63 patients with moderate and severe head injury with either intra-cerebral haemorrhage (or) contusion was studied. The following features were studied: age, GCS score, midline shift, basal cisterns and mortality index. There was no difference in outcome between between ICH and contusion with regard to age and GCS score when the GCS score less than 8. When the GCS score was more than 8, when the midline shift was present, when the basal cisterns were obliterated there was a statistically significant difference between both the groups.

Key Words: Cerebral contusion - head injury - intracerebral haemorrhage - outcome.

INTRODUCTION

A spectrum of lesions can occur in patients with head injury. The outcome in patients with head injury depends not only on the severity of injury but also on the type of pathology. This has been borne out by a number of studies[1,2,3]. The present study was conducted to find out the difference in outcome in patients with post-traumatic intracerebral hemorrhage and contusion.

AIM OF THE STUDY

The aim of the study was to find out the outcome in patients with intracerebral hemorrhage and contusion due to head injury.

MATERIALS AND METHODS

63 patients admitted to the head injury unit of Government Rajaji Hospital, Madurai were included in the study. The criteria for inclusion were 1. definite evidence of injury and 2.CT scan showing either intracerebral hemorrhage or contusion or both. The following cases were excluded from the study: 1. Patients with known hypertension, 2. known bleeding disorders, 3. multiple injuries 4. cases which could not be placed in either category due to observer differences in interpretation of the type of lesion and 5. cases where the contusions were due to depressed fractures. 6. cases with associated significant EDH, SDH, IVH.

Patient Management

All patients were evaluated after initial cardiopulmonary resuscitation. X-rays of the head and neck were taken and an emergency CT scan was done. Depending on the findings on the CT scan, the patients were either taken to the operating room or to the neurosurgical intensive care unit. The outcome was divided into two groups: 1. those who survived and 2. Those who expired.

Statistical Methods used

The Chi square test was used to find out the statistical significance of the two variables.

RESULTS

1.   **Mode of injury:** The mode of injury was almost similar in both the groups.

2.   **Outcome in patients with ICH:** When the outcome was compared in patients with ICH, it was found that 82% of patients with single ICH survived in contrast to 56% of patients with multiple ICH. (Fig.1)

3.   **Outcome in patients with contusion :** In the contusion group, 46% of patients with single contusion survived, where as only 16% of patients with multiple contusions survived (Fig.2).

4.   **Outcome in ICH VS Contusion:** The overall mortality rate in our series is 50.7%. The mortality rate in the ICH group was 30% and in the contusion group was 63.4%. Patients with multiple lesions fared worse than those with single lesions. Patients with multiple contusions fared worse than those with multiple ICHs (Fig.3).

5.   **Midline shift vs outcome in ICH vs Contusion:** When the midline shift was absent, the ICH group had a mortality rate of 15% and the contusion group had a mortality rate of 40%. When the midline shift was present, the ICH group had a mortality rate of 56% whereas the contusion group had a mortality rate of 100%. This was found to be statistically significant (Fig.4).

6.   **Basal cisterns vs outcome in ICH vs Contusion:** When the basal cisterns were normal, the mortality rates were 0% and 35% in the ICH and contusion groups. When the basal cisterns were obliterated, the mortality rates were 60% and 100% in the ICH and contusion groups respectively. This was found to be statistically significant (Fig.5).

7.   **Glasgow Coma Scale and outcome in patients with ICH vs contusion:** The patients were then divided into three groups on the basis of the GCS scores. Group one consisted of patients with a GCS score of 3-4, Group two consisted of patients with a GCS score of 5-7 and Group three consisted of patients with a GCS score of 8 and more. The outcome was then compared in these three groups with respect to ICH and contusion. It was found that there was no statistically significant difference between the ICH group and contusion group in the GCS 3-4 and 5-7 groups. In patients with a GCS of 8 or more, a statistically significant difference was found between ICH and contusion groups (Figs.6 and 7)

8.   **Age and outcome in ICH Vs Contusion:** The patients were divided into four groups depending on their age viz: less than 20, 20-40. 40-60 and more than 60. There was no statistically significant difference between both the groups as far as the age was concerned (Fig.8).

9.   **Mortality Index:** The importance of a single lesion among the entire spectrum of lesions caused by head injury depends not only on the mortality rate for that particular lesions but also on how frequently that lesion occurs. For example, a lesion may be associated with a very high mortality rate but may occur so infrequently that when a series of 100 head injury patients are considered it may account only for a small number of deaths. On the other hand there may be another lesion that may be associated with a moderate mortality rate but it may occur frequently enough to cause a significant number of deaths when a series of 100 head injured patients are considered. Hence, Generalli et al evolved the mortality index which is a product of the mortality rate and the frequency. We applied this mortality index to our series of patients and found that ICH had a mortality index of 6 and contusions had a mortality index of 28.1. Thus, contusions are four times more important than intracerebral hemorrhages in head injured patients as far as outcome was considered.

CONCLUSIONS

1.   Single ICH has the best prognosis.
2.   Multiple contusions have the worst prognosis
3.   Single ICH has a better prognosis than single contusion
4.   Multiple ICH has a better prognosis than multiple contusions.
5.   Midline shift: If the midline shift is absent, ICH has a better prognosis than contusions. When midline shift is present, the prognosis is equivocal in ICH but definitely worse in contusions.
6.   Basal cisterns: If the basal cisterns are normal, ICH has a better prognosis than contusions. If the basal cisterns are obliterated, the prognosis is equivocal in ICH but definitely worse in contusion.
7.   Age: There was no significant difference between both the groups.
8.   GCS Scores: When the GCS score is less than 8, there is no significant difference in the outcome in patients with ICH and contusion. This implies that in lower GCS scores, it is the severity of injury as measured by the depth of coma that determines the outcome than the type of lesion. Whereas when the GCS score is more than 8, ICH has a better prognosis than contusion.

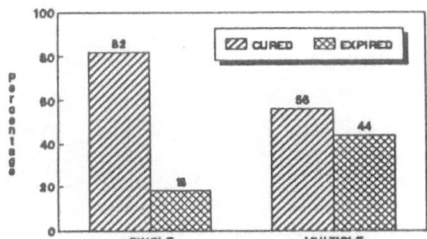

Fig.1 OUTCOME RELATED TO
INTRACEREBRAL HAEMORRHAGE (ICH)

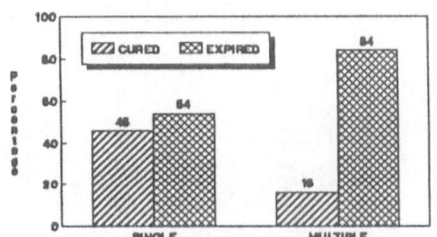

Fig.2 OUTCOME RELATED
TO CONTUSION

OVERALL MORTALITY : 50.7%
MORTALITY : ICH : 30% CONTUSION : 83.4%

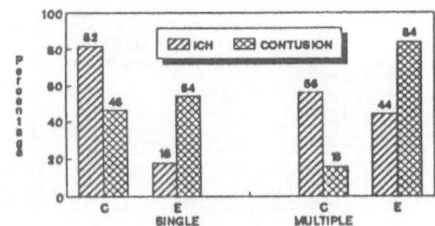

Fig.3 OUTCOME IN ICH VS
CONTUSION

C-CURED E-EXPIRED

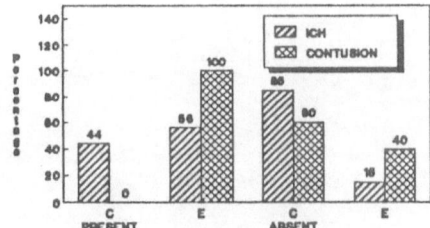

Fig.4 MIDLINE SHIFT V OUTCOME
V ICH/CONTUSION

C-CURED E-EXPIRED

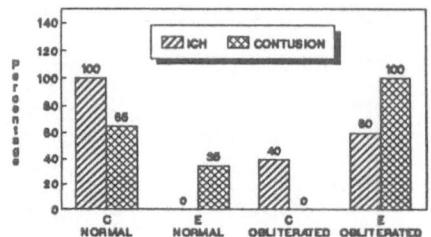

Fig.5 BASAL CISTERN V OUTCOME
V ICH/CONTUSION

C-CURED E-EXPIRED

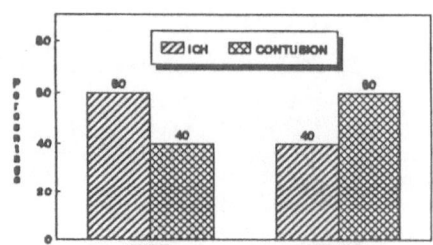

Fig.6 GCS 3-4 V OUTCOME
V ICH/CONTUSION

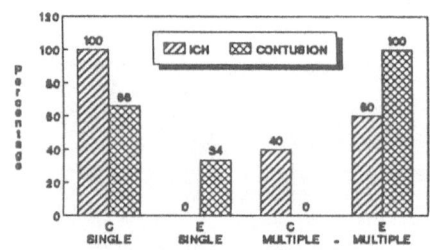

Fig.7 GCS >=8 V OUTCOME
V ICH/CONTUSION

C-CURED E-EXPIRED

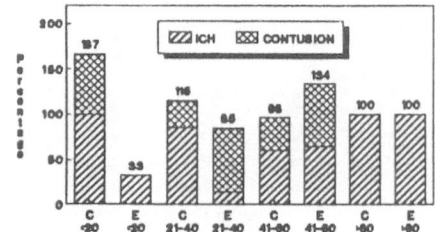

Fig.8 AGE V/S OUTCOME
V/S ICH/CONTUSION

C-CURED E-EXPIRED

References

1. Gennarelli TA, Spielman GM, Langfitt TW (1982): J Neurosurg 56: 26-32.
2. Gennarelli TA, Langfitt TW (1982): J Neurosurg 19-25.
3. Lobato RD, Cordobes F, Rivas JJ, Fuente M, Montero A, Barcena A, Perez C, Cabrera A, Lamas E (1983): J Neurosurg 59: 762-774.

Head Injury Deaths – Intracranial, Extracranial: What Is Unavoidable Death?

S.B. Marshall, R. Chesnut, M. Klauber, M. van Berkum-Clark, J. Piek, and L.F. Marshall

University of California, San Diego, CA 92103, USA

SUMMARY

We describe the causes of death in 717 patients entered into the Traumatic Coma Data Bank of the United States. Approximately 40% of all head injury deaths in potentially salvageable survivors could be avoided under ideal circumstances. The role of shock, both in the pre-hospital and in-hospital phase, as well as that of pneumonia, septicemia, and coagulopathy are described. Mechanisms by which these presently potentially catastrophic complications could be avoided or mitigated are discussed and the need for novel approach is emphasized.

KEY WORDS

Head injury, extracranial complications, intracranial complications, potentially avoidable death.

INTRODUCTION

During the years 1984 through 1988 the Traumatic Coma Data Bank, (TCDB), enrolled 1,030 consecutive patients suffering severe head injury [1]. Patients were enrolled from four centers in the United States. Details regarding their overall outcome, as well as many other aspects of these patients, can be found in the November, 1991 supplement to the Journal of Neurosurgery.

The TCDB database offered a unique opportunity to ask a number of questions regarding mechanisms by which patients succumb or are left severely irreversibly damaged from brain injury.

In the past, a rather nihilistic attitude toward head injury characterized world neurosurgery. The work of Becker et al. [2] and other groups however, indicated that a rapid systematic approach to such patients could produce a substantially better outcome than simple non-directed care. As resource allocations have become a greater and greater issue in health care, it becomes increasingly important to identify those who are unsalvageable and those who might have made a good, or at least independent recovery, but in whom unexpected complications or events occurred, which resulted in a mortal or morbid outcome.

Because the Traumatic Coma Data Bank collected extensive data in all phases of the care of these patients and, in addition, graded complications in such a way so as to determine their importance in the outcome of the patient, a unique opportunity existed to determine the frequency of what one might call "unavoidable deaths" and also those deaths that were   clearly potentially avoidable, had these complications not occurred or if they had been rapidly reversed.

MATERIALS AND METHODS

Of the 1,030 patients entered into the Traumatic Coma Data Bank, 717 remained after eliminating those patients who died prior to resuscitation, those suffering from gunshot wounds, or those in whom data was incomplete during their hospital course (N=35). This report, therefore, details the causes of death in these 717 patients and attributes mortality to the patient's brain injury if the patient was over age 60 and admitted in coma without a hematoma, in patients admitted who were flaccid with one unreactive pupil or more without a hematoma, and in those patients with surgical mass lesions who have at least a decorticate or worse following resuscitation and in whom the surgeon decided not to operate despite of a mass lesion in excess of 25 cc. Causes of death in patients in whom the post-resuscitation Glasgow Coma Scale, (GCS), score was at least 6, 7 or 8, and in whom a surgical mass lesion was not present, were attributed to an extracranial complication unless evidence of deterioration on a subsequent CT scan could be clearly attributed to the presence of increased brain swelling or other indicators of increased intracranial volumes such as new parenchymal contusions, etc..

A large number of extracranial complications were identified and coded during the patient's course. These are shown in Figure 1 [3]. Multiple regression equations were used to determine whether or not a specific complication made any appreciable contribution to the patient's course, based on the nurses grading of the complication. Multiple complications occurring in the same patient were rated independently because of difficulties in assigning a relative weight to one complication versus another.

RESULTS

Thirty-six percent of the 717 patients died during the first year following data collection. Of these deaths, employing the criteria enumerated in the Methods and Material section, 60% could be directly attributed to the overall impact injury and not to a subsequent intracranial or extracranial complication which was potentially avoidable. Of the remaining deaths, 40% could be attributed to either an extracranial complication alone or the interaction of extracranial complications with the development of an intracranial complication, for example coagulopathy leading to a delayed intra-parenchymal hematoma or shock and hypoxia leading to an increased frequency of diffuse brain swelling. The incidence of diffuse brain swelling, using the new CT classification in the data bank, doubles in patients who have an identifiable episode of shock or hypoxia or both in the pre-hospital phase.

The most important complications and their relative contribution to a reduction in mortality are shown in Table 2. Note the tremendous influence of shock. More than half of all the potentially avoidable deaths are a result of shock. Of particular interest is our observation that shock, defined as a systolic blood pressure of 90 or less, is frequent within hospital complication often occurring during intensive treatment for intracranial hypertension. In over 100 salvageable patients, shock occurred nine or more hours following hospitalization. When these patients were compared to hospitalized patients who had never had an episode of shock, there was a trebling of mortality and vegetative survivorship. Significant contributions to preventable mortality and morbidity were also made by pneumonia, coagulopathy, and septicemia.

DISCUSSION

This study clearly demonstrates that substantial improvements in head injury mortality and morbidity could be obtained if complications, both intracranial and extracranial, could either be avoided or more rapidly responded to. Better rehydration of patients being treated with Mannitol, for example, or the earlier use of pressors to maintain a much higher cerebral perfusion pressure in patients receiving drugs such as barbiturates or propophol are likely to have a significant salutary influence. The use of monoclonal antibody technology for the treatment of septicemia, a therapy now being introduced in the

United States, while expensive, if targeted properly might also have a significant beneficial effect. In addition, clinical trials which are aimed at preventing colonization of the upper gastrointestinal tract with organisms which later are aspirated into the lung, or the application of gamma interferon, for example, to the lung by inhalational installation are novel approaches now being tested. While obviously it is naive to assume that all complications could be expeditiously treated or avoided, nevertheless, their contributions to head injury mortality and morbidity have been grossly underestimated and it is likely that with a few relatively simple steps and with the introduction of agents to protect the brain acutely in the pre-hospital and early-hospital setting that significant progress can be made in this area prior to the end of the century.

REFERENCES

[1] Foulkes MA, Eisenberg HM (Eds.): Report on the Traumatic Coma Data Bank, Supplement to the Journal of Neurosurgery, November, 1991.

[2] Becker DP, Miller JD, Ward JD, Greenberg RP, Young HF, and Sakalos R (1977) J Neurosurg 47:491-502.

[3] Piek J, Marshall LF, Blunt BA, Klauber, MR, van Berkum-Clark M (In Press) J Neurosurg.

FIGURE 1

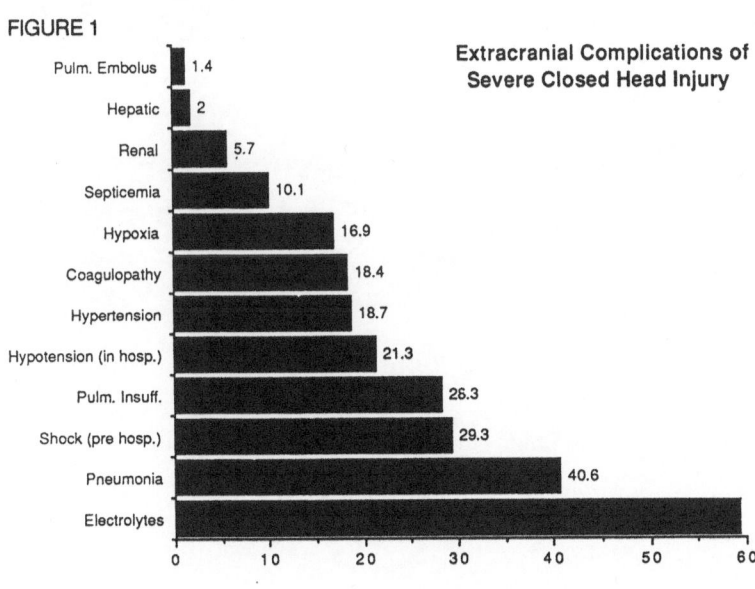

Extracranial Complications of Severe Closed Head Injury

Percent

TABLE 1

CAUSE OF DEATH

Overall Mortality	36%
Primary Injury	(20%)
Avoidable Deaths*	16%
Shock	10%
Pneumonia	10%
Coagulopathy	03%
Sepsis	02%
*Potentially	(01%)
	0%

351

10—Acute Epidural and Subdural Hematoma

Temporal Tip Acute Epidural Hematoma –
Its Diagnosis and Clinical Features

TAKEHIDE ONUMA, MOTONOBU KAMEYAMA, YASUKO SHIMOSEGAWA,
GENZOH SHIINA, and MASAHIRO YOSHIDA
Department of Neurosurgery, Sendai City Hospital, Sendai, Japan

SUMMARY

In the past 9 years, we have experienced 10 cases of acute epidural hematoma located at the temporal tip (TTEH). Mechanism, diagnosis, associated skull fractures and prognosis of TTEH were clinically analyzed. As results, TTEH is a rare occurrence (3.5% among acute epidural hematomas) and is noticed predominantly in the young, in traffic accidents and in the blow on the face. Diagnosis might be sometimes missed without careful observation of the temporal tip. MRI was the most effective means for diagnosis. Fractures of the ala major were mostly involved, and frequent associations of facial bone fractures such as zygoma, maxilla, orbital roof were also characteristic. TTEH itself did not extend to life threatening hematoma as other portion of acute epidural hematoma. TTEH has special clinical features and should be distinguished from so called " temporal acute epidural hematoma ".

KEY WORDS: temporal tip, acute epidural hematoma, diagnosis , pathogenesis, head injury

INTRODUCTION

Since the introduction of CT scan, even a small sized hematoma has become easily be diagnosed. This time we focused on the acute epidural hematoma localized to the temporal tip (TTEH) having special clinical features which is sometimes difficult to make a correct diagnosis unless careful attention was made (Fig. 1). The pathogenesis of TTEH together with diagnostic problems, clinical features, and the prognosis are discussed.

CLINICAL FEATURES OF TTEH

In the pasts 9 years, we have experienced 10 cases of TTEH accounting 3.5 % among 288 consecutive cases of acute epidural hematoma. The patients ranged in age from 8 to 74 years with an average of 27 years. Eight patients were male and 2 were female (Table 1). The mechanisms of injury were traffic accidents in 7 cases, fall in 2 and face injury by gas explosion in 1. Sites of injury were faces including anterior part of temporal region in 9 cases, temporal region in 1. In 9 cases, abrasions or swelling of cheek or peri-orbital region were observed.

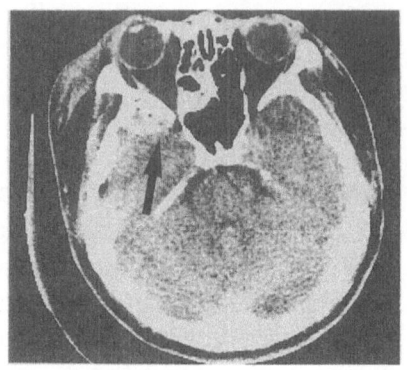

Fig. 1 CT scan showing a typical TTEH (arrow).

No. of Cases	10
frequency	3.5% (10 / 288)
age	8 ~ 74 (27)
sex	M : 8 F : 2

Table 1

GCS scores on admission were 15 in 2 cases, 14 in 4, 12 in 1, 10 in 2, and 7 in 1 respectively. Neurological signs responsible for TTEH were found in only 2 cases; oculomotor palsy in 1 case and sensory disturbance of the 2nd branch of the trigeminal nerve with anosmia in 1 .

Plain skull X-P or bone image CT disclosed nine cases (90%) of fractures. Plain skull X-P showed linear fractures of frontal bone in 4 cases, parietal bone in 1, and maxillar fracture in 1, however, in other 3 cases, fractures could not be detected. On the other hand, bone image CT disclosed fractures in all nine cases. Those were ala major in 8 cases, zygoma in 6, maxilla in 4, orbital roof in 4, ethmoid bone in 4, and ala minor in 2 (Table 2).

Locations of TTEH were unilateral in 8 cases and bilateral in 2 . Associated intracranial lesions were acute epidural hematomas of other regions in 3 cases and callosal injury in 1. Hemorrhages in the paranasal sinus were found in 6 cases. MRI were taken in 4 cases on the 2nd to 16th day after injury. TTEH was demonstrated clearly in T1 image as high signal intensity. No findings of brain edema nor contusion were found in the vicinity of TTEH.

All cases were treated conservatively regarding TTEH except one case in which concomitant temporoparietal epidural hematoma was removed surgically. Outcomes evaluated by Glasgow outcome scale were good recovery in 9 cases, moderate disability in 1 case due to associated diffuse brain injury.

location of fr.	No. of cases
ala major	8
zygoma	6
maxilla	4
orbital roof	4
ethmoid bone	4
ala minor	2

Table 2   Location of fractures defined by bone image CT

DISCUSSION

The temporal tip is a small hollow formed by posterior border of ala minor of the sphenoid, ala major and superior orbital fissure. Before CT era, it was virtually impossible to make a diagnosis of epidural hematoma localized to the temporal tip due to its unusual location and small size. Even in CT era, however, this diagnosis might be sometimes missed without careful observation of the temporal tip. Hitherto, no detailed reports about TTEH has been appeared in the literature.

In our series, frequency of TTEH is rare (3.5% of acute epidural hematomas).

Diagnosis can be made by CT scan as a biconvex high density area at the temporal tip . But sometimes, high density of TTEH was masked by the skull base. In this point, MRI was very effective means to diagnose TTEH, since it was clearly demonstrated as high signal intensity in T1 weighed image without artifacts produced by bone as seen in CT scan (Fig. 2).

Although fractures in the ala major were mostly involved, frequent associations of facial bone fractures such as zygoma, maxilla, orbital roof were characteristic, which suggests that the fracture of temporal tip might often occur secondary to facial injury.

The volume of TTEH is usually small and did not enlarge to life threatening lesion

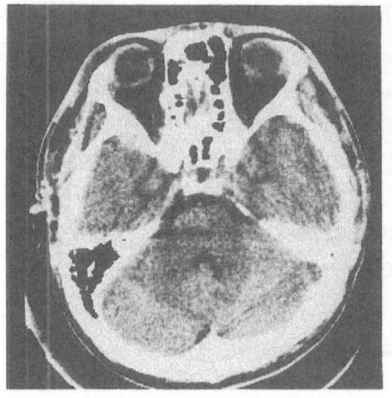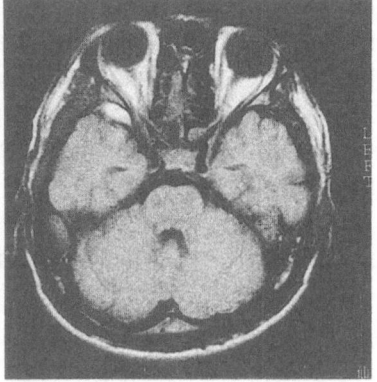

Fig. 2 CT scan (left) showing a small TTEH , which was more clearly visible on MRI (right).

like temporal epidural hematoma. This may be due to the fact that the temporal tip was under the guards of the thick temporal muscles, zygomatic arch and facial bones which plays an important role in preventing the tearing of the meningeal arteries, and thus resulting in minor dural detachment and slight meningeal vessel injuries following direct impacts to the head. Moreover, even if a anterior branch of middle meningeal artery is injured, enlargement of hematoma would be hindered by strong adhesion of the dura to the skull base.

Neurological signs related to TTEH was seen in only 2 cases and TTEH disappeared spontaneously by 2 month after injury. Outcome of TTEH was dependent of other associated intracranial lesion and the prognosis was thought to be good (Table 3).

- rare occurrence (3.5%)
- predominant in the young, in traffic accidents
- frequent association of facial bone fractures
- MRI is effective for diagnosis
- good prognosis

Table 3 Clinical features of TTEH

From an unusual location and clinical features, TTEH should be distinguished from the " temporal epidural hematoma " which sometimes enlarges and requires an emergent evacuation.

Preliminary Results of Sequential Scans Tc-HM-PAO (SPECT) and CT in Patients with Post-Traumatic Asymptomatic Extradural Hematoma Who Have Been Operated Versus Patients Who Have Not Been Operated. A Multicentre Randomized Study in Northern Italy

P. Fachinetti[1], A. Fachinetti[2], F. Servadei[3], M. Agostini[4], G. Moscatelli[4], G. Faccani[5], G. Castellano[6], R. Datti[7], G. Villavecchia[8], S. Pasetti[9], and B. Calbiani[10]

[1]Neurosurgery and [2]Nuclear Medicine Departments, Circolo Hospital, Varese, [3]Neurosurgery and [4]Nuclear Medicine Departments, Bufalini Hospital, Cesena, [5]Neurosurgery Department, CTO Torino, [6]Nuclear Medicine Department, S.G. Battista Hospital, Torino, [7]Neurosurgery and [8]Nuclear Medicine Departments, Galliera Hospital, Genova, [9]Neurosurgery and [10]Nuclear Medicine Departments, Parma, Italy

SUMMARY

22 patients with post-traumatic asymptomatic extradural hematoma (APEHs) were randomized in two groups: 11 operated versus 11 not operated. After CT scan controls all patients were submitted to HM-PAO[1] cerebral SPECT at 2.5 and 6 months. We found that 8 (73%) non operated patients showed hypoperfusion areas at the first SPECT control and 3 (27%) of these remained positive at the second SPECT control. In the operated group 3 were SPECT positive at the first control but nobody at the second one. There is a correlation between thickness, volume reabsorption time and SPECT control findings .

KEY WORDS: asymptomatic extradural hematoma, cerebral SPECT, 99mTC-HM-PAO

INTRODUCTION

The management of APEHs is still controversial . Some authors are in favour of surgical evacuation of hematoma, while others recommend awaiting its spontaneous reabsorbtion.

In a previous study, based on the use of SPECT with 99mTc-HM-PAO in two groups of 5 patients each who had a APEH of comparable site and volume 1 to 8 years before, we found a reduced cerebral perfusion in non operated patients, while other parametres such as EEG, CT and NMR appeared to be normal. This finding could mean that the compressive action of hematoma upon the brain during the time required for reabsorption was able to cause an impairment of perfusion: an event which was not apparent if the hematoma had been early operated.

To confirm these preliminary findings and to determine a "treshold volume" beyond which the patients with non operated APEH may reveal a defect of cerebral perfusion, we have carried out the present multicentre randomized study.

MATERIALS AND METHODS

22 patients with APEHs (average GCS 13.77) were randomized: 11 were operated within 48 hours of injury and 11 were kept under observation by CT scan until reabsorption of their hematomas.
Eligible patients were either male or female subjects between 10 and 65 years of age, affected by pure post traumatic hematoma thicker than 5 mm and confirmed by CT scan within 48 hours of injury.

Exclusion criteria were the coexistence of dementia, HIV sieropositivity, epilepsy, acute or chronic cerebrovascular disease, migrane or other abnormalities detectable by CT.

The operated patients underwent a post-surgical control CT to verify the complete removal of their hematoma and a normal brain. The non operated patients were followed by serial CT scans (from 3 to 6) until reabsorption.

---

1 Ceretec TM - Amersham International plc

Table 1 : BASELINE EVALUATION Individual data are reported in Table 1A (non operated patients) and Table 1B (operated patients). The two groups are significantly different for the values of maximal thickness and volume of hematoma, which are higher in the operated patients (see Table 2: Comparison between groups).

Tab. 1A . Baseline evaluation of non operated patients.

Case No.	Centre	GCS	Site*	Extent (mm)	Thick ness (mm)	Volume (cc)	Compres sion (score)	Shift (score)
1	VARESE	15	FL	50	12	15	0	0
2	VARESE	15	TL	20	9	4	0	0
4	VARESE	14	TR	30	10	4	0	0
7	VARESE	14	PR	60	20	25	0.5	0
1	PARMA	15	TL	61	18	14	1	0.5
3	PARMA	15	PR	68	17	32	1	1
2	CESENA	15	TL	32	8	10	1	0
3	CESENA	15	FL	20	10	12	1	0
4	CESENA	15	TR	32	28	27	1	0
7	CESENA	15	FR	18	10	9	0	0
8	CESENA	14	FR	35	10	5	0	0
Mean		14.73		38.73	13.82	14.27	0.50	0.14
S.D.		0.47		18.01	6.21	9.70	0.50	0.32
S.E		0.14		5.43	1.87	2.92	0.15	0.10
Min.		14		18	8	4	0.00	0.00
Max.		15		68	28	32	1.00	1.00
N.		11		11	11	11	11	11

Tab. 1B . Baseline evaluation of operated patients.

Case No.	Centre	GCS	Site*	Extent (mm)	Thick ness (mm)	Volume (cc)	Compres sion (score)	Shift (score)
3	VARESE	15	TL	25	15	18	0	0
5	VARESE	14	TL	50	18	10	0	0
2	PARMA	14	TL	45	12	6	0	0
1	GENOVA	10	OL	50	16	12	0	0
1	TORINO	15	TR	70	20	40	1	0
2	TORINO	14	TR	60	24	22.5	0	0
6	CESENA	14	PR	65	20	37	2	0
9	CESENA	10.5	TL	60	22	44	1	1
10	CESENA	15	TL	50	15	27	1	0
11	CESENA	15	TR	35	20	32	1	0
12	CESENA	15	TR	50	22	38	1	1
Mean:		13.77		50.91	18.55	26.05	0.636	0.182
S.D.		1.81		13.00	3.67	13.23	0.674	0.405
S.E.		0.55		3.92	1.11	3.99	0.203	0.122
Min.		10.00		25	12	6.00	0.00	0.00
Max.		15.00		70	24	44.00	2.00	1.00
N.		11		11	11	11	11	11

* F = frontal; T = temporal ; P = parietal; O = occipital; R = right; L = left

Table 2 : COMPARISON BETWEEN GROUPS

Variable	Statistical test *		p
GCS	t (d.f. 20)	= 1.696	N.S.
Extent	t (d.f. 20)	= 1.819	N.S.
Thickness	t (d.f. 20)	= 2.173	< 0.05
Volume	t (d.f. 20)	= 2.380	< 0.05
Compression	U (n1=11 n2=11)	= 55.000	N.S.
Shift III	U (n1=11 n2=11)	= 59.500	N.S.

* t = Student's t test for independent samples
U = Mann - Whitney's U test

Each patient was submitted to two successive SPECT scans 2.5 and 6 months after; cerebral tomoscintigraphy was performed by using 99mTc-HM-PAO at the dose of 1110 MBq.For each patient 8 orbital-meatal sections of 2 pixel (12mm) thickness were considered.Firstly, a qualitative analysis of all sections (orbital-meatal, sagittal, coronal) was carried out by giving them a severity score as follows: 1+ = slightly reduced, 2+ = moderately reduced, 3+ = markedly reduced captation. On the most significant OM sections a semiquantitative analysis was also made by delimiting 3 equal and simmetrical ROIs and then calculating for each pair the ratio of the affected to unaffected side counts. We have also identified additional ROIs on the more marked lesions, determinig their ratio to equivalent and simmetrical areas in the controlateral hemisphere. For a semiquantitative evaluation we considered as normal a right to left ratio (or vice versa) equal to 1+ 0.01.

RESULTS

The non operated patients had the following average values for their hematomas: maximal diameter 38.73 mm,thickness 13.88 mm, volume 14.27 cc. The corresponding values in the operated group were 50.9 mm for maximal diameter, 18.55 mm for thickness and 26.0 cc for volume. The site most often involved in both groups was the temporal one, although the non operated patients showed a more omogeneous distribution.

Tab. 3A : Site of initial injury and SPECT findings (severity and site) in non operated patients.

Case	Site of initial injury	1st SPECT severity	1st SPECT site	2nd SPECT severity	2nd SPECT site
1	FL	slight	FL	negative	-
2	TL	slight	PR	slight	PR
4	TR	slight	TR	negative	-
7	PR	marked	PL	slight	PL
1	TL	slight	TR	negative	-
3	PR	slight	PL	negative	-
2	TL	negative	-	negative	-
3	FL	slight	FL	slight	FL
4	TR	negative	TR	negative	-
7	FR	slight	FR	negative	-
8	FR	negative	FR	negative	-

Tab. 3B : Site of initial injury and SPECT findings (severity and site) in operated patients.

Case	Site of initial injury	1st SPECT severity	1st SPECT site	2nd SPECT severity	2nd SPECT site
3	TL	negative	-	-	-
5	TL	negative	-	-	-
2	TL	slight	TL	negative	-
1	OL	slight	NBL	negative	-
1	TR	negative	-	negative	-
2	TR	negative	-	negative	-
6	PR	negative	-	negative	-
9	TL	slight	TL	negative	-
10	TL	negative	-	-	-
11	TR	negative	-	-	-
12	TR	negative	-	-	-

There were no significant differences between groups in the frequency and extent of ventricular compression and in the shifting of the median line. The mean time to complete reabsorption of non operated hematomas in CT scans has been 49.4 days. In all 11 operated patients a SPECT examination at 6 months appeared to be normal. In this group 3 patients (27%) were positive at the first control (. 2.5 month).

In the non operated group 8 patients (73%) were SPECT positive at the first control : the degree of positivity was rated one plus (+) in 7 (64%) and two plus (++) in 1 patient (9%). Fig.1.

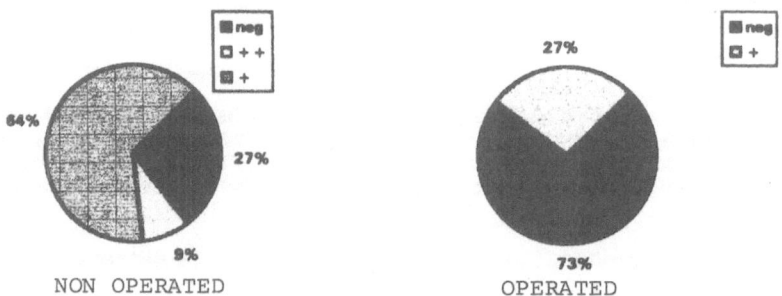

NON OPERATED   OPERATED

Fig. 1 Results of the 1st SPECT examination

Subsequently 5 patients went back to normal, so that 3 patients (27%) retained a positive SPECT (+) at 6 months . Fig.2.

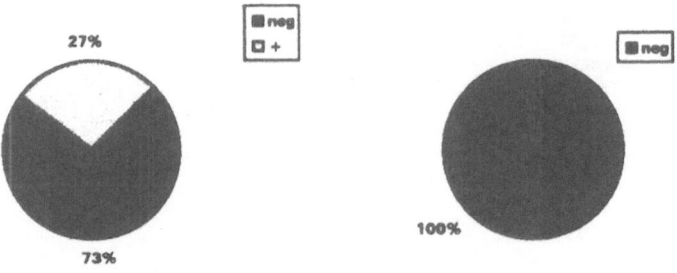

NON OPERATED

Fig. 2 Final evaluation of SPECT findings

362

Of these 3 patients the area of reduced perfusion was located at the site of the hematoma in one case, while it was controlateral in the remaining two (Table 9) In the non operated patients there was a correlation both between the extent of hematoma and the ratio non-injuried/injuried side at the first SPECT control and between the hematoma reabsorption time and the first SPECT control .

The following variables did not appear to be correlated with the SPECT findings: patient's age , site, initial thickness and volume of hematoma, though the observed volumes were relatively small, i. e. less than 30 cc in 10 patients.

Table 4 : CORRELATION OUTCOMES : the outcomes of the correlation estimates between pairs for a number of parameters in the non operated patients are shown below in table 5. Significant correlations were found between : volume and extent , volume and thickness , 1st SPECT findings and disappearance time , radioactivity ratio at the 1st SPECT control and extent of lesion.

Parameter	Disappear ance time	Extent	Thick ness	Volume	1st SPECT	Ratio 1st SPECT
Age	-0.012ns	0.335ns	0.348ns	0.422ns	-0.412ns	-0.226ns
Disapp.time	-	0.320ns	0.483ns	0.558ns	0.620*	0.598ns
Extent	-	-	0.473ns	0.665*	0.129ns	0.720*
Thickness	-	-	-	0.795*	0.256ns	0.198
Volume	-	-	-	-	0.128ns	0.354
spect	-	-	-	-	-	0.146

* $p<0.05$

DISCUSSION

The aim of this prospective , randomized study, carried out in a sample of 22 patients, was to evaluate the outcome of operated versus non operated APEHs , as judged by SPECT 2.5 and 6 months after the injury. While all the 11 operated patients proved to have normal SPECT scans, 3 of the 11 non operated patients appeared to be still positive at the second SPECT control .

This finding, though only approaching statistical significance , points to a clearly different trend in respect of the operated patients. In 2 subjects the site of SPECT positivity was controlateral to that of the past hematoma: we have no explanation of this finding, already observed in 1 out of the 4 patients belonging to the previous series. In the third patient the site of SPECT positivity was the same as that of the hematoma. The present study could not demonstrate a correlation between the volume of hematoma and SPECT positivity for hematomas greater than 25cc. This is likely due to the relatively small number of patients studied and to the limited size of the non operated hematomas; however the significant correlation of the SPECT findings with both the maximal extent and reabsorption time of hematomas makes it reasonable to assume a direct relationship in the above direction.

The SPECT technique which appears to be a highly sensitive diagnostic tool in the management of patients with cerebral hematomas has shown that areas of reduced perfusion persist in 27% of the non operated APEHs, whereas this event does not occur in the operated patients. The clinical significance of the above finding is not clear, nor there is evidence of its relationship with the development of epileptogenic foci, so that sure rules of treatment cannot be dictated. We feel, however, that the results of the present study justify the surgical option in those APEHs having a volume greater than 25 cc or a maximal extent greater than 50mm or showing an abnormal course in the reabsorption time.

Rapid Spontaneously Disappearance of Acute Subdural Hematomas: Analysis of 31 Cases

MOTOAKI FUJII, YOICHI KATAYAMA, HIROAKI TANAKA, YASUHIDE MAKIYAMA, TAKAMITSU YAMAMOTO, and TAKASHI TSUBOKAWA

Department of Neurological Surgery, Nihon University School of Medicine, Tokyo, 173 Japan

SUMMARY

We reviewed 31 cases of acute thin subdural hematomas including those reported in the literature and our own which had disappeared spontaneously within 72 hours post-trauma. The subdural hematomas in these cases were detected mostly within 60 min after injury. A significant decrease in hematoma size was demonstrated at as early as 2 hours after injury. It seems therefore that the earlier the initial CT scan was taken, the more frequently acute thin subdural hematomas which rapidly disappeared could be detected. The hematomas did not explain clinical conditions on admission. Brain swelling and cardiorespiratory failure appeared to be responsible for poor outcome. Repeated CT scans and careful observation of the neurological changes is recommended before undertaking surgical intervention in such cases.

KEY WORDS: CT - acute subdural hematoma - traumatic intracranial hematoma - cerebral swelling

INTRODUCTION

Since our initial reports [4,5], we have experienced 10 cases of acute thin subdural hematomas detected in the very early period following trauma which had disappeared spontaneously within a day. It seems that the earlier the initial CT scan is taken, the more frequently such hematomas are encountered [1-8]. Recognition of this entity has raised a dilemma in the clinical setting as to whether the given hematoma should be operated on or not [1,2], since some acute thin subdural hematomas do, on the other hand, increase in size rapidly and could therefore lead to disastrous neurological deterioration [9]. We reviewed in the present study 31 cases of such hematomas including those reported in the literature and our own.

MATERIALS AND METHODS

We analyzed cases of acute thin subdural hematomas with thickness of more than 4 mm which had disappeared within 72 hours. Although their ages ranged from 3 to 84 years, most cases were between 15 and 30. Injury had often been induced by traffic accidents, suggesting high velocity injury. The Glasgow coma scores (GCS) on admission were highly variable, ranging from 3 to 15.

RESULTS

Acute thin subdural hematomas were detected mostly within 60 min after injury. A significant decrease in hematoma size was demonstrated at as early as 2 hours after injury. It seems therefore that the earlier the initial CT scan was taken, the more frequently acute thin subdural hematomas which rapidly disappeared could be detected.

Although hemiparesis and pupillary abnormality were sometimes observed, these abnormalities were not related to a bad outcome. In contrast, the presence of respiratory disturbance (4 cases) was always associated with subsequent death (Table 1).

Table 1. Summary of fatal cases

Age /Sex	Trauma	GCS	Clinical findings	Initial CT (min)	Second CT (hour)
5/M	traffic accident	6	respiratory disturabance pupil abnormality	120	2
19/M	downfall	6	hypotension shock respiratory disturbance	60	2
61/F	downfall	4	respiratory disturabance pupil abnormality	60	72
65/M	traffic accident	5	hemiparesis pupil abnormality respiratory disturbance	60	21

Cases with GCS values of 8 or less frequently demonstrated early development of unilateral hemispheric swelling or diffuse brain swelling on their CT scans, although only diffuse brain swelling was associated with a high mortality rate. Since hematomas did not explain the low GCS values on admission as well as poor outcome, brain swelling and cardiorespiratory failure appeared to be responsible for these clinical conditions.

Intracranial pressure (ICP) was monitored in 5 cases. The ICP initially ranged from 15 to 30 mmHg. It remained below 20 mmHg in 3 cases with moderate hyperventilation ($PCO_2 > 23$ mmHg). In 2 cases, the ICP was controlled at below 30 mmHg with intense hyperventilation ($PCO_2 < 23$ mmHg) and barbiturate administration. Even with intense hyperventilation, the oxygen saturation of the jugular vein was maintained at above 65%. The hematomas disappeared within 36 hours and good recovery was achieved in all of the 5 cases.

DISCUSSION

It does not seem uncommon for acute thin subdural hematomas detected in the very early period following injury disappear spontaneously [1-8]. Repeated CT scans and careful observation of the neurological changes have therefore been recommended before undertaking surgical intervention in such cases [1,2]. ICP monitoring provides an alternative means in cases with a low GCS for deciding whether or not surgical removal of the hematomas is required.

This group of hematomas may constitute part of the so-called "benign" acute subdural hematomas [10]. Their clinical course, however, is not always benign, which suggests that co-existent intraparenchymal lesions may play a significant role in deciding the clinical conditions and outcome. A review of 31 cases of spontaneously disappearing acute thin subdural hematomas indicated that low GCS values are often associated with early development of unilateral hemispheric or diffuse brain swelling [4,5]. The present study revealed that such hemispheric swelling is associated with an elevated ICP. Intensive medical control of the ICP is apparently more important than surgical removal of the hematomas in such patients.

Based on the above characteristics of spontaneously disappearing acute thin subdural hematomas, such hematomas can be treated conservatively with following criteria: (1) the hematomas were detected within 60 min after injury; (2) the GCS value on admission is more than 8; and (3) hematoma does not explain the clinical conditions.

REFERENCES

1. Aoki N (1990) Acute subdural haematoma with rapid resolution. Acta Neurochir (Wien) 103:76-78
2. Fujioka S, Hamada J, Kaku M et al (1990) Rapid resolution of acute subdural hematoma. Report of two cases. Neurol Med Chir (Tokyo) 30:827-831 (in Japanese)
3. Joki T, Hashimoto T, Akachi K, Boku M, Suzuki K, Nakamura N (1992) Neurol. Surg. 20: 915-919 (in Japanese).
4. Katayama Y, Fujii M, Tsubokawa T, Miyazaki S, Yamamoto T, Kinoshita K (1992) Spontaneously disappearing acute subdural hematomas: conservative treatment with intracranial pressure monitoring. Intracranial Pressure VIII in press.
5. Makiyama Y, Katayama Y, Tsubokawa, T (1987) Rapid, spontaneous disappearance of acute subdural hematoma. Neurosurgery 21:429
6. Nagao T, Aoki N, Mizutani H et al (1986) Acute subdural hematoma with rapid   resolution in infancy. Case report. Neurosurgery 19:465-469
7. Niikawa S, Sugimoto S, Hattori T et al (1989) Rapid resolution of acute subdural hematoma. Report of four cases. Neurol Med Chir (Tokyo) 29:820-824
8. Polman CH, Gijsbers CJ, Heimans JJ et al (1986) Rapid spontaneous resolution   of an acute
9. Seelig JM, Becker DP, Miller JD et al (1981) Traumatic acute subdural hematoma. N Engl J Med 304:1511-1518.
10. Singounas EG, Sfakianos G, Sourtzis I et al (1990) "Benign" acute subdural hematomas. Acta Neurochir (Wien) 106:140-144.

Treatment of Acute Subdural Hematoma

TAKASHI TOKUTOMI, MINORU SHIGEMORI, NAOMI KIKUCHI, TATSUO YUGE, KIMIHIRO NAKAHARA, and SHINKEN KURAMOTO
Department of Neurosurgery, Kurume University School of Medicine, Kurume, Japan

SUMMARY

Three types of surgical treatment and adjunctive barbiturate therapy were evaluated by analyzing their outcome in patients with traumatic acute subdural hematoma. From June, 1982 to December, 1990, 120 patients underwent surgery for acute subdural hematoma at Kurume University Hospital. Of these, 108 patients admitted to the hospital with a Glasgow Come Scale (GCS) score of 8 or less, and 75 with a GCS score of 5 or less. Removal of the hematoma with craniotomy (RH), removal of the hematoma with decompressive hemicraniectomy (DH) and hematoma irrigation with trephination therapy (HITT) were performed in 42, 51 and 27 patients, respectively. Of those with uncontrolled intracranial pressure over 30 mmHg, 23 were treated with barbiturates. The overall mortality rate was 51.7 %, and the rate of good outcome was 26.7 %. The rate of good outcome was singnificantly higher in the patients who underwent RH (47.6 %), although the mortality rate of them was higher than that of the patients who underwent DH when the GCS score was 5 or less. Among the patients with a GCS score of 8 or less, the mortality rate was significantly higher in those who underwent HITT (74.1 %). In patients with barbiturate therapy, RH had the best result. This study suggests that RH is preferable for acute subdural hematoma, although DH appears to be better for improving the mortality rate. HITT is not recommended in patients with a GCS score of 8 or less.

KEY WORDS : subdural hematoma, head injury, treatment, outcome

INTRODUCTION

Traumatic acute subdural hematoma remains a difficult challenge for neurosurgeons because of the high mortality rate and limited functional recovery, We have reported a good correlation between raised intracranial pressure (ICP) and severe morbidity and mortality in patients with acute subdural hematoma [2], and have adopted aggressive treatment by decompressive hemicraniectomy and barbiturate therapy to control high ICP level which may associate with good outcome [3]. In this study, we investigated the effectiveness of different surgical treatment and adjunctive postoperative barbiturate therapy for acute subdural hematoma.

MATERIALS AND METHODS

We treated 910 patients with closed head injury between June, 1982 and December, 1990. Of these, 120 patients underwent surgery for acute subdural hematoma. The patients ranged in age from 4 to 92 years, with mean age of 54.5 years. Twelve patients had a Glasgow Coma Scale (GCS) score [4] of 9 or above, 33 had a score of 6 to 8, and 75 had a score of 3 to 5. Removal of the hematoma with craniotomy (RH) for 42 patients, removal of the hematoma with decompressive hemicraniectomy (DH) for 51 and hematoma irrigation with trepphination therapy (HITT) for 27 were performed immediately after admission. Of those with uncontrolled postoperative ICP over 30 mmHg, 23 were treated with barbiturate. Outcome was evaluated based on the Glasgow Outcome Scale [1]. The patients with good recovery and moderate disability were classified as 'good' and those with severe disability and persistent vegetative state as 'poor'. Associated intracranial lesions on CT scans was also evaluated.

RESULTS

The overall mortality rate was 51.7 % and the rate of good outcome was 26.7 %. As seen in Table 1, there was statistically

Table 1 Outcome in 120 patients in relation to type of surgery.

Type of Surgery	No. of Cases	Outcome		
		Good	Poor	Death (%)
RH	42	20 (47.6)[*1]	7 (16.7)	15 (35.7)
DH	51	9 (17.6)	15 (29.4)	27 (52.9)
HITT	27	3 (11.1)	4 (14.8)	20 (74.1)[*2]
Total	120	32 (26.7)	26 (21.7)	62 (51.7)

RH : removal of the hematoma by craniotomy, DH : removal of the hematoma with decompressive hemicraniectomy, HITT : hematoma irrigation with trephination therapy, *1 : significant difference from DH and HITT (p < 0.01), *2 : significant difference from RH (p < 0.01)

significant difference in good outcome in the RH group
(47.6 %) and in death in the HITT group (74.1 %). However,
in the patients with GCS scores of 9 or above, five patients
underwent HITT had good outcome, and all of them were
over 66 years, In 75 patients with GCS scores of 3 to 5
on admission, the mortality late was 64.0 % and the rate
of good outcome was 12.0 %. In these patients, the mortality
rate was significantly higher in the HITT group (84.2 %).
and the rate of good outcome was significantly higher
in the RH group (22.2 %). By age, however, mortality rate
tended to be lower in the DH group in the patients aged
65 years or younger.
In 23 patients with barbiturate therapy, the mortality rate
was 56.5 % and the rate of good outcome was 17.4 %. Those
with RH had the best result ; 37.5 % mortality and 37.5 %
good outcome rates, but, the patients aged over 65 years
had no good outcome and high mortality rate (80.0 %).
Thirty eight patients had associated intracerebral hematoma.
The incidence of postoperative development of intracerebral
hematoma was higher in the DH group, but there was no
significant change in outcome associated with the presence
of intracerebral hematoma. Diffuse subarachinoid hemorrhage
around the brainstem on intial CT scans associated significantly
with high mortality rate (76.9 %).

DISCUSSION

Control of ICP is one of the most important factor in the
management of acute subdural hamatoma [2,5], and surgical
therapy is still a principal part of the management of
elevated ICP influencing on the outcome. The findings in
this study indicate that HITT dose not favorably affect
the outcome of the patients with acute subdural hematoma
with a GCS score of 8 or less. This therapy will remain
for elderly patients with a GCS score of 9 or above, or
urgent decompression in emergency room prior to craniotomy.
The patients with a GCS score of 8 or less are preferably
treated by craniotomy with evacuation of the hamatoma.
Decompressive hemicraniectomy with hamatoma evacuation
must be considered for young patients with a GCS score
of 5 or less.
Barbiturate thrapy was not to be effective for elderly patients,
and even in young patients, further reseach needs to be
done. This study has also confirmed the importance of associated
subarachnoid hemorrhage around the brainstem, which suggests
the severe impact damege as primary brain injury, significantly
correlated with high morbidity and mortality rates.

REFERENCES

1. Jennet B, Bond M (1975) Assesment of outcome after severe

brain damage. A practical scale. Lancet 1 : 480 − 484

2. Shigemori M, Shojima K, Nakayama K, Kojima T, Ogata T, Watanabe M, Kuramoto S (1980) The outcome from acute subdural hematoma following decompressive hemicraniectomy. Acta Neurochir 58 : 61 − 69

3. Shigemori M, Tokutomi T, Yamamoto F, Kobayashi S, Nakashima H, Watanabe M, Kuramoto S (1989) Treatment of acute subdural hematoma with a low GCS score. Neurosurg Rev 12 : 198 − 200

4. Teasdale G, Jennent B (1974) Assement of coma and impaired consciousness, A practical scale. Lancet 2 : 81 − 84

5. Wilberger JF, Harris M, Diamond DL (1991) Acute subdural hematoma : morbidity, mortality, and operative timing. J Neurosurg 74 : 212 − 218

Outcome of Acute Subdural Hematoma – Large Decompressive Craniectomy Vs Hematoma Irrigation with Trephination Therapy

Tohru Aruga, Tetsuya Sakamoto, Kazuya Kiyota, Yasufumi Miyake, Tohru Mizutani, Hiroshi Tanaka, Masaru Sasaki[1], Koji Mii[1], and Kintomo Takakura[2]

Critical Care Center, Showa General Hospital, Kodaira, Tokyo, 187 Japan and Departments of [1]Emergency Medicine and [2]Neurosurgery, University of Tokyo Hospital, Bunkyo-ku, Tokyo, 113 Japan

SUMMARY

The clinical comparison was instituted between large decompressive craniectomy (LDC) and hematoma irrigation with trephination (HIT) therapy for 120 cases suffering from the complicated hematoma type of traumatic acute subdural hematoma. The medical management of increased intracranial pressure (ICP) included osmotherapy, hyperventilation and barbiturate induced coma post-operatively equally in these two strategies. LDC proved superior to HIT in patients with severely disturbed consciousness (30 to 200 /Japan coma scale) on admission. The parenchymal lesion associated with the complicated type of acute subdural hematoma should be regarded as the severest entity of diffuse cerebral injury. For the present, the surgical removal of subdural clot with large external decompression and the intensive medical decompression with continuous ICP monitoring, containing barbiturate administration, if necessary aré both recomended for the management of this clinical entity.

KEYWORDS: acute subdural hematoma, extrnal decompression, barbiturate therapy, intracranial pressure, outcome

INTRODUCTION

Acute subdural hematoma is categorized into two different types; a simple hematoma type and a complicated hematoma type. The former is acute subdural hematoma caused mostly by laceration of cortical vessel or bridging vein with little amount of parenchymal injury, if any. The latter is complicated with parenchymal pathological process which consists of cerebral contusion, diffuse axonal injury as primaly injuries and brain edema, swelling, hypoxic and ischemic lesions as secondary insults. The autors advocated and applied HIT therapy to the management of the complicated type of acute subdural hematoma from theoretical and practical points of view. HIT therapy with aggressive medical control of intracranial hypertension, which proved not inferior to other classic or conventional methodologies[1] should be compared with the strategy of large external decopressive surgery with such equal conditions other than operative prosedures as the timing of operaton, tactics of ICP control etc. This article is on the clinical control study of making a comparison between HIT and LDC for the management of the complicated type of acute subdural hematoma, performed co-operatively by two institutions.

MATERIALS AND METHODS

Clinical entry of this study was as follows; 1) Acute subdural hematoma compatible with the complicated hematoma type was the main finding of computerized tomography and no other intracranial hematoma was evident. 2) HIT or LDC was performed within 24 hours after trauma. 3) The patients was 15 years of age or more. HIT therapy is composed of the removal of the subdural clot with manual injections of saline and the medical aggressive management of intracranial hypertension including barbiturate administration[1]. Another strategy of LDC included subtemporal decompression and dural plasty. During the ten years from January, 1982 to December, 1991, 68 cases were treated with HIT therapy in University of Tokyo Hosipital and 52 cases with LDC in Showa General Hospital. The age distribution and its average in each group are shown in Table 1. Each group was classified into 3 subgroups according to Japan coma scale (Table 2). Post-operatively ICP was continuously monitored for all with the catheter inserted into subarachnoid or dubdural space[2]. When ICP increased more than 20 mmHg, the upper half of the body elevated to 15 though 20 degrees and osmotherapy was induced. Then mild hyperventilation (25 to 30 mmHg of $PaCO2$) was used with endotracheal intubation and mandatory ventilation. If ICP was not controlled with these tactics and got to 35 mmHg or more, the barbiturate coma therapy was induced with the method described in Table 3, which maintained 25 to 35 μ g/ml of the serum concentration of pentobarbital[3]. The outcomes of the two strategies and postoperative courses of ICP were analized statistically with χ -square test.

RESULTS

The clinical outcome of all the materials according to Glassgow outcome scale is demonstrated in Table 4. The barbiturate therapy was induced not only in HIT (53%) but also in LDC group (41%). As is shown in Table 5, in Group II, HIT was found to be inferior to LDC because of its statistically higher rate of mortality. In Group I or III no statistical difference was verified betwen HIT and LDC. The initial ICP which was measured just after HIT proved higher than that immediately after LDC in Group II (Table 6). As to the Maximum ICP, which was the most increased level throughout bedside minitoring after LDC or HIT, because of the fact that the maximum ICP of the dead equalled the value of mean arterial pressure, with cerebral perfusion pressure decreasing to null, the maximum ICP of survivors was compared and the statistically significant difference was verified in Group II (Table 7). But no significant difference was found in initial ICPs between HIT and LDC survivors.

DISCUSSION

It has been reported that the mortality rate of traumatic acute subdural hematoma is about 50 through 80%, which suggests acute subdural hematoma for one of the most difficult clinical entities to manage. Acute subdural hematoma is often complicated with parenchymal lesions of cerebral contusion, diffuse axonal injury as primary injuries and brain edema, swelling, hypoxic and ischemic lesions as secondary insults. Even if the subdural clot is removed appropriately enough, its parenchymal involvements still remain unsolved. The authors ever categorized acute subdural hematoma into two different types and reported that the mortality rates of the simple hematoma type and the complicated hematoma type were 44% and 71%, respectively[4]. The materials of this study suffered from the latter. Generally

Table 1: Material and surgical therapy

	HIT	LDC	
Cases (male/female)	68 (47/21)	52 (36/16)	p = N.S.
Age (years, average)	17~91 (53.4)	16~78 (49.7)	p = N.S.

Table 2: Consciousness on admission and surgical therapy

Group (Japan coma scale)	HIT	LDC	
I (3~ 20)	8 cases	11 cases	
II (30~200)	47 cases	37 cases	
III (300)	13 cases	4 cases	
Total	68 cases	52 cases	p= N.S.

Table 3: Method of pentobarbital administration for adults
Initial dosage: 400 mg/hr × 5 hrs or 200 mg/hr × 10 hrs   ; intravenously
Maintenance dosage: 50 mg/hr; ditto
(up to maximum of 200 mg/hr if the serum concentration of pentobarbital less than 25 μg/ml)

Table 4:

1) HIT and outcome

JCS	D	PVS	SD	MD	GR	Total
3	1				2	3
10	1			2(1)		3 (1)
20	1					2
30	3 (3)		1			4 (3)
100	2 (2)	1(1)		1	2(1)	6 (4)
200	33(19)	2(1)	1(1)	1		37(21)
300	13 (7)					13 (7)
	54(31)	4(2)	2(1)	2	6(2)	68(36)

2) LDC and outcome

JCS	D	PVS	SD	MD	GR	Total
3	2(1)			1	4	7 (1)
10	1					1
20	1			2(1)		3 (1)
30	1				4(1)	5 (1)
100	4(2)	1	3(3)	5(3)	5(3)	18(11)
200	8(4)	2(2)		2	2	14 (6)
300	3(1)	1				4 (1)
	20(8)	4(2)	3(3)	10(4)	15(4)	52(21)

Abbreviations: D; death, PVS; persitent vegetative state, SD; severe disability,
MD; moderate disability, GR; good recovery (Glasgow outcome scale)
No. of cases in parentheses had barbiturate therapy induced.

Tabel 5: Surgical therapy and outcome

Group I	HIT	LDC
dead	3(2)	4(2)
alive	5	7
total	8	11

p = N.S.

Group II	HIT	LDC
dead	38(4)	13(4)
alive	9	24
total	47	37

p <0.001

Group III	HIT	LDC
dead	13(2)	3(0)
alive	0	1
total	13	4

p = N.S.

No. of cases in parentheses indicate dead cases due to systemic complications

Table 6: Initial ICP (average ± standard deviations, mmHg)

Group	HIT	LDC	
I	14.1±19.2 (N=8)	18.8±35.9 (N=11)	p = N.S.
II	39.7±33.8 (N=47)	8.9±13.9 (N=37)	p < 0.0001
III	33.2±23.5 (N=13)	22.0±15.2 (N=4)	p = N.S.

Table 7: Maxmum ICP of survivors

Group	HIT	LDC	
I	37.2±23.9 (N=5)	18.6± 6.3 (N=7)	p = N.S.
II	33.6±14.7 (N=9)	19.2±12.3 (N=24)	p < 0.05
III		41.0 (N=1)	

Table 8: Initial ICP of survivors

Group	HIT	LDC	
I	18.2±23.1 (N=5)	2.3± 4.4 (N=7)	p = N.S.
II	10.1± 8.8 (N=9)	4.0± 9.6 (N=24)	p = N.S.
III		41.0 (N=1)	

decompressive craniectomy in the management of acute subdural hematoma has been advocated for the treatment of brain edema or swelling associated with it. The bony decompression with dural plasty seems successful in some cases but enhances cerebral swelling and exacerbates edema in others, often follwing excessive changes in systemic aterial pressure. Such clinical experiences are supported by experimental facts[5,6]. And besides cerebral contusion or diffuse axonal injury complicated with acute subdural hematoma is regarded essentially far from indicative of operative resection. In HIT group the parenchymal lesions were managed medically within the physiological cranial vault. In this meaning, LDC and HIT are located in two opposite poles. According to the results of this study although LDC might have induced possibly more amount of hydrostatic edema, it was certificated that LDC proved superior to HIT except for in relatively less severe (3-20 /JCS) cases and deeply comatose (300 /JCS) cases. The results on ICP monitorings coresponded well to the clinical outcomes. Enlarged external decompression and barbiturate administration added if necessary could aford effective intracranial space against tentorial herniation in accordance with the pressure-volume response curves before and after external decompression[7].

On the other hand, the outcome of HIT therapy whose mortality was 79% of the total was worse than the generally recognized prognosis of diffuse cerebral injury. The traumatic coma data bank in U.S.A. reported that the mortality of the severest diffuse injury was 56%[8]. According to the theory of rotational acceleration-decceleration mechanism producing diffuse cerebral injury, severest shearing strains are observed in brainstem and brain surface[9]. It is reasonable that the diffuse shearing injury induces acute subdural hematoma and even acute brain swelling at its maximum as well as diffuse parenchymal lesions. Therefore the complicated type of acute subdural hematoma revealed not solely the simple sum of subdural clot and diffuse cerebral injury but should be regarded as more serious and also as the severest clinical entity out of diffuse cerebral injuries. In Group I no statistically significant difference was recognized between initial ICPs or clinical outcomes of the two strategies, but the mortality of LDC was 38% of the total, which is the supreme that has ever been reported. For the present the surgical removal of subdural clot with large exteral decompression and the aggressive medical decompression containing barbiturate administration with continuous ICP monitoring are both recommendedfor the management of this clinical entity.

REFFERENCES

1. Aruga T, Mii K, Sakamoto T, Yamashita M, Sasaki M, Tsustumi H, Toyooka H, Takakura K (1984) Brain & Nerve 36: 709-716
2. Yano M, Aruga T, Kobayashi S, Hiranuma N, Yamamoto Y, Hennmi H, Nishimura N (1981) Jap J Anesthesiol 30: 395-400
3. Nishihara K, Kohda Y, Tamura Z, Tsutsumi H, Sasaki M, Aruga T, Toyooka H, Mii K (1987) Neurol Med Chir (Tokyo) 27: 617-622
4. Tsutsumi H, Fuchinoue T, Aruga T, Mii K, Manaka S (1982) Neurotraumatology 5: 235-242
5. Cooper PR, Hagler H, Clark WK, Barnett P (1979) Neurosurgery 4: 296-300
6. Koike J (1983) Neurol Med Chir (Tokyo) 23: 325-335
7. Hase U, Reulen HJ, Menig G, Schürmann K (1978) Acta Neurochirurgica 45: 1-13
8. Marshall LF, Gautille T, Klauber MR, Eisenberg HM, Jane JA, Luerssen TG, Marmarou A, Foulkes MA (1991) J Neurosurg 75: S28-S36
9. Nakamura N (1990) Head injury. 1st ed. Bunkodo. Tokyo. pp601-616

Re-Evaluation of Acute Subdural Hematomas by Using Recent Neuro-Imaging Studies

Takeki Ogawa[1], Yoshio Taguchi[2], Yoshitarou Yamaguchi[2], Tatsuo Hayashi[2], and Hiroaki Seikino[2]

[1]Department of Neurosurgery, St. Marianna University Yokohama City Seibu Hospital, Yokohama, Kanagawa, 241 Japan and [2]Second Department of Surgery, Division of Neurosurgery, St. Marianna University School of Medicine, Kawasaki, Kanagawa, 213 Japan

SUMMARY

Acute subdural hematoma (ASDH) appears to have masquerade in its clinical feature. Since the recent advances in neuro—imaging allowed us to know the real—time pathological process in the head injured patients, we evaluated the patients with ASDH again to clarify the effect of diffuse shearing force. Except for a small number of patients, multi—focal lesions frequently seen in diffuse brain injury were identified in the follow up CT scan and/or MRI. The patients who had acompanied lesions in the central brain showed a poor outcome. We concluded that the diffuse shearing force may play a major role to worse the clinical condition of ASDH. We discuss the new classification system of ASDH.

KEY WORDS: acute subdural hematoma(ASDH), neuro — imaging, diffuse axonal injury (DAI), central brain structure

INTRODUCTION

Although brain injuries are simply divided into two categories: focal and diffuse brain injuries[1], several pathohistological reports suggested the overlaps of these two categories especially in ASDH. While, progress in recent neuro — imaging provided us with many useful informations in the clinical study of neurotraumatology. We studied the neuro — imaging of 54 patients with ASDH experienced the past five years to evaluate the effect of diffuse shearing force on their pathological process.

MATERIALS AND METHODS

All 54 patients were admitted to our hospital within 30 minutes after the head injury. They underwent on evacuation of hematoma immediately after the neurological evaluation followed by a CT examination. They were treated intensively by using ICP and SJO_2 (saturation of oxygen of internal jugular vein) monitoring to maintain intracranial homeostasis. According to Glasgow Coma Scale score(GCS) on admission, they were classified into three groups; mild (GCS 13 — 15), moderate

(GCS 9 — 12), and severe (GCS 3 — 8). CT examination were made sequantially after the surgical treatment and MRI(1.5 Tesla) was taken several days after the admission.

RESULTS AND DISCUSSION

Over a half of patients were comatose on admission. Table 1 and 2 show patient's profile of ASDH. The type of injury was mostly road traffic accident. They include 31 males and 23 females. The outcome (Glasgow outcome scale) of 54 patients with ASDH was summarized in Table 3 in relation to GCS. This revealed that the patients who had better GCS score tended to have the better outcome. Table 4 and 5 show the accompanied lesions recognized by neuro— imaging study in the acute and subacute stages respectively. The classificaton was refered to TCDB[2]. In fifty — four cases, only 6 cases are thought to be simple hematoma type (11.1%). In the other patients, Neuro — imaging frequerntly showed a disproportional midline shift, small hemorrhagic or non — hemorrhagic lesions both in the subcortex and the central part of the brain. These findings were quite similar to the lesions seen in pathological reports of diffuse axonal injuries (DAI). It is clear that MRI has a far superiority to CT scan to visualize traumatic lesions in the brain, especially in the deep white matter. As we reported before, most patients who has a "pure" traumatic subarachnoid hemorrhage around the mesencephalon shown on CT scan should be classified into diffuse brain injury, because a lot of small traumatic lesions were visualized in MRI[3]. Similiarly, in most of our patients of ASDH, associate lesions suggesting DAI were shown. Therefore, we conclude that a diffuse shearing force may play a major role to yield a serious state in the patient with ASDH. According to the ordinary classification of ASDH[4], this was divided into two types; the simple hematoma type, and complicated hematoma type. This simple hematoma type is thought to be a focal brain injury. This must be caused by an injury on the bridging veins. The complicated hematoma type however, whould not be accepted as simply a multiplication of focal injury, that is, cerebral contusion plus subdural blood collection. Based on the real — time visualization of injured brain, these must be a considerable effect of diffuse shearing force in the complicated hematoma type. Hence, we advocated new classification of ASDH that includes a simple hematoma type, a type of multiplication of focal injuries, and a type of associated diffuse brain injury (Figure).

Abbreviation. ped, pedestrian; bicy, bicyclist; moto, motorcyclist; driv, driver; pas, passenger; GOS, Glasgow Outcome Scale; GR, good recovery; MD, moderately disabled; SD, severely disabled; PVS, persistent vegetative state; D, dead; DI, diffuse injury; TCDB, traumatic coma data bank.

Table 1 Types of injury in relation to patient's age.

CAUSES	fall	slip	blow	ped.	bicy.	moto.	driv.	pas.	unknown
AGE 0 − 14	2	1	1	1				2	1
15 − 59	4	1	1	4	3	10	2	3	3
60 − 84	2	5	1	6	1				

Total 54 cases

Table 2 GCS and patient's age.

AGE	0 − 14	15 − 59	60 − 84
GCS severe	6	18	5
moderate	2	6	6
mild	2	5	4

Table 3 GOS in relation to GCS.

GOS	GR	MD	SD	PVS	D
GCS severe	2	3	3		22
moderate	4	1	2		6
mild	9	1		1	

Table 4 accompanied lesions detected by CT scan refered CT category[2] in the acute stage.

CT CATEGORY	DI I	DI II	DI III	DI IV	evacuated mass lesion	non-evacuate mass lesion
GCS severe	2	11	5		(8)*	6
moderate	1	1	1	1	(3)	4
mild	6				(1)	4

( )*:including other hematomas

Table 5 Detected number of lesions by CT/MRI on 22 cases of ASDH in the subacute stage.

		central Brain Structure*1	Cortical/ Subcortical*2
GOS	severe	8	8
	moderate	4	12
	mild	0	4
			total 36 lesions

*1 Central Brain Structure includes; basal ganglia, thalamus, midbrain cerebellar peduncle, pons, corpus callsum

*2 Subcortical:including centrum semiovale

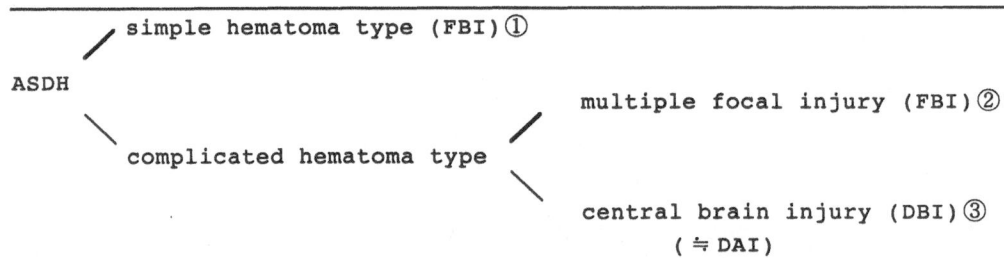

Fig. New neuro－imaging concept of ASDH.
ASDH may be divided into three types(①,②,③) by neuro－imaging.

REFERENCES
1. Adams JH (1984) In: Adams JH, Corsellis JAN, Duchen LW (eds) Greenfield's Neuropathology. Edward Arnold, London, pp 86－124
2. Marshall LF, Eisenberg HM, Jane JA, Luerssen TG, Marmarou A, Foulkes MA (1991) J Neurosurg 75: 14－19
3. Ogawa T, Katabami T, Ozawa T, Shinomiya H, Sakamoto T, Sekino H, Uzura M, Taguchi Y, Yamaguchi Y, Hayashi T, Yamashita K, Okada M, Yamanaka I, Ohhama N, Imaki S (1991) St Marianna Med J 19: 282－287
4. Jamieson KG, Yelland JDN (1972) J Neurosurg 37: 137－149

11—Diffuse Axonal Injury and Severe Head Injury

Diagnostic Significance of Serum Neuron-Specific Enolase and Myelin Basic Protein Assay in Patients with Acute Head Injury

YOSHINORI YAMAZAKI[1], HIROTOSHI OHTAKA[1], SEIJI MORII[2], TAKAO KITAHARA[3], TAKASHI OHWADA[3], and KENZOH YADA[2]

[1]Department of Neurological Surgery, Higashiyamato Hospital, Higashiyamato, Tokyo, 207 Japan, Departments of [2]Neurological Surgery and [3]Critical Care and Emergency Medicine, Kitasato University School of Medicine, Sagamihara, Kanagawa, 228 Japan

SUMMARY

Serum levels of neuron-specific enolase (NSE) and myelin basic protein (MBP) in the internal jugular venous blood were measured in 25 patients with acute head injury and related to both the initial levels of consciousness and the clinical outcome. There was not a significant relationship between either NSE or MBP values and the GCS score on admission. If the final outcome was related, however, it was noted that the levels of NSE and MBP were significantly higher in patients who died than in those survived. In the survivors, concentrations of serum NSE and MBP were 17.6±11.4 ng/ml and 1.4±1.5 ng/ml, while in the patients who died the both levels were elevated as 51.3±27.3 ng/ml ($p < 0.005$) and 11.3±9.5 ng/ml ($p < 0.01$) respectively. Measurement of serum NSE and MBP concentrations is a useful laboratory adjunct to clinical assessment for judging the outcome of head injured patients.

KEY WORDS: neuron-specific enolase, myelin basic protein, head injury, prognosis

INTRODUCTION

The early assessment of the severity of brain damage and the prognosis of patients after head injury is difficult. It has depended mainly on clinical criteria such as Glasgow Coma Scale (GCS) score [1][2]. After severe head trauma, neuron-specific enolase (NSE) and myelin basic protein (MBP) derived from injured brain tissues are considered to appear in the systemic circulation [3][4][5]. The levels of NSE and MBP in the internal jugular venous blood possibly reflect tissue damages of the brain. In the present study, therefore, serum concentrations of NSE and MBP in the internal jugular venous blood were measured during an acute stage of head injury, and correlated with the initial levels of consciousness and the clinical outcome. Significance of serum NSE and MBP assay was validated to estimate the prognosis of patients.

MATERIALS AND METHODS

Twenty-five patients with acute head injury were entered in this study. There were 20 males and 5 females, ranging in age from 14 to 91 years (mean 45 years). The initial level of consciousness of the patients at the time of admission varied from 3 to 15 scored by Glasgow Coma Scale. Cases associated with hypoxia, systemic hypotension, epidural or subdural hematomas were excluded from this series of patients, because it is well known that those major complications themselves cause poor prognosis. Blood samples were taken from the internal jugular vein within 24 hours after injury. The mean time period before sampling was 4.3 hours. Subsequently, the serum was separated, and concentrations of NSE and MBP were measured by disequilibrium radioimmunoassay. NSE was measured in 17 cases and MBP in 25 cases. The level of consciousness was continuously evaluated during follow-up periods from 3 to 82 days.

Protocol of Analyses

First, the patients were divided into two groups according to the initial GCS score obtained at the time of admission. Serum concentrations of NSE and MBP were compared between the two groups. Secondly, the same patients were again grouped into two by their outcome. The levels of NSE and MBP were compared between the two groups. Finally, those patients were classed in accordance with particular levels of NSE and MBP with which their clinical outcome was correlated.

Statistics

All data were expressed as mean±SD. The differences of NSE and MBP values between two groups were assessed by 2-tailed Student's t test for unpaired data. The relationship between the outcome of patients and the levels of NSE and MBP was evaluated by Chi-square test using Yates' correction. The statistical significance was determined with $p < 0.05$.

RESULTS

As indicated in Table 1, the mean level of NSE was 24.1±23.2 ng/ml in patients with GCS 8 or more, and in those with GCS less than 8, the mean value was 39.8±26.0 ng/ml. The difference was not statistically significant. If the outcome was related to the levels of NSE, there was a significant difference between survived patients and the dead. In the survived patients, the mean level of NSE was 17.6±11.4 ng/ml, whereas in the patients who died the mean was 51.3±27.3 ng/ml. As Table 2 shows, when the patients·were again divided by GCS as in Table 1, the mean values of MBP were 2.3±1.8 ng/ml and 8.6±10.6 ng/ml in the two groups respectively. There was not a statistical difference. When the levels of MBP were compared with the outcome, however, there was a statistical difference. The mean level of MBP was 1.4±1.5 ng/ml in the survivors, while in the dead the mean was significantly elevated as 11.3±9.5 ng/ml.

Table 1. Difference of the serum levels of neuron-specific enolase (NSE) between two groups of patients divided by the Glasgow Coma Scale (GCS) score on admission and by the outcome

	number	NSE (ng/ml)		number	NSE (ng/ml)
GCS ≥ 8	9	24.1±23.2	survived	10	17.6±11.4
GCS < 8	8	39.8±26.0	dead	7	51.3±27.6**

Values are mean±SD. The mean levels of neuron-specific enolase were not statistically different between the two groups divided by GCS, but significantly higher in the dead than in the survived (** $p < 0.005$).

Table 2. Difference of the serum levels of myelin basic protein (MBP) between two groups of patients divided by the Glasgow Coma Scale (GCS) score on admission and by the outcome

	number	MBP (ng/ml)		number	MBP (ng/ml)
GCS ≥ 8	16	2.3±1.8	survived	17	1.4±1.5
GCS < 8	9	8.6±10.6	dead	8	11.3±9.5*

Values are mean±SD. The mean levels of myelin basic protein were not statistically different between the two groups divided by GCS, but significantly higher in the dead than in the survived (* $p < 0.01$).

Table 3. Relationship between the outcome of patients and the levels of neuron-specific enolase (NSE) and myelin basic protein (MBP)

	survived	dead		survived	dead
NSE<20 ng/ml	6 cases	none	MBP<4 ng/ml	17 cases	1 case
NSE≥20 ng/ml	4 cases	7 cases†	MBP≥4 ng/ml	none	7 cases††

The mortality was significantly worse if the levels of neuron-specific enolase were above 20 ng/ml or if those of myelin basic protein were above 4 ng/ml († $p < 0.05$ and †† $p < 0.005$).

As Table 3 indicates, 6 patients in whom the NSE concentrations were less than 20 ng/ml all survived and rather recovered, but 7 out of 11 patients whose concentrations were more than 20 ng/ml finally died. Furthermore, 17 out of 18 patients were alive when the levels of MBP were less than 4 ng/ml. In contrast, if those of MBP were more than 4 ng/ml, there were no survivors. Thus, high levels of NSE and MBP indicated poor outcome of the patients.

DISCUSSION

In the present study, a possible advantage of measuring serum levels of NSE and MBP for early estimation of prognosis after head injury was evaluated. It was demonstrated that the levels of serum NSE and MBP were significantly higher in patients who died than in those alive. High concentrations of NSE and MBP in the serum are considered to be derived directly from severely damaged brain tissues. Therefore, when the levels of NSE and MBP are elevated in the internal jugular venous blood after acute head injury, it is suggested that the patients substantially have poor prognosis even though their initial GCS score is more than 8. It is concluded that assay of serum NSE and MBP levels provides reliable laboratory means for early prediction of the prognosis in patients with acute blunt head injury.

REFERENCES

1. Braakman R, Gelpke GJ, Habbema JDF, Maas AIR, Minderhoud JM (1980) Neurosurgery 6: 362-370
2. Jennett B, Bond M (1975) Lancet 1: 480-484
3. Thomas DGT, Palfreyman JW, Ratcliffe JG (1978) Lancet 21: 113-114
4. Scarna H, Delafosse B, Steinberg R, Debilly G, Mandrand B, Keller A, Pujol JF (1982) Neurochemistry International 4: 405-411
5. Thomas DG, Rabow L, Teasdale G (1979) Acta Neurochirurgica 28: 93-95

Is Diffuse Axonal Injury a Clinical Entity?

TAISUKE KIKUCHI, MINORU SHIGEMORI, TAKASHI TOKUTOMI, and
SHINKEN KURAMOTO

Department of Neurosurgery, Kurume University School of Medicine, Kurume, Japan

SUMMARY

Traumatic injury of the axons is a subjacent damage of the brain in head injury. But the clinical concept of diffuse axonal injury (DAI) has still remained unclear. We autopsied 27 cases of head injury in order to clarify this concept of DAI. They included following lesion types ; 10 cases of diffuse brain injury (DBI), 16 cases of focal brain injury (FBI), and three cases with other pathological lesions. We also examined the brains of three monkeys sacrificed two hours after inflation of an epidual balloon. In the postmortem examination, attension has been focused on pathologic features of DAI ; macroscopic lesions in the corpus callosum and dorsolateral quadrant of the upper brainstem and histological evidence of axonal retraction balls. Lesions in the corpus callosum were found in four cases of DBI (40.0 %) and in eight cases of FBI (50.0 %). All cases of DBI and 10 cases of FBI (62.5 %) had the brainstem lesions. Axonal retraction balls were found in five of DBI (50.0 %) and eight of FBI (50.0 %). Axonal retraction balls were also verified in a case died of hemorrhagic shock, malignant glioma or aneurysmal subarachnoid hemorrhage. There were numerous axonal retraction balls in the experimental animals. This study indicates that diffuse and focal brain injuries commonly have pathologic features of DAI, and that axonal retraction balls does not necessarily mean axonal damage by shearing force generated at the moment of impact.

KEY WORDS : head injury, axonal injury, autopsy,

INTRODUCTION

Axonal injury has been regarded as a primary impact damage in head injury [1]. Clinical concept of diffuse axonal injury (DAI), however, still remained unclear [2,3]. We autopsied the brains of fatal head injured patients and other clinical and experimental lesions to clarify the clinical problem of DAI in severe head injury.

MATERIALS AND METHODS

Neuropathological examination was undertaken in 27 brains from head injured patients who admitted to our hospital within six hours after injury and had a Glasgow Coma Scale score of 8 or less. They were 10 of DBI, 16 of FBI and a case with multiple injury died of hemorrhagic shock. DBI included two of DAI, six of traumatic subarachnoid hemorrhage and two of diffuse cerebral swelling. FBI subdivided into eight of acute subdural hematoma and eight of traumatic intracerebral hematoma with cortical contusion. We also examined the brains from the patients died of malignant glioma or aneurysmal subarachnoid hemorrhage and the brains of monkeys. In the experimental animals, cerebral perfusion pressure was reduced to zero level for 10 minutes by inflating epidural balloon, and sacrificed.

The brains were fixed in 10% formol saline solution at least 3 weeks before dissection. After transecting midbrain, the cerebral hemispheres were cut in the coronal plain and cerebellar hemispheres and brainstems were also cut in horizontal section. Blocks of cerebrum, cerebellum and brainstem were embedded in paraffin and 10μ sections were stained with hematoxylin and eosin, Luxol fast blue, Nissl and Bodian techniques. We then paid an attension to pathological features of DAI; macroscopic lesions in the corpus callosum and dorsolateral quadrant of the upper brainstem and histological evidence of axonal retraction balls in the cerebral white matter. The pathological changes of the brainstem with transtentorial herniation were also evaluated.

RESULTS

Lesions in the corpus callosum were found in four cases (40.0%) of DBI and eight (50.0%) of FBI. All cases (100%) of DBI and 10 cases (62.5%) of FBI had lesions in dorsolateral quadrant of the upper brainstem. Axonal retraction balls were found in five (50.0%) of DBI and in eight (50.0%) of FBI (Table 1 - a,b). Traumatic subarachnoid hemorrhage, hemorrhage in the right basal ganglia and numerous axonal retraction balls were found in the case with multiple injury died of hemorrhagic shock, Axonal retraction balls were also found in the case died of malignant glioma or aneurysmal subarachnoid hemorrhage. Even in the brains of monkeys, axonal retraction balls were found. The brainstem lesions could not be differenciated either primary or secondly injury.

DISSCUSION

DAI is now a clinical entity widely accepted in neurotrauma [4]. This neuropathological study revealed that DBI and FBI have pathological features of DAI in common. One question

Table 1 − a. Pathological evidence in diffuse brain injury

Case No.	CT	Age	Sex	Tentorial herniation	Lesions in corpus callosum	Lesions in brainstem	Axonal retraction balls
1.	DAI	34	M	yes	yes	yes	yes
2.	DAI	46	M		yes	yes	yes
3.	TSAH	20	M	yes		yes	
4.	TSAH	43	M			yes	
5.	TSAH	52	M		yes	yes	
6.	TSAH	66	F			yes	
7.	TSAH	53	M	yes		yes	yes
8.	TSAH	72	M		yes	yes	yes
9.	DCS	6	M	yes		yes	
10.	DCS	54	M	yes		yes	yes
				5 (50%)	4 (40%)	10 (100%)	5 (50%)

Table 1 − b. Pathological evidence in focal brain injury

Case No.	CT	Age	Sex	Tentorial herniation	Lesions in corpus callosum	Lesions in brainstem	Axonal retraction balls
11.	SDH	69	M	yes	yes	yes	yes
12.	SDH	55	F				
13.	SDH	39	M	yes		yes	yes
14.	SDH	78	M	yes	yes	yes	
15.	SDH	29	M	yes			yes
16.	SDH	17	M	yes			
17.	SDH	16	M	yes	yes	yes	
18.	SDH	46	M	yes	yes	yes	yes
19.	ICH	41	M	yes		yes	
20.	ICH	25	M	yes			
21.	ICH	57	M	yes		yes	yes
22.	ICH	59	F	yes	yes		yes
23.	ICH	50	M	yes	yes	yes	yes
24.	ICH	78	M		yes		
25.	ICH	59	M	yes	yes	yes	yes
26.	ICH	47	M	yes		yes	
				14 (87.5%)	8 (50%)	10 (62.5%)	8 (50%)

DAI : diffues axonal injury, TSAH : traumatic subarachnoid hemorrhage,
DCS : diffuse cerebral swelling, SDH : acute subdural hematoma,
ICH : traumatic intracerebral hematoma with cortical contusion

is also remained if the pathologic features of DAI is primary damage by shearing force generated at the moment of impact or secondary insult. In the cases with transtentorial herniation, lesions in the brainstem were quite variable and we could not differentiate them primary lesions or secondary lesions exactly. Axonal retraction balls were found not only in head injured patients but also in patients with other pathological lesions. Even in the brains of monkeys with complete ischemia by intracranial hypertension, there were numerous axonal retraction balls. These results therefore indicate that "DAI" should not be used as a clinical entity and axonal retraction balls dose not necessarily means primary axonal injury.

REFERENCE

1. Adams JH, Mitchell DE, Graham DI, Doyle D (1977) Diffuse brain damege of immediate impact type : Its relationship to primary brainstem damege in head injury. Brain 100 : 489 − 502
2. Shigemori M, Tokutomi T, Kuramoto S, Moriyama T, Kikuchi N, Sasaguri Y (1991) Diffuse axonal injury and early intracranial sequelae in severe head injury. Neurol Med Chir 31 : 390 − 395
3. Sahuquillo-Barris J, Lamarca-Ciuro J, Vilaita-Castan J, Rubio-Garcia E, Rodriguez-Pazos M (1988) Acute subdural hamatoma and diffuse axonal injury after severe head trauma. J Neurosurg 68 : 849 − 900
4. Gennarelli TA (1987) Cerebral concussion and diffuse brain injuries. Willams & Wilkins. Baltimore, pp 108 − 124

Analysis of 260 Cases of Severe Head Injury – Did an Aggressive Treatment Improve the Functional Outcome?

JUN-ICHI ONO, TAKAO NAKAMURA, KATSUMI ISOBE, and AKIRA YAMAURA

Department of Neurosurgery, Chiba University School of Medicine, Chuo-ku, Chiba, 260 Japan

SUMMARY

Two-hundred and sixty consecutive patients of severe head injury (GCS ≤ 8) were retrospectively analyzed in regards to the efficacy of the aggressive treatment (AT). Those were divided into two groups: group A; 131 patients treated without AT and group B; 129 treated with AT. The patient transfer time was significantly shorter in group B (p<0.001), but the outcome at 6 months after injury did not differ in two groups. The mortality rate in the patients under 20 years of age was significantly lower in group B (p<0.05). In addition, the earlier transfer and the younger age were related to better outcome in the patients, who talked prior to deterioration.

In the management of severe head injury, AT was successful to reduce the mortality of the patients under 20 years of age, but not to improve their functional outcome. It was stressed that quick transfer and resuscitation are crucial to achieve better outcome, especially in young patients who talked prior to deterioration.

KEY WORDS: severe head injury, aggressive treatment, age, outcome, talk and deteriorate

INTRODUCTION

Aggressive treatment (AT), such as hyperventilation and barbiturate coma therapy, has been adopted in the management of severe head injury for the last 15 years, but it is still unknown whether AT might have improved the functional outcome. The AT consisted of hyperventilation, perioperative barbiturate therapy, a large amount of osmotic agents and surgical internal decompression in our institute. This study is designed to evaluate the outcome in pre-AT and in post-AT period and to elucidate the problems in the management.

CLINICAL MATERIALS AND METHODS

Two hundred and sixty consecutive patients with Glasgow Coma Scale (GCS) score 8 or less were analyzed. The age ranged from 3 to 86 years (mean: 36 years). Those were divided into two groups: group A; 131 patients treated without AT, and group B; 129 treated with AT. The factors analyzed were age, cause of injury, GCS score, CT findings, such as extraparenchymal hematoma and paren- chymal lesion. The parenchymal CT findings were classified into 5 categories: no abnormality, hemispheric swelling, hemorrhagic lesion, diffuse cerebral swel- ling or low density. The outcome was evaluated at 6 months after injury using Glasgow Outocme Scale: A good outcome was defined as good recovery or moderately disabled, and a poor outcome ás severely disabled, vegetative or dead. In addi- tion, 29 patients (11 %), who talked prior to deterioration, were analyzed. The significance of difference was evaluated by chi-square test.

RESULTS AND DISCUSSION

The mean age and the GCS score did not statistically differ in two groups. As a cause of injury, traffic accident was most frequently observed in both groups. The incidence of the traffic accident was 61 % and 81 % in group A and group B, respectively. This difference was statistically significant ($p<0.001$). The mean transfer time of the patients was 5.5 hours in group A and 2.3 hours in group B. Sixty-four percent of the patients in group B was transferred earlier than 1 hour of injury, whereas only 15 % in group A arrived hospital within 1 hour (Table 1). This difference was statistically significant ($p<0.001$). In the CT findings, two groups did not differ in the incidence of the extraparenchymal hematoma, such as epidural or acute subdural hematomas, and the parenchymal lesions. The mortality rate was 57 % and 48 % in group A and group B, respectively, but the difference was not statistically significant (Table 2). The number of the patients, who recovered well, did not differ in two groups. However, in 86 patients under 20 years of age, the mortality rate was 47 % and 26 % in group A and group B, res- pectively. The mortality had been significantly reduced by AT in this age group ($p<0.05$). Furthermore, in the patients whose CT disclose diffuse cerebral swel- ling, 47 % had poor outcome in group A, whereas only 26 % in group B (Table 3). This difference was noteworthy, but statistically insignificant.

Twenty-nine patients, who talked prior to deterioration, were analyzed. Sixty-two percent of these patients were transferred to our hospital later than 3 hours of injury. In 6 patients who talked prior to deteriorating and had good outcome, 5 patients were under 20 years of age, and 5 were transferred earlier than 2 hours of injury. On the CT findings, 2 patients had diffuse cerebral swelling and 4 had acute subdural hematoma, as a cause of deterioration (Table 4). AT has been widely accepted in the management of severe head injury, since Becker, et al.[1] reported its efficacy. However, Ward, et al.[2] recently stated that prophylactic hyperventilation resulted in a poorer outcome at 3 and 6 months. In fact, it has not exactly evaluated whether AT could improve the outcome, and the true effect of AT is still controversial. Our results suggested that AT might had reduced the mortality in the young patients with diffuse cerebral swelling and that it could improve the outcome in the young patients who talked prior to deterioration. It is stressed that AT should be indicated in the restricted cases, as Nakamura, et al.[3] had documented.

Table 1. Patient transfer time in two groups.

Group	No. of Patients	Transfer Time (hours)			
		≦1	1~2	2~6	>6
Without AT	131	15%†	27%	37%	21%
With AT	129	64%†	18%	8%	10%

† $p < 0.001$

Table 2. Outcome at 6 months after injury.

Group	No. of Patients	Outcome				
		GR	MD	SD	PVS	Dead
Without AT	131	21%	11%	5%	6%	57%
With AT	129	19%	18%	11%	5%	48%

N.S.

cf. GR: good recovery, MD: moderate disability
SD: severe disability, PVS: persistent vegetative state

Table 3. Outcome at 6 months in 86 patients under 20 years of age.

Group	No. of Patients	Outcome				
		GR	MD	SD	PVS	Dead
Without AT	43	40%	12%	0%	2%	47%†
With AT	43	42%	19%	12%	2%	26%†

† P<0.05

cf. GR: good recovery, MD: moderate disability
   SD: severe disability, PVS: persistent vegetative state

Table 4. Summary of 6 cases, who talked prior to deterioration, and had good outcome (good recovery and moderate disability).

Age Sex	GCS on Admission	Transfer Time (hrs)	Cause of Deterioration
16 M	7	2.0	Diffuse cerebral swelling
19 F	8	1.5	Diffuse cerebral swelling
15 M	7	1.75	Acute subdural hematoma
17 M	5	7.5	Acute subdural hematoma
18 M	8	1.0	Acute subdural hematoma
40 M	5	1.75	Acute subdural hematoma

cf. GCS: Glasgow Coma Scale

REFERENCES
1. Becker DP, Miller JD, Ward JD, Greenberg RP, Young HF, Sakalas R (1977) J Neurosurg 47: 491-502
2. Ward JD, Choi S, Marmarou A, Moulton R, Muizelaar JP, DeSalles A, Becker DP, Kontos HA, Young HF (1989) In: Hoff JT, Betz AL (eds): Intracranial Pressure VII Springer-Verlag, Berlin Heiderberg, pp 630-633.
3. Nakamura H, Watanabe Y, Sato A, Kobayashi S, Kageyama Y, Hirai S (1987) Neurotraumatology 10: 40-48 (in Japanese).

Difficulties in Modelling Criteria Predicting Intracranial Hypertension in Severe Closed Head Injury

IOANNIS BALTAS[1], MAKEDOS FYLAKTAKIS[1], NIKOS BASKINIS[1], KOSTAS POLYZOIDIS[1], KOSTAS KOLETSOS[2], and SPYROS ANDREADIS[1]

[1]Department of Neurosurgery G. Hospital G. Papanikolaou, Thessaloniki, Macedonia, Greece and [2]Department of ICU G. Hospital G. Papanikolaou, Thessaloniki, Macedonia, Greece

SUMMARY

In an attempt to discover criteria predicting intracranial hypertension in severe closed head injury, we studied retrospectively the highest ICP in the first 3 days after injury, the pupillary condition and the CT findings in 48 patients with GCS less than 8. Patients were divided into 2 groups of ICP<20mmHg and ICP>20 mmHg. Unilateral pupillary dilatation was not found in the first group, but was increased in the later. The statistical difference of the CT findings between the two groups were not of predictive value. We coclude that in all head injured patients with GCS less than 8, ICP measuring is mandatory in spite of the reported risks of the monitoring techniques.

KEY WORDS: head injury, intracranial hypertension, pupillary condition, computerized tomography

INTRODUCTION

Although it is becoming increasingly acceptable among the neurosurgeons that the measurement of intracranial pressure is necessary in patients with severe head injury, nevertheless, there is still some hesitation among the ICU physicians due to reported complications of the ICP monitoring techniques[1,2].

This study is an attempt to model practical and easily used criteria, concerning the intracranial pathology, which will distinguish those patients who are likely to develop intracranial hypertension and should be monitored, from those who are not likely to develop hypertension and need not to be monitored, thus avoiding the potential risks of the monitoring techniques. The criteria we used were the pupillary condition and the findings of the computerized tomography.

MATERIALS AND METHODS

The study includes 48 patients aged 15-65 years, suffering from severe closed head injury with a Glascow Coma Scale (GCS) of 8 or less, who were treated conservatively. After the initial resuscitation in the emergency room, the patients were evaluated according to the GCS and the pupillary condition was recorded. Patients with bilateral dilatation of the pupils, with CSF leak and oligemic shock due to major extracranial injuries were excluded. In all patients the ICP was measured with the use of a Camino 110-4B fiberoptic intraparenchymal transducer. The catheter of the transducer was inserted at the side of the major lesion defined by the CT. The mesurements were done under sedation (fentanyl+midazolam) and artificial respiration. The duration of ICP monitoring was 3-5 days. Intracranial hypertension was defined as an ICP higher than 20mmHg persisting for more than 5 min. No complication due to the monitoring technique was recorded.

The patients were divided into two groups according to the highest ICP they presented during the first 3 days after the injury: Group of ICP<20mmHg and group of ICP>20mmHg.

The CT scan was perfomed 4 to 8 hours after the injury. The findings were classified as following: 1.Normal CT, 2.Single contusion without shift of the midline structures, 3.Multiple con-- tusions without shift, 4.Contusion(s) with shift, 5,Abnormal ventricular system: distorted, collapsed or absent, 6.Abnormal basal cisterns: collapse or abscense of the ambient and/or the perimesenchephalic cisterns, 7.Blood within the ventricles and/or the subarachnoid space.

The CT findings along with the condition of the pupils of the two groups were statistically compaired retrospectively.

RESULTS

6 patients (12.5%) out of the total of 48 presented unilateral pupillary dilatation. All belonged to the high ICP group (22.2%) and none to the normal ICP group. The statistical difference is significant (p<0.05).

The results of CT findings are seen in table 1. Significant difference is seen in the normal CT and the contusion with shift. In the other findings the differences are not significant.

Table 1 Comparisons between the groups

ICP	<20mmHg n=21	>20mmHg n=27	"P" values -Fishers' test-
Pupillary dilatation	0%	22%	<0.024
Normal CT	19%	0%	<0.030
Single contusion without shift	38%	25.9%	not significant
Multiple contusions without shift	14.2%	14.8%	not significant
Contusion(s) with shift	14.2%	40.7%	<0.044
Abnormal ventricles	23.8%	18.5%	not significant
Abnormal basal cisterns	26.5%	29.6%	not significant
Blood within the ventricl. and/or the sub/noid space	19%	18.5%	not significant

DISCUSSION

It is well known that the unilateral pupillary dilatation is indicative of intracranial hypertension, leading to transtentorial herniation. The normal pupils, nevertheless, do not guarantee normal intracranial pressure. Consequently, the pupillary condition does not have predictive value.

In our material the normal CT is indicative of normal intracranial pressure but Becker[3] reported that 13% of patients with normal CT developed intracranial hypertension.

There is agreement among several authors that the midline shift is not of predictive value for ICP[4,5,6]. In our study the difference between the two groups regarding the midline shift is significant. This alone,could lead us to suggest that the midline shift could have predictive value, but the fact that in our material almost 26% of the patients who had contusion without shift and almost 15% of patients with multiple contusions without shift developed finally intracranial hypertension, leads to the coclusion that the absence of midline shift does not guarantee normal ICP.

High ICP was recorded by Toutant et al[7] in all patients who presented abnormal basal cisterns. Sadhu[5] regarding the same CT finding recorded low and high ICP's as well. In our material the difference between the two groups is not statistically significant, which means that abnormal basal cisterns do not necessarily correlate with intracranial hypertension.

From our results and the above discussion we can say that the CT findings can not be used as criteria for ICP prediction.

The aim of the treatment of itracranial hypertension is to prevent the secondary damages. Since this therapy does not lack adverse reactions it should be administered only when indicated.

We conclude that practically it is impossible to model criteria predicting which patients will develop intracranial hypertension and which will not. Consequently all head injured patients with GCS of 8 or less should be ICP monitored. The fact that we didn't have complications from the monitoring technique we used, strengthens this concept.

REFERENCES

1. Narayan RK, Pulla RSK, Becker DP, Ward JD, Enas GG, Greenberg RP, Da Silva AD, Lipper MH, Choi CS, Mayhall CG, Lutz HA and Young HF (1982) Intracranial pressure: to monitor or not to monitor? J Neurosurgery 56: 650-659
2. Rosner MJ, Becker DP (1976) ICP monitoring: Complications and associated factors. Clin Neurosurg 23: 494-519
3. Becker DP (1983) Selecting Patients for Intracranial Pressure Monitoring in Severe Head Injury. In: Ishii et al (eds) Intracranial Pressure V. Springer. Berlin Heidelberg New York Tokyo. pp 512-516
4. Klauber MR, Toutant SM and Marshall LF (1984) A model for predicting delayed intracranial hypertension following severe head injury. J Neurosurg 61: 695-699
5. Sadhu VK, Sampson J, Haar FL, Pinto RS and Handel FS (1979) Correlation between computerized tomography and intracranial pressure monitoring in acute head trauma patients. Radiology 133: 507-509
6. Tabaddor K, Danziger A, Wissof HS (1982) Estimation of Intracranial Pressure by CT Scan in Closed Head Trauma. Surg Neurol 18: 212-215
7. Toutant SM, Klauber MR, Marshall LF, Toole BM, Bowers SA,

Seeling SM and Varnell JB (1984) Absent or compressed basal cisterns onfirst CT scan: Ominous predictors in severe head injury. J Neurosurg 61: 691-694

A Mathematical Model for Outcome Prediction in Severe Head Injury

U.S. Srinivasan, N. Muthukumar, R. Gajendran, and
M. Mohan Sampath Kumar

Department of Neurosurgery, Government Rajaji Hospital, Madurai-625 020 Tamil Nadu, India

SUMMARY

A prospective study was conducted using ten clinical parameters in prediction of outcome in hundred patients with severe head injury who satisfied the criteria adopted by the International Data Bank. Results of the first fifty patients showed a combination of glasgow coma scale, fronto-orbicular reflex and vertical oculocephalic response can provide a reliable prediction of outcome in severe head injury. Based upon this, a mathematical model was constructed giving a value for the above mentioned three factors. It was used prospectively in the next fifty patients to determine the type of outcome. The mathematical model was "Glasgow coma scale x (Fronto-orbicular reflex + Vertical oculocephalic response) x 5". The results obtained by use of this model was compared with the logistic regression model. The accuracy of this mathematical model when used on third post traumatic day was above 90%.

KEY WORDS

Frontoorbicular reflex, Glasgow coma scale, Prognosis, Severe head injury, Vertical oculocephalic response.

INTRODUCTION

Over the past 20 years, features of prognostic significance have been identified in patients with severe head injury. Relatively complex statistical formulae and charts have been proposed for prediction of prognosis in severe head injury, incorporating various clinical parameters and sophisticated investigations (1,2,3,4,5,6). Most of them are too complicated and require the use of computers and calculators. Hence a study was conducted to develop a simple mathematical model based upon clinical parameters and to test its accuracy in predicting the outcome in severe head injury.

CLINICAL MATERIALS AND METHODS

The analysis is based upon hundred consecutive patients admitted with severe head injury in the Head Injury Unit in Government Rajaji Hospital, Madurai after January 1990. Patients who satisfied the criteria for coma adopted by the International Data Bank only were chosen for study (7). The study did not include patients who were apneic on admission. Those with multiple injuries and whose impaired consciousness was due to alcoholic intoxication were also excluded. Their mean GCS score and age were 5.85 and 38.69 respectively. Conscious level was graded using glasgow coma scale (8) after resuscitation. Skiagrams of head and neck and cranial CT scan were obtained. Standard protocol was observed in the management of these patients. Survivors were reviewed at 1, 3 and 6 months intervals. Glasgow outcome scale (9) was used to assess the final outcome at the end of 6 months.

In this study, outcome was grouped into 3 categories. "Good outcome" indicated those patients with good recovery and moderate disability. "Poor outcome" implied patients with severe disability and vegetative state and the third category "death".

The usefulness of the following ten clinical parameters were studied in predicting the outcome: 1.Age, 2.Glasgow coma scale, 3.Fronto-orbicular reflex, 4.Vertical oculocephalic response, 5.Horizontal oculocephalic response, 6.Pupil reaction, 7.Pupil size, 8.Pulse, 9.Respiratory rate and 10.Blood pressure. Logistic regression analysis was used on various combinations of two or more prognostic data taken on first and third post traumatic days. Based upon the results of the first fifty patients, a mathematical model was constructed. The model was used prospectively in the next fifty patients and its accuracy in predicting the outcome was analysed.

RESULTS

Among the variables considered, glasgow coma scale, fronto-orbicular reflex and vertical oculocephalic response were found to be the three clinical factors that could be used in combination to predict the outcome. A value was given for each parameter depending upon the prognostic importance of the clinical factor in predicting the outcome. A simple equation was developed which is given in Table - 1 and the results of the accuracy of it in first fifty patients were reported in our previous paper (10). Results were also compared with that obtained using logistic regression model.

TABLE - 1: THE MATHEMATICAL MODEL WITH VALUES FOR THE THREE VARIABLES AND THE FINAL OUTCOME

EQUATION : Probability of Survival = Glasgow come scale score X (Frontoorbicular reflex + Vertical oculocephalic response) X 5

Variable	Score
Glasgow coma scale	
3 - 4	1
5 - 7	2
8 - 11	3
12 - 15	4
Frontoorbicular reflex:	
Present	3
Absent	1
Vertical oculocephalic response	
Present	2
Impaired	1
Absent	0

Final Value	Outcome
Less than 15%	Death
15 - 40%	Vegetative State/Severe disability
More than 40%	Good recovery/Moderate disability

The same mathematical model was used prospectively in the next fifty patients. Accuracy of the model in predicting the outcome in all the hundred patients was calculated, the results of which are shown in Table 2.

TABLE - 2: ACCURACY OF THE MATHEMATICAL MODEL IN PREDICTING THE OUTCOME IN HUNDRED PATIENTS ON THIRD DAY

Outcome Group	Patient Number	True Prediction %	False Prediction	
			Actual Outcome	Percentage
Good Outcome	34	97	Death	3
Poor Outcome	19	79	Death	16
			Good Outcome	5
Death	20	95	Poor Outcome	5

(Number of patients died before third day: 27)

In order to illustrate the use of equation, consider for example a patient with a GCS Score of 6 with presence of both frontoorbicular reflex and vertical oculocephalic response. Using this mathematical model by substituting the value for the response from the table it was 2 x (3+2) x 5 = 50% which indicated that he will have a good outcome.

DISCUSSION

Recovery of frontoorbicular reflex and vertical oculocephalic response within 72 hours in comatose patients indicated a good prognosis, even when the patient GCS was less than 8. (10). In Glasgow liege scale, vertical oculocephalic response was given a higher value than horizontal oculocephalic response (11,12). Similar results were obtained in our preliminary study in which the vertical oculocephalic response ranked the third most important factor (10).

A fundamental question regarding the mathematical model is its accuracy in prediction. It was observed that a true prediction was made in 97% of cases in the good outcome group, 79% in the poor outcome group and 95% in the death category (Table 2). A sharp prediction of outcome above 95% could be made in the "good outcome" and "death" groups. The multimodality evoked potentials and ICP monitoring were stated to be the strongest predictors of outcome with a prediction value of 90% (4) while with the clinical parameters mentioned above the accuracy of prediction was of same degree. This mathematical model can be used by the bed side and it helps the clinician to confidently predict the outcome in 90% of cases with severe head injury and aids him in objective counselling of patient's relatives.

REFERENCES

1.   Jennett B, Teasdale G, Braakman R, Minderhoud JM, Knoll Jones R (1976) Lancet 1:1031-1034.
2.   Braakman R, Gelpke GJ, Habbema JDF, Maas AIR, Minderhoud JM (1980) Neurosurgery 6:362-370.
3.   Stablein DM, Miller JD, Choi SC, Becker DP (1980) Neurosurgery 6:243-248.
4.   Narayan RK, Greenberg RP, Miller JD, Enas GG, Choi SC, Kishore PRS, Selhorst JB, Lutz III MA, Becker DP (1981) J Neurosurg 54:751-762.
5.   Choi SC, Ward JD, Becker DP (1983) J Neurosurg 59:294-297.
6.   Choi SC, Muizelaar JP, Barnes TY, Marmarou A, Brooks DM, Young HF (1991) J Neurosurg 75:251-255.
7.   Miller JD, Butterworth JF, Gudeman SK, Faulkner JE, Choi SC, Selhorst JB, Harbison JW, Lutz HA, Young HF, Becker DP (1981) J Neurosurg 54:282-299.
8.   Teasdale G, Jennett B (1974) Lancet 2:81-83.
9.   Jennett B, Bond M (1975) Lancet 1:480-484.
10. Srinivasan US, Muthukumar N, Gajendran R, Mohan Sampath Kumar M (1992) Neurology India (In Press).
11. Born JD, Albert A, Hans P, Bonnal J (1985) Neurosurgery 16:595-601.
12. Born JD, Hans P, Albert A, Bonnal J (1987) Neurosurgery 20:513-517.

12—Pediatric Head Injury

Neuropsychological Aspects of Severe Brain Contusions and Diffuse Axonal Damages in Children

NATALIA GOGITIDZE[1] and ANATOLIY BANIN[2]

[1]Burdenko Neurosurgical Institute, Moscow, Russia and [2]Advanced Training Central Institute for Doctors, Moscow, Russia

SUMMARY

The two group of children aged 4 to 15 with severe brain contusions and diffuse axonal damages were the subject of neuropsychological investigation. The obtained results demonstrated that each of two type of trauma was characterized by its own specific structure of neuropsychological syndromes. The correlation between their components determined the severity of mental state in acute period and following outcome of patients.

KEY WORDS: Severe brain contusions, diffuse axonal damage, structure of neurological symptom, outcome.

INTRODUCTION

The problem of systematization of clinical symptoms of severe head injury (SHI) is actual because of variety of primary impairments of brain tissues,as well as the accompanying pathophisiological reactions,intra- and extracranial complications.Prognosis of the outcome after different types of the traumatic brain damages and choice of the most effective set of the rehabilitation means are of great interest as well.A number of studies have showed,that patients inability after SHI is caused by the defects of mental sphere as well as by neurological disorders[1,2,3,].Due to that in the perspective of mentioned problem, the comparative neuropsychological exploration of the children with different types of SHI turns out to be of the big importance.

MATERIALS AND METHODS

44 kids aged 4 to 15 were included in this study.On the basis of examination by means of the whole complex of modern diagnostic methods 2 main types of SHI in children were selected: 22 kids with severe brain contusions and 22 - with diffuse axonal damages.The main method of the investigation was the neuropsychological method,worked out by A.R.Luria.The patients underwent the complete neuropsychological axploration during the acute period as soon as they have become open to the extensive contact,, and in a year after trauma, too.Proceeding from worked out criteria - mild,moderate and severe degrees of neuropsychological deficits - were distiguished out.Dependig on there role in formation of the syndrome in the acute period and there influence on the further recovery and compensatory processes,all the symptoms were subdivided into 3 main blocks: I - nonspecific desturbances of mental activity (inactivity, aspontaneity, sluggishness, exhaustibility, impulsivness and so on); II - personality and emotional disorders (disorientation,a range of emotional aberrations, motivation disorders); III - specific defects

of mental functions (initial impairments of praxis,gnosis,speach, optico-spatial functions,memory,itelligance).

RESULTS AND DISCUSSION.

The data of the comparative neuropsychological exploration closely correlate with the character of brain damage and clinical picture.

Severe Brain Contusions

In the case of the local contusion the patients were open for the carrying out of the examination in 1-2 weeks after injury.The neuropsychological syndroms in this category of patiens have the following typical features in this period (Fig 1).
I block.
Only a half of patients had nonspecific disturbances of mental activity in a form of exhaustibility, elements of sluggishness, aspontaneity, more seldom - impulsiveness , which in none of cases exceeded the moderate degree.
II block.
Emotional-personal disfunctions were mild.As a rule chidren were easy to build up contacts,adequate in their reaction to examination situation, demonstated their interest in the results of the testing.
III block.
Specific initial defects of highest mental functions ,such as praxis,gnosis,speach,optico-spatial processes,memory and thinking were clearly observed.The concrete set and the manifestation degree of those defects varied depending of severity and localization of brain damage,presence of complications,age,individual peculiarities.In some cases disorders exeeded up to the decay degree.However,observed in this group of patients defects never had global chareter but concerned a limited number of components of highest mental functions selectively,leaving others intact.Presence of safe links in the system of psychological functions is of great value for the following rehabilitation.
Catamnestic observation afer 1 year after trauma showed good outcome in most of cases.Neuropsychological examination demonstrated the corresponding normalization of highest mental functions:full recovery of nonspecific parametres of mental activity(I block), good condition of emotional-personal sphere (II block),sagnificant regress of initial specific praxic,gnostic,speach,optico-spatial ,mnestic and intellectual defects.

Diffuse Axonal Damages.

THe severety of the condition, caused by prolonged unconciousness and vital disorders made the patients of these group available for the exploration essentially later, usually 1-1,5 months after SHI (Fig 1).
I block.
First of all rude non-specific disorders of mental activity were observedin all patients:severe exaustibility,aspontaneity,inactivity, sluggishness.They manifast in the form of absence of spontaneous disires,difficulties in involving in test programm and changing one type of the activity to another,lowering of productivity and efficiency.
II block.
Half of kids in addition to above mantioned disorders had a compex of emotional-personal disfunctions, leading to sagnificant difficulties of working out of the direction for fulfilling the examination task,

non-critical attitude to themselves and their results,"fild"
behavior,negativism.All kinds of disorientation were typical for
present contingent of patients.
III block.
The present contingent of children revealed various specific initial
impairments of mental functions: two-sided complex dispraxias,
polymodal gnostic defects,elements of all kinds of apraxias, severe
optico-spatial disturbancies, massive polymodal and complex memory
disorders and intellectual disability. Typically, almost the whole
range of disorders was present. As a rule the pathological process
spreaded on the majority of the components of the functions. But,
inspite of extremely massive and frequint optico-spatial and mnestic
impairments, functional disorders rare exceeded moderate degree.
So, severeness of the neuropsychological picture in this type of SHI
was caused by noncpecific disorders of mental activity coming out in
the first row in the syndrome structure in cmplex with motivational
changes.

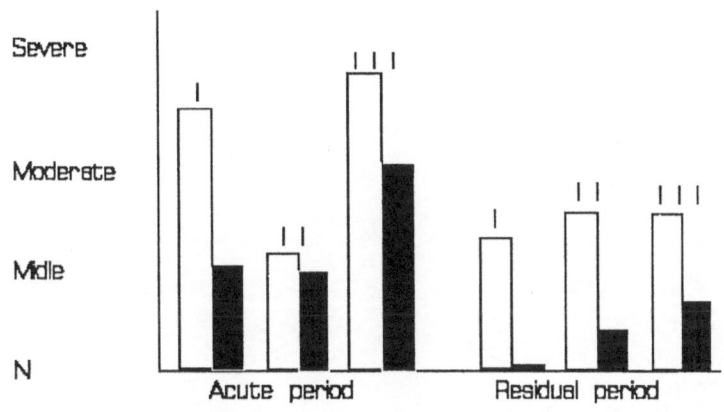

Fig 1.The structure of neuropsychological syndromes
in patients with severe brain contusions ▆▆▆ and
diffuse axonal damages ▭

After 1 year and even more after SHI these children demonstrated the
poor outcome: most of them became invalids anable to return to school
and premobrbid social invironment. Neuropsychological examination
showed the residual elements of noncpecific activity disfunctions (I
block). Beside this the growth of the part of the II block disorders
was showed. Many of the kids formed out complexes of emotional-
personal disorders, developed negative personal features,
difficulties with their friends and parents, episodes of asocial
behavior. Comparatively slower regress was found in the III block
defects.
So,one had to state the stability of the neuropsychological
impairments and low efficiency of rehabilitation measures.

CONCLUSIONS
As a matter of fact results of the investigation showed,that the main
difference between two kinds of SHI layed in the different structures
of neuropsychological syndromes in acute period and their following
dynamics.
Comparative safeness of nonspecific parameters of mental activity and
emotional-personal sphere in the patients with severe brain

contusions permit them to take active part in rehabilitation process and to fasten it. Availability of intact components in the system of mental activity gave possibility to compensatoric reconstructions of functions and good outcome.

On the contrary, the structure of neuropsychological syndrome, in which the significant place belongs to noncpecific disorders of mental activity in acute period and emotional-personal changes, forming during the posttraumatic period,essentially hardened the rehabilitation and caused unfavourable outcome with distinguished signs of invalidization.

REFERENCES

1.Harvey S.Levin and Howard M.Eisenberg (1979) Childs Brain 5:281-292
2.Harvey S.Levin,Hovard M. Eisenberg and Michael E.Miner (1983) In: Ed. K.Shapero, New York, Pediatric head trauma, pp 223-239
3.R.J.McClelland (1988) British Journal of Psychiatry 153: 141-146

Assessment of Cerebral Contusion of Acute Subdural Hematoma in Children by MRI

HIROSHI TAKAHASHI[1], SHOZO NAKAZAWA[1], and HIROYUKI YOKOTA[2]

[1]Department of Neurosurgery and [2]Department of Critical Care Medicine, Nippon Medical School, Bunkyo-ku, Tokyo, 113 Japan

SUMMARY

Recent surgical cases with acute subdural hematoma in children were comparatively examined with such surgical cases in adults, paying attention to the presence of cerebral contusion.
The subjects consisted of 43 children cases with an operation of acute subdural hematoma recently experienced in our hospital and of 141 adults cases with an operation at the same period. These cases were divided into 2 groups by the presence of cerebral contusion on the basis of computed tomography (CT) or surgical findings, and clinical studies were performed. Also, magnetic resonance imaging (MRI) was conducted as far as possible in recently experienced cases with head trauma in children.
Results were as followed; 1) The type of hematoma without cerebral contusion was developed more in children with significant difference, as shown in 37% of the children and 19% of the adults. 2) The operative mortality in the children showed a lower rate of 33% as compared with 42% of the adults, but this seemed to be caused by that the mortality of the group without cerebral contusion showed a far lower rate of 19% in the children than 37% in the adults. 3) In cases with head trauma where cerebral contusion was not clearly shown by CT, there were present cases showing contused changes by MRI.

KEY WORDS: acute subdural hematoma, children, cerebral contusion, MRI

INTRODUCTION

We have already reported the characteristics of head injury in infant and children [1,2]. However, in this study, we tried to clarify that the diagnosis of cerebral contusion is most important factor in acute subdural hematoma in children, again. On the other hand, magnetic resonance imaging (MRI) is thought to be superior to computed tomography (CT), but the usefulness of MRI in acute head injury has not yet to be fully explored. In this paper, we describe the usefulness of MRI in acute head injury, especially in evaluating parenchymal cerebral contusion.

MATERIALS AND METHODS

Recent surgical cases with acute subdural hematoma in children were comparatively examined with surgical cases in adults, paying attention to the presence of cerebral contusion, and it was attempted to clarify those characteristics of infant cases.
The subjects consisted of 43 children cases with an operation of acute subdural hematoma recently experienced in our hospital and of 141 adult cases with an operation at the same period. These cases were

divided into 2 groups by the presence of cerebral contusion on the basis of CT or surgical findings, and clinical studies were performed. Furthermore, MRI which may detect cerebral contusion more precisely than CT was conducted as far as possible in recently experienced cases with head trauma in children.

RESULTS

The type of hematoma without cerebral contusion was developed more in children with significant difference, as shown in 37% of the children and 19% of the adults (Fig. 1).

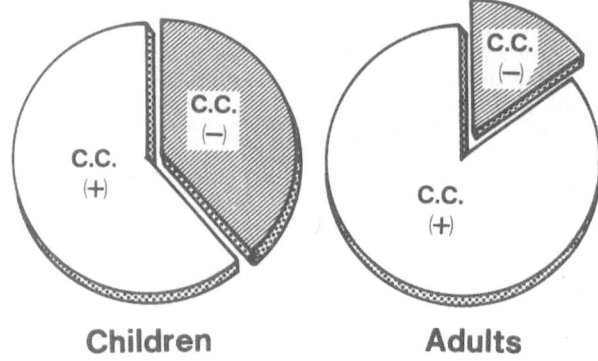

Children   Adults

Fig. 1 Acute subdural hematoma with or without cerebral contusion in children and adults.
C.C.=cerebral contusion

We also studied on mortality of acute subdural hematoma, paying attention to the presence of cerebral contusion. The operative mortality in the children showed a lower rate of 33% as compared with 42% of the adults, but this seemed to be caused by that the mortality of the group without cerebral contusion showed a far lower rate of 19% in the children than 37% in the adults.
Two interesting cases, in which MRI could detect cerebral contusion more clearly than CT, will be demonstrated.

Case 1

This patient is a 14-year-old girl whose GCS was 9 at admission. Although the CT revealed no clear abnormal findings as shown in Fig. 2 (left), T2-weighted MRI revealed thin epidural hematoma and small cerebral contusion at the right temporo-parietal lobe as shown in Fig. 2 (right).

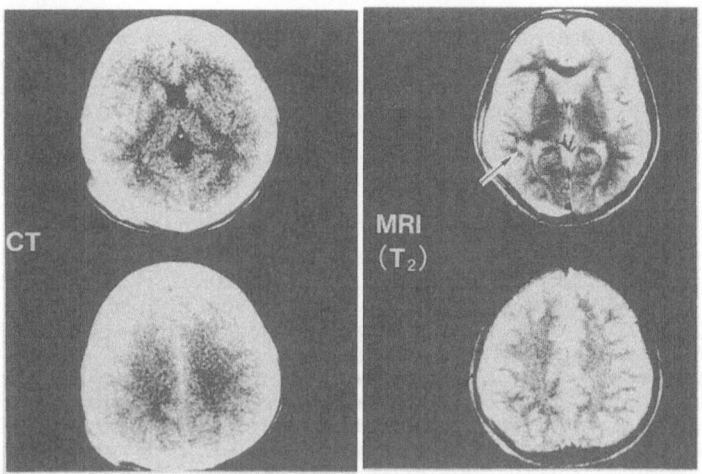

Fig. 2 Case 1. CT was performed on admission (left). MRI was performed just after CT (right).

Case 2

This is interesting head injury case in adult whose GCS score was 10 at admission. At that time, CT showed only traumatic subarachnoid hemorrhage, but T2 weighted MRI revealed thin subdural hematoma at left temporal lobe and cerebral contusion at right temporal lobe as shown in Fig. 3 (left). We performed conservative therapy because of a little mass effect.

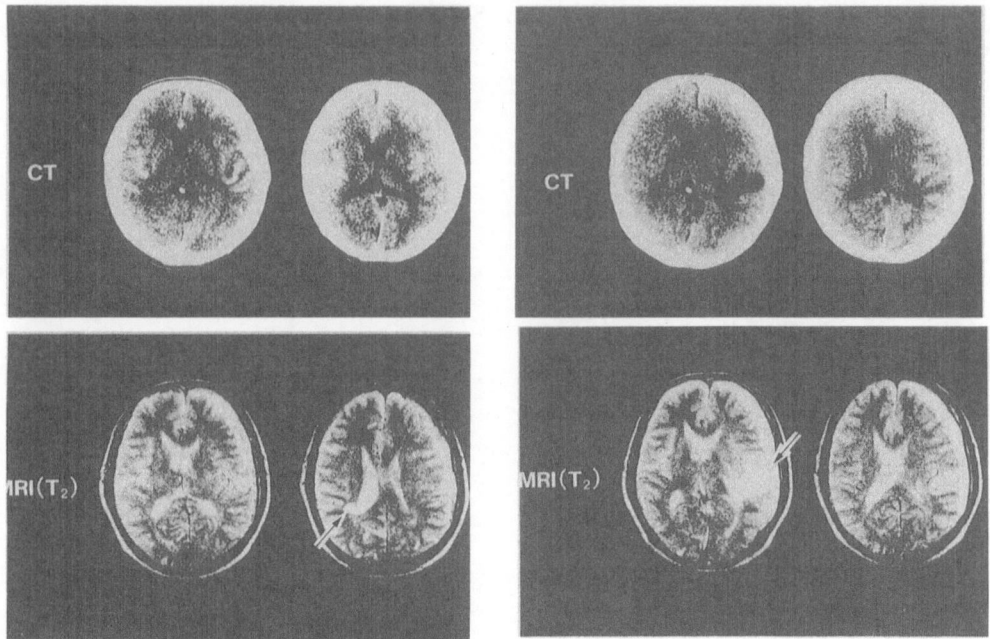

Fig. 3 Case 2. CT and MRI were performed on admission (left). CT and MRI performed 7 days after admission (right).

When the patient's consciousness became worse, one week after admission, CT and MRI examinations were performed again. CT revealed low density area at left temporal lobe and T2 weighted MRI clearly visualized severe cerebral contusion and increased subdural hematoma in left temporal lobe. We performed operation at that time, and he got very good recovery.

DISCUSSION

As we already reported, we divide cases of acute subdural hematoma into three groups from CT findings, and basically we select different treatment for each group [3]. This grouping is depending on the extent of cerebral contusion. So, it is very important to make a diagnosis of precise cerebral contusion.
Our study suggests that the greatest factor to decide the prognosis of acute subdural hematoma is the degree of cerebral contusion and the main reason of the favorable prognosis in children seems attributable to the less frequency of causing cerebral contusion in children. We previously reported that MRI is clearly more sensitive than CT in detecting traumatic brain damage and MRI is useful to evaluate the severity of acute head injury [4]. In our study, this matter was proved especially in children's acute head injury cases.
MRI may be able to predict the prognosis of these pediatric patients, and the introduction of MRI may improve the outcome of head injured children.

REFERENCES

1. Takahashi H, Nakazawa S (1980) Child's Brain 7: 124-131
2. Takahashi H, Nakazawa S (1981) Neurol Surg (Tokyo) 9: 51-57
3. Takahashi H, Nakazawa S, Okada T (1986) Nissai Ikai Shi 34: 291-295
4. Yokota H, Kurokawa A, Otsuka T, Kobayashi S, Nakazawa S (1991) J Trauma 31: 351-357

Diffuse Brain Injury in Children

Hiroshi Nakamura[1], Yoshiro Watanabe[1], Kazumasa Fukuda[2], Yusuke Kageyama[1], Shigeki Kobayashi[1], Masaru Odaki[1], Akira Sato[1], and Akira Yamaura[2]

[1]Department of Neurological Surgery, Chiba Emergency Medical Center, Chiba, Japan and [2]Department of Neurological Surgery, Chiba University, Chiba, Japan

SUMMARY

Factors that might have influences on the outcome of children with diffuse brain injury (DBI) were analyzed and compared with those of adult cases. One hundred and twelve patients with DBI, 24 children and 88 adults, were studied. This study indicated that children had a better outcome than adults. Traffic accident was the predominant cause of injury both in children and adults. Pedestrian-injuries were more frequent in children (71%) than in adults (23%). Most patients with hypotension by systemic trauma or severe brainstem injury had a poor outcome, but shocked victims were significantly fewer in children (4%) than in adults (26%). Initial computed tomographic findings were divided into 3 categories proposed by Marshall in 1991. Correlation between types of DBI and outcome was not significant in children, but significant in adults. The relationship between outcome and neurological status on admission was studied in 88 patients without hypotension. Children had a better Glasgow coma scale score and better neurological status than adults. Outcome in adults correlated with GCS and abnormalities of posturing, pupils, and brain stem reflex. But in children, this relationship was not significant except for GCS. These findings suggest that the pathophysiology of DBI in children is different from that in adults.

KEY WORDS: diffuse brain injury, children, outcome, computed tomography, neurological status

INTRODUCTION

It has been pointed out that children with severe head injury have a better outcome than adults because of a low incidence of intracranial hematoma and a high incidence of diffuse brain injury [1, 2, 3]. In this study, we analyzed the factors that might have influences on the outcome of children with diffuse brain injury (DBI) in comparison to that of adults.

MATERIALS AND METHODS

One hundred and twelve patients with DBI, 24 children and 88 adults, were studied. Children were aged from 3 to 14 years, and adults from 15 to 76 years. Initial GCS scores on admission were 8 or less in all and they were comatose for more than 24 hours after injury. Computed tomography (CT) revealed DBI in all and some cases had co-existing small focal lesions such as contusion, subdural hematoma or epidural hematoma. Excluded were the cases who had showed hemispheric swelling or marked brainstem hemorrhage on CT, and had failed to recover from shock in spite of resuscitation. Initial CT findings were classified into 3 categories proposed by Marshall in 1991 [4]. Type 1 means no visible intracranial pathology. Type 2 shows lesion densities such as multifocal hemorrhages on CT scan. Type 3 means diffuse cerebral swelling (DCS). Hypotension or shock was defined as arterial systolic blood pressure less than 80 mm Hg within 6 hours of injury. Outcome was assessed according to Glasgow Outcome Scale (GOS) at 3 through 6 months after injury. Initial neurological status was evaluated by Glasgow Coma Scale score (GCS), posturing of extremities, and pupillary and brain stem reflexes. Chi-square test or two-sample Wilcoxon test was used for statistical analysis.

RESULTS AND DISCUSSION

Children had a better initial GCS score than adults (p <0.05). More than a half of adults became vegetatives or died, while any children did not remain in vegetative state and only two children died (p <0.05). Traffic accident was a common cause of injury; all in children, and 93% in adults. Pedestrian-injuries were significantly more frequent in children (71%) than in adults (23%). On the other hand, driver's injury was a common cause in adults. Both children and adults were frequently accompanied with multiple injuries, while severe multiple injury, i.e., chest, abdominal or pelvic injury, was not common in children (25%), but common in adults (46.5%). Cases with hypotension were significantly fewer in children than in adults. Few patients with hypotension could recover, and the only one pediatric case in this group died. Massive hemorrhage by multiple trauma and/or severe brain stem damage was a cause of hypotension. There were six cases (all in adults) in shock obviously sustaining severe lower brain stem damage (Table 1).

There was no significant difference between children and adults in types of DBI on CT scan. In adults, type 3 had a poorer outcome than remaining 2 types of DBI, while in children, difference in outcome between type 2 and type 3 was not significant (Table 2).

The relationship between initial neurological status and outcome was analyzed in cases without hypotension. Children had a significantly better initial GCS score than adults. Dividing the patients into two GCS groups, that is, 3 to 5 and 6 to 8, outcome was significantly better both in children and adults. Findings of abnormal posturing of extremities were divided into two categories; complete and incomplete posturing. Bilateral extensor or bilateral abnormal flexor response was defined as complete posturing. Unilateral abnormal posturing or posturing mixed with withdrawal was as incomplete posturing. Incomplete posturing was significantly more common in children. There was no correlation between posturing and outcome in children. But in adults, incomplete posturing led to a significantly better outcome. Impaired pupillary light reflex was seen less frequently in children than in

Table 1. Summary of Cases

	Children No.	Children %	Adults No.	Adults %	Total No.	Total %
No. of cases	24		88		112	
GCS score 3-5	9	37.5	52	59.1	61	54.5
6-8	15	62.5	36	40.9	51	45.5
GOS:PVS or Dead	2	8.3	49	55.7	51	45.5
Cause of injury						
Pedestrian	17	70.8	20	22.7	37	33.0
Bicylcle/motorcycle	7	29.2	37	42.0	44	39.3
Automobile	0	0.0	25	28.4	25	22.3
Fall/other	0	0.0	6	6.8	6	5.4
Multiple trauma	16	66.7	52	59.1	68	60.7
Hypotension	1	4.2	23	26.1	24	21.4
GOS:PVS or Dead	1	100.0	17	73.9	18	75.0

Table 2. Type of DBI on Computed Tomography and Outcome

CT type	Children (n=24)				Adults (n=88)			
	GR/MD	SD	V/D	total	GR/MD	SD	V/D	total
Type 1	2	1	0	3	2	2	1	5
Type 2	5	3	1	9	8	20	16 ⌉*	44
Type 3	4	7	1	12	2	5	32 ⌋	39

GR:good recovery, MD:moderately disabled, SD: severely
disabled, V: vegetative, D: dead, *$p < 0.01$

Table 3. Initial Neurological Status and Outcome
            (Cases without hypotension)

Neurological status	Children (n=23)				Adults (n=65)			
	GR/MD	SD	V/D	total	GR/MD	SD	V/D	total
GCS score								
3-5	1	6	1 ⌉*	8	2	7	25 ⌉**	34
6-8	10	5	0 ⌋	15	9	15	7 ⌋	31
Posturing								
complete	3	3	1	7	2	8	21 ⌉*	31
incomplete	4	6	0	10	2	11	5 ⌋	18
Pupillary reflex								
abnormal	5	6	1	12	7	16	27 ⌉*	50
normal	6	5	0	11	4	6	5 ⌋	15
Brain stem reflex								
abnormal	4	3	1	8	4	10	24 ⌉**	38
normal	7	8	0	15	7	12	8 ⌋	27

*$p < 0.05$, **$p < 0.01$

adults. Correlation between pupillary abnormality and outcome was not found in children, while in adults abnormal pupillary reflex meant poorer outcome. Brain stem reflexes were less frequently impaired in children, but the difference between children and adults was not significant. The relationship between brain stem reflex and outcome was not significant in children, but significant in adults (Table 3).

It is well known that hypotension is one of causes of poor outcome in severe head injury. Extracranial insults are less frequent and do not have influences on the outcome of children with severe head injury [3]. Gennarreli demonstrated that severe diffuse axonal injury (DAI) was predominant in vehicle occupant (80%), and moderate DAI was more common in pedestrian [5]. DCS is a common cause of neurological deterioration and a reversible hyperemic syndrome in children, while cases with DCS and a low GCS score suffer from more severe direct impact injury [6]. In pediatric DBI, reason of better outcome would be due to less occurrence of hypotension, severe DAI and untreatable DCS. The reasons of infrequent hypotension are low incidence of severe multiple injuries and less occurrence of severe DAI or lower brain stem damage. In this study, all the children except one case with DCS survived, while most of adults with DCS became vegetatives or died. DCS in most of children may not play a significant role in determining the outcomes, though may deteriorate neurological status. Moreover, the present study demonstrated that initial neurological status of DBI was less severe in children than in adults, and was not a good predictor of prognosis in children but in adults as previously reported by some authors [7, 8]. These results suggest that the pathophysiology of DBI in children is different from that in adults.

REFERENCES

1. Alberico AM, Ward JD, Choi SC, Marmarou A, Young HF (1987) J Neurosurg 67: 648-656
2. Bruce DA, Schut L, Bruno LA, Wood JH, Sutton LN (1978) J Neurosurg 48: 679-688
3. Berger MS, Pitts LH, Lovely M, Edwards MSB, Bartkowski HM (1985) J Neurosurg 62: 194-199
4. Marshall LF, Marshall SB, Klauber MR, Clark MB (1991) J Neurosurg 75: S14-20
5. Gennarelli TA (1983) Acta Neurochir Suppl 32: 1-13
6. Bruce DA, Alavi A, Bilaniuk L, Dolinskas D, Obrist W, Uzzell B (1982) J Neurosurg 54: 170-178
7. Becker DP, Miller JD, Ward JD, Greenberg RP, Young HF, Sakalas R (1977) J Neurosurg 47: 491-502
8. Facco E, Zuccarello L, Pittoni G, Zanardi L, Chiaranda M, Davia G, Giron GP (1986) Child's Nerv Syst 2: 67-71

13—Spinal Cord Injury

Electrophysiological and Biochemical Study in the Acute Stages of Experimental Spinal Cord Injuries

KATSUMI YAMASHIRO[1], HIROSHI MIYAZATO[1], KAZUHIKO SUYAMA[2],
TERUAKI KAWANO[2], KATSUTOSHI HIRATA[2], JIRO MUKAWA[1], and KAZUO MORI[3]

[1]Department of Neurosurgery, University of the Ryukyus School of Medicine, Nishihara, Okinawa, 903-01 Japan,
[2]Department of Neurosurgery, Nagasaki University School of Medicine, Nagasaki, 852 Japan and [3]Department of
Neurosurgery, Hamamatsu Rosai Hospital, Hamamatsu Shizuoka, 430 Japan

SUMMARY

Monitoring the spinal cord function with the use of evoked potentials have been extensively used in experimental spinal injuries and during operative monitoring. The purpose of this experiment is to compare the electrophysiological and biochemical changes in acute spinal cord injuries of rats. Male Wistar rats were anesthetized and a laminectomy was performed at T1-T3. A microdialysis tube was placed into the T2 spinal gray matter. Somatosensory evoked spinal cord potential(SESP) and motor evoked potential(MEP) recordings were at the level of T1 and T3. Monoamines, monoamine metabolites and amino acids were measured by using the HPLC-ECD technique. After electrophysiological and biochemical control data had been obtained, spinal crush injuries were made by a Sugita's curved aneurysm clip which was applied extradurally for 5 seconds. Data was collected for a 120 min. after the spinal injury.

Most of the rats showed increased amplitude of MEP and SESP within 10 min. after the spinal injury, then amplitude decreased gradually. Dopamine(DA), DOPAC, HVA, 5-HIAA could also be measured after the spinal injury. All of them showed decreased gradually after the spinal injury. On the other hand, excitatory amino acids(aspartate, glutamate) showed a temporary increase, then showed a gradual decrease up until 120 min. after the spinal injury. These results suggested that temporary increase of MEP and SESP in amplitude after the spinal crush injury may correlate with the increase of excitatory amino acids.

KEY WORDS: evoked potentials, monoamine, monoamine metabolites, excitatory amino acids, GABA

INTRODUCTION

Monitoring spinal cord functions with the use of somatosensory evoked potentials and motor evoked potentials have been extensively used in experimental spinal injuries and during operative monitoring[1][2][3]. Chemical substances were also measured before and after the spinal cord injury[4][5][6]. The purpose of this experiment was to compare the electrophysiological and biochemical changes in acute spinal cord injuries of rats.

MATERIALS AND METHODS

Male Wistar rats weighing 250-300g were anesthetized with ketamine hydrochloride and placed in a rodent stereotactic frame. A total laminectomy was performed from T1 to T3 thoratic region with the use of a microscope.

A microdialysis tube was placed into the T2's spinal gray matter for analysis of amine, amine metabolites and amino acids[7]. Percutaneous needle electrodes were placed along the course of the right sciatic nerve for elicitation of somatosensory evoked spinal cord potentials (SESP). Transcortical stimulation of motor evoked potentials (MEP) was achieved using screw electrodes placed epidurally over the left motor complex. SESPs and MEP were recorded via a 1 mm silver ball electrode from dorsal and lateral part of the spinal cord. The stimulation rate was 1 Hz. Thirty-two responses were summated and analysis time 10-20 msec was used. Monoamine, Monoamine metabolites and amino acids were measured from the perfused Ringer solution of microdialysis system by using the high performance liquid chromatography (HPLC-ECD) technique. Chemical substances were collected every 20 minutes. After electrophysiological and biochemical control data had been obtained, spinal crush injuries were made at the T2 level by a Sugita's curved aneurysm clip. The clip, with 120 grams of pressure, was applied extradurally for 5 seconds. Electrophysiological and biochemical data were collected for 120 minutes after the spinal injury.

RESULTS

MEPs and SESPs were recorded at the level of T1 and T3. An example of the changes of MEP were recorded before and after the spinal cord crush injury and are shown in figure 1.

These responses were recorded at the T1 level. Control responses consisted of first positive-negative wave and were followed by small waves. We focused on the first negative-positive wave for analysis. It showed a remarkable increase of amplitude 2 minutes after the spinal injury. This increase continued for about 2-5 minutes, then gradually decreased(Fig.1). Interanimal variability in signal amplitude does exists. Percent amplitudes as compared to the control value were examined at each recording. Figure 2 shows the results of MEP percentage amplitude change at T1 and T3. Both T1 and T3 amplitude recordings showed a temporary increase for 2 to 5 minutes after the spinal injury. A remarkable reduction was seen at the T3 recording. Thirty minutes after the injury, the T1 recording also showed a reduction of amplitudes. However, this reduction was small compared to T3 s amplitude changes. SESPs were also showed a similar pattern of changes.

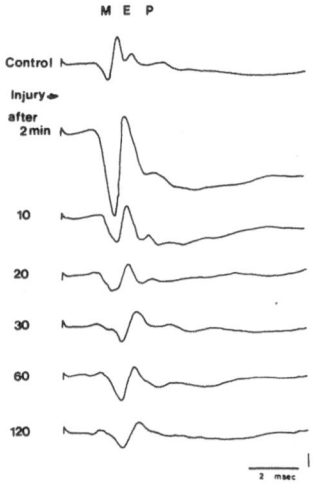

Fig. 1 An example of MEP changes before and after the spinal cord injury

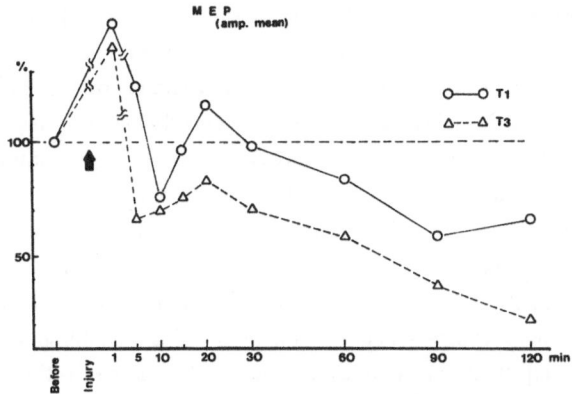

Fig. 2 The changes of percent amplitudes which were recorded at the T1 and
T3 spinal cord level.

There was no increase in DA, DOPAC, HVA and 5-HIAA in relation to the spinal injury. On the other hand, amino acids showed different patterns of changes after the spinal injury.

Figure 3 showed the changes of excitatory and inhibitory amino acids. Excitatory amino acids, aspartate and glutamate showed a remarkable increase as compared to the control value at 20 minutes after the spinal injury. Then, these two amino acids continued to increase more than 150% until 120 minutes after the spinal injury. Inhibitory amino acid, GABA, showed a slight increase until 40 minutes after the injury.

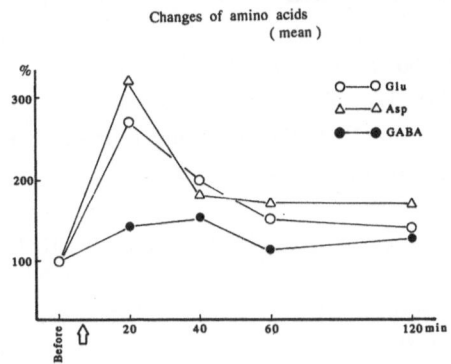

Fig. 3 Changes of amino acids around the spinal cord injury

DISCUSSION

Relating to the spinal injury, Salzman et al[4] reported that turnover and utilization of NE was increased at the injury site, while the dopamine function was not affected. Trauma resulted in rapid and sustained

419

elevations in 5-HT concentration at and around the injury site. Sharma et al [5] also reported that the serotonin concentration in the traumatized segment had increased. We did not measure the serotonin; however, 5-HIAA, DA, DOPAC, and HVA showed a decrease for a short period after the spinal cord injury. In correlation between amino acids and spinal cord injury, Demediuk et al[6] reported that the excitatory amino acids, glutamate and aspartate were significantly decreased by 5 min post-trauma, and remained low at 4 hours and 24 hours. The inhibitory amino acid, GABA also decreased.

On the other hand , Panter et al[8] reported extracellular concentration of excitatory and inhibitory amino acids increased after trauma, with the degree of increase related to the severity of the injury. These results were very similar to our results. Evoked potentials were a useful tool in assessiing the spinal cord's function. Somatosensory and motor evoked potentials were used to examine the spinal cord functions. Baskin and Simpson[9], Zileli et al[10] stated motor evoked potential is more sensitive than SESP. We couldn't detect a difference in sensitivity between MEP and SESP. However, MEP and SESP had showed a temporary increase of amplitude after the spinal cord crush injury, and excitatory amino acids increased at almost the same time. These results suggest the change of amplitude of evoked potential may correlate with the increase of excitatory amino acids.

REFERENCES

1. Li C, Houlden DA, Rowed DW (1990) J. Neurosurg 72: 600-609
2. Rivlin AS, Tator CH (1978) Surg Neurol 10: 39-43
3. Tsubokawa T, Katayama Y, Maejima S, Hirayama T, Yamamoto T (1987) Neuro-Orthopedics 3: 82-89
4. Salzman SK, Hirofuji E, Llados-Eckman C, MacEwen GD, Beckman AL (1987) J. Neursurg 66: 431-439
5. Sharma HS, Olsson Y, Dey PK (1990) Neuroscience 36: 725-730
6. Demediuk P, Daly MP, Faden AI (1989) J Neurochem 52: 1529-1536
7. Kawano, T, Miyake H, TsutsumiK, Mori K (1987) Spinal Surgery 1: 128-131
8. Panter SS, Yum SW, Faden AI (1990) Ann Neurol 27: 96-99
9. Baskin DS, Simpson RK (1987) Neurosurg 20: 871-877
10. Zileli M, Taniguchi M, Cedzich C, Schramm J (1989) Acta Neurochir 101: 141-148

Modern Concepts in the Neurosurgical Treatment of Severe Thoraco-Lumbar Spine Injuries

THOMAS PENTELÉNYI, SÁNDOR ZSOLCZAI, LASZLÓ TUROCZY, and RÓBERT VERES

National Institute of Traumatology, Department of Neurosurgery VIII, Budapest, Hungary

SUMMARY

Most of the severe thoraco-lumbar spinal injuries need emergency surgery. Operation must be done by well defined indications. Primary complete neurological lesion is not contraindication for emergency surgery. Reduction, decompression and stabilization have to be performed in the primary neurosurgical treatment. The stabilization method must be chosen with neurorehabilitation aspect. That is why segmental stabilization methods seem to be the best ones. Primary neurosurgical operation is one of the most important first steps of the complex, long-lasting rehabilitation, and has basic role both in neurological and motor-system improvements of the patient.

KEY WORDS

Fixateur Interne, Steffee plates, Eger plates, Emergency treatment, Segmental stabilization.

INTRODUCTION

Up-to-date treatment of spinal injuries must be done with 5 aims:
1/ Restoration of impaired neurology functions.
2/ Conservation of unhurt neurology functions.
3/ Restoration and conservation of spinal stability.
4/ To assure patient's comfort.
5/ To assure conditions of early physical, psychical and vocational rehabilitation.
If we wish to fulfill all these demands 70-80 per cent of severe spinal injury cases are to be operated on. It means that very wide neurosurgical activity is wanted on one side, but we must not forget the good and reliable methods of conservative treatment for the other 20-30 per cent of patients on the other side.

INDICATIONS FOR SURGERY

There are 3 groups of indications: emergency, absolute and relative indications.

Emergency indications

1/ Time interval between trauma and neurology symptoms.
2/ Progression in the symptoms of primary incomplete neurology lesion.
3/ Compound injuries.

Absolute indications

1/ Spinal block, partial or complete.
2/ Bone or disc fragment in the spinal canal.
3/ Irreducible spine.
4/ Unstable spine.

Relative indications

1/ Age.
2/ Polytrauma.
3/ Special conditions.
4/ Chronic diseases.

It is very important to take into consideration that the clinical picture of primary complete neurology lesion is not contraindication for surgery.

LOCAL NEUROSURGICAL TREATMENT

It consists of 3 important actions: reduction, decompression and stabilization. All three of them are achieved mainly by segmental stabilization methods: Fixateur Interne, AO-ASIF /1,2/ or angle-stable plate fixation, Steffee or Eger plates /3,4/. By this trans-pedicle screw-fixation technique most of the acute cases can be treated by posterior approach which is much smaller load for the patient than the ventral or combined ventral and dorsal approach. Classical long rod systems - i.e. Harrington /5/, Luque /6/, Jacobs /7/ - and those posterior plate instrumentations in which there is no fix angle between the plate and screws are not the best for trauma cases /8/. Ventral or combined ventro-dorsal approaches are rarely used in acute thoracolumbar trauma cases, they are applied rather in inveterated trauma and tumor cases.

TIMING

There are pathology changes of three origins in acute traumatic spinal cord lesions: primary mechanical lesion at the time of trauma, secondary circulatory-metabolic lesion during 2-6 hours, and persisting compressive lesion from the first hours till days or weeks /if not decompressed/. We can not do anything with the first one. But we can do very much in preventing or treating the second and third ones if our intervention is on time. That is why these cases have to be considered as emergency cases, and operative treatment must be performed possibly in the first 6 hours, or as soon as possible after six hours if there is no vital contraindication for surgery. Also megadoses of corticosteroids are to be given from the first hour till 24 hours with the same reason.

PATIENTS, OPERATIONS AND RESULTS

During 5 years between 1986 and 1990 163 severe thoraco-lumbar spinal trauma cases were treated by surgery. 102 were operated on by Fixateur Interne, and 61 by angle-stable Steffee or Eger plates. 66 per cent of the patients had neurology lesions of different severity, 34 per cent of them were without neurology symptoms. 15 per cent of the Frankel A, 55 per cent of the Frankel B, and 90 per cent of the Frankel C neurology-lesion-patients improved to useful neurology grades /Frankel D and E/ after surgery and long-lasting rehabilitation /9/. No neurological deterioration were seen at the end of rehabilitation period, compared with the primary state.
In 92 per cent of the cases solid union in good position was seen after 6-12 months. Removal of the metal implants was done after 10-12 months in the first period, and after 6-8 months in the second period /10, 11, 12/.

REFERENCES

1. Dick W /1984/ Innere Fixation von Brust- und Lendenwirben-brüchen. Huber, Bern Stuttgart Wien.

2. Dick W, Kluger P, ... erl F, Wörsdörfer O, Zäch G /1985/ A new device for internal fixation of thoracolumbar and lumbar spine fractures: the "fixateur interne". Paraplegia 23: 225-232.

3. Arthur D. Steffee, Sitkowski Daniel J. /1988/ Posterior Lumbar Interbody Fusion and Plates Clin Orthop Rel Res 227: 99-102.

4. Arthur D. Steffee /1989/ The Variable Screw Placement System with Posterior Lumbar Interbody Fusion. In: P.M. Lin /ed/ Lumbar Interbody Fusion: Principles and Techniques in Spine Surgery. Aspen Publishers, Inc. pp. 81-93.

5. Harrington PR, Dickson JH /1973/ The development and further prospects of internal fixation of the spine. Isr J Med Sci 9: 773-781.

6. Luque E, Cassis N, Ramirez-Wiella G /1982/ Segmental spinal instrumentation in the treatment of fractures of the thoraco-lumbar spine. Spine 7: 312-320.

7. Jacobs RR, Schlaepfer F, Mathys R Jr, Nachemson A, Perren SM. /1984/ A locking hook spinal rod system for stabilization of fractur-dislocations and correction of deformities of the dorsolumbar spine. Clin Orthop 189: 168-177.

8. Roy-Camille R, Saillant G, Berteaux D, Salgado V /1976/ Osteosynthesis of thoracolumbar spine fractures with metal plates screwed through the vertebral pedicules. Reconstr Surg Traumatol 15: 2-17.

9. Frankel HL, Hancock DO, Hyslop G, Melzak J, Michaelis LS, Ungar GH, Vernon JDS, Walsh JJ /1969/ The value of postural reduction in the initial management of closed injuries of the spine with paraplegia and tetraplegia. Paraplegia 7: 179-186.

10. Pentelényi T, Zsolczai S. /1988/ First Hungarian Neurosurgical Experiences with "Fixateur Interne" in the treatment of Thoracolumbar Spine Injuries. Acta Neurochir. 93: 104-109.

11. Pentelényi T /1986/ Up-to-date operative treatment of spine injuries. Magy Traumat Orthop 29: 198-214.

12. Pentelényi T, Zsolczai S. /1988/ Fixateur Interne - New Method for Segmental Stabilization of the Thoracolumbar Spine. Acta Chir Hung 29: 373-383.

Late Results of Surgical Management of Thoraco-Lumbar Injuries with Kluger's Fixateur Interne

A. KARIMI-NEJAD

Neurosurgical Clinic, University Cologne, 5000 Köln 41, Germany

SUMMARY

Since 1987 all thoracolumbar injuries with fractures, fracture dislocations with or without neurological deficits are treated in an
early stage. This surgical management is performed with a dorsal
access only. The reconstruction of fractured vertebrae is achieved
by intercorporal and in some patients also by interbody bone grafting.

The bone grafting has been done with small chips taken by laminectomy
or from spinous and not as usual with cancellous bone. After reduction in anatomical shape with special instruments and clearance of
the spinal canal by replacement of bone fragments into the fractured
vertebral body the best achievable position was fixed with KLUGER's
fixateur interne. The radiological and neurological evaluation of
6o patients who have been followed up for at least 1 year after
surgery have been reviewed. The late results especially in patients
with bone grafting are excellent. The correction loss at followup
is less than 5°. None of 6o patients suffered a constant neurological
deterioration. 17 out of 33 patients with preoperative neurological
deficits improved significantly.

KEY WORDS: Thoracolumbar injuries. Spine. Fixateur interne.
KLUGER's fixateur. Vertebral bone grafting.

INTRODUCTION

The advantages of surgical treatment versus non-operative treatment
of thoracolumbar fractures do not seem to be controversial anymore.
The main goals of surgery are reduction in anatomical shape, reconstruction of fractured vertebrae, clearance of the spinal canal,
stability, prevention of late correction loss and complications as
well as early painless mobilization. In the last few years the surgical management has been subject to many changes. The HARRINGTON (1)
dual-distraction rods were initially most accepted as a standard
spinal fixation system. Sublaminar wires were later added to
reinforce the rods (2). The transpeduncular plate fixation developed
in 1963 by ROY-CAMILLE (3) were a new device for surgical treatment
of thoracolumbar injuries too in 197o. The AO DICK's spinal internal
fixateur system as a pedicle screw system with "spanning rods" (4)
allowed stable and accurate reduction with limited segmental fixation.
KLUGER (5) designed the internal fixateur system with a variable
hypomochlion in the length as a further development of fixateur

interne devices. This fixateur device led to a more precise reduction and reconstruction of fractured vertebrae with possibilities
of correction at any stage of surgical procedures. Since 1987 we
used this fixateur system for surgical management of thoracolumbar
injuries. A number of other internal plate fixation devices using
posterior instrumentation and/or using anterior procedures are
available. They will be not the subject of discussion in this presentation.

PATIENTS AND METHOD

From 1987-1991 6o patients with major fractures and fracture disloc-
cations of thoracic and lumbar spine were treated with KLUGER's fixateur system. The injuries were classified according to the three-
column spine concept of DENIS (6) and related to the level of
fracture i.g. fracture dislocation (Fig. 1).

Fracture typ according to DENIS classification		Level of fractures No.	%
A: 5	8 %	D_5 2	3
B: 39	63 %	D_{11} 2	3
C: 3	5 %	D_{12} 16	26
D: 6	1o %	L_1 24	39
E: 9	14 %	L_2 1o	16
		L_3 3	5
		L_4 5	8

Two patients suffered fractures $L_3 + L_1$ respectively $L_1 + L_2$

Fig. 1: Distribution and classification of fracture types.

Surgery was performed as early as possible with an average interval
time between accident and operation of 2 days. Only in 2 cases who were
initially operated on abroad the second surgery has been performed
8 weeks e.g. 1 year after accident. The neurological examination were
classified on an modified FRANKEL scale (7). With grade "motor useful"
it is distinguished between "able to walk with support" and "able to
walk without support". Due to instability, pain and combined injuries
the preoperative neurological findings were estimated concerning able
to walk with or without support according to the neurological status.
The radiological examination at follow up and the correction loss
were evaluted by using the Cobb method. All patients with neurological
involvement besides having X-rays underwent CT examination to realize
the displacement of the bony fragments in the spinal canal. Depending
on the CT-scan findings a hemilaminectomy or laminectomy were made to
achieve a fully replacement of fragments into the fractured vertebrae.
For transpedicular fixation for the thoracic and lumbar parts of the
spine usualy Schanz screws of 6-6,5 mm diameter were used. However

in the upper thoracic part Schanz screws of 5-5,5 mm diameter were inserted. After the reduction 4 mm canals in the pedicle of fractured vertebrae were reamed. A 6 mm pin with collar was introduced into the same canal through the pedicle. The top of DANIAUX (8) funnel with impactor was placed in the body of the fractured vertebrae as far as possible ventraly. After intercorporal extending of fractured vertebral body the displaced fragments in the spinal canal were replaced and compressed into the vertebral body. In the beginning of our activities in 8 patients with dislocations and 18 patients with burstfractures we did not perform additional interbody bone grafting. After some disappointing results in 9 patients with early screw breakage and correction loss at follow up about 8° intercorporal bone grafting were done in remained 38 patients. For bone grafting the bone taken by laminectomy or from spinous which were broken in small chips, has been used. Obviously the compact bone chips provide more firmness. The bone chips were gradually placed ventrally as far as possible. This technique enhanced an early ventral ossification and subsequent stability without correction loss at follow up (Fig. 2). Multiple injuries of non-adjacent vertebrae were fixed with 2 devices. However burst fractures of two adjacent vertebrae were stabilized only by one fixateur device (Fig. 3).

An additional mechanical device for dynamic reduction produced good results both in the realignment and in the stabilization still of old fracture dislocation (Fig. 4). Postoperative mobilization time were 1-2 weeks on average only with a brace for the first 6 months. Fixateur were removed 1-1 1/2 years after surgery. This time was extended only by patient's wishes.

RESULTS

The surgical management was performed in 6o patients. Two patients suffered two vertebral fractures ($L_1 + L_2$; $L_1 + L_3$). All patients were followuped 4-1 years after surgery (average 2,1 years). 33 out of 6o patients showed preoperative neurological involvement. The neurological dysfunction was classified on a modified FRANKEL scale (7). The preoperative neurological status included 7 patients with complete, 2 patients with sensory only, 6 patients with motor useless, 5 patients with able to walk with support, and 13 patients able to walk without support. 27 patients showed no neurological involvement. At follow-up examination 17 patients out of 33 patient (51 %), with preoperative neurological dysfunction were improved significantly. Fig. 5 shows follow up with individual neurological improvment of all patients. None of patients suffered constant neurological deterioration after surgery. 6 patients with complete paraplegia remained unchanged. Two patients who were classified preoperatively as "able to walk with support" improved. But they remained in the same category at follow-up examination because of combined leg and pelvic injuries. Three patients with severe preoperative neurological deficits as "motor useless" improved up to recovery i.g. "able to walk without support. In all 3 patients the

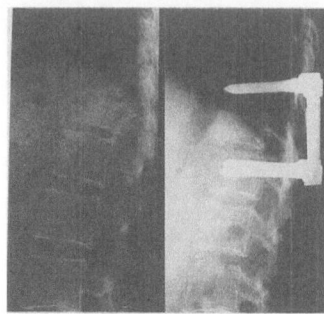

Fig. 2: Bone grafting with small compact chips placed ventrally as far as possible.

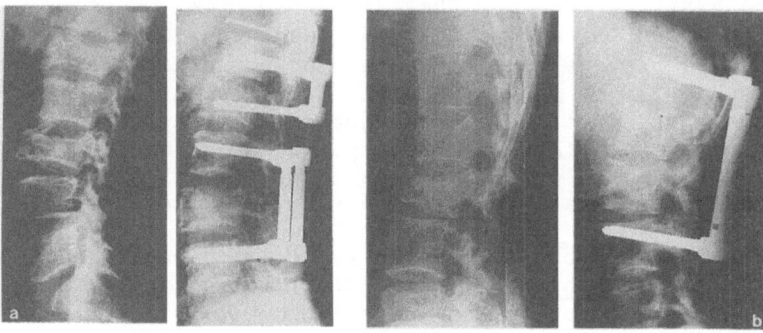

Fig. 3
a) Multiple injuries of non-adjacent vertebrae were fixed with 2 devices.

b) Fixation of two adjacent vertebrae with one fixateure device.

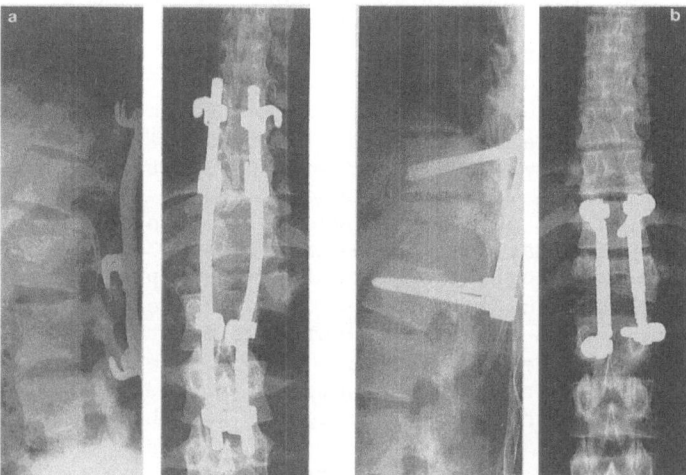

Fig. 4:
a) Severe fracture dislocation D_{12} after abroad treatment with HARRINGTON-rods. There was still an enormous dislocation in length and axis.

b) Realignment and fixation in anatomical shape 8 weeks after first surgery.

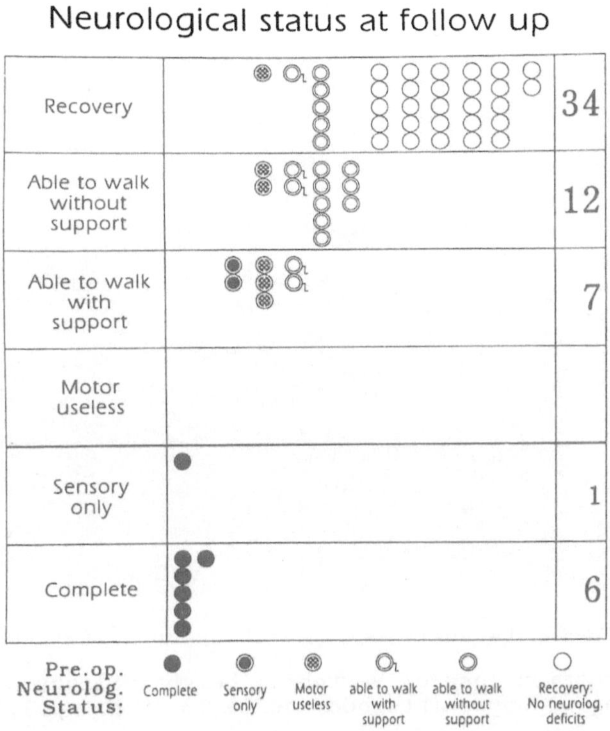

Neurological status at follow up

Recovery		34
Able to walk without support		12
Able to walk with support		7
Motor useless		
Sensory only		1
Complete		6

Pre.op. Neurolog. Status:	Complete	Sensory only	Motor useless	able to walk with support	able to walk without support	Recovery: No neurolog. deficits

Fig. 5: Neurological findings pre-operative and at follow up (60 patients).

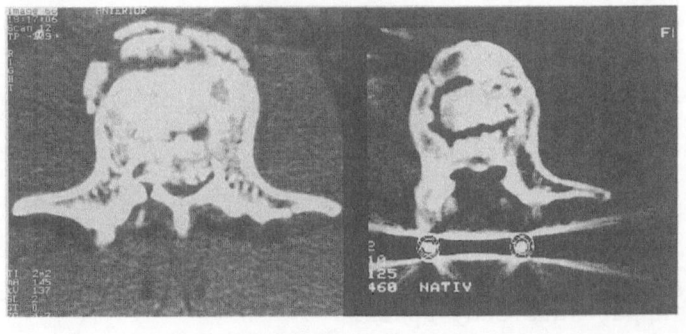

a   b

Fig. 6: a) Pre-op CT scan of a 3o j. old patient with neurological deficits "motor useless". Spinal canal narrowing by bone grafts.

b) CT scan post. op.
Spinal canal clearance by replacement of bone grafts back into the fractured vertebral body. Patient improved to "recovery".

429

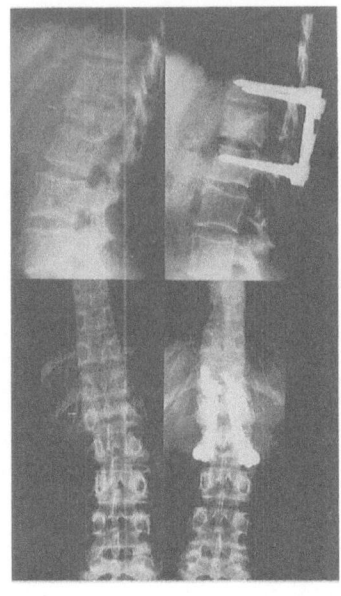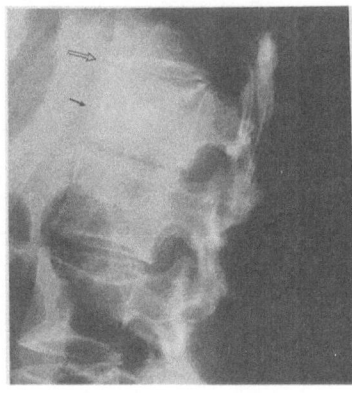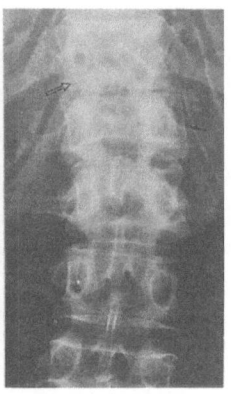

Fig. 7: a) Severe burst fracture. Bone grafting and fixation.

b) Non-correction loss of vertebral height. Slight narrowing of upper interbody space (3 j. p. op.).

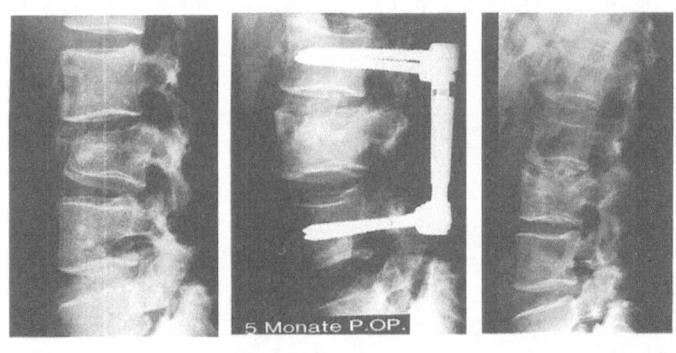

Fig. 8: a) Fractur of vertebral body. Bone grafting and fusion of upper interbody space.

b) Follow up after 3 j., non-correction loss of interbody space.

430

spinal canal was extremly narrowed with bone fragments. A total reduction of the spinal canal was accomplished in all 3 patients (Fig. 6). One patient were regarded as technical failure with misplaced Schanz-Screw. She experienced severe temporary neurological deterioration. Reoperation with correction was performed 6 hrs after first surgery. She improved entirely and was free from neurological symptoms.

The preoperative and postoperative kyphotic deformities were measured using the Cobb method on the lateral röntgenogram, taking the superior end-plate of the vertebral body one level above and the inferior endplate of the body one level below. The rate of correction loss at follow-up was most frequent with patients without bone grafting. In this group correction loss averaged 6,3°. However in patients with intercorporal and/or interbody grafting the correction loss averaged less than 5°.

In most cases the vertebral body height has remained unchanged. But in few cases a collapse prodominantely of the upper intervertebral space has been occurred (Fig. 7). This was the reason for resection of damaged disks and subsequent interbody grafting to achieve a stable interbody fusion (Fig. 8). None of the patients showed a fracture instability at follow-up.

COMPLICATIONS

The number of complications of clinical importence was low. The single Case of temporary neurological deterioration was caused by false screw position. We experienced one superficial wound infection without sequelae. Screw breakage 19(31 %) was most frequent in patient without bone grafting. This did not cause any instability or collapse of fractured vertebral body. In 9 patients (15 %) complete extraction of the fractured screws were not done and short segments were left embedded in pedicles.

REFERENCES

1. Harrington PR. (1962) J. Bone Joint Surg. 44 A: 591-6o2
2. Luque E.R; Cassis N.; Ramirez-Wiella G. (1982) Spine 7: 312-317
3. Roy-Camille R; Berteaux D.(1976) Montpellier Chir. 22: 3o7-315
4. Dick W. (1987) Spine 12: 882-9oo
5. Kluger P. (1989) in: Stuhler Th. (Ed.) Fixateur externe-Fixateur interne. Springer-Verlag Berlin Heidelberg PP 36-58
6. Denis F. (1983) Spine 8: 817-821
7. Frankel HL, Hancock DO, Hyslop G, Melzak J, Michaelis LS, Ungar GH, Vernon JDS, Walsch JJ.(1969) Paraplegia 7: 179-192
8. Daniaux H. (1986) Unfallchirurg 89: 197-213

Lumbosacral Selective Posterior Rhizotomy for Lower Limb Spasticity in Adults

A.K. Purohit, D.P. Bedekar, G.S. Alexander, B.N. Prasad, A.K. Singh, S. Mohandas, and I. Dinakar

The Nizam's Institute of Medical Sciences, Panja Gutta, Hyderabad-500 482, India

SUMMARY: Lumbosacral Selective Posterior Rhizotomy(SPR) is routinely performed at our centre for the spastic cerebral palsied. The indications of this surgical procedure have been extended to spinal injury, head injury and some other cases who have non-progressive severe painful spasticity in their lower limbs. Five cases have been operated in the last 4 years. The age ranged from 25 to 45 years. Three patients were bed ridden and two had some mobility. In all of them rehabilitation even in wheel chair was not possible. Following Lumbosacral SPR spasticity has subsided in all the cases. They have partial relief in lower limb spasms also. One patient is able to walk with crutches and is back to his previous occupation. All others are able to lead comfortable wheel chair life. Improvement in spastic urinary bladder problem has also been noticed in 3 patients. Lumbosacral SPR can be of considerable benefit to nonprogressive spastic paraplegics like spinal trauma, head injury etc, patients.

KEY WORDS: Cerebral palsy, Selective posterior Rhizotomy, Spasticity, Spinal injury, Trauma.

INTRODUCTION: Selective Posterior Rhizotomy is indicated for relief of spasticity in cerebral palsied children who have nonprogressive spasticity. Lot of work has been done in U.S.A, Europe and India on this surgical procedure. In the last 16 years more than 1000 cerebral palsied cases have undergone this operation all over the globe. All the reports have consistently shown relief in spasticity, no recurrence, and improvement in motor functions (1,2). The encouraging results of our own as well as Laitinena etal (3) have prompted us to extend the indications of this surgical procedure for patients suffering from nonprogressive painful disabling spasticity in the lower limbs resulting from spinal or head trauma, myelities etc.

MATERIAL AND METHODS: Five patients underwent Lumbosacral Selective Posterior Rhizotomy. There were 4 males and one female. The age ranged from 25-45 year. They were followed for a maximum of 4 years and minimum of 10 months.

The causes of development of neurological deficits were various. There were two cases of neurotrauma. One sustained # dislocation of D12 vertebra and another one had severe head injury. There was one each of Encephalomyelitis and myelities. The only female patient of the series had Tuberculosis of upper Thoracic spine. She underwent multiple upper thoracic Laminectomies and decompression 1 year prior to SPR. All the cases had 6 to 18 months of static neurological picture prior to SPR. This was suggestive of presence of nonprogressive disorder.

All the 5 cases had severe spasticity in both the lower limbs and the head injury patient had the same in upper limbs also. There was some element of rigidity in his all the limbs. Three cases had severe spasms, one had moderate spasms and the head injury patient had minimal spasms. All the cases had some amount of sensory impairment which ranged from 10-50%. Four cases had urgency incontenance and one had minimal urgency.

One case was walking a few steps with heavy support. Another case had mobility in squatting position because of inability to straighten the lower limbs. Other 3 cases were bed ridden. All the cases underwent Peacock's procedure of Selective Posterior Rhizotomy. Under endo tracheal general anaesthesia, the patient was positioned prone. The lower limbs were kept exposed for applica tion of electrodes and clinical observation of movements. Surface electrodes were tied on the limbs and connected to EMG machine. Lumbar 2 Lumbar 5 limited laminectomy was performed. Dura was opened. Cauda equina was exposed. $Lumbar_2$ to $sacral_2$ roots were defined on either sides. The posterior roots were lifted on two hooked micro neurosurgical electrodes and were split into their constituent rootlets. The electrode were connected to EMG machine. Each posterior rootlet was stimulated to findout threshold of its excitation and then a train stimulus of 50 CPs for one second was given. Response of stimulation was observed visually and was registered on EMG machine. The procedure was performed on all the rootlets of each posterior root from Lumbar 2 to sacral 2 on either side. Rootlets which were showing hyperactive response were sectioned. Phasic, sustained, incremental and spread of stimulus were considered as hyperactive responses responsible for carrying the impulses to generate spasticity. Four months later one patient had to undergot T_{11}-L_1 limited laminectomy and T_{11}-L_1 bilateral SPR with the idea to reduce residual spasms and spasticity by reducing the diffusion from above. The patient showed definite reduction in spasms and spasticity involving the lower limbs. The same patient 6 months later underwent bilateral Hamstring release. Later developed bladder calculi which were removed by cystolithotomy.

RESULTS: Spasticity has subsided completely in all the cases. There is almost total relief in spasms in 2 cases some disability is occuring in one case and in 2 cases, the spasms are quite disabling in performing motor functions. Both of them have shown significant reduction in spasms with Baclofen therapy. Three cases have almost total relief in discomfort, agony and pain. Two patients still have some discomfort. In all the cases nursing and handling have improved, rehabilitative therapy has become easier and energy consumption during the motor activities have also reduced significan tly. SPR has also helped them in preventing the further worsening of complications of spasticity like development of contractures etc.

Following 6 months of SPR one patient started walking for short distances with the help of crutches, 4 cases started bottom shuffling and all could be put into a comfortable wheel chair sitting. Preoperatively one patient had persistent 3 tier supine position and 3 had this sort of posture intermittently. In this posture thighs used to touch the chest and legs used to get flexed at knees. Postoperatively allof them are able to lie straight in supine position.

Prior to SPR only two patients could sit hanging the legs on the sides of cot with considerable difficulty. But following SPR all the patients could sit in this position with great ease.

Three cases had urgency incontinence and prior to surgery itself were put on indwelling catheter drainage. There was reduction in urgency in 3 patients, one is on indwelling catheter, and another one is on intermittent catheter drainage. The one severe head injury case who has very poor higher motor functions is intermittently automatically passing the urine. One patient who had severe urgency incontinence developed retention of urine and is on intermittent catheterization, an another patient has slight urgency which is persisting post-operatively. Our patients have preferred the intermittent catheterization according to socially acceptable timings compared to urgency incontinence. There was minimal worsening of sensations in lower limbs in all the cases. One patient developed vesical stone one year following SPR and the same patient developed plaster sore which was applied for 3 months after 1 1/2 years of SPR. This has completely healed in 3 weeks time.

All the cases are still showing improvement in their motor functions. It would take a few years before final results could be established.

DISCUSSION: Lumbosacral Selective Posterior Rhizotomy (SPR) is a functional neurosurgical procedure which has been designed to relieve spasticity. Till date around 1000 spastic cerebral palsied cases have undergone this operation all over the globe and well established results of the procedure have been published. But firm indications of this procedure for non cerebral palsied cases have not been established. We have operated 5 cases and have followed them for sufficient period of time.

We have taken following main criteria for selection of cases for SPR.

1. Non-progressive spasticity: The clinical picture should have been stable for atleast 6 months and the primary disease should have been cured.

2. Presence of painful agonizing disabling spasticity: The spasticity should be severe enough to be responsible for pain, agony and should be disabling him to perform motor functions.

3. Resistant spasticity: The patient should have undergone physiotherapy and should have taken pharmacotherapy to claim that there is no significant relief in his symptoms.

The following are the goals of the surgery:

1. Complete relief in spasticity and maximum possible relief in spasms so as to provide comfortable resting hours and sleep.

2. To provide comfortable wheel chair sitting and further management

3. To facilitate rehabilitation therapy for all motor activities of a) daily routine activities; b) pertaining to suitable job.

4. Walking with or without device.
5. Prevention of complications of spasticity like contractures etc.

<u>The following are the relative contra-indications:</u>

* Presence of severe frequent spasms with only minimal or no spasticity.
* Fixed lumbosacral spinal pathologies like kyphoscoliosis.
* Multiple severe contractures and myositis ossificans.
* Unstable spine:
a) Extensive damage of **the** lower thoracic spine by the primary disease or
b) Presence of multiple level laminectomies of the lower thoracic spine.

We feel that following factors play a major role in the ultimate poor motor outcome of these patients:
1. Underlying poor muscle power
2. Presence of severe spasms
3. Presence of spastic bladder symptoms.
4. Major sensory loss.
5. Presence of contractures, deformities etc.

It is mandatory to explain the goals of surgery in detail to the patient and his or her relatives prior to the surgery.

References :
1. Peacock WJ, Arens LJ, Berman B (1987) Cerebral Palsy spasticity, Selective posterior rhizotomy, Pediatr Neurosci 13: 61-66.
2. Fasano VA, Broggi G (1989) Functional Posterior Rhizotomy State of the Art Reviews, Vol 4, No.2, 409-412.
3. Laitinen LB, Nilsson S, Fugl-Meyer AR (1983) Selective Posterior Rhizotomy for treatment of spasticity J.Neurosurg 58: 895-899.

Role of Birth Injury in Syringomyelia

TOSHIAKI ABE, NORIO NAKAMURA, KOICHI TASHIBU, HISASHI ONOUE, and HIROYASU NAGASHIMA

Department of Neurosurgery, The Jikei University School of Medicine, Minato-ku, Tokyo, 105 Japan

SUMMARY

The role of birth injury was evaluated in different pathological types of syringomyelia by assessing the history of 74 patients with syringomelia. According to the intraoperative findings and magnetic resonance imaging (MRI), these syringomyelias were classified into three types; type 1; hindbrain-related syringomyelia without basal arachnoiditis (52 cases), type 2; hindbrain-related syringomyelia with basal arachnoiditis (10 cases), type 3; primary spinal syringomyelia (12 cases). As the results, 41% of patients, in type 1 had a history of difficult labor and 7 of them was due to breech delivery. In type 2, all patients with idiopathic basal arachnoiditis had a history of difficult labor and a half of them was due to breech delivery. The disturbance of cerebro-spinal fluid (CSF) circulation around the craniovertebral junction is the most important factor in the pathogenesis of hindbrain-related syringomyelia. A difficult labor may aggravate the disturbance of CSF circulation by further impaction of the cerebella tonsils due to an excessive moulding of the foetal head and/or traumatic subarachnoid hemorrhage (SAH) produced basal arachnoiditis.

KEY WORDS; birth injury, syringomyelia, basal arachnoiditis, Chiari malformation

INTRODUCTION

A difficult labor has been suggested to be a factor in the pathogenesis of syringomyelia.[1][2] However, pathological findings related evaluation has not been done. And also it has not been discussed that either increased intracranial pressure during the difficult labor or SAH due to birth injury is mainly related with pathogenesis of syringomyelia.

So we evaluated the role of birth injury in different types of syringomyelia.

MATERIALS AND METHODS

FROM 1982 TO 1992, 74 patients with syringomyelia documented by MRI

436

were evaluated. The obstetric history of these patients was obtained by direct interview or by postal questionnaire.

Table 1   classification of syringomyeliain in 74 cases

Type 1 :	Hindbrain-related syringomyelia without basal arachnoiditis	52
	(with Chiari malformation 51)	
	(with occlusion of F. Magendie 1)	
Type 2 :	Hindbrain-related syringomyelia with basal arachnoiditis	10
	(idiopathic arachnoiditis 8)	
	with Chiari malformation 6	
	(post meningitic arachnoiditis 2)	
Type 3 :	Primary spinal syringomyelia	12
	(with spinal arachnoiditis 9)	
	(with spinal cord tumor 3)	

According to MRI and intraoperative findings, these cases were classified into following three types, type 1: hindbrain-related syringomyelia without basal arachnoiditis (52 cases), type 2: hindbrain-related syringomyelia with basal arachnoiditis (10 cases), type 3: primary spinal syringomyelia (12 cases).

In type 1, 51 of 52 cases had a Chiari malformation. The character-istic feature of MRI in type 1 revealed that the herniated tonsils were wedge-shaped and occupied the cisterna magna, the rostra end of the intraspinal syrinx was pencil-shaped and the caudal part of the fourth ventricle was obliterated (Fig 1). These findings suggested that the herniated tonsils produced significant pressure against the lower brain stem and the upper cervical cord, and the disturbance of cerebro-spinal

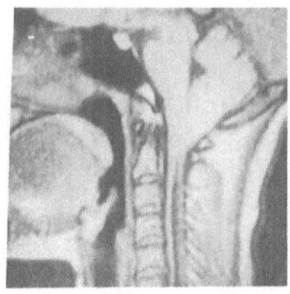

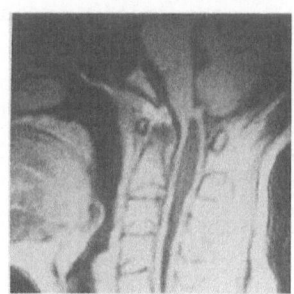

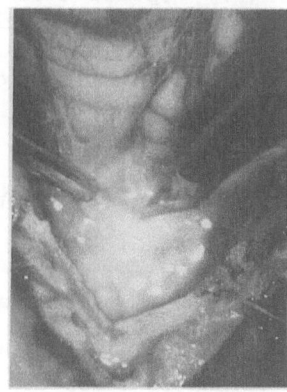

Fig.1 MRI in hindbrain-related syringomyelia without basal arach-noiditis (type 1)

Fig.2 MRI in hindbrain-related syringomyelia with basal arach-noiditis (type 2)

Fig.3 Intraoperative findings of type 2 syringomyelia

fluid (CSF) circulation at the foremen magnum by impacted into it. Intraoperative findings showed that the arachnoid membrane overlaying the herniated tonsils was normal and the foramen Magendie was patent, and also the central canal seemed to be opened at the obex.

In type 2, two of 10 cases had a past history of bacterial meningitis and tuberculous meningitis respectively, and both cases were unassociated with Chiari malformation. Other 8 cases were associated with so called idiopathic basal arachnoiditis, among them 6 cases were associated with Chiari malformation. The characteristic feature of MRI in these 6 cases revealed that the tip of the herniated tonsils was round in shape, and a triangular space was

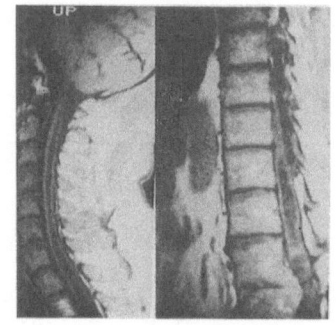

Fig.4 MIR in primary spinal syringomyelia (type 3)

identified between the herniated tonsils and the upper spinal cord. In addition, the rostral end of the intraspinal syrinx was round in shape and the caudal part of the fourth ventricle was well visualized (Fig 2). These findings revealed that the herniated tonsils produced less pressure against the brain stem and the spinal cord than that of type 1. Because the main cause of CSF circulatory disturbance was thought to be a basal arachnoiditis around the foremen magnum in type 2 instead of impacted tonsils in type 1.

Intraoperative findings showed that the triangular space between the herniated tonsils and the upper cervical cord in MRI was filled with thick adhesive arachnoid membrane which occluded the foremen Magendie (Fig 3). In addition, the central canal was not opened at the obex in our all cases of type 2.

In type 3, each case had a past history of minigitis, spinal cord injury, spinal cord surgery, SAH, or vascular accident, and no cases were associated with Chiari malformation. MRI revealed adhesions of arachnoid membrane around the spinal cord or intraspinal cord tumor in association with normal cranio-vertebral junction. Intraoperative findings confirmed spinal arachnoiditis or tumor.

RESULTS AND DISCUSSION

Forty-one of 52 patients with type 1 and all patients with type 2 and 3, knew correct data about their birth by direct information from their parents or other members of their family. Seventeen of 41 type 1 patients with Chiari malformation, 8 of 8 type 2 patients with idiopathic basal arachnoiditis, none of 2 type 2 patients with post meningitic basal arachnoiditis and none of 12 type 3 patients underwent a difficult labor-in 7 cases of type 1 and in 4 cases of type 2 having a history of breech delivery.

Table 2 Birth injury and syringomyelia: results

Type 1 :	Difficult labor (Breech delivery 7)	17/41	(41%)
Type 2 :	Difficult labor (Breech delivery 4)	8/8	(100%) in idiopathic cases
	Difficult labor	0/2	(0%) in postmeningitic cases
Type 3 :	difficult labor	0/12	(0%)

All 8 patients with an idiopathic basal arachnoiditis and syringomyelia had a history of difficult labor. It suggested that SAH due to a traumatic birth was probably responsible for the basal arachnoiditis. Forty-one percent of the type 1 patients who had no basal arachnoiditis, had a history of difficult labor and all of them were associated with Chiari type 1 malformation. However, Newman[3] reported no increase in traumatic birth in patients with the Chiari malformation but no syringomyelia.

These fact suggested that if the labor of patients who had the Chari anomaly from faulty embryogenesis, is traumatic, then a combination of prolonged and forceful exclusive pressures in an obstructed birth canal and excessive moulding of the foetal head or squeezing the foetal neck in case of breech delivery may be associated with impaired venous return from the head of the infant. These factors may cause further impaction of the cerebella tonsil. The disturbance of CSF flow around the craniovertebral junction is the most important factor in the pathogenesis of hindbrain related syringomyelia. A difficult labor may aggravate the CSF circulatory disturbance by further impaction of the cerebella tonsils and/or basal arachnoiditis due to the traumatic SAH.

REFERENCES

1. Williams B (1977) Difficult labor as a cause of communicating syringomyelia. Lancet 2:51-53
2. Vaquero J, Santos H, Martinez R (1985) Traumatic birth and syringomyelia. Neurology 35:137-138
3. Newman PK, Terenty TR, Foster JB (1981) Some observations on the pathogenesis of syringomyelia. J Neurol Neurosurg Psychiatry 44:964-969

Effect of Methylpredonisolone on Spinal Cord Blood Flow After Spinal Cord Injury in Rats

HIROYUKI IMAMURA, YOSHINOBU IWASAKI, KAZUTOSHI HIDA, and HIROSHI ABE
Department of Neurosurgery, Hokkaido University School of Medicine, Kita-ku, Sapporo, 060 Japan

SUMMARY

The effect of methylpredonisolone (MP) on spinal cord blood flow (SCBF) was investigated after spinal cord clipping injury in rats. The injury was produced at T7/8 level by clipping force of 140g for 3 seconds, which resulted in transient paraplegia but 50% recovery of motor function in 3 weeks after injury. MP or saline was injected at 30 minutes after ninjury, and SCBF was measured by 14C-iodoantipyrine autoradiography at 2 hours after injury.
In the normal control group, in which only laminectomy was performed at T7,8 level, SCBF of gray matter and white matter were 96.0±3.3 ml/100g/min and 22.9±4.1 ml/100g/min, respectively. In the injury groups, SCBF were mostly decreased at the injury level and preserved with distance from that level. SCBF of MP 30mg/kg group was not different from that of saline group in gray matter and white matter at the injury level. However, the decrease of SCBF in the white matter was observed at the rostral and caudal to the injury level in MP group more than in the saline group. We thought that in the acute phase, the effect of MP is the suppression of white matter SCBF at rostral and caudal to the injury level.

KEY WORDS: spinal cord blood flow, spinal cord injury, methylpredonisolone, autoradiography

INTRODUCTION

It is said that the symptom of spinal cord injury is progressd by the spinal cord ischemia secondary to primary damage. And recently some studies have reported lipid peroxidation takes part in this progression[1]. National Acute Spinal Cord Injury Study II (NASCIS II) reported that after six months the patients who were treated with megadose methylpredonisolone (MP) within eight hours of their injury had significant improvement as compaired with those given placebo in motor function and sensation[2]. And experimentally spinal cord blood flow (SCBF) at the injury level was preserved in MP group more than in the control group[3]. But the effect for the rostral and caudal area has not been studied yet. This study reports the change of SCBF at the rostral and caudal to the injury level and the effect of MP by means of 14C-iodoantipyrine (IAP) autoradiogrphy technique.

MATERIALS AND METHODS

Seventeen female Wister rats weighning 215-330g were used. The animal
was anesthetized with the inducing diethyleter and then aspiration of
1.5% Halothane , and a catheter was inserted into the femoral artery
for continuous recording of the mean arterial blood pressure and for
blood sampling, and into the femoral vein for infusion of MP or saline
and isotope. A dorsal laminectomy was performed at the Th 7-8 level
under microscopic guidance, leaving the dura intact. And then epidural
clipping injury at Th7/8 level was made by 140g clipping force for 3
seconds.　After removal of the clip the muscle and skin were closed
and the animal was placed on the heating mat and allowed to wake
up.This injury made a complete paraplegia just after injury, but
recovered 50% motor function at 3 weeks after injury by the assesment
of the inclined plane method as descrived preveously by Rivlin and
Tator[4].(Fig.1)
Experimental groups were devided to four groups. Normal SCBF was
assesed in five animals at the T7/8 level and at every 1mm rostral and
caudal to that level. Four animals were injected 1ml saline at 30
minutes after injury and 2 hours after injury SCBF was measured at the
injury level and at every 1mm rostral and caudal to that level as far
as 5mm. One ml of 30 or 60 mg/kg MP was injected to every four animals
and SCBF was measured at the same levels as saline group.
Tow hours after injury, animals received 75 μCi/kg of 14C-IAP in 2.5
ml saline over a 60-second interval. Arterial blood was sampled from
the femoral artery every 5 seconds during the isotope injection. At
the end of the 1-minute isotope injection, animals were sacrificed and
spinal cords were removed. Sections were   then cut at 20 μm in the
cryostat at -20 °C. They were placed on microscope slides and dried on
a hot plate at 60°C. Slides were placed with a standard on a Kodak SB-
5 X ray film for 1 week. Following the development of the film, the
densities were determined by means of quantitive autoradiography
system MCID (Imaging Research Cooporation, Canada). SCBF calculation
was according to the Sakurada's method[5],in which partition
coefficient of 0.8 was used in the present study. In addition, frozen
20 μm sections were taken from each segment and stained with
hematoxylin and eosin.

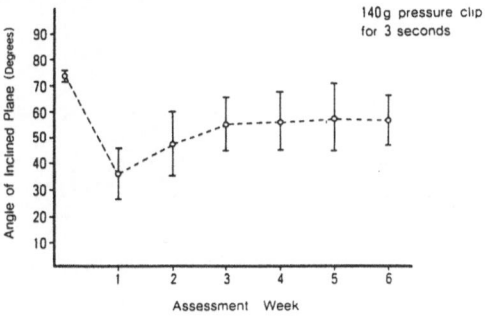

Fig.1 The average maximum angles attained by rats subjected to injury

RESULTS

Mean arterial blood pressure just before isotope injection was

441

102.5±2.2 mmHg. Arterial blood gases were as follows:
Pao2,138.9±14.6;Paco2,37.1±0.9;and pH,7.415±0.022. Hematocrit was
42.9±1.1% and body temperature was 36.8±0.1 °C.
Normal SCBF of gray matter and white matter were 96.0±3.3 and 22.9±4.1
ml/100g/min, respectively.

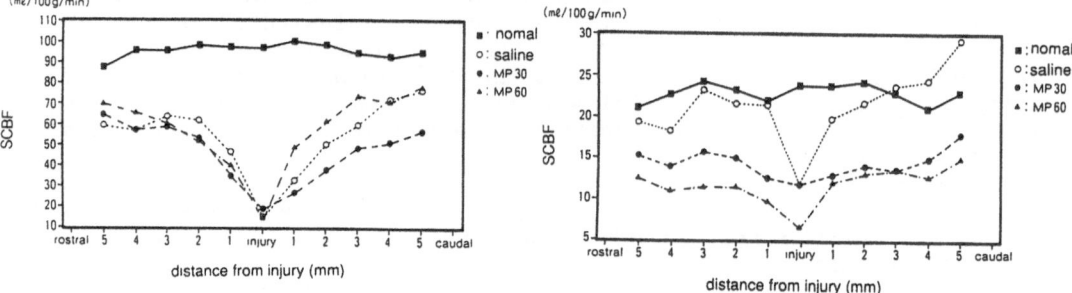

Fig.2 SCBF(gray matter)   Fig.3 SCBF(white matter)

a   b

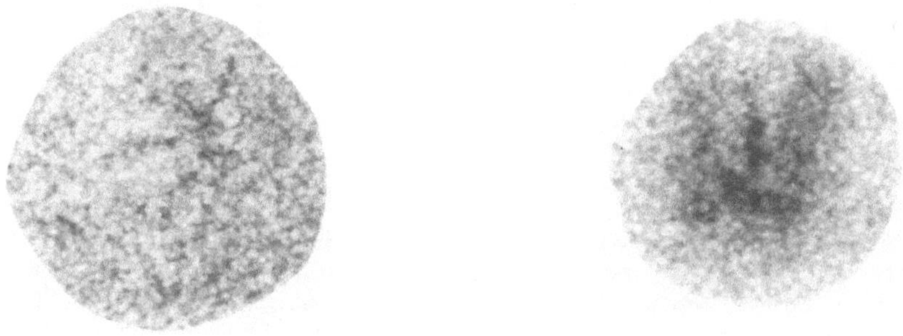

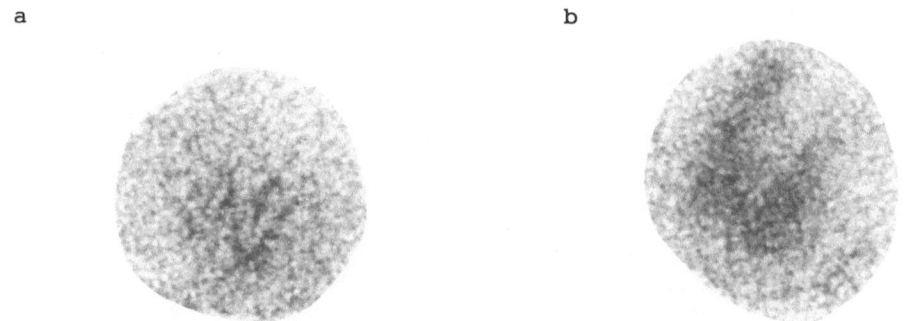

Fig.4 Autoradiography of saline group a:injury level
      b:5mm rostral to injury level

a   b

Fig.5 Autoradiography of MP 30mg/kg group a:injury level
      b:5mm rostral to the injury level

In the injury groups, SCBF were mostly decreasd at the injury level
and preserved with distance from that level. SCBF of MP 30mg/kg or

60mg/kg group was not different from that of saline group in the gray matter. And also in the white matter SCBF of MP group was not different from saline group at the injury level. However, the decrease of SCBF in the white matter was observed at the rostral and caudal to the injury level in MP group more than in the saline group. And in the saline group increase of SCBF was obsereved at more than 3mm caudal to the injury level.(Fig.2,3,4,5)

Pathologically gray and white matter were destroyed at the injury level and at 5mm from that level neurons were preserved in the gray matter and mild edema was found in the white matter. Those findings were not so different in the saline and MP groups.

DISCUSSION

Steroid therapy after spinal cord injury was used from yeras ago, but the effect of it was not always definite. However NASCIS II reported the clinical effect of megadose therapy of MP[2]. Experimentally it is reported lipid peroxidation would be supressed [6] or SCBF of dorsolateral white matter would be preserved at the injured level [3] by 30mg/kg of MP not by 60 mg/kg. In our study there was no difference of SCBF in the gray matter between saline group and MP group at the injury level. And also in the white matter there was no difference between saline group and MP 30mg/kg group, though there was decrease in MP 60mg/kg group. Consequently there was no effect for SCBF by MP at the injury level. SCBF was preserved with distance from injury level. We could not find the difference between the saline group and MP groups about SCBF in the gray matter. In the white matter SCBF was decreased from rostral to caudal of the injury level in MP groups but in the saline group SCBF was not so decreased and at the point of 3 to 5mm caudal of the injury level SCBF were increasd more than normal control group. We thought that at 2 hours after injury SCBF of the white matter was preserved or white matter was hyperemic around the injury level,and the secondary damage would progressed in that condition. Maybe megadose of MP would protect this phenomenon.

CONCLUSION

Effect of megadose therapy of MP was thought to suppress the SCBF of the white matter around the injury level at 2 hours after injury and to protect the secondary damage which was produced by hyperemia or such conditions.

REFFERENCES

1.Hall ED, Braughler JM, McCall JM (1988) J Neurotrauma 5:81-89
2.Bracken MB, Shepard MJ, Collins WF, Holford TR, Young W, Baskin DS, et al (1990) N Engl J Med 322:1405-1411
3.Hall ED, Wolf DL, Braughler JM (1984) J Neurosurg 61:124-130
4.Rivlin AS, Tator CH (1977) J Neurosurg 47:577-581
5.Sakurada O, Kennedy C, Jehle J, Brown JD, Carbin GL,Sokoloff L (1978)   Am J Physiol 234(1):H59-H66
6.Hall ED, Braughler JM (1982) J Neurosurg 57:247-253

14—Epidemiology, Miscellaneous

III Epidemiology, Mechanisms

Neurotraumatology in West Africa – Burkina Faso's Experience

A. Bou-Salah[1], J. Ilboudo[2], R.M. Ouiminga[2], and J. Richard[2]

[1]Department of Neurosurgery BP.23 98 Ouagadougou Burkinia Faso and [2]Department of Surgery, Hospital Yalgado Ouedraogo Ouagadougou BKF

Summary : Neurotraumatology in Burkina Faso started only two years ago. After two years of activities, the authors describe the situation in developing countries having other priorities. The authors attempt to pinpoint problems particularly in neurosurgery and to propose solutions adopted to their specific conditions.

Burkina Faso, a former French colony, is situated in the Sahel area in West-Africa, covering an area of 274,200 km2. The country became independent in 1960 and has a population of approximately 8 million inhabitants. There are two main cities: Ouagadougou, the capital: 800,000 inhabitants, Bobo Dioulasso: 400,000 inhabitants, both cities having general hospitals.

However, neurosurgery in Burkina Faso only started two years ago in Ouagadougou. During these last two years we have received 2,200 head traumas and about 200 spinal traumas. These patients have been coming from all over the country and even from surrounding nations. Some patients come from neighbouring countries where there is no practice of neurosurgery.

What are our working conditions? and what conclusions can be drawn from them? Yalgado OUEDRAOGO Hospital is equipped with 714 beds of which 182 are for surgery. The patients are followed by surgeons and anesthesiologists but their relatives take care of them 24 hours a day, including looking after them in the intensive care unit.

Because of the reduced number of the staff (nurses, paramedical personnel), this formula is the most appropriate to the situation since the population of the Country have kept alive the traditional solidarity relations in the family.

Before 1990, there was no practice of neurosurgery, and this activity was included in other surgical specialities. The Department of General Surgery: 2,955 surgical operations have been carried out by the 12 surgeons (including 3 foreigners). 9,178 patients suffering from trauma were admitted in emergency. Among these, 2,000 suffered from a central nervous system trauma with head injuries and spinal cord injuries. The causes of head or spinal trauma are different from those caused in the developed countries.

Here, most of road accidents are caused by "two-wheel drivers", cyclists or motor-cyclists. Cases of assaults, work accidents (by agricultural workers), falls from trees such as the baobab tree, karitea (shea nut tree) and "papaya" or people falling in wells come next.
The problems we encountered when we arrived were related to:
1) The lack of neurosurgery tradition,
2) The lack of specialized training in neurology and neurosurgery. The students in medicine were taught by foreign specialists, during short periods of time. There was no practical training.
3) The lack of a specialized unit.
4) Lastly, the lack of specialized means for diagnosis or therapy.
We started from the following principle; "If the mortality and morbidity caused by head and spine injuries are to be reduced, it is essential that all physicians understand the physiopathologic aspects of head or spinal cord trauma, and the appropriate treatment of injuries of the scalp, skull, brain and medulla".
The results achieved have eventually convinced the students, and the para-medical staff and our colleagues from other specialities as well.
Our two year-work in Burkina has led us to draw some conclusions which I submit to your attention:

1) Neurosurgery and especially neurotraumatology is a necessity in the least developed countries.
2) But neurosurgery is very expensive.
3) That is why it would be unrealistic to try to train people to practice this speciality as they do in developed countries.
4) We must find the means:
   - to help physicians become more familiar with the pathology, and mainly the traumatology of the brain and the medulla.
   - to initiate programs that address this objective, taking into account, the specificities of each country.
   - to postpone the training of neurosurgeons according to classic scheme.
5) Though it seems difficult for the least developed countries to contemplate a national coverage of neurotraumatology because of their economic predicament, I believe it is essential that at least one or two units be set up, otherwise, thousands of patients will be left to deal with their sad lot on their own.

This is why I completely agree with the great initiative taken by our Subcommittee on Education in Neurotrauma concerning the organization of regional courses and seminars in developing countries.

Epidemiological Aspect of Chronic Subdural Haematoma

KEIICHI KUWAMURA[1], HIROSHI KUDOH[1], HIROSHI TOMITA[1], ICHIRO IZAWA[2], and NORIHIKO TAMAKI[2]

[1]Department of Neurosurgery, Hyogo Prefectural Awaji Hospital, Sumoto, Hyogo, 656 Japan and [2]Department of Neurosurgery, Kobe University, School of Medicine, Kobe, Hyogo, 650 Japan

SUMMARY

The epidemiological study for chronic subdural haematoma (CSH) in the elderly over 65 years old, was done in Awaji Island having about 170,000 inhabitants. Since the Island is surrounded by inland-sea and our department is the only one neurosurgical service, we could make the statistical analysis for occurences of CSH.
The overall incidence of CSH was 13.1 per 100,000/year, 3.4 in people under 65 year old, and 58.1 in the elderly. The elderly over 65 years old in Awaji Island in 17.7% of all inhabitants at the time of this study.
If these incidences of CSH are extrapolated to all of Japan in the year 2020 when the elderly over 65 years old will acount 23.6% of whole population, incidence will be 16.3 per 100,000/year. This analysis suggests that CSH may become the most popular neurosurgical disease in near future.

KEY WORDS: chronic subdural haematoma, epidemiology, elderly people

INTRODUCTION

Chronic subdural hematoma (CSH) occurs especially frequently among old people[1,3]. The number of old people is increasing steadily in Japan. A Ministry of Health and Welfare Survey found that the elderly who are 65 years old or elder accounted for 11.2% of all people in 1988[2]. In 2020, the population of Japan will be 135,304,000, of which 23.6% will be the elderly[2]. Awaji Island in Hyogo prefecture presently has a population of 168,000, of which 17.7% is the elderly. We investigated the present incidence of CSH on Awaji Island and discuss the epidemiological problems.

MATERIALS AND METHODS

Sixty-six patients (54 males and 12 females) with CSH were admitted to our institute from January, 1986 through December, 1988. Fifty-two patients (43 males and 9 females) were the elderly. The incidences of CSH in the towns and city on Awaji Island were calculated to assess the epidemiological trends.

RESULTS AND DISCUSSION

Awaji Island consists of one city (Sumoto) and ten towns. The incidence of CSH per 100,000/year in the elderly ranged from 8.6 to 153.5, with a mean of 58.1. Figure 1 shows that some areas (the towns of Goshiki and Ichinomiya: white) had high incidences, while

dotted area (the towns of Awaji, Hokutan, Higashiura, Seitan, and
Nantan) had low incidences. Fourteen patients under 65 years old
were treated for CSH at our hospital. The incidence of CSH patients
under 65 years old was a mean of 3.4 per 100,000/year. The total
incidence of CSH was a mean of 13.1 ranging from 4.0 to 36.1 per
100,000/year (Fig. 2). The mean was 13.6 in the dashed area (the
towns of Tsuna, Midori, and Mihara, and Sumoto city) and 34.0 in the
white areas. The elderly were 33-100% (mean, 79%) of all cases.
The population contains 21.4% elderly in the white areas and 15.8%
in the dashed areas.
The epidemiological trends can be assessed, if the incidences of
CSH on Awaji Island are applied to Japan until the year 2020. The
incidence of CSH in the elderly as a part of the total population
will be: 58.1 x 23.6/100 = 13.7 per 100,000/year. The incidence of
CSH in people under 65 years old in the total population will be:
3.4 x 76.4/100 = 2.6 per 100,000/year. Therefore, the total incidence of CSH will be 16.3 (= 13.7 + 2.6) per 100,000/year in Japan
in 2020.

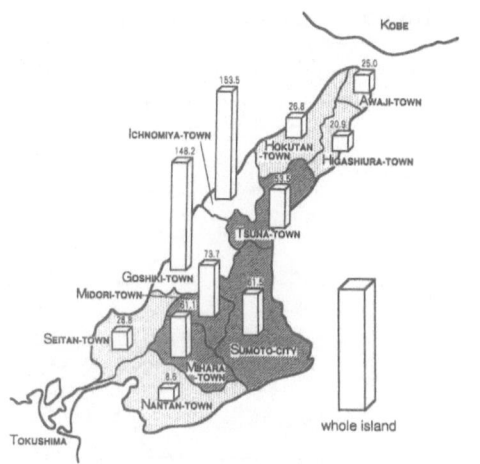

Fig. 1 Incidences of CSH in the
elderly who are 65 years old or
elder on Awaji Island (/100,000
people/yr).

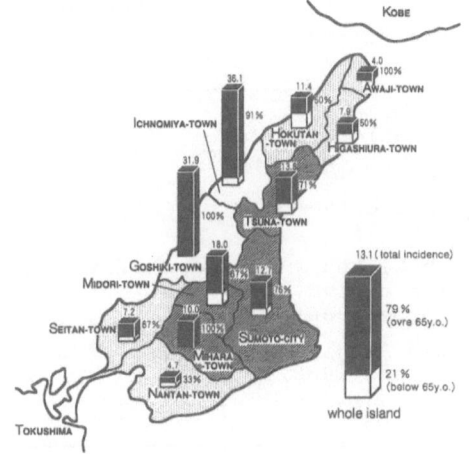

Fig. 2 Incidences of CSH in
total population on Awaji
Island (/100,000 people/yr).
Over 65 y.o. includes 65
years old.

The epidemiological study of Awaji Island shows that the incidence of
CSH was lower in the dotted areas, compared with other areas.
Although our neurosurgical service covers the whole island, people
in these areas facing Kobe or Tokushima areas, may consult with other
clinics in these areas, because of easy access. People in the white
and dashed areas are more likely, therefore, to form a representative
sample. The white areas had a much higher incidence of CSH in the
elderly than the dashed areas. Two reasons may be considered: age
distribution and environment. The elderly are 15.8% of all inhabitants in the dashed areas, but 21.4% in the white areas. Furthermore, the white areas are mountainous and the dashed areas flat
plains. People in the white areas, therefore, have more opportunities
for accidents than people in the dashed areas.
Very few papers discuss the incidences of CSH (Fig. 3). Fogelholm
et al[1] reported 1.72 per 100,000/year in all people and 7.4 per

100,000/year in people over 70 years old in Helsinki. Weber[3] reported 1 or 2 per 100,000/year in all people in Switzerland in 1968. The incidences in our series are much higher than in the Helsinki and Switzerland series. The mean incidences for the whole island were 13.1 per 100,000/year in all people, 3.4 per 100,000/year in people under 65 years old, and 58.1 per 100,000/year in the elderly. At present, the elderly are 17.7% of the entire population of Awaji Island.

In Japan, the elderly will account for 23.6% of the population in 2020[2]. If the incidence of CSH on Awaji Island can be extrapolated to Japan in 2020, the incidence of CSH in the elderly will be approximately 13.7 per 100,000/year and the total incidence will be 16.3 per 100,000/year. However, these figures may not be accurate, because the dotted areas are included in these calculations. If the dotted areas are excluded, the incidence of CSH will be much higher. However, the approximate data indicate that CSH will become more frequent and may be the most common neurosurgical condition.

Place (Year)	Ratio of the elderly ($\geq$65y.o.) (%)	Incidence (/100,000 people/yr)		
		<65y.o.	$\geq$65y.o.	All people
Switzerland (1968)[3]	-	-	-	1 or 2
Helsinki(1975)[1]	-	-	7.4#	1.72
Sumoto city (1988)*	15.8**	3.6	61.5	12.7
Goshiki and Ichinomiya towns(1988)*	21.4	2.1	150.8	34.0
Whole Awaji Island(1988)*	17.7	3.4	58.1	13.1
Japan (2020)[2]	23.6	(3.4)	(58.1)	16.3*

*Present study. **Mean value in Sumoto city and Tsuna, Midori, and Mihara towns. #70-79 years old. y.o.: years old.

Fig. 3 Summary of incidences

REFERENCES

1. Fogelholm R, Heiskanen O, Waltimo O (1975) Chronic subdural hematoma in adults. Influence of patient's age on symptoms, signs, and thickness of hematoma. J Neurosurg 42:43-46
2. A Ministry of Health and Welfare in Japan (1989) Kokumin Eisei No Doukou (Jinkou Seitai), pp42-47 (in Japanese)
3. Weber G (1969) Das chronische Subduralhematom. Schweiz Med Wschr 99:1483-1488

Management in Multitraumatized Patients with Head and Spine Injuries

R. KALFF, J. POSPIECH, U. OBERTACKE[1], and B. HOFFMANN

Department of Neurosurgery and [1]Traumatology, Medical Center, University of Essen, Germany

SUMMARY

The management of polytraumatized patients makes great demands on the medical staff as well as on its technical or organizing qualification.From the neurosurgical point of view head and spine injuries might be problematic considering the time of treatment.Especially in unconcious patients there is a relatively high frequency of 6-39 % with accompaniing spine injuries.A severe head injury you can see in 50-72 % of multiinjured patients.

We present our kind of management and the results of treatment regarding to the time of neurosurgical treatment in 986 multitraumatized patients between 1975 until 1990 .

In our opinion only rapid removal of epidural and subdural haematomas and reposition of dislocated spine fractures are necessary for neurosurgical treatment in the acute phase. All other injuries of the neurosurgical special field might be done with postponed priority.

KEY WORDS : polytrauma , head injury , spine injury

The management of multitraumatized patients makes great demands on the medical staff as well as on its technical or organizing qualification. In our opinion the following conditions are necessary for most favourable treatment of these seriously injured patients.

A *helicopter landing field* should be available in the hospital area.The most important central institution is the *emergency-room* , an operation-theatre for primary urgent treatment around the clock. A *specialist* , either a traumatologic surgeon or an anaesthetist, must lead and coordinate the further therapeutical and diagnostical steps responsibly. He may be supported, depending on the kind of injury, by heart-, ENT- or general surgeon as well as by neurosurgeon , maxillar surgeon or ophthalmologist. Nearby the emergency-room a *bloodbank* and *radiological unit* , inclusive computerized tomography and angiography , should be situated. After primary treatment transmission to an *intensive-care-unit* must be guaranted (Fig.1).

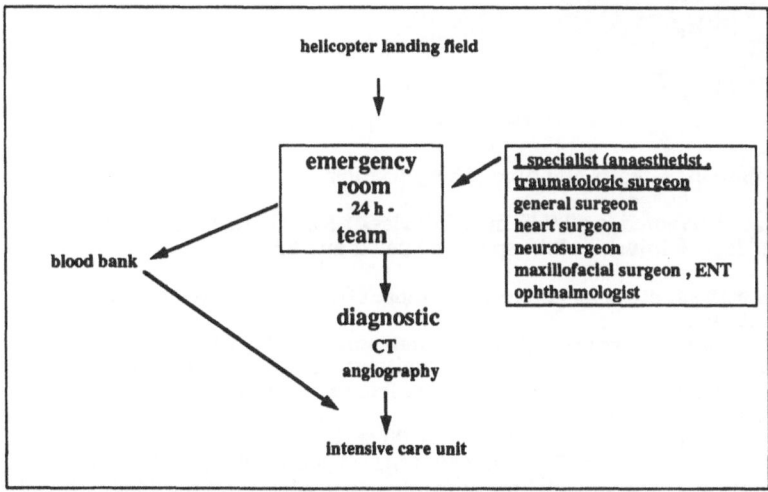

Fig. 1 Conditions for treatment of polytraumatized patients

From the neurosurgical point of view, head and spine injuries may be problematic in primary treatment of multitraumatized patients.

Especially you have to look on the large number, up to39 %, of accompanying cervical spine injuries in unconcious patients (6,13.17,21).Because of this, all these patients get a stiff-neck until neuroradiological examination is done.

Head injuries are basicly classified into *open* and *closed* ones. Protrusion of damaged brain points to a *penetrating , open head injury* , often associated with a lesion of an intracranial artery or venous sinus just as *oto- or rhinoliqourrhoea* . Also *intracranial air* in x-ray or computerized tomography shows a communication between the intradural space and outside.

In *closed head injuries* we must mention *generalized edema, contusions* with accompanying edema, an *impressed skull fracture* as well as *epidural hematomas* and *subdural hematomas* , mostly an enormous space occupying lesion , because of additional brain edema.

Retrobulbar hematomas , mostly in fronto-basal injuries , are extremely rare but need immmediate decompression to provide loss of vision.

Spine injuries must be classified into *stable* and *unstable spine fractures* .It is important to assess an exact *neurological examination* initially because further treatment depends on the evidence and / or progression of neurological deficits.We know that because of accompanying injuries it is often difficult to get a primary neurological status.

In multitraumatized patients you can notice a head injury in 50 - 85 % (2,6,13,16,17,20), in our clinic in 68 % of these patients, including 9,7 % epidural and 15,3 % subdural haematomas. Between 1975 and 1990 we treated 986 polytraumatized people with an average age of 36 years. 72 % were men and 28 % women.The average hospilization time was 16 days. The overall lethality was 19,4 %, in case of accompanying head injury 20,2 % (Fig.2).

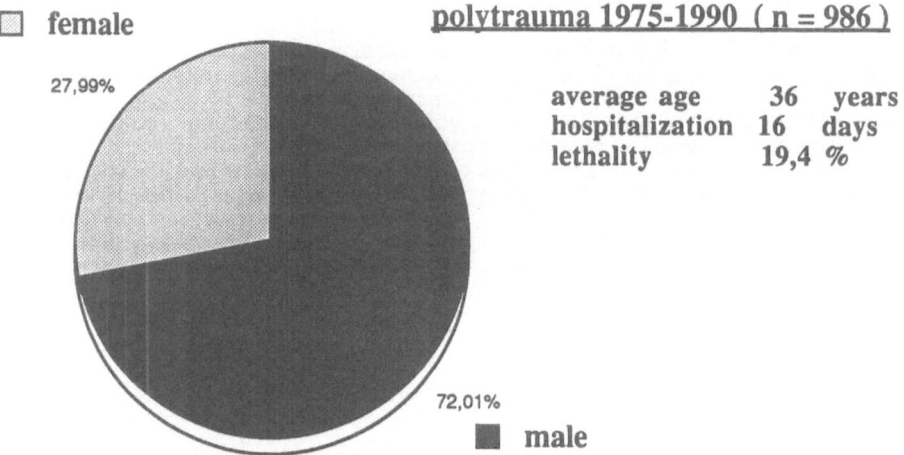

Fig. 2 Age and sex distribution , lethaliy and time of hospilization

The different lesions were distributed to 67,8 % head injuries,47,5 % thoracic-and 22,4 % abdominal lesions and in 36,9 % injuries of the spine and pelvis and 83,4 % of the extremities (Fig.3).

We noticed that patients with subdural hematomas had more often accompanying lesions than those with epidural hematomas.

Initial coma score and patient`s age are essential for the outcome after head injury.

The *Brussel `s coma score* has been established in our hospital to classify patients with head injuries.The *lethality-rate* rised with increasing coma score from 12-18 % in coma I, up to 30-49 % in coma II, and 40-62 % in coma III. Nearly nobody survives in coma IV (8,9,11,14,15). In patients older than 6o years of age the mortality is 64-100 %, in 30-60 years old patients 40-52 %; in 20-30 years old people 33-41 % and in children and young adults between15-33% (1,4,10,11,12,14).When have the before mentioned injuries to be treated from the neurosurgical point of view ?In our opinion the classification of polytrauma management into different phases of treatment has been established (22,23).

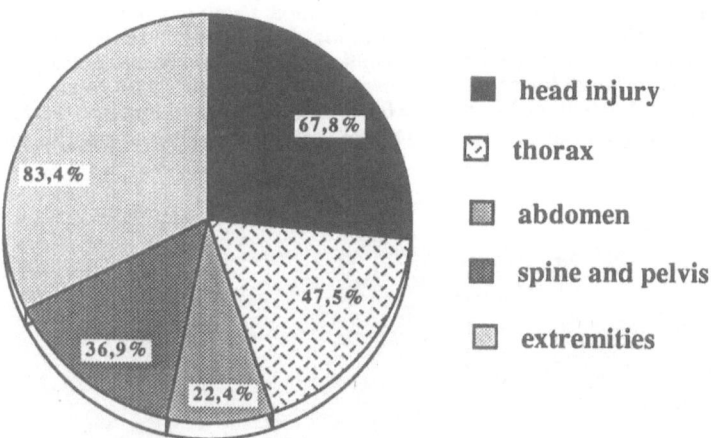

- ■ head injury
- ☑ thorax
- ▓ abdomen
- ■ spine and pelvis
- ▦ extremities

67,8%
83,4%
47,5%
36,9%
22,4%

Fig.3 Kind of lesion in polytraumatized patients

In the **acute phase** (Fig.4) all massive bleedings into the thoracic or abdominal cavity must be treated with priority (7,22,23). Profuse bleeding out of nose or mouth can be stopped mostly by plugging . In this stage of treatment *radiological examinations* are limited to x-ray of the chest and cervical spine, inclusive the lower part , as well as sonography of the abdominal cavity. In suspicion of an intracranial mass lesion is suspected computerized tomography has to be done, too. An acute*epidural hematoma* has been also operated in this stage. Sometimes, if thoracic or abdominal bleeding is combined with an epidural hematoma, a simultaneous operation is necessary (3). Evacuation of *subdural hematomas* and operation of *penetration injuries* should be done rapidly too.The medical *therapy of brain edema* with elevated upper body , controlled hyperventilation and osmodiuresis has to be also started in this phase.If there are signs of progressive transverse section, *decompression of the spinal cord* must be done immediately. E.g. this can be achieved in case of dislocated cervical spine fracture by anatomical reduction with axial traction (7). The definitive stabilizing operation can be done later.

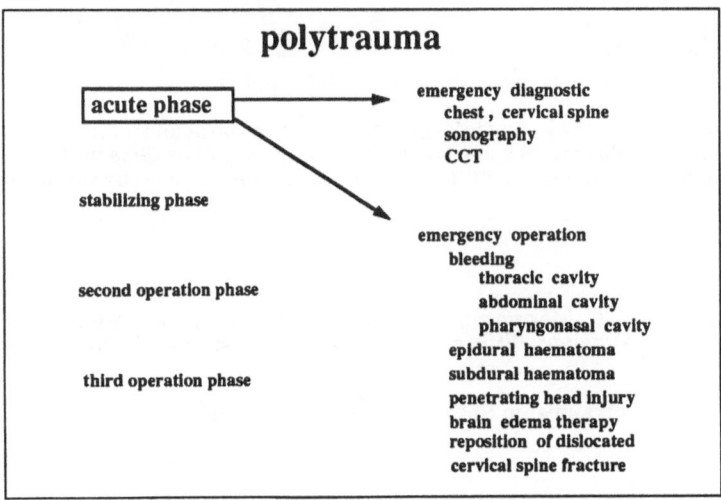

Fig.4 Neurosurgical operations in the acute phase after polytrauma

The place of further radiological examination should be in the stabilizing phase whereby only examinations of clinical interest should be done.

In the second operation phase all other operations are performed. From our point of view there are trepanations for evacuating *space occupying contusions*, elevation of a *skull impression fracture* above functional important brain areas as well as *optic nerve decompression* in case of a *retrobulbar hematoma* and *monitoring of intracranial pressure* to control osmotic therapy. In case of progressive neurological deficit reduced spine fractures now are stabilized (7,Fig.5)

If the neurological status is unchanged this is to be done in the third operation phase. In this stage also *covering of a liquor - fistula* has its place.

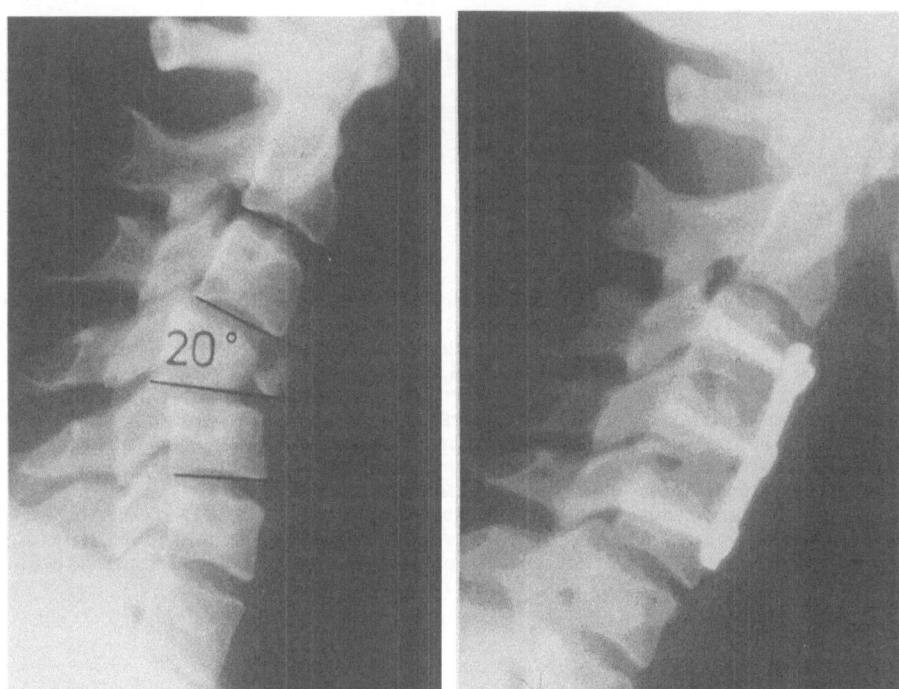

Fig.5 left: compression fracture of C4   right: anterior plate stabilization

From the neurosurgical point of view only immediate operation of an epidural and subdural hematoma as well as reposition of a dislocated spine fracture are necessary to be done in the primary phase in multitraumatized patients. All other neurosurgical injuries might be carried out with postponed priority.

REFERENCES

1. Alberico, A M, Ward, J D, Choi, S C, Marmarou, A,Young, H F(1987) Outcome after severe head injury.Relationship to mass loseions, diffuse injury, and ICP course in pediatric and adult patients.J Neurosurg 67: 648-656

2. Arnold, K (1985) Das Schädelhirntrauma im Rahmen der Mehrfachverletzung.Beitr. Orthop. Traumatol. 32:282-286

3. Bakay L(1983) Brain Injuries in Polytrauma.World J. Surg. 7:42-48

4. Berger, M S, Pitts, L H, Lovely, M,Edwards, M S B, Bartkowski, H M (1985) Outcome from severe head injury in children and adolescents.J Neurosurg 62:194-199

5. Brihaye J, Frowein, R A, Lindgren S, Loew, F, Stroobandt, G (1978) Report on the Meeting of the W.F.N.S .Neuro-Traumatology Committee, Brussels, 19-23 September 1976, Acta Neurochirurgica 40:181-186

6. Dittmer, H, Faist, E, Lauterjung, K L, Heberer, G (1983) Die Behandlung des Polytraumatisierten in einem Klinikum.Chirurg 54: 260-266

7. Frowein, R A, Reichmann, W, Terhaag, D, Rosenberger, J (1978) Die Schädel-Hirnverletzung beim Polytraumatisierten.Chirurg 49: 663-667

8. Frowein, R A, Schiltz, F, Firsching, R, Stammler, U (1982)Verlaufskontrolle und Prognose beim prolongierten Koma.In: Schädel-Hirn-Trauma, Herausgeber K H Bushe, Melsunger Med Mitteilung 103-109

9. Frowein, R A, Reichmann, W, Firsching, R (1985)Das Polytrauma aus neurochirurgischer Sicht In: Schürmann: Der cerebrale Notfall.Urban/Schwarzenberg-Verlag 58-63,

10. Heiden, J S, Small, R, Caton, W, Weiss, M H, Kurze, T H (1979) Severe Head Injury and Outcome: A Prospective Study.In: Neural Tauma, ed.: A J Popp et al. Raven Press, New York 181-193,

11. Kalff, R, Kocks, W, Pospiech, J, Grote (1989) Clinical outcome after head injury in children Child's Nerv Syst 5:156-159

12. Karimi-Nejad, A, Tritz, W (1984) Sequelae and Prognosis of Craniocerebral Trauma in Elderly People.Advances in Neurosurgery 12:212-215, Springer-Verlag Heidelberg

13. Kaukinen, L, Pasanen, M. Kaukinen, S (1984) Outcome and Risk Factors in Severely Traumatised Patients.Annales Chirurgiae et Gynaecologiae 73: 261-267

14. Kocks, W, Kalff, R, Pospiech J, Grote W (1989) Klinischer Verlauf bei Schädelhirntraumen in höherem Lebensalter Verhandlungen der Deutschen Gesellschaft für Neurologie5

15. Peters, R. Richard, K E, Frowein, R A (1989) PrognosticValue of Factors Affecting Outcome After Severe Head Injury.Advances in Neurosurgery 17:73-77 Springer-Verlag

16. Silva, J F (1984) Review of Patients with Multiple Injuries Treated at University Hospital, Kuala Lumpur.The Journal of Trauma 24:526-531

17. Sinclair, D, Schartz, M, Gruss, J, McLellan, B (1988) A Retrospective Review Of The Relationship Between Facial Fractures, Head Injuries, And Cervical Spine Injuries The Journal of Emergency Medicine 6:109-112

18. Sollmann, W P , Hussein, S. Stolke D (1985) Behandlungsergebnisse von schweren Schädel-Hirn-Traumen mit und ohne Dexamethasontherapie.Neurochirurgia 28:46-50

19. Schmit-Neuerburg, K P, Joka, T H (1985) Principles of treatment and indications for surgery in severe multiple trauma.Acta chir.belg. 85:239-249

20. Schwartz, M L (1983) Head Injury in Multiple Trauma.The Canadian Journal Of Surgery 26 (1) 23-36

21. Schwarz, R, Usbeck, W (1983) Luxationsfrakturen der Halswirbelsäule in Verbindung mit einem Schädelhirntrauma.3. Wissenschaftliche Tagung der Sektion Neurotraumatologie der Gesellschaft für Neurochirurgie der DDR, Berlin

22. Tscherne, H, Oestern, H.J. Sturm, J (1982) Operative Versorgung bei Schädel-Hirn-Trauma und Mehrfachverletzungen.Chirurgische Aspekte bei Verletzungen des Bewegungsapparates In: Schädel-Hirn-Trauma.Herausgeber: K H Bushe 54:61-69, Melsunger Med. Mitteilungen

23. Tscherne, H (1985) Das Polytrauma aus chirurgischer Sicht.In: Schürmann: Der cerebrale Notfall, 53-57 Urban und Schwarzenberg

Decline in Mortality Following Head Injury: Results of a Better Treatment on the Scene of Accident and of New Indication for CT Scanning

F. SERVADEI, M. GRILLI, G. CIUCCI, MT. NASI, G. VERGONI, and A. ARISTA

Division of Neurosurgery and Department of Neuroradiology Ospedale M. Bufalini Cesena and
EMS Helicopter Service/Division of Neurology Ospedale S.M. Croci Ravenna, Italy

SUMMARY

Two prospective epidemiological studies on head injury were conducted in our region in 1985 and in 1989; in the first period there were 370 admission following head inury/100000 pop./year and a mortality of 26 cases /100000 pop./year with 83% of patients dieing on the scene of accident or on admission to the first hospital.Since then, in 1986 we adopted a new protocol for management of head injury over the entire area (all patients asymptomatic but with a skull fracture were submitted to CT scanning);in 1987 an emergency medical service with helicopter was organized and in 1988 an ambulance with a Casualty doctor became available to treat trauma patients on the scene of accident.In 1989 the hospital admission rate decreased to 250 cases/100000 pop./year.The mortality was reduced to 18 cases /100000 pop./year with only 56% of prehospital mortality.In conclusion, as in other experiences,a significant reduction in head injury mortality was obtained with a better prehospital organisation of trauma care and with a more aggressive diagnostic approach to minor head injury

.
KEY WORDS
prehospital mortality-minor head injury-epidemiology-emergency medicalservice

INTRODUCTION

The availabilty of CT scanner in the eighties made it possible to extend the indication for this examination to a part of patients admitted in clinical conditions of minor head injury(9).
The result of these new protocols is a reduction of hospital admission following head trauma toghether with an increase of CT examinations in the patients admitted.In the same period (from 1985 to 1989) in our area we introduced an emergency medical service both with ambulance and helicopters. A prospective epidemiological study of head injury mortality was conducted in1985(8) and repeated in 1989 to see whether the improvement in diagnostic techniques and prehospital treatment had resulted in a decrease of mortality following head injuries in the area.

MATHERIAL AND METHODS

A well circumscribed region ,corresponding to the comune of Ravenna (172000 pop. in 1985,168000 pop. in 1989) was taken as the geographical area of the epidemiological study.All head injured patients in this area admitted to the hospital were prospectively

followed with a computer compatible form in the periods: from
1/4/84 to 31/3/85 and from 1/1/89 to 31/12/89.In the same periods
all patients who were dead either on arrival or on the scene of
accident were included in the study if autopsy showed head injury
as the principal cause of death.In the first period
(1984/1985)patients admitted in the clinical condition of a minor
head injury (9) were submitted to CT scanning only in the case of
clinical deterioration ;indication for hospital admission was
simple loss of consciussness ,even doubtful.In the second period
patients were submitted in adult age to CT scannig if skull x-ray
revealed a skull fracture, even in an asymptomatic
phase;furthermore hospital admission was regulated by a protocol
similar to that of british neurosurgeons (1)and simple loss of
conscioussness was not enough to warrant hospitalization.Other
improvements in the care of head injured patients occurred between
1984/85 and 1989:in 1987 an emergency medical service with
helicopters was established;in 1988 the system was improved: an
ambulance service with a casualty department doctor beacame
avilable for trauma care in connection with the helicopter
service.

RESULTS

Country	year	admission rate	mortality rate	authors
Norway	1974	236	12(69%)*	Netsvold (7)
USA	1978	208	25	Jagger (4)
USA(S.D)	1978	200	24(65%)*	Klauber (5)
USA(S.D.)	1982		17(60%)*	Klauber (6)
USA(N.Y)	1983	249	28(78%)*	Cooper (2)
ITALY(RA)	1985	372	24(83%)*	Servadei (8)
ITALY(RA)	1989	257	18(57%)*	this report

Table1:mortality rate and hospital admissions following head
injury per 100000 population per year of different prospective
epidemilogical studies in different countries;*percentage of
patients dead on arrival or on the scene of accident.
Concerning then the use of advanced emergency systems the
helicopter on scene of accidents was involved in a pure head
injury case in 16% of flights and in 41% of cases the head injry
was a part of a severe politrauma.In 1987 60% of flights were
interhospital transfer with only 40%of flights to the scene of
trauma.In 1989 the flights to the accident location increased up
to 82% of the total.We then reviewed 100 consecutive cases of
severe head trauma (initial GCS<8) assisted on the scene of
accident either by the helicopter team or by a doctor-ambulance.In
51 cases the patient was intubated and ventilated on the scene,in
26 there was only intubation and in 23 patients the oral airways
were protected.On arrival to the first regional Center only 4
cases were ipoxic and 5 were ipotensive.

DISCUSSION
The epidemiological study we published concerning our data of 1985
showed,in comparison with other countries, the high number of both
hospital admissions (372) and of deaths (24).Even more important
the excessive deaths on the scene of accident and on arrival
(83%,the highest on table 1).The institution of new protocols for
hospital admission and for minor head injury management produced a

reduction in hospital admission rate which became comparable with other studies(4,5,6,7).No adverse effect was seen on mortality which showed a similar decline.The reduction from 83% to 56% of prehospital mortality°can only be explained by the better care on the scene of accident.The study of the 100 consecutive cases of severe head injury treated in the prehospital phase show how infrequent were in these patients ipotension and ipoxia as compared with Gentleman series(4).We also found that an emergency medical service needs an advanced ground transportation to be used in cases of urban accidents, in case of bed wheather or in the cases of a trauma occurring in the night.As shown by Klauber with the reduction in mortality in San Diego from 23.8 to 17.5 (6), the possibilty to intubate and initiate the fluid therapy on the scene of accident decreases the influnce of secondary brain damage on outcome.Our experience conferms that a decline in mortality depends mainly on a better prehospital care and the assumption "a few patients could have been saved with better initial care"(3) is, in our experience,unjustified.

REFERENCES

1)BriggsM,Clarke P ,Crokard A.and the britsh neurosurgeons group:Guidelines for initial manegement after head injuries in adults. Br Med J 288:983-985,1988
2)Cooper DK,Tabbador KD,Harsner WA,Shulman K,Feiner C,Factor PR:The epidemiology of head injury in the Bronx.Neuroepidemiology 2:70-88,1983
3)Gentlemen G,Jennett B:Audit of transfer of unconscious head injured patients to a neurosurgical unit Lancet 335:330-334,1990
4)Jagger J,Levine JI,Jane JA,Rimel RW:Epidemiological features of head injury in a predominantly rural population J of Trauma 24:40-44,1984
5)Klauber MR,Marshall LF,Connor EB,Bowers SA:Prospective study of patients hospitalized with head injury in San Diego county,1978 Neurosurgery 9,3:236-241,1981
6)Klauber MR,Marshall LF,Toole BM,Knowlton SL,Bowers SA:Cause of decline in head injury mortality rate in San Diego County J Neurosurg 62:528-531,1985
7)Netswold K,Lundar T,Blirka G,Lonnum A:Head injuries during one year in acentral hospital in Norway: a prospective study Neuroepidemiology 7:134-144,1988
8)Servadei F,Ciucci G,Piazza G,BianchediG,Rebucci G,Gaist G,Taggi F:A prospective clinical and epidemiological study of head injuries in northern Italy:the comune of Ravenna Itl J Neurol Sci 9:499-457,1988
9)Servadei F,Ciucci G,Morichetti A,Pagano F,Burzi M,Staffa G,Taggi F:Skull fracture as a factor of increased risk in minor head injuries Surg Neurol 30:364-369,1988

Coagulation and Fibrinolysis in Head Injury: An Analysis with New Molecular Markers

S. Ayuzawa[1], A. Matsumura[1], I. Mitsui[2], S. Takeuchi[2], Y. Yoda[2], and T. Nose[1]

[1]Department of Neurosurgery, University of Tsukuba, Institute of Clinical Medicine, Tsukuba, Ibaraki, 305 Japan and [2]Departments of Neurosurgery and Hematology, Moriya Daiichi General Hospital, Kitasoma, Ibaraki, 302-01 Japan

SUMMARY

Coagulation and fibrinolytic abnormality is a frequent complication in head injury patients. Fibrin and fibrinogen degradation products (FDP), D-dimer (DD), alpha 2-plasmin inhibitor (a2PI), plasmin-alpha 2-plasmin inhibitor complex (PIC), antithrombin III (AT-III), and thrombin-antithrombin III complex (TAT) were measured sequentially and hemostatic abnormality was analyzed in detail. The result indicate that coagulation and fibrinolytic activity is markedly accelerated in severe head injury patients with high FDP, DD, PIC, TAT, and with low a2PI, AT-III. Monitoring these markers is beneficial for early diagnosis of the hemostatic abnormalities. In the cases of delayed traumatic intracerebral hematoma, fibrinolytic activity are progressively accelerated in several hours immediately after the injury. From our results, early administration of anti-thrombin drug is strongly recommended to normalize the coagulation and fibrinolytic activity and to prevent hemostatic complications in severe head injury, and we also proposed the necessity of anti-thrombin for brain protection.

KEY WORDS: head injury, fibrinolysis, D-dimer, plasmin-alpha 2-plasmin inhibitor complex, thrombin-antithrombin III complex

INTRODUCTION

Severe head injury frequently complicates hemostatic abnormality based on accelerated thrombin proteolysis which is commonly monitored with the value of FDP. Recent advance of laboratory technology made it possible for us to monitor DD, AT-lll, TAT, a2PI and PIC which could reflect the dynamic state of coagulation and fibrinolysis more accurately. This clinical study is to evaluate the significance of those values and to analyze the pathophysiology of coagulation and fibrinolytic abnormality especially in acute phase of head injury.

MATERIALS AND METHODS

Coagulation and fibrinolytic dynamics was analyzed in 24 cases of head injury patients. 11 patients of cerebrovascular disease (CVD)(8 cases of intracerebral hemorrhage, 3 cases of subarachnoidal hemorrhage) and 6 cases of non-head injury (NHI)(1 case of hemothorax, 3 cases of extremity fracture, 1 case of chest contusion , and 1 case of renal injury) were also investigated as control group. Head injury patient, who are all without other systemic trauma, are classified in two groups; severe head injury group (SHI)(Glasgow coma scale 8 or less) and mild head injury group (MHI)(Glasgow coma scale 9 or more). Mild head injury group is classified in two groups; positive intracranial radiological finding group (PRF) and negative radiological finding group (NRF).

Computerized tomography (CT) was carried out in all patients. Magnetic resonance imaging was performed especially in mild head injury patients to detect minimal brain damage which could not be detected by CT. In all patients, FDP(≤10 μg/ml), DD(≤150 ng/ml), a2PI(85-115 %), PIC(≤0.8 μg/ml), AT-III(79-121 %), and TAT(≤3.0 ng/ml) were measured sequentially in acute stage.

RESULT

Coagulation and fibrinolytic activity in severe head injury
Coagulation and fibrinolytic activity is more accelerated in severe head injury than mild head injury with statistical difference, especially in high level of DD, TAT, PIC, and low AT-III. PIC has the highest significance in this study (Table 1).

Table 1 Peak level of molecular markers during clinical course in head injury and non-head injury patient.

		FDP	DD	AT-III	TAT	a2PI	PIC
SHI	Mean	106.3[s]	10384.0[¶]	75.2[¶]	60.0[*†]	55.7[s]	12.7[*]
(n=11)	±SD	±118.9	±10260.6	±22.0	±0.0	±29.1	±9.3
MHI	Mean	19.6	1665.7	96.3	31.2	78.9	2.4
(n=13)	±SD	±43.4	±3640.2	±14.8	±24.2	±23.8	±3.5
CVD	Mean	2.3	99.3	95.6	14.1	95.2	0.6
(n=11)	±SD	±1.4	±61.7	±22.4	±16.4	±16.5	±0.2
NHI	Mean	9.6	1161.2	89.2	50.8	78.3	3.2
(n=6)	±SD	±6.0	±799.9	±17.0	±22.5	±16.7	±3.1

(*p<0.001, ¶p<0.01, ^{s}p<0.05)
(† TAT was cut off at 60 ng/ml in this study)

Relationship between DTICH and hemostatic abnormality
Delayed traumatic intracerebral hematoma (DTICH) occurred in 3 of 11 cases of severe head injury group, in which coagulation and fibrinolytic activity progressively accelerated within several hours after injury. In contrast, acceleration of these activity was comparatively mild in the cases without DTICH and was normalized immediately.

Coagulation and fibrinolytic dynamics in clinical courses
Two representative cases, which is with DTICH (case 1) and without DTICH(case 2), are described.

Case 1; 38 year old, male, traffic accident. GCS on arrival was 4-4-6. Initial CT showed thin acute subdural hematoma and mild cerebral swelling (Fig. 1-A), however, his consciousness gradually deteriorated. CT 5 hours after injury showed multiple DTICH (Fig. 1-B). The level of FDP on arrival was only 10 μg/ml, while TAT and PIC were already high. All markers deteriorated at the time when DTICH had appeared. Administration of Gabexate Mesilate (FOY®; ONO Pharmaceutical Co. Ltd., Japan) was started and these abnormalities gradually improved, but this patient died 5 days after injury.

Case 2; 16 year old male, traffic accident. GCS on arrival is 1-2-5. Initial CT showed thin acute subdural hematoma (Fig. 3-A). Gabexate Mesilate (FOY®) administration was started soon after arrival. Hematoma removal and insertion of ICP monitor were performed. Following CT showed a small cerebral contusion on the right temporal lobe (Fig 3-B). The level of TAT on arrival was high, however, accerelation of coagulation and fibrinolytic activity are normalized immediately under administration of anti-thrombin drug (Fig. 4). This patient made a good recovery.

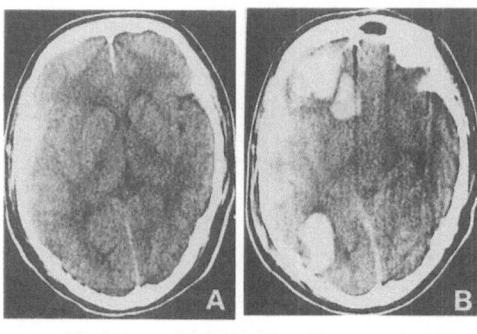

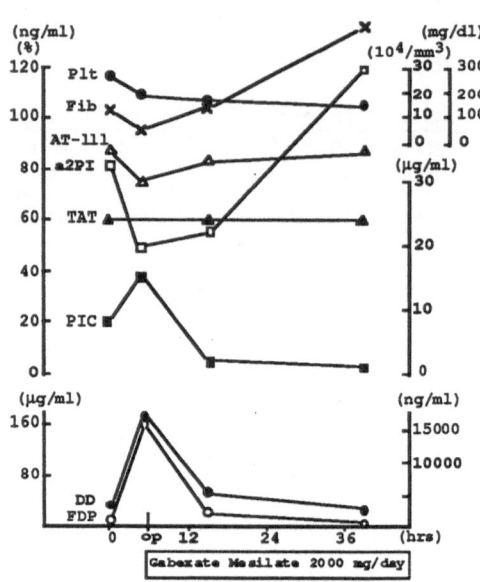

Fig. 1(↑) Case 1. A: CT on arrival. B: Multiple DTICH appeared 4 hours after injury.

Fig. 2(→) Changings of the markers in case 2. TAT and PIC were already high on arrival. Coagulation and fibrinolytic activity markedly accelerated when DTICH occurred.

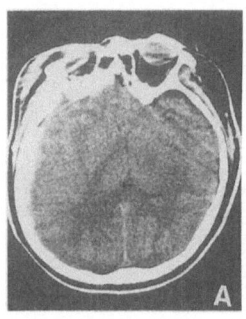

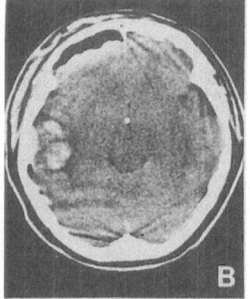

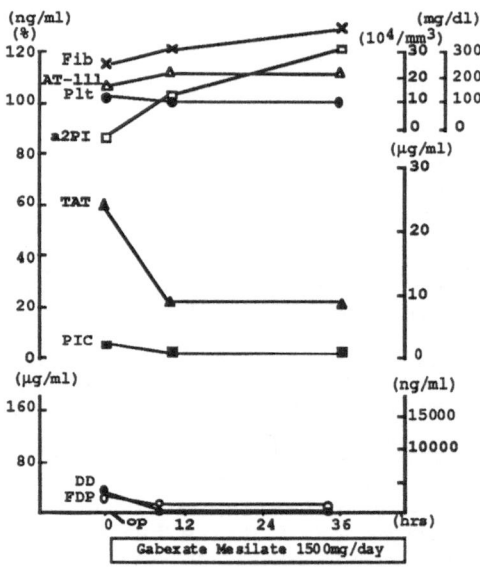

Fig. 3(↑) Case 2. A: CT on arrival. B: Following CT after operation. Small cerebral contusion appeared in the right temporal lobe 9 hours after injury.

Fig. 4 (→) Changings of the markers in case 2. Coagulation and fibrinolytic activity soon decreased.

Fibrinolytic activity in mild head injury

In mild head injury, acceleration of coagulation and fibrinolytic activity is seen in positive intracranial radiological finding group when compared with negative finding group, but these are statistically not significant (Table 2).

Table 2 Molecular markers in mild head injury

		FDP	DD	AT-III	TAT	a2PI	PIC
PRF	Mean	30.6	2640.0	95.9	40.6	81.9	3.6
(n=8)	±SD	±53.6	±4460.0	±16.7	±19.7	±26.1	±4.2
NRF	Mean	2.0	106.0	97.0	16.1	74.1	0.5
(n=5)	±SD	±2.1	±57.9	±13.1	±24.8	±21.5	±0.1

Discussion

Coagulation and fibrinolytic abnormalities in head injury has been often reported. Some reports suggest that concentration of FDP correlates to the prognosis [1], degree of brain damage [5] or the incidence of DTICH [2]. FDP, which is commonly monitored as the marker of disseminated intravascular coagulation(DIC), indicates only thrombin proteolysis, however, by monitoring several molecular markers we can evaluate the dynamics of coagulation and fibrinolysis more accurately. Monitoring these markers is also beneficial for early diagnosis of hemostatic abnormalities which may precede the hemorrhagic or thrombotic events. These data suggest high thrombin activity and high coagulation and fibrinolytic activity in acute phase of severe head injury. From these results, early administration of anti-thrombin drug is strongly recommended to normalize the coagulation and fibrinolytic activity and to prevent hemostatic complications in severe head injury.
In addition, acceleration of coagulation and fibrinolytic activity was seen even in patients of mild head injury, especially with positive intracranial radiological findings. These data suggest that the organic brain damage may exist in cases with clinical diagnosis for "cerebral concussion". In fact, intravascular coagulation is found in small vessels of the brain in experimental concussion model [4]. Additionally in clinical cases of severe head injury which complicate DIC, the high incidence of microthrombi in the brain vessels are identified at autopsy [1]. In the point of view, we also proposed the necessity of early administration of anti-thrombin as brain protective drug in head injury, of which usefulness require further clinical investigation.

Refernces

1. Kaufman HH, Hui K-S, Mattson JC, Borit A, Childs TL, Hoots WK, Bernstein DP, Makela ME, Wagner KA, Kahan BD, Gildenberg PL (1984) Neurosurgery 15: 34-42
2. Kaufman HH, Moake JL, Olson JD, Miner ME, duCret RP, Pruessner JL, Gildenberg PL (1980) Neurosurgery 7: 445-449
3. Olson JD, Kaufman HH, Moake J, O'Gorman TW, Hoots K, Wagner K, Brown CK, Gildenberg PL (1989) Neurosurgery 24: 825-832
4. van der Sande JJ, Emeis JJ and Lindeman J (1981) J Neurosurg 54: 21-25
5. van der Sande JJ, Veltkamp JJ, Boekhout-Mussert RJ, Vielvoya GJ (1981) J Neurosurg 55: 718-724

Opioid Peptides and SP as Growth Factors for Neurons and Glial Cells CNS: Experimental Model in Culture

SVETLANA KASUMOVA[1], MARINA KOZLOVA[2], VIACHESLAV KALENTCHUK[2], ALEXANDER POTAPOV[1]

[1]Burdenko Neurosurgical Institute, Moscow, Russia and [2]Institute of Experimental Cardiology, National Cardiology Research Center, Moscow, Russia

SUMMARY

Organotypic and dissociated CNS and PNS tissue are a wery convenient model to test biological activity of factors in neural regeneration. Endogenous opioid peptides and synthetic analogue of [Leu]-enkepha- lin and substance P (SP) were shown to stimulate neurite outgrowth, survival and adhesion properties of CNS neurons in the dissociated culture model by aggregation assay. Peptides change the properties of CNS glial cells (astrocytes and oligodendrocytes), increase the rate of migration, adhesion, survival and degree of differentiation.

KEY WORDS: opioid peptides, substance P, regeneration,nervous tissue

INTRODUCTION

For many years, the biology of nerve regeneration has been of the special province of neurosurgical investigators interested in peri- pheral nerve and spinal cord injuries.
The growing evidence that the primary lesion in head injury is me- chanical damage to neurons, resulting in axonal degeneration was shown now by different investigators [1].
The results of 160 cases of fatal craniocerebral trauma dealt in the Burdenko Research Institute and literature data show evidence of the different means of structural and functional restoration of the cen- tral nervous system tissue following localized and diffuse axonal head injury [2].
Intracellular reparative processes in the neurons of the pericontu- sion zone may lead to the compensatory changes in localized head in- jury.
Structural and functional recovery of the brain following diffuse axonal injury is determined to a certain extent by the regenerative possibilities of partly damaged axons.

RESULTS AND DISCUSSION

To study of regeneration in vitro we used organotypic and dissocia- ted cultures of the central nervous system (CNS) and peripheral ner- vous system (PNS) tissues.
According to the recent studies opioid peptides [3,4] and substance P [5] can be referred as the growth-promoting factors on neuronal tissue.
According to our studies opioid peptides (endogenous, but also syn- thetic analogues) and SP increase not only the survival neurons, the

intensity of neurite outgrowth of neurons CNS and PNS on organotypic
culture. Last time we performed experiments on rat spinal cord dissociated cell culture,as a model of neuron survival,neurite outgrowth
and cell adhesion.
This kind of peptide activity was measured in dissociated culture of
rat spinal cord by aggregation assay [6]. It was found that the aggregation place during opioid peptides and personaly dalargin action
had increased on average by 1,7 - fold compared to control), thus
altering cell adhesion and increasing survival of neurons and
glial cells of CNS.
Opioid peptides and SP change non only neuron survival, outgrowth of
neurites, adhesion of neurons,but also the properties of glial cells
CNS and PNS in culture. The rate of migration of Schwann cells and
astrocytes of human spinal cord in organotypic cultures increased
under the effect of opioid peptides and SP, altering their adhesion
and survival.
The analysis of the effect of opioid peptides on CNS glial cells,
considering the change in the activity of PNS glial cells was performed in dissociated cultures obtained according to the method of
McCarthy and de Vellis [7]. The addition of opioid peptides (10 M)
changes the culture growth pattern (Fig.1). The confluent layer of

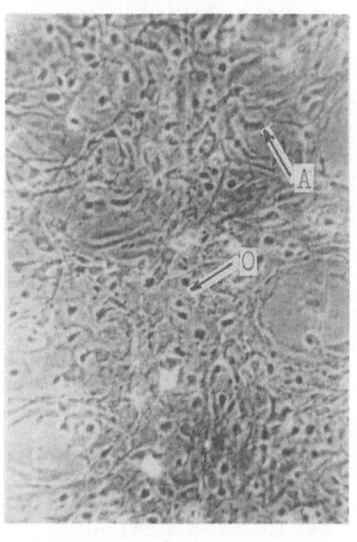 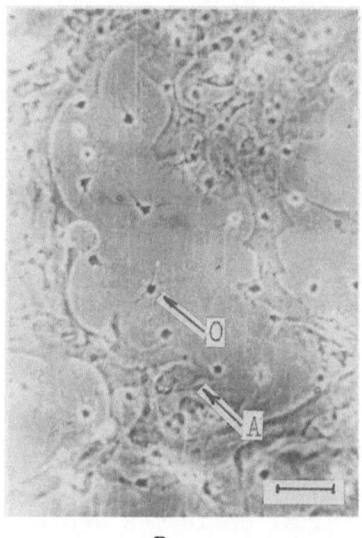

A   B

Fig.1. Effect of dalargin (10^{-9} M) on dissociated culture
of rat CNS glia (20 DIV)
Fig.1A - confluent layer astrocytes with oligodendrocytes
in control.
Fig.1B - collapsed monolyer (confluent layer and increasing outgrowth of oligodendrocytes by action of dalargin.
Phase optic micrograph. A - astrocytes, O - oligodendrocytes. 50 - μm.

astrocytes collapses. This may be explained by changes in the astro-

cyte adhesion. The phenotype of oligodendrocytes also changes - peptides increased the maturation of oligodendrocytes, since the kind of oligodendrocytes processes is a differentiation marker.
Present studies of opioid peptides effect on CNS cells in culture we have made on the model of human brain glial cells (Fig.2). We have

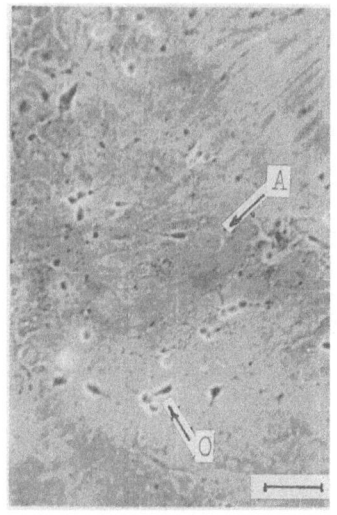
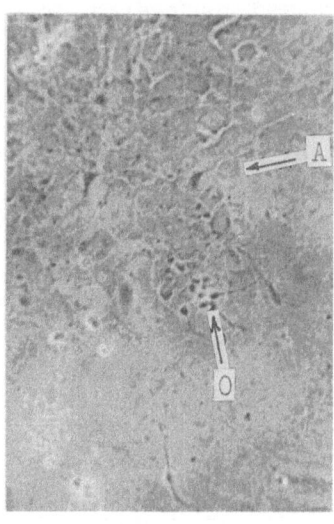

A   B

Fig.2. Culture of human glial cells from brain region after operation. Monolayer of astrocytes with oligodendrocytes. A - astrocytes, O - oligodendrocytes. 50 - μm.

astrocytes and oligodendrocytes in dissociated culture, as a model to screening of neurogrowth activity opioid peptides and personaly dalargin on glial cells of human brain. Our experiment data allow us to assume that dalargin (Tyr-D-Ala-Gly-Phe-Leu-Arg) - a synthetic analogue of [Leu]-enkephalin is the factor which promoted the regeneration of nervous tissue.
These results were the basis of patients with amyotrophic lateral sclerosis [8]. Stabilization of the process for 3-6 months was noted in 30% of patients under injection of dalargin.
Thus endogenous opioid peptides, SP and dalargin change the properties of glial cells CNS and PNS and posible have action on myelinogenesis.
The results obtained on the CNS and PNS tissue and cell cultures indicated that endogenous opioid peptides, dalargin, SP specifically exhibited novel biological activity; they act as nonspecific growth factors for nervous tissue.These peptides may play a role in the development and regeneration of CNS and PNS tissue,and dalargin is the most active agent.
Possible these experimental results may be used in a clinical practice for the treatment of the destructions of human CNS and PNS tissue of patients.

REFERENCES

1. Genarelli J.A., Adams H., Graham D.S. (1986) Mechanisms of secondary brain damage. New York, pp 27-28
2. Kasumova S.Yu. (1992) J.Vopros Neurochirurg 1:17-19 (in Russian)
3. Ilynsky O.B., Kozlova M.V., Kondrikova E.S., Kalentchuk V.U., Titov M.I., Bespalova Zd.D. (1987) Neurosciense 22: 719-735
4. Zagon I.S., McLaughlin P.J. (1987) Brain Res 412: 68-72
5. Kozlova M.V., Andjan A.S., Slepko N.G. (1991) In: Signal molekules and behavious. W.Winlow et al., ads. Manchester University Press. Manchester and New York, pp 255-258
6. Kalentchuk V.U., Kozlova M.V. (1992) Citology. 34:94-99 (in Russian)
7. McCarthy K.D. and De Vellis J. (1980) J.Cell Biol 85: 890-902
8. Kozlova M.V., Zavalishin J.A., Kalentchuk V.U., Nevskaya O.M. (1990) J.Neuroil.Sci. 98 Suppl: 316

Frozen Autograft Cranioplasty After Decompressive Craniectomy – Medical and Economical Benefits

Hiroshi Nihei, Shinya Manaka, Makoto Hirakawa, Jun Sashida, and Seiji Noguchi

Department of Neurosurgery, Ichihara Hospital, University of Teikyo School of Medicine, Ichihara, Chiba, 299-01 Japan

SUMMARY

A simple method of cranioplasty using frozen autograft is reconsidered. Since 1986, 42 cases have undergone cranioplasty using methyl methacrylate, and 14 cases used a frozen autograft. Operation times were 46 min. shorter when a frozen autograft was used reducing operation costs by an estimated 48,500 yen, which is the sum of anesthesia and methyl methacrylate costs. The cosmetic results were also superior in the former, and postoperative infection occurred at the same ratio. It is concluded that frozen autografts have more medical and economical benefits compared to methyl methacrylate, and should be reconsidered as a material for cranioplasty.

KEY WORDS : cranioplasty, frozen autograft, economy, operation time

INTRODUCTION

Large decompressive craniectomy still remains one of the important surgical procedures to reduce intracranial pressure when medical therapy fails, and is frequently employed in cases of acute subdural hematoma. Thereafter, cranioplasty should be performed when an intracranial pressure becomes normal. Although there is no ideal material for cranioplasty, it is rarely discussed probably because it is considered to be a rather simple surgical procedure.

At present, methyl methacrylate is generally used as a substitute for the removed skull flap[1]. However, it has some disadvantages such as difficulties in shaping, a rejection reaction, and poor resistance against infection. A frozen autogeneic skull flap was used for cranioplasty in 1953 with good results[2].

We employed their method and reconsidered the suitability of frozen autogeneic bone as a material for cranioplasty.

PATIENTS AND METHODS

Since 1986, 56 patients have undergone cranioplasty at our hospital. Methyl methacrylate was used in 42 of these patients (Group M: age 3 to 65), and frozen autogeneic bone in 14 patients (Group A: age 10 to 66). The underlying disease varied and included penetrating injury, acute subdural hematoma, and hypertensive intracerebral hematoma. Operation times, operative complications, and esthetic quality were analyzed retrospectively. Operative costs were estimated by operation time according to the tables of medical remuneration provided by the Japanese Department of Health. Some cases from group A were followed up to investigate how the reabsorption of the bone graft occurred.

OPERATIVE TECHNIQUES

Cranioplasty using methyl methacrylate was performed according to the textbook conventional method[3], with the exception that stainless steel wire mesh is not applied in our institution. Autogeneic bone flap was soaked in 100% ethanol and stored sterile at -70℃ immediately after it was removed during the decompressive craniectomy. The frozen bone flaps were thawed at room temperature, and used in the same way as methyl methacrylate flaps. Postoperative prophylactic antibiotics was used routinely in both groups.

RESULTS

As shown in Table 1, the average operation time was 46 min. shorter in Group A than in Group M(89 min. vs. 135 min.). Operation costs were calculated according to the mean operation time. The cost was 48,500 yen (anesthesia 10,500 yen, Cranioplasty Kit 38,000 yen) less expensive in Group A. Epidural abscess was the main complication, and occurred in 4 patients(1 in Group A and 3 in Group M). The ratio of infection was identical. The cosmetic results were, of course, superior in Group A, because the autogeneic bone grafts have a natural curvature.

Table 1. Summary of patient data by operative material

Group	Numbers	Operation Time (Average)	Infection Rate	Cost (yen)
A	14	89 min.	3 cases(7%)	-----
M	42	135 min.	1 case (7%)	+48,500
Difference		46 min.		48,500

Reabsorption of the frozen bone graft was investigated in three cases out of the 14 group A patients, and found to be negligible in all cases, including that from a ten years old boy(Fig. 1).

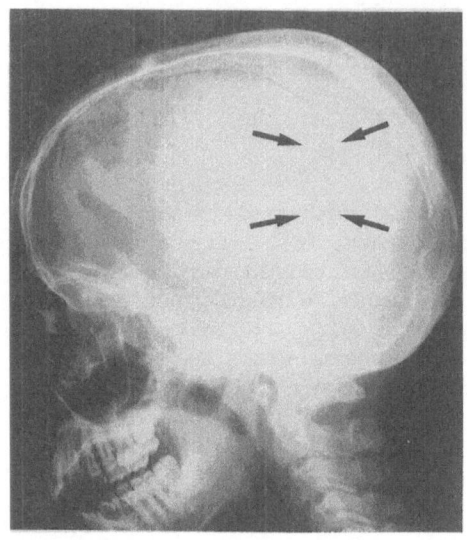

Figure 1. Lateral craniogram of ten years old boy 3 years after cranioplasty using frozen autograft. The frontotemporal lucent area is the portion rongeured out during the decompressive craniectomy. Arrows indicate the reabsorbed portion.

DISCUSSION

There is no ideal material for cranioplasty, such as vital autografts. Beginning with coconut shells, a number of materials have been tried as replacements for the removed skull flap, including various kinds of metal plates, allo- or autografts, and various alloplastics. Since methyl methacrylate was introduced to cranioplasty in 1940, the one-stage acrylic method has become the most widely used method[1]. The acrylic resins provide favorable properties, including strength, esthetic qualities, inertness, availability, thermal nonconductivity, and ease of application. However, it has problems, such as risks of infection, brittleness[4], and difficulties in shaping.

Successful use of frozen autografts was first reported in the early 1950's by Odom[2]. It has many benefits compared to acrylic resins, including availability, low cost, esthetic quality, radiolucency, and lower rejection reactivity. The weak points of frozen autografts are lack of viability, lower resistance against infection and reabsorption. At this time, the only generally accepted method of preserving exteriorized skull flaps is by freezing at -70℃. The reabsorption within these frozen plates is considerable, however, although restoration of the skull with frozen autogeneic skull is reported to be generally successful, except in individuals under 13 years[5].

In our series of patients, frozen autografts were considered superior to methyl methacrylate in esthetic quality, economy, and operation time. Shortening of the operation time is very important because it may reduce not only surgical complications, but also anesthesiological complications and medical costs. Complications from cranioplasty, especially infection, was similar in both groups at 7%. Reabsorption, the weakest point of autografts, was not apparently significant and appeared negligible even in a 10 year old boy. In contrast, erosion of the scalp over the acrylic resin was observed in one patient, and another patient, in whom methyl methacrylate was used, complained about the cosmetic results which led to a second operation.

Ceramic is reported recently to be a new material for substitution of skull flaps with a lower rejection reaction, and enough strength, and affinity to the surrounding bone. However, ceramic flaps are extremely expensive, costing more than 1,000,000 yen each, and require several weeks to prepare the flap prior to operation

CONCLUSION

We conclude that frozen autogeneic skull flaps are a more useful material than methyl methacrylate for cranioplasty from both a medical and economical point of view.

REFERENCES

1. Spence WT (1954) Form-fitting plastic cranioplasty. J Neurosurg 11:219-225
2. Odom GL, Woodhall B, Wrenn FR Jr (1952) The use of refrigerated autogenous bone flaps for cranioplasty. J Neurosurg 9:606-610
3. Prolo DJ (1985) Cranial defects and cranioplasty. In: Wilkins RH, Rengachary SS(eds.) Neurosurgery. McGrawhill. New York. pp1646-1656
4. Galicich JH, Hovind KH (1967) Stainless steel mesh-acrylic cranioplasty. J Neurosurg 27:376-378
5. Hancock DO (1963) The fate of replaced bone flaps. J Neurosurg 20:983-984

Indirect Traumatic Optic Neuropathy – Visual Outcome of Transcutaneously Electrostimulated Cases

SERGEY YEOLCHIJAN, NATALIJA SEROVA, NATALIJA ELISEEVA, and LUDMILA LASAREVA

Burdenko Neurosurgical Institute, Russian Academy of Medical Sciences, 125047 Moscow, Russia

SUMMARY

From 1989 till 1991 52 patients (64 eyes) with indirect traumatic optic neuropathy were treated with the method of transcutaneous optic nerve electrostimulation. Patients' age varied from 5 to 56 years. All the patients received conservative treatment. Period after trauma varied from 1 month to 5 years. Optic atrophy was revealed in all patients up to the moment of stimulation. Electrostimulation was carried out in pack-regime by monophase right-angled impulses, feding on eyelid by means of active electrode. The treatment course included 6-8 procedures. In 12 eyes with amaurosis and in 3 eyes with light perception no visual improvement could be seen. In 29 of 46 eyes (63%) visual acuity improvement was revealed. Significant correlation between the degree of vision improvement after the first course of electrostimulation and the initial visual acuity was found (P < 0,001). In 26 of 29 eyes (89,6%) the therapeutic effect was stable during the follow-up period. Partial visual field defect reduction was observed in 14 of 49 eyes (28,6%). Neither complications no change for the worse in visual functions were observed.The follow-up period ranged from 2 months to 2 years. Transcutaneous optic nerve electrostimulation is effective method of indirect traumatic optic neuropathy treatment long after trauma, when medicine treatment fails. Visual functions improvement and stable preservation of the therapeutic effect achieved testify to functional restoration of the anatomy-preserved optic nerve fibres.

KEY WORDS: head injury, indirect traumatic optic neuropathy, conservative treatment, transcutaneous electrostimulation, optic nerve

INTRODUCTION

Indirect traumatic optic neuropathy has been estimated to be 0,5 - 1,5% of patients with head injury [1,2]. Walsh and Hoyt define this as traumatic loss of vision, which occurs without external or initial ophthalmoscopic evidence of injury to the eye or its nerve [3]. If there is to be an improvement this is usually evident within the first 2 - 4 days and may continue for up to 4 - 6 weeks after the injury after which the condition becomes stationary [2,4,5]. In rare cases improvement has been reported several months after the injury, especially following decompressive operations [6,7]. This report deals with the results of non-invasive method's of the transcutaneous optic nerve electrostimulation application to visual functions restoration long after trauma.

MATERIALS AND METHODS

From 1989 till 1991 52 patients (64 eyes) were treated with optic nerve transcutaneous electrostimulation. The age distribution of the patients ranged from 5 to 56 years with an average of 24 years. There were 41 males and 11 females. Period after trauma varied from 1 month to 5 years (mean 11 months). All the patients were managed conservatively without high-dose steroids use. In 40 cases there was one-side optic neuropathy and in 12 - both optic nerves and chiasm were involved. In 12 cases visual acuity was zero, in 3 - light perception, in 46 of 49 eyes it varied from hand motion to 0,6. In 3 cases with chiasm involvement visual acuity in one eye was 1,0 and electrostimulation was carried out with the purpose of visual field defects reduction. Optic athrophy resulted in each case up to the moment of stimulation. We used non-invasive method of electrostimulation developed by Rostov University researchers [8]. Electrostimulation was carried out by monophase right-angled impulses with the frequency of 20 - 30 cycles per second in pack-regime. Electric impulses parameters were selected individually for each eye depending on phosphens (elementary visual sensations) origin threshold. The stimulating current strength ranged usually from 300 to 600 mcA with the maximum value of 1000 mcA, that lies within physiological safe limits. An active electrode was fixed on patient's upper eyelid. Each procedure lasted for 15-20 minutes. The treatment course included 6-8 procedures. It took 8-10 days to complete it. Transcutaneous method allows optic nerve electrostimulation without any discomfort of the subject. Visual acuity and visual fields were examined before and after each procedure. The EEG were recorded in each patient before and after the stimulation course. EEG epileptic focuses or anamnestic epilepsy were regarded as contraindications for electrostimulation treatment. Patients follow-up ranged from 1 month to 2 years, with an average of 8,4 months.

RESULTS

Electrostimulation therapeutic effect was evaluated according to visual acuity and visual field changes. The criteria for visual acuity improvement, set separately for various visual acuity initial levels, are presented in Table 1. The results exeeding these criteria were considered as marked improvement. Totally 64 eyes were stimulated. In 12 eyes with amaurosis and in 3 eyes with light perception no visual improvement could be seen. Omitting these, 49 eyes visual outcomes were further analized.

Table 1   Criteria for visual acuity improvement.

Visual initial	Acuity final
less than LP	HM
less than FC	0,01
less than 0,01	0,02
less than 0,1	2 times as much but not less than 0,05
0,1 and more	rise by 2 steps

LP - light perception, HM - hand motion, FC - finger count.

The over-all improvement rate constituted 63% (29 of 46 eyes).The improvement rate of 67% (24 of 36 eyes) was found in cases, where electrostimulation started within 1-12 months after trauma, but the impovement rate of 50% (5 of 10 eyes) was found in cases where electrostimulation started later than 12 months after trauma. The observed difference was statistically significant. For details see Table 2.
Significant correlation between the degree of vision improvement after the first course of electrostimulation and the initial visual acuity were revealed (P < 0,001). In 26 of 29 eyes (89,6%) therapeutic effect was stable during follow-up period. In 3 of 13 eyes underwent the second

Table 2   Results of electrostimulation application in different periods after trauma depending on initial visual acuity levels.

Period after Trauma	Visual Acuity					
	HM & CF	0,01-0,09	0,1-0,3	0,4-0,6	Total	Improvement
1 - 3 m	4 (3)	7 (5)	3 (1)	1 (1)	15 (10)	67%
3-12 m	4 (3)	6 (3)	6 (3)	5 (5)	21 (14)	67%
> 12 m	1	6 (4)	3 (1)		10 (5)	50%
Total	9 (6)	19 (12)	12 (5)	6 (6)	46 (29)	63%

HM - hand motion, FC - finger count, m - months, ( ) - number of eyes with improvement

electrostimulation course in 3-6 months intervals the improvement was achieved. Only 1 of 6 eyes underwent the third course showed the further rise of visual acuity level. As a whole, marked improvement was found in 19 of 46 eyes (41,3%). In 14 of 49 cases (28,6%) visual fields' improvement was attained. In 1 case visual field improvement started during the first course and went on. In 3 cases visual field defects' reduction was observed both after the first and the second courses of electrostimulation. Hemianopsy never reduced. Visual functions improvement had spasmodic development. In some cases visual acuity levels rised 2 times as much after only one electrostimulation procedure. The longest trauma to treatment interval in cases with improvement was 5 years. There were no changes for the worse in visual acuity levels or visual fields in any case. We observed neither complications, no neurological deficiency aggravation after electrostimulation courses.

DISCUSSION.

Visual disturbances in indirect traumatic optic neuropathy patients are very difficult to treat with the help of medicine in periods long after trauma [9,10]. Fujitani et all reported that in 13 eyes where conservative treatment started later than 3 weeks after trauma improvement was seen only in 15% [9].During the last few years invasive (direct) and non-invasive (transcutaneous) methods of anterior visual pathway electrostimulation were adopted for visual functions restoration in low -vision patients with optic nerve partial athrophy of different genesis [11,12]. Some authors reported quite high visual functions improvement rate of 60-70% in patients with low vision of different origin treated with electrostimulation [12,13]. As for our report, it first presents numerous selected seria of indirect traumatic optic neuropathy patients where improvement was evaluated according to definite strict criteria. The mechanism of visual functions restoration in electrostimulated patients has not been clarified yet. The spasmodic development of visual functions improvement allows to conclude that functional visual analyzer changes take place.These changes may be conditioned by polarising current effect and synchronized retinal cells electrostimulation [14].Side by side with this, it was suggested that long-term posttetanic potentiation mechanism developing in deprived visual cortex, was also involved in visual functions improvement [15]. As our investigations demonstrated,in some cases the injuired optic nerves possess definite functional reserve long after trauma.Transcutaneous electrostimulation is quite effective method for this reserve realization in comparison with conservative medicine treatment.Visual functions improvement degree is determined by optic nerve reversible and irreversible structure-functional changes correlation. We consider, that there is an urgent necessity for further clinical and experimental researches of electrostimulation application for visual functions restoration in indirect traumatic optic neuropathy patients because of encouraging results achieved.

REFERENCES

1. Brandle VK (1955) Confin Neurol 15: 169-208
2. Turner JWA (1943) Brain 66: 140-151
3. Walsh FB, Hoyt WF (1969) Clinical Neuro-ophtalmology. Williams and Wilkins. Baltimore, p.2376
4. Rodger FC (1943) Brit T Ophthalmol 27: 23-33
5. Huges B (1962) Bull John Hopk. Hosp. 111: 98-126
6. Fucado Y (1975) Mod. Prob. Ophtalmol. 14: 474-481
7. Niho S, Niho M, Niho K, (1970) Canad J Ophthalmol: 22-39
8. Gingihashwili SJ, Kompaneetz EB, Petrovsky VV (1988) In: 4-th All-Union Neurosurgical Congress. Moscow pp 219-220
9. Fugitani T, Inoue K, Takahashi K, Asai T (1986) Jpn J Ophthalmol 30: 125-134
10. Matsusaki H, Kunita M, Kawai K (1982) Jpn J Ophthalmol 26: 447-461
11. Khilko VA, Shandurina AW, Matveev YK, Kondratyeva MI, Lyskov EB, Panin AV, Nykolsky AV (1984) Zh Vopr Neirokhir 3: 35-45
12. Shandurina AN, Panin AV, (1990) Phyziologiya cheloveka 16-1: 53-59
13. Khilko VA, Gaidar BV, Kondratyeva MI, Nikolskaya IM, Usanov EI, Shandurina AN (1989) Zh Vopr Neirokhir 3: 17-20
14. Faber DS, Korn H, (1989) Physiol. Rew 69: 821-863
15. Polyansky VB, Ruderman GL, Kompaneetz EB, Borovkov BB, Forofonova TI, Efimova MN (1992) Sensornye Sistemy 6-2: 67-77

A Case of Traumatic Aneurysm of the Lenticulostriate Artery Associated with Basal Ganglia Hemorrhage

Takashi Takase, Hiroshi Kajikawa, and Shogo Fujii

Department of Neurosurgery, Suiseikai Kajikawa Hospital, Naka-ku, Hiroshima, Japan

SUMMARY

Traumatic hematoma localized in the basal ganglia has been attributed to the shearing force to the perforating arteries. However, there have been only a few reports demonstrating the resultant pseudoaneurysm of the lenticulostriate artery. A rare case of traumatic aneurysm of the lenticulostriate artery is presented in this report. A 16-year-old boy was forcefully struck in the right frontal region in an automobile accident, and CT scans revealed a left putaminal hemorrhage. The left carotid angiography, on the 11th day, demonstrated an aneurysm of the lenticulostriate artery, which corresponded well to the location of the hematoma. This aneurysm remained but decreased in size two months later on the second angiography, but disappeared five months later on the third angiography. The patient recovered fully and now works for a company. The pertinent literature on the traumatic aneurysm and the traumatic basal ganglia hemorrhage is briefly reviewed.

KEY WORDS: traumatic intracranial aneurysm, traumatic basal ganglia hemorrhage

INTRODUCTION

Traumatic basal ganglia hemorrhage is probably secondary to rupture of the lenticulostriate or anterior choroidal arteries. However, there have been only a few reports demonstrating the resultant pseudoaneurysm of the lenticulostriate artery, as described below.

CASE REPORT

On August 14, 1990, a 16-year-old boy was admitted to our hospital 30 minutes after a motorcycle accident. He couldn't be aroused with any forceful mechanical stimuli but could respond with movements to avoid the stimulus (Japan Coma Scale; 100 [1]). There were right facial and right frontal skin contusions and an apparent right hemiparesis was present. X-ray films of the skull did not reveal any fracture. Plain CT scans showed a left putaminal hemorrhage (Fig.1). Left carotid angiograms on the 11th posttraumatic day demonstrated a pseudoaneurysm of the left lenticulostriate artery (Fig.2). MRI showed no abnormal intensity area except the left putaminal hemorrhage. Under conservative management, he recovered gradually. In the second angiograms taken on October 4, the 52nd posttraumatic day, the aneurysm was still visible but had decreased in size (Fig.3 Upper). And, in the third angiograms on January 25, 1991, no aneurysm was demonstrated (Fig.3 Lower). He was discharged on February 3. On a follow-up one year later, CT scans showed a low density area of left putamen and slight dilatation of left lateral ventricle (Fig.4), but on neurological examination he was alert and the condition of his right hemiparesis had fully improved. He was enjoying a normal life and worked for a company.

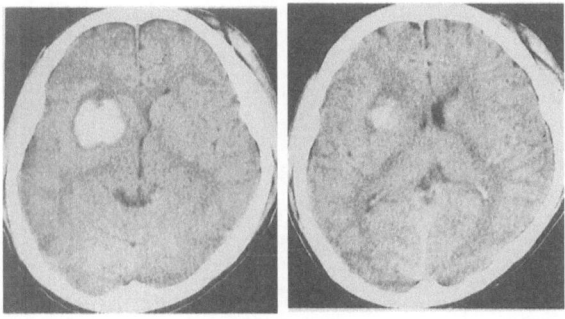

Fig.1: Plain CT scans on admission showed the left putaminal hemorrhage and also showed the right frontal subcutaneous hematoma.

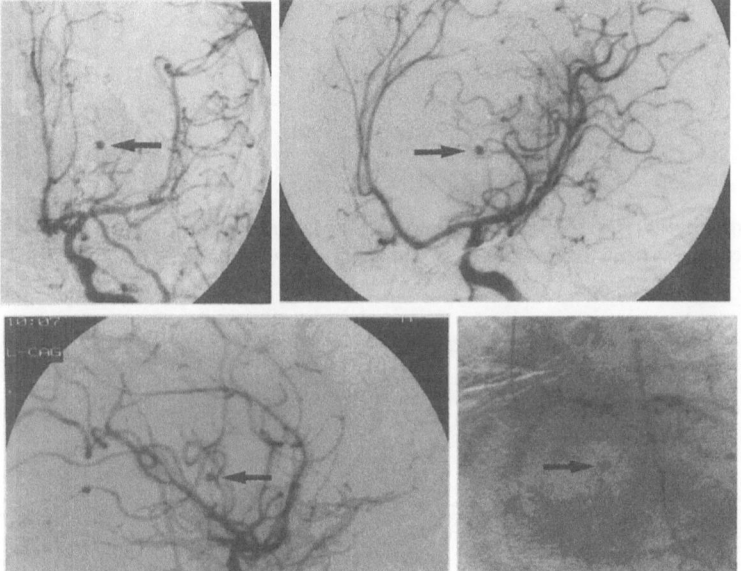

Fig.2: Left carotid angiograms on the 11th posttraumatic day demonstrated a pseudoaneurysm of the left lenticulostriate artery (arrows). Upper left; A-P view. Upper right; lateral oblique view. Lower left; lateral view. Lower right; lateral view, the capillary phase.

DISCUSSION

Traumatic intracranial aneurysm

Traumatic intracranial aneurysms usually result from a severe head injury. They are characterized by the following features: 1) the patient has had an evident head injury; 2) traumatic aneurysms are usually shown histologically to be pseudoaneurysms with an indistinct aneurysmal neck; 3) compared with so-called congenital aneurysms, traumatic ones often involve distal arteries and usually do not develop at a branching point; 4) patients with traumatic aneurysms are often young; and 5) sometimes, they are spontaneously obliterated, and in such cases, they are visualized irregularly and still

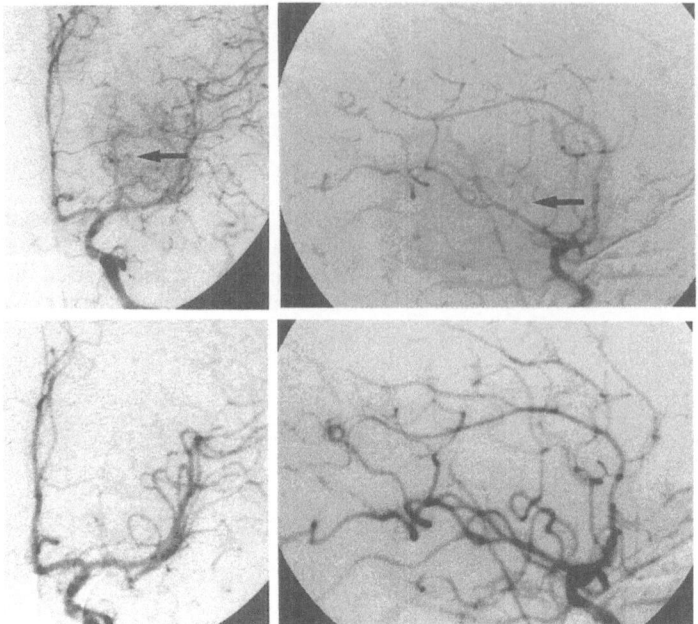

Fig.3: Upper; The second angiograms. The aneurysm was still visible but had decreased in size (arrows). Lower; The third angiograms five months later. No aneurysm was demonstrated.

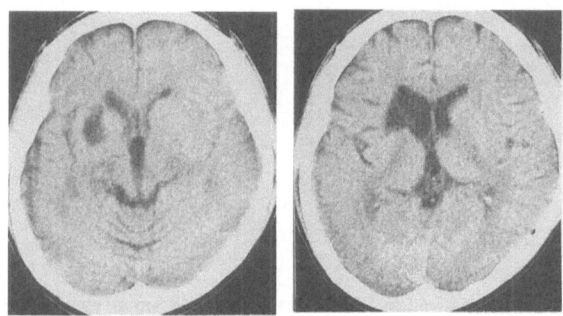

Fig.4: Follow up CT scans one year later showed a low density area of left putamen and slight dilatation of left lateral ventricle.

visualized on the venous phase on angiography [2, 3]. Traumatic intracranial aneurysms secondary to nonpenetrating trauma occur commonly at the skull base or in the periphery [4]. Their pathogenesis is usually either direct vessel injury by the bony structures of the sphenoidal wing, the falcine edge, or fracture of the overlying skull. Traumatic aneurysm of the lenticulostriate artery is very rare. We have found only one report by Akimoto et al, which describes a 10-year-old boy with a low density area in the left basal ganglia on CT scan, showing poor filling of lenticulostriate arteries and a vague microaneurysmal shadow at their distal part on the left carotid angiography [5].

Traumatic basal ganglia hemorrhage

Traumatic basal ganglia hemorrhage is probably secondary to rupture of the lenticulostriate or anterior choroidal arteries. According to Mosberg, with an impact to the vertex which shifts the hemisphere in a caudal direction, the firm edge of the tentorium may cause pronounced stress on the anterior choroidal artery and its branches [6]. But, in general, the role of shearing forces is more important. Holbourn indicated that shearing forces resulted at the juncture between the white and gray matter from the rotation of the skull by an external force [7]. It can be assumed that tearing of small arteries, such as lenticulostriate arteries, caused by shearing forces among the different tissues may bring about a basal ganglia hemorrhage [8]. Macpherson et al suggested that patients with basal ganglia hemorrhages shared many features with patients with severe diffuse white matter injuries, and they stressed the role of shearing forces [9]. There have been only a few reports demonstrating vessel injury on angiography [10, 11], but in their reports extravasations were shown but aneurysm itself was not. We could not find other reports of cases of traumatic aneurysms of the lenticulostriate artery associated with basal ganglia hemorrhage. In our case, the shearing forces which were brought about by right frontal impact are thought to cause tearing of the lenticulostriate artery and the formation of the pseudoaneurysm.

REFERENCES

1. Ohta T, Kikuchi H, Hashi K, Kudo Y (1986) Nizofenone administration in the acute stage following subarachnoid hemorrhage. J Neurosurg 64: 420-426
2. Yuge T, Shigemori M, Tokutomi T, Kuga S, Kuramoto K (1990) Diffuse axonal injury associated with multiple traumatic aneurysms of the distal anterior cerebral artery. -Case report-. Neurol Med Chir (Tokyo) 30: 412-416
3. Tsubokawa T, Kotani A, Sugawara T, Moriyasu N (1975) Treatment for traumatic aneurysm of the cerebral artery -Identification between deteriorating type and spontaneously disappearing type-. Neurol Surg (Tokyo) 3: 663-672 (In Japanese)
4. Buckingham MJ, Crone KR, Ball WS, Thomas TA, Berger TS, Tew JM (1988) Traumatic intracranial aneurysms in childhood: Two cases and a review of the literature. Neurosurgery 22: 398-408
5. Akimoto H, Maki Y, Hasue M, Tajima K, Shirai S, Tosa J (1979) Injuries of basal ganglia following head trauma in children. Nervous System in Children (Tokyo) 4: 215-224 (In Japanese)
6. Mosberg WH Jr, Lindenberg R (1959) Traumatic hemorrhage from the anterior choroidal artery. J Neurosurg 16: 209-221
7. Holbourn AHS (1945) The mechanics of brain injuries. Br Med Bull 3: 147-149
8. Shigemori M, Tokutomi T, Shirahama M, Hara K, Yamamoto F (1981) Massive traumatic hematoma localized in the basal ganglia. Neurol Med Chir (Tokyo) 21: 697-700
9. Macpherson P, Teasdale E, Dhaker S, Allerdyce G, Galbraith S (1986) The significance of traumatic haematoma in the region of the basal ganglia. J Neurol Neurosurg Psychiatry 49: 29-34
10. Aoki N (1979) In: Hiroyasu Makino (ed) Proceeding of the 2nd conference of Japanese society of neurotraumatology. Tokyo, Japan, p 187 (In Japanese)
11. Ikeda H, Kagawa S, Kuwayama N, Sonobe M, Takahashi S (1984) Angiographic extravasation in contrast medium in traumatic intracerebral hematoma. Iryo (Tokyo) 38: 1064-1068 (In Japanese)

Author Index

First-mentioned author only